Mainstreaming Midwives

The Politics of Change

Edited by
Robbie Davis-Floyd and Christine Barbara Johnson

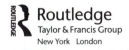

Routledge
Taylor & Francis Group
New York   London

Routledge is an imprint of the
Taylor & Francis Group, an informa business

Published in 2006 by
Routledge
Taylor & Francis Group
270 Madison Avenue
New York, NY 10016

Published in Great Britain by
Routledge
Taylor & Francis Group
2 Park Square
Milton Park, Abingdon
Oxon OX14 4RN

Printed in the United States of America on acid-free paper
10 9 8 7 6 5 4 3 2 1

International Standard Book Number-10: 0-415-93150-9 (Hardcover) 0-415-93151-7 (Softcover)
International Standard Book Number-13: 978-0-415-93150-2 (Hardcover) 978-0-415-93151-9 (Softcover)
Library of Congress Card Number 2005031271

Library of Congress Cataloging-in-Publication Data

Mainstreaming midwives : the politics of change / edited by Robbie Davis-Floyd and Christine Barbara Johnson.
    p. cm.
  Includes bibliographical references and index.
  ISBN-13: 978-0-415-93150-2 (hardback : alk. paper) -- ISBN-13: 978-0-415-93151-9 (pbk. : alk. paper)
  1. Midwifery--United States--History. 2. Midwives--United States--History. I. Davis-Floyd, Robbie. II. Johnson, Christine Barbara, 1952-   . [DNLM: 1. Nurse Midwives--history--United States. 2. Mid-wifery--history--United States. 3. Politics--United States. 4. Professional Autonomy--United States.   WY 11 AA1 M225 2005]

RG950.M34 2005
362.198'2--dc22
    2005031271

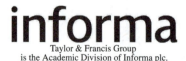

informa
Taylor & Francis Group
is the Academic Division of Informa plc.

Visit the Taylor & Francis Web site at
http://www.taylorandfrancis.com

and the Routledge Web site at
http://www.routledge-ny.com

This book is dedicated to the midwives of America, in the belief and hope that one day they will realize their full potential to be the primary care providers for the majority of American birth-giving women, and that in so doing, they will continue to uphold their ideals and practices of woman-centered care.

Table of Contents

GLOSSARY OF FREQUENTLY USED ACRONYMS

ABM — Alternative birth movement.

ACC — American College of Nurse-Midwives Certification Council, the body responsible for testing and certifying CMs and CNMs. (In late 2005, the ACC changed its name to the American Midwifery Certification Board (AMCB). This change came too late in the publication process for us to be able to include it in this book.)

ACNM — American College of Nurse-Midwives.

CfM — Citizens for Midwifery, a consumer organization supporting the Midwives Model of Care™.

CM — Certified Midwife, a national certification granted by the ACC (and a state certification granted in Michigan and New Hampshire by those state's direct-entry midwifery associations).

CNM — Certified Nurse-Midwife, a national certification granted by the ACC.

CPM — Certified Professional Midwife, a national and international certification granted by NARM.

CTF — Certification Task Force, a coalition of MANA members who advised the NARM board on many aspects of creating the CPM.

DEM — Direct-entry midwife (in the U.S., a professional midwife who enters midwifery without passing through nursing first).

DOA — The Division of Accreditation of the ACNM, the body responsible for evaluating and accrediting programs that graduate students eligible to become ACC-certified CNMs and CMs.

DOE — The United States Department of Education.

Homebirth — In this volume we use "homebirth" both as an adjective ("a home-birth midwife") and a noun ("Susan had a homebirth"). Our dual usage of this fused word reflects the way women and midwives often employ it; it seems to them and to our scociocultural view that a certain unifying ethos forms around this uniting of two words into one—an ethos that

ix

encompasses midwives' and women's felt sense that "homebirth" constructs as one the place that shelters and shapes the birth and the acts and emotions of people engaged in the birth.

IWG — Interorganizational Work Group, a group sponsored by the Carnegie Foundation for the Advancement of Teaching, consisting of ACNM and MANA representatives and charged with trying to unify American midwifery, 1989–1994.

LM — Licensed Midwife, a midwife who achieves state licensure.

MANA — Midwives Alliance of North America.

MEAC — Midwifery Education and Accreditation Council, the body responsible for evaluating and accrediting programs that graduate students eligible to become CPMs.

MMOC — Midwives Model of Care, a definition trademarked by the Midwifery Task Force (a coalition of MANA members and consumers) in 2000.

NACPM — National Association of Certified Professional Midwives.

NARM — North American Registry of Midwives, the body responsible for testing and certifying CPMs.

NHCM — New Hampshire Certified Midwife.

NM — Nurse-midwife.

RM — Registered Midwife (licensed in her state but called a Registered Midwife instead of a Licensed Midwife).

VBAC — Vaginal birth after cecarean.

INTRODUCTION

Why Are Social Scientists Studying the Development of Direct-Entry Midwifery in the United States?: Politics, Identity, Professionalization, and Change

Robbie Davis-Floyd and Christine Barbara Johnson

• **From Robbie Davis-Floyd: Research, Methodology, and the National Context** • **From Christine Barbara Johnson: Research, Methodology, and Findings on Home Birth Consumers** • **Overview of the Book**

CNMs think DEMs have copped out, and DEMs think CNMs have sold out.

—**Joyce Roberts, President of the American College of Nurse-Midwives, 1999**

One group needs to tighten up, and the other group needs to lighten up!

—**Katherine Camacho Carr, President of the American College of Nurse-Midwives, 2005**

FROM ROBBIE DAVIS-FLOYD: RESEARCH, METHODOLOGY, AND THE NATIONAL CONTEXT

Research and Methodology

This book builds on my twenty years of research on American childbirth, which have included since 1991 a growing fascination with

1

midwives and midwifery. My first book, *Birth as an American Rite of Passage* (1992, reissued in a second edition in 2004), analyzes the responses of 100 women to their medical and social treatment during pregnancy and birth. In subsequent studies I comparatively investigated the self- and body-images of pregnant professionals and home-birthers (Davis-Floyd 1994 a, b) and the worldviews and values that underlie their birth choices (1992b). This research brought midwives to the forefront of my attention, as they are the only childbirth practitioners who seek to span the spectrum of women's choices, from highly technological hospital birth to relatively untrammeled birth at home. It is that spectrum of choice with which I have been primarily concerned.

In May 1996 I began a study of the politics and problematics involved in the professionalization and legitimation of *direct-entry (non-nurse) midwives.* The two major midwifery organizations in the United States—the American College of Nurse-Midwives (ACNM) and the Midwives Alliance of North America (MANA)—were in the early stages of designing and implementing two different routes to national certification for midwives who do not pass through nursing training (direct-entry midwives [DEMs]). For both organizations, this process is revolutionary: *lay midwives* who had in the past maintained their autonomy largely outside the system were now professionalizing within it, and *nurse-midwives* were seeking to move their profession away from its embeddedness in nursing and toward greater independence and autonomy. The desire of both groups is to move midwifery from the margins into the mainstream of American society.

Both new types of direct-entry midwifery certification will undoubtedly affect the evolution of the spectrum of choice for childbearing women in the United States, shaping the extent and style of midwifery care (read: birth options) that will be available in the future. Thus the investigation of these processes has formed a logical next step in the evolution of my research in the anthropology of reproduction.

My research for this study of the development of direct-entry midwifery in the United States was multi-sited, consisting of participant observation at nine ACNM national and regional conferences, fifteen MANA national and regional conferences, twenty national or international *Midwifery Today* conferences (*Midwifery Today* both publishes an international magazine and puts on conferences that bring together midwives of all types from many countries), and the conferences of numerous other birth-related groups, including the Maternity Center Association, Lamaze International, the International Childbirth Education Association (ICEA), the Association of Women's Health, Obstetrical, and Neonatal Nurses (AWHONN), Doulas of North America (DONA), and the

Coalition for Improving Maternity Services (CIMS). I played multiple roles at these conferences—I gave talks at all of them, served on various committees and one board, attended many workshops and presentations, engaged in countless conversations about midwifery, took copious notes, and conducted extensive tape-recorded interviews with over two hundred midwives.

Seventy of these were leaders and educators in nurse- and direct-entry midwifery; my interviews with these leaders focused on their motivations for developing these new certifications, the practical and philosophical issues that divide them, and the legislative processes in various states. I also interviewed eighty midwifery students (forty-five nurse-midwifery students, thirty direct-entry students in the process of becoming certified professional midwife [CPMs], and five direct-entry students in the process of becoming certified midwife [CMs]) about their educational processes, seeking to understand the relative benefits and disadvantages of each. I traveled throughout New York, California, and Washington state conducting interviews with midwives, consumers, and public officials about midwifery legislation and regulation in those states. To date, results of this work have been published in twelve chapters and articles (Benoit et al. 2001; Davis-Floyd 1998 a, b, c, 1999, 2003 a, b, 2004a, b, 2005; Davis-Floyd and Davis 1997). This volume represents the culmination of this work.

The National Context of My Research

Obstetrics as a medical specialty accounts for a disproportionate share of the rising costs of health care in the United States, as a result of over reliance on costly technological interventions and frequent lawsuits. Fear of being sued and the high costs of malpractice insurance are driving many obstetricians out of the field. Those who remain tend to cluster in cities, leaving many rural areas without obstetrical services. In contrast, midwives are rarely sued, many serve rural areas, and their expertise in facilitating normal birth results in fewer interventions and less costly care (Rooks 1997, chap. 10–11; MacDorman and Singh 1998; Perkins 2004; Johnson and Daviss 2005). In 2002, approximately 6,000 certified nurse-midwives (CNMs) practicing in the United States attended 8.6 percent of U.S. births. Around 3,000 lay and direct-entry (non-nurse) midwives (no one knows for sure exactly how many non-nurse homebirth midwives are out there) attended approximately less than one percent (0.6 percent) of American births. In contrast, approximately 40,000 obstetricians (and some family practitioners) attended ninety percent of American births, ninety-nine percent of which took place in hospitals.

The United States and Canada are the only two industrialized nations in which professional midwives do not attend the majority of births. As the direct result of a campaign by physicians, nurses, and public health officials from the early 1900s on, by the 1960s midwives in North America had been almost completely eliminated. During this period, birth moved into the hospital and became medically managed and technologically controlled as the obstetrical branch of medicine developed (Oakley 1984; Leavitt 1986). It is therefore quite remarkable that midwives have generated their own renaissance since that time. In achieving this rebirth, midwives have undergone a transformation from the illiterate grannies and rural midwives who served specific ethnic groups in bounded communities (Susie 1988; Logan and Clark 1989; Fraser 1992) to full participants in the postmodern world. Thousands of midwives across North America have become educated, articulate, organized, political, and highly conscious of their cultural uniqueness and importance—a phenomenon that I have labeled *postmodern midwifery* (Davis-Floyd and Davis 1997; Davis-Floyd 2005).

> With this term, I am trying to highlight the qualities that emerge from the practice, the discourse, and the political engagement of a certain kind of contemporary midwife—one who often constructs a radical critique of unexamined conventions and univariate assumptions. Postmodern midwives as I define them are relativistic, articulate, organized, political, and highly conscious of both their cultural uniqueness and their global importance. . . . Postmodern midwives are scientifically informed: they know the limitations and strengths of the biomedical system and of their own, and they can move fluidly between them. These midwives play with the paradigms, working to ensure that the uniquely woman-centered dimensions of midwifery are not subsumed by biomedicine. They are shape-shifters, knowing how to subvert the medical system while appearing to comply with it, bridge-builders, making alliances with biomedicine where possible, and networkers . . .[with a sense of mission around preserving and growing midwifery] and an understanding that *for a midwife, the professional is always political*: midwives and their colleagues must have an organized political voice if they are to survive. So postmodern midwives work to build organizations in their communities, join national and international midwifery organizations, and work within them for policies and legislation that support midwives and the mothers they attend. (Davis-Floyd 2005:13)

This book brings together various social scientific analyses of the efforts of postmodern American midwives and their consumer supporters to achieve sociocultural recognition and acceptance for the two new types of direct-entry midwifery created by their national organizations almost simultaneously in the mid-1990s.

Postmodern American midwifery is far from constituting a unified social movement. Disparate factions have emerged, each of which employs competing discourses of desire for, appropriation of, and resistance to the authority of technomedicine and mainstream professionalization. These separate factions provide an opportunity for the ethnographic tracking of multiple conflicting relationships to each other and to medical authority from within what is still widely regarded by American consumers as a culturally marginal, "alternative" practice. In the United States, the two major organizations that represent the majority of practicing midwives constitute the sometimes competing, sometimes cooperating factions addressed by my research.

The ACNM represents certified nurse-midwives (CNMs), who are recognized in all fifty states; in some they may operate independently in hospital and private practice, while in others they must work under (or cooperatively with) physicians. Their training consists of nursing plus one or two years of in-hospital midwifery (sixty percent of nurse-midwifery programs also offer some out-of-hospital clinical experience for their students, usually in birth centers [Katherine Camacho Carr, personal communication, 2005]). ACNM also now represents the new certified midwife (CM), who receives both midwifery education and "the equivalent" of nursing training as it relates to midwifery (see chapter 2).

The Midwives' Alliance of North America (MANA) primarily represents direct-entry midwives, who were formerly known as lay midwives—an appellation they came to resent as their commitment to professionalization increased. Founded on ideals of "sisterhood" and "inclusivity," MANA welcomes as members all midwives who support its nonmedicalized, holistic approach to birth, including CNMs and both new types of direct-entry midwives—the CM and the certified professional midwife (CPM), a designation created by the North American Registry of Midwives (NARM), a sister organization of MANA.

Members of ACNM and MANA often sharply disagree over the nature of midwifery and the definition of what constitutes appropriate midwifery education and competent care. Most divisive is the issue of apprenticeship, which many CNMs devalue because they believe that not tying midwifery to a college degree is disempowering to women and that university education is fundamental to becoming a healthcare professional. On the other hand, the members of MANA highly value apprenticeship for the connective and embodied experiential learning (Jordan 1989) it provides, as well as for the deep trust in women and in birth that apprenticeship training builds (see chapters 1 and 3). Accordingly, the new national direct-entry certification process developed by NARM honors "multiple routes of entry," including apprenticeship, to becoming a CPM. In contrast, ACNM's new process of direct-entry certification (the CM) recognizes primarily programs affiliated with universities. ACNM recognizes the value of apprenticeship learning—indeed, the *preceptorship* is an integral part of ACNM-accredited training programs—but insists that it be only one component of an education that should be equally grounded in formal university-type didactic training. MANA members link university training to medical/technocratic co-option of the midwifery emphasis on the normalcy of pregnancy and birth, insisting that apprenticeship training, private vocational direct-entry schools, and small direct-entry college programs provide a less medicalized, more holistic, and more woman-centered approach to care—one that is not based on a sense of danger and risk in birth, but rather on trust in the birth process and the birthing woman. They affirm that an attitude of trust on the part of the midwife fosters and facilitates the mother's ability to trust and believe in herself, noting that many hospital-trained midwives prefer to rely on the information generated by the electronic fetal monitor and the sense of security that if a crisis arises, full-scale assistance is right around the corner.

After the creation of the CM (described in chapter 2), the ACNM's Division of Accreditation (DOA) immediately set about establishing a framework and set of guidelines for the creation of university-affiliated CM training programs. These could potentially have included schools (such as the Seattle Midwifery School) that are already formally accredited by MANA's other sister organization, the Midwifery Education Accreditation Council (MEAC), but the DOA set its standards beyond the reach of such schools (the major impediments are university affiliation and the requirements that key faculty members be CNMs or CMs), clearly intending to keep these two direct-entry certification processes separate and distinct.[1] Larson (1979) identifies the core of the professionalizing project as the attempt to secure a structural linkage between education and occupation; between *knowledge* as the negotiation of cognitive exclusiveness and *power* in the form of a market monopoly. While ACNM members have sought to create and strengthen such linkages, homebirth midwives have tried to weaken them, ensuring that midwifery knowledge is available to anyone who wishes to attend births as an apprentice, and rejecting monopolistic moves that tie the necessary knowledge to a particular form of education.

Professionalization is a contentious issue not only between these organizations, but within each of them. Although the CPM national certification process enjoys strong support from most members in MANA, it is a source of tension and polarization for others who have found great benefit in uncertified, nonprofessional, unregulated status. To professionalize is to accept a level of regulation and bureaucratic conformity that can compromise independence of practice (Torstendahl and Burrage 1990; Witz 1992). For example, in every state where direct-entry midwives seek licensure, they find that along with the benefits come limitations (including prohibitions on attending certain kinds of births at home, such as vaginal birth after cesarean [VBACs], breeches, and twins). Some in MANA fear that even the self-regulation that accompanies self-designed national certification will be too constraining. Likewise, in ACNM there is ongoing tension between those who wish to preserve nursing as the primary route of entry to midwifery and those who dream of being freed from the restrictions placed on nurses and of "getting out from under the thumb" of state nursing boards, to be regulated instead under newly established state midwifery boards.

Central to many professionalization processes (in addition to credentialing, the development of practice standards, a code of ethics, and accredited educational routes) is the attempt to gain legalization and state licensure (MacDonald 1985; Witz 1992). NARM and many MANA members have been actively lobbying in various states for recognition of the CPM credential and for state adoption of the NARM exam as the state licensing exam for direct-entry midwives; these efforts have been successful in twenty-one states to date. Active lobbying of state legislatures by local ACNM chapters in favor of their own direct-entry certification (the CM) and adoption of their exam and their standards has but recently begun or is yet to materialize in most states; there is no national plan. In some places the local chapters of ACNM and the state organizations of homebirth midwives (many of whose members belong to MANA and/or have become CPMs) are coordinating their lobbying efforts; in others they have been or may become directly opposed. New York state constitutes the clearest example to date of the bitterness and havoc that can be created by such opposition, as Maureen May and I describe in chapter 2. In contrast, the nurse- and direct-entry midwives of Massachusetts are working together on joint legislation in a very conscious effort to counteract the divisive and distrustful legacy of the New York legislation, as Christine Barbara Johnson describes in chapter 9.

A dangerous set of problematics arises from these new kinds of professionalization, which includes not only internal dissensions and divisions and legislative turf wars between MANA and the ACNM, but also very real possibilities for the co-option of homebirth midwifery, including the chance that the autonomous niche in the system that midwives are seeking to establish through licensure and certification could backfire into increased dependence on physicians (Reid 1989). (Indeed, in the 1990s this became a danger in New York and California, where current legislation requires that midwives have practice agreements with physicians.) An enticing set of possibilities accompanies these problematics, including the growth and expansion of both organizations and thus of midwifery itself, mutual cooperation between them to create a birth care system in which CNMs and CMs work in tandem with CPMs, offering more options and a more complete range of choice to birthing women, and pooling of resources and efforts in state legislatures around the country to work for bills that benefit both CMs and CPMs. There is much to recommend this sort of cooperative approach; whether or not it develops will depend to a great extent on the motivations of the prime movers in both organizations—motivations I have tried to identify and clarify through my research.

My specific objectives have been: (1) to identify the goals and motivations of those women[2] in both organizations who are most influential in setting future-oriented directions and policies in the brand new field of non-nurse midwifery certification; (2) to examine the dynamics of the relationships between the ACNM and MANA; (3) to identify and analyze within each organization the tensions generated around the direct-entry certification process, as well as its design and implementation; (4) to study the attitudes of key members of both organizations toward professionalization and all that it entails; and (5) to synthesize a clear and useful holistic overview of the future directions in midwifery now emerging in North America and their implications for birth care and women's reproductive choices. (A part of this endeavor has been my editorial participation in the recently published volume *Reconceiving Midwives*, which describes the development of direct-entry midwifery in Canada [Bourgeault, Benoit, and Davis-Floyd 2004]).

As an anthropologist, I have made every effort to maintain a neutral stance toward the political differences between MANA and the ACNM, so that I can work fluidly with both groups. I fully support midwives who practice both in and out of the hospital; my focus as a birth activist has always been on keeping open the full spectrum of choice for birthing women, and I see midwives as absolutely essential to that endeavor. (While it is not hard to find an obstetrician who will willingly schedule a cesarean at his and the mother's convenience, it is almost impossible to find an obstetrician who will attend a homebirth—there are probably only about fifty in the country.)

At present, the status of direct-entry midwives fluctuates wildly from state to state. In some states, like Missouri and Alabama, direct-entry midwifery is explicitly illegal. In others, such as Pennsylvania, it is *alegal.* This is a misleading term that means that the practice of midwifery is not legally secure. When alegal, midwifery is not specifically addressed in statutes, but the actions involved in midwifery practice are considered the practice of medicine and/or nursing; these midwives are left vulnerable to criminal prosecution whenever anyone cares to pursue such action. (For a full discussion of *alegality,* see www.fromcalling-tocourtroom.net.) In others states, such as Florida, Washington, and New Mexico, midwifery is completely legal and even supported by the system; licensed midwives in these states can obtain not only medical backup but also third-party insurance reimbursement. Many are now looking to these states to see what kind of market will be generated over time by the increased availability of homebirth. Any significant jump would generate awareness nationwide of the availability of a huge new market niche for insurers and HMOs. (But where these institutions are deeply involved with hospitals, they often act to stop midwifery and out-of-hospital birth because these take income away from hospitals [Hodges 2004]).

Planned, midwife-attended home and birth center births have been repeatedly shown to be as safe as hospital birth. Such births are far more woman-empowering, and far more baby- and family-friendly. They are also much cheaper—a homebirth and home midwifery care cost an average of one-third that of a hospital birth. If this information, third-party reimbursement, and professional midwives were widely available around the country, many women who now enter alternative birth centers in the hospital might wish to choose freestanding birth centers or homebirth instead.

In 2005, the newly created CMs could be licensed in three states (New York, New Jersey, and Rhode Island), while the newly created CPMs are licensed in twenty-one states. Now the consumer must deal with CNMs, CMs, CPMs, LMs, and RMs (many homebirth midwives are licensed in their states and called either Licensed Midwives or Registered Midwives) and "plain" midwives who refuse to professionalize. Are you confused yet? You would think it would be simpler for the ACNM and MANA to work something out together—one type of professional non-nurse-midwife that everyone could agree on. They tried for three years during the early 1990s, in intense meetings of the

Interorganizational Work Group (sponsored by the Carnegie Foundation for the Advancement of Teaching), during which ACNM did agree with MANA's establishment of NARM and that NARM-certified midwives and CNMs would have similar scopes of practice (a similarity that later vanished as CNMs moved into gynecological care). But that's as far as they could get; their differences over the issue of higher education were just too deep. ACNM insists that midwives have college degrees and graduate from formal training programs; effectively, their programs require a master's degree (see chapter 1). MANA insists that degrees do not a good midwife make. While many MANA members do graduate from formal training programs, the membership agrees that apprenticeship should remain a valid route to midwifery.

So for the foreseeable future, there will be three national certification processes for midwifery, with three titles obtainable—CNM, CPM, and CM. And there will be five kinds of midwives: CNMs, CMs, CPMs, midwives licensed in their states who have no national certification (such as LMs and RMs), and the plain midwives who work and wish to stay completely outside the system. Many bridge-builders want to make midwifery into one profession with one flexible set of educational standards on which everyone will (eventually) agree. But those on opposing sides insist on the utter impossibility of that. ACNM will continue to insist on formal educational programs leading to advanced degrees. NARM and MANA will continue to insist that a college degree has nothing to do with one's competence as a midwife,[3] and will go on validating multiple routes of entry into their profession, including apprenticeship, self-study, private midwifery schools, and university programs. In some states these groups may fight each other in the legislatures for legitimation of their version of direct-entry midwifery, when their energies would be much better spent fighting the medical system and the insurance companies for greater public access to midwifery care. The public will have to deal with five kinds of midwives. And the future of homebirth and of freedom of choice for the childbearing women of North America—which only midwives can guarantee—will hang in the balance. In some states members of both MANA and ACNM will cooperate to write legislation that legitimates both certifications, as some midwives belong to both organizations and are aware of the benefits of making common cause. When they do fight each other, it will likely be because their differences are real: many CNMs see homebirth as irresponsible and think that other midwives are poorly trained; many MANA members see CNMs as sellouts to the medical establishment—"physician extenders" more interested in making money than in serving women. ACNM is determined to set the standard for midwifery in the United States. MANA and NARM are just as determined to set a strong standard for nonmedicalized midwifery and their independent Midwives Model of Care™ (see chapter 3).

I was thrilled when I met Christine Barbara Johnson, informally known as Barbara, who is an experienced and accomplished sociologist and has been a birth activist for many years. She lives and breathes the cultural treatment of childbirth and of midwives and midwifery politics as deeply, on a daily basis, as I do. Her outstanding editorial skills have contributed substantially to the excellence of every chapter in this book, and her deep and lengthy involvement in midwifery politics in her home state of Massachusetts has given her not only local ethnographic understanding but also a broad and informed perspective on the national midwifery scene. It is that broad and informed perspective that we try to bring to you, our readers. *We declare our complete support for the survival and prospering of all types of midwives and midwifery models of care in the United States,* and we refuse to take sides in the debates and disagreements between midwives of differing philosophies and educational backgrounds. Midwives in general give more nurturant, more woman-centered, more compassionate, and often more effective care than obstetricians (see Rooks 1997; Davis-Floyd 2004c; chap. 13 of this volume), and so we wish to make clear from the beginning that *our bias is in favor of midwives,* period. We contribute this analysis of the philosophical, practical, and political divisions and disagreements, as well as the areas of accord among American midwives, not in the interest of tarnishing midwifery's image in any way, but rather in the spirit of social scientists who wish, through their critical and comparative analyses, to contribute to healing the traumas and pain and political prices of the divisions that we analyze in these pages.

FROM CHRISTINE BARBARA JOHNSON: RESEARCH, METHODOLOGY, AND FINDINGS ON HOMEBIRTH CONSUMERS
Research and Methodology

My contributions to this book have been shaped by over twenty years of experience (Johnson 1987, 2000, 2001; Johnson and Galvin 2001), including extensive interviews with homebirth consumers. I have been actively involved in studying and supporting midwifery since 1983 and became so engrossed by the subject that I decided to focus my Ph.D. thesis entirely on midwifery in Massachusetts, *Normalizing Birth* (1987, unpublished). The themes that captivated my interest at that time and have continued to mature and evolve over the years involve, first, the relationship between the individual/small groups and institutions, micro- and macro-configurations, structure and agency. In particular, I have been fascinated to uncover the process through which nascent and pioneering social movements gain social legitimacy and widespread public acceptance while maintaining their identity and autonomy. With regard to midwifery, I have been most interested in how this model of care, through networking and public outreach, has the potential to transform medical, legal, and political institutions. Second, I have been equally interested in the chasm between the reality of who the homebirth consumer is and the public misperception.

From the beginning, the more I studied the homebirth consumer, the more I became amazed at the conscientious and well-thought-out research most of them undertook in deciding to have a homebirth. In addition, their willingness to be proactive birthgivers, and the level of responsibility they were willing to assume constantly impressed me. The more I have learned about the homebirth consumer, the more I have become dedicated to doing everything I can to correct the erroneous public image of homebirth consumers as irresponsible and reckless. In addition to my research on homebirth consumers,[4] I have interviewed over one hundred midwives and have presented and advocated the midwifery model of care in talks around the country, as well as throughout the New England region.

In my dissertation I observed firsthand how homebirth midwifery in Massachusetts was transformed almost overnight. One moment it appeared very likely that this option would be deemed the practice of medicine and thus outlawed. The next moment homebirth had the support of all three branches of state government: judicial, administrative, and legislative (see chapter 9 on Massachusetts midwifery, "Creating a Way Out of No Way"). This series of events made a lasting impression on me with respect to how individuals can change the fabric of our societal institutions through their sustained and committed actions. This realization in turn has fostered in me an avid interest in exploring how institutions are transformed and altered at their core through social action.

As a social activist I served many years on the board of directors of the Massachusetts Friends of Midwives (MFOM) and was one of the six original members of the Massachusetts Coalition for Midwifery (MCM), a group dedicated to representing the interests of certified nurse-midwives, direct-entry midwives, and homebirth consumers. This coalition was created in large part to support the Massachusetts midwifery legislation effort. This is a joint legislative bill, the first of its kind in the United States that would license both CNMs and CPMs under a single board (see chapter 9). In addition to these activities, I have publicly supported midwifery in university classrooms, professional conferences, state houses, courtrooms, and on many occasions have agreed to meet with couples wanting to learn more about midwifery so they could evaluate it as a viable option. My evolving research has been motivated by my social activist concerns and the desire to use a disciplined and grounded research methodology to further investigate viable ways to disseminate information about the midwifery model of care to the wider public.

To this end, I jumped at the chance to be an "expert consultant" on the prenatal care module of the United States National Library of Medicine's Information Infrastructure Program (contract NO-LM-6-3539) and write a report based on these findings (Johnson and Galvin 2001). This project explored how the dissemination of online health care information creates new health care spaces by influencing ideas and behaviors. In addition, I have completed in-depth interviews with seventy homebirth mothers and over 100 direct-entry midwives, with the express purpose of writing a thoroughly researched and accessible book conveying an accurate profile of homebirth consumers and their midwives. Findings from this research have been incorporated in this book in chapters 9, 11, 12, and 13. Findings from the National Library of Medicine's Information Infrastructure Program are encapsulated below.

Informing the Public about Midwives through the Internet: Results of the National Library of Medicine Study

The National Library of Medicine Information Infrastructure Program was set up to fund empirically-based evaluations assessing the impact of Internet-based health care information. Prenatal care was one of the five preventive health-care topics that were targeted for in-depth study. The research team agreed that I could include a research component assessing the effectiveness of the web for disseminating midwifery information to the wider public. Previous to this, I had hypothesized that the web would be an effective tool for informing the public about the midwifery model of care. Here was my chance to find out how powerful the web could be as a communication tool for disseminating information not usually available through official channels.

Our health-care research team produced a specially designed webpage and the respondents answered two online questionnaires, one taken before viewing the prenatal care (PNC) webpage and the other after exploring the PNC site. In addition to the questionnaires (both closed and open-ended questions were included), we designed and facilitated three focus groups to gain more in-depth data about process, especially to determine whether women change their ideas about using midwives when they learn more about them. When the PNC webpage went online, the midwifery portion of the project had not yet been completed. As soon as this section was finished, we e-mailed all participants offering this information along with extensive links explaining the philosophy behind the midwifery model of care. In addition, two types of midwives were described: the certified nurse-midwife and the direct-entry midwife. Extensive links describing the philosophical tenets of the midwifery model in general and the specific differences between the two types of midwives augmented this information. Our Information Infrastructure sample consisted of one hundred women of childbearing age at a prominent Northeastern university who were pregnant or planned on a future pregnancy and had ready access to webpage technology. The sample included representative members of the staff, faculty, graduate students, and a selected subset of undergraduate students.

When asked if their ideas about midwives had changed as a direct result of viewing the webpage, a significant minority (twenty-eight percent) said "yes." When the respondents were asked to elaborate on how their ideas about midwives changed, the women answered that they were more positively inclined to think of midwives as a viable option. This sample population highlighted three major dimensions that they felt were involved in creating a new health-care practitioner narrative—in this case, a new midwifery narrative. First, clear and easily understandable information must be available to counteract stereotypes and vague, uncertain knowledge. Second, this information must contain enough substance to directly challenge negative images. Third, the source of the information must be viewed as legitimate. When these three criteria were satisfied, the respondents become more open to redefining who is and is not an appropriate health care professional.

The focus group participants provided more in-depth access to their redefinition process. The following quotes illustrate this reconstruction process:

> Before [reading the webpage] midwives didn't seem as reputable as being in a hospital, so it was really interesting to see that some insurance does cover it and it is an option, not that I'm personally ready to have this baby now, but [using a midwife] actually became an option and before [the webpage] it wasn't. Midwifery was demystified on the webpage. I have had no other

experience of midwifery except through this webpage; it would definitely be an option now whereas before I don't think I would have used it.

The webpage answered a lot of questions that I had that I wouldn't necessarily ask anyone just because everyone starts assuming that you want to get pregnant. For example, the thing I would call the most [enlightening] was the whole issue of the midwives vs. the doctors and the hospital, it really opened my eyes and made choosing a midwife something that I want to do.

Through the midwifery links I learned about all the categories of prenatal care providers—physicians and midwives. I found this very useful because I didn't know anything about that. Usually, you just go to the physician and that is it. Now I have more options.

I found the part of the webpage on midwives the most interesting. It has really opened my mind, something I've never had to consider before, especially the differences between them and the physician. Whether the physicians are male or female, it just blew me away. It is definitely good to know that midwives exist.

As a direct result of the website I would consider using a midwife now; I never would have considered a midwife before.

I'm probably a little more aware of questions I should be asking. For me it was just that everyone in my family has always used a physician. I have never even considered a midwife. It was always something that other people do, alternative people do, people that do alternative medicine. It wasn't something that I would necessarily do…so I have never really investigated it. And perhaps it makes me more comfortable with asking the question, is using a midwife an option that I want to choose?

After viewing the webpage I think I do know more about midwives. I think I have an open mind to probably learning as much as I can when I do become pregnant or when I want to become pregnant. I think it is good that the information about midwives is out there because I think people will be more open and curious, including me.

Now as a result of the webpage I am more curious about midwives. Although it probably won't be an alternative that I would pick in the near future, it could be. I would probably ask more about it, especially when I hear people say that they have used a midwife. I will be more interested to hear their decision making process and what went into it, rather than writing it off. It's like you have a certain predisposition almost and the webpage might lead you to question your position and what you feel comfortable with more than before.

The webpage made me rethink the idea of using midwives (this woman has had two children with doctors).

The webpage made me open to midwives; it just gave me another cue to be open when I get to that point in my life.

Despite extensive information detailing the difference between certified nurse-midwives and direct-entry midwives, the women in the study were not able to discriminate between them, but rather combined them into one indistinguishable category. We found that the idea of actually using a midwife was so novel that the difference between the two types of midwives described on the prenatal care webpage was not retained. This was a big surprise to us since our study population was highly educated and able to readily grasp conceptual information. We hypothesized that the novelty of seeing midwives as a viable option caused the majority of women in our study to reach saturation at this point, and the differences between the two kinds of midwives became excess data.

As the United States moves increasingly toward a market-driven managed health-care industry, health-care consumers will turn to the Internet with greater frequency as they are required to act more as consumers than as patients. Under these conditions the Internet will become an innovative medium for constructing new narratives about midwives. In fact, a little over one-fifth of the seventy women I interviewed for my forthcoming book reported having based their choice to pursue a homebirth on information gleaned from the web. In this environment it becomes more important than ever for midwives to settle their differences. If *two* types of midwives were confusing to a highly educated segment of the population, then *five* types of midwives will most certainly confuse the wider public about the midwifery model of care. Resolving the midwifery differences of opinion at this historical juncture will do much to promulgate the proliferation of midwifery.

Our ardent hope is that this book may contribute in some small measure to midwifery unity.

OVERVIEW OF THE BOOK

Part I, Developing Direct-Entry Midwifery in the United States

The three chapters in Part I of this book take a national perspective on the development of direct-entry midwifery, offering a comparative overview of MANA and the ACNM and descriptions of the creation of the CM by ACNM members and of the CPM by MANA members.

Many midwives have questioned the existence of two national midwifery organizations in the United States, suggesting that unifying under one organizational banner would do a great deal more to promote midwifery and improve women's health. In chapter 1, the comparative overview of ACNM and MANA, Robbie analyzes points that could have led to convergence, explains the very real reasons (some of which were briefly described above) why they have not, and points to some very positive contemporary convergent trends that hold promise for mutual respect and effective collaboration between these two national organizations—one large, the other small, but both equally committed to growing midwifery in the interests of better care for women.

Another central question often posed by midwives has been, why would ACNM, an organization whose members took twenty-five years to attend one percent of American births (by the late 1970s), and another thirty years to reach close to ten percent and to get its members legal, licensed, and regulated in all fifty states, challenge its own gains with a new certification not based on nursing, which at least is already a culturally accepted and respected profession? Maureen May and Robbie Davis-Floyd seek to answer this question in chapter 2, which describes and analyzes the creation of the CM. It might seem more logical to have separated this chapter, which is by far the longest one in the book, into two, one describing the national creation of the CM and the other focusing on the legalization of the CM in New York. These chapters would have most properly fit into Part II of this book, which consists of state-based case studies in the legalization of direct-entry midwifery. But the CM's national creation and state legitimation are inseparable: they are really one story and that story is all about the history, politics, and culture of nurse-midwifery in New York.

New York was formative in the development of both nurse- and direct-entry midwifery in the United States, and an understanding of that history is essential to an understanding of why the CM was created and the ramifications of the law that allowed its creation, the 1992 New York Midwifery Practice Act. The development of direct-entry midwifery is our main focus in this book, and the history, culture, and politics of nurse-midwifery have been intimately tied to this process. Much of this history unfolded in New York, along with a particular kind of midwifery politics and a particular type of culture, which the authors characterize in that chapter as one of pragmatism, showing how that culture influenced the political decisions the New York nurse-midwives made as they created and fought to legalize the CM. This hefty chapter must also treat the history of MANA-style lay and direct-entry midwifery in New York—a history that unfolded sometimes in synchrony with, and sometimes in opposition to, the efforts of the New York CNMs to create their own version of direct-entry midwifery, the CM. The battles fought in New York over the type of direct-entry midwife that should exist in that state have had long-standing national ramifications, both for relations between CNMs and DEMs in other states, and for the creation of the CPM described in chapter 3.

Thus we ask our readers to stick with the authors through all the pages of the New York story because it is so central to understanding (1) the creation and legalization of the CM; (2) the history, politics, and culture of nurse-midwifery in the United States; (3) the history, politics, and culture of direct-entry (formerly lay) midwifery in the United States; and (4) the essence of the differences and struggles between these groups as they were played out on New York's political terrain. The New York story is told and retold among midwives around the United States, usually as a story of betrayal and exploitation of one side by the other, and as an example of why the groups don't trust each other and what was so awful about one group or the other, with little understanding of what really happened there and why. We hope that you will find the information in this chapter enlightening, the stories fascinating, and the politics revealing, and that you will become engaged as you read in understanding the motivations and ideals of the two competing groups—the group that lost the battle (homebirth DEMs) and the group that won.

Another question midwives sometimes pose is: Why would lay midwives, who fought hard and long to stay independent, autonomous, and often, unregulated, drop the term "lay" in favor of "direct-entry," create a national certification for direct-entry midwives who practice out-of-hospital, and work extremely hard to get it legalized (entailing licensure and regulation) in most states? Robbie addresses this question in chapter 3, in which she describes the creation of the CPM in terms of what she calls *qualified commodification*—a successful effort to commodify and market midwifery within the legal system without compromising its essential ideals of autonomy and woman-centeredness.

Part II, State-Based Case Studies in the Legalization of Direct-Entry Midwives

The six chapters in Part II document the efforts of direct-entry midwives (successful and unsuccessful) to become legal, licensed, and regulated in six states: Florida, Minnesota, Colorado, Virginia, Iowa, and Massachusetts. Although we wish for more, in this book we cannot hope to deal with the complexities of midwifery politics in every U.S. state. Because this book is a work of social science, our decisions about which states to include as case studies stemmed from our discoveries that particular social scientists were actively engaged in studying midwifery politics in their states, and that the states they were studying provided the full spectrum of the legal struggles and situations of homebirth direct-entry midwives in the contemporary United States.

We were fortunate to find that Melissa Denmark, at the time an anthropology masters' student at the University of Florida (and now a graduate of Seattle Midwifery School), was willing to conduct an extensive study of midwifery history and legislation in Florida. Rhetorician Mary Lay had long been both participating in and observing the proposed direct-entry midwifery legislation in Minnesota and had formed a professional friendship with Kerry Dixon, a direct-entry midwife who became chapter coauthor. A similar relationship formed between anthropologist Susan Erickson and midwife Amy Colo, coauthors of the Colorado chapter. Anthropologist Christa Craven spent years studying and participating in midwifery legislative efforts in Virginia, as did Carrie Hough (also an anthropologist) in Iowa, and Christine Barbara Johnson (sociologist) in Massachusetts. Collectively, these six chapters offer profound lessons about what works and what does not in attempts to legalize midwifery.

With enormous effort over several years, DEMs had achieved legalization in Florida before Melissa Denmark began her research. In Minnesota, they achieved it toward the end of Mary Lay's research process through combined legislative and grassroots efforts, as also happened for Susan Erickson and Amy Colo in Colorado and Christa Craven in Virginia, who had to rewrite portions of her chapter to record legislative success shortly before this book went to press! Legalization efforts remain ongoing in Iowa and Massachusetts. Salient successful strategies that emerge from the analyses in these chapters include organization, communication, savvy lobbying, education of consumers and legislators, collaborative efforts among midwives and related groups, cultivation of particular officials and physicians, effective consumer support, perseverance over many years, and occasional serendipitous doses of luck. (We offer much more detail about successful strategies in the Introduction to Part II.) The foundational basis of the success of all of these strategies is the midwives' documentation of, and the consumers' testaments to, the excellent, evidence-based, and woman-centered care they provide.

As part of her original research project, Robbie conducted extensive interviews in California and Washington state on the history of midwifery in those states, direct-entry midwives' successful legislative efforts in both, and the problematics resulting from their achievement of legalization, licensure, and regulation. She originally intended to include chapters on these states in this volume, but space limitations intervened, along with her discovery that sociologist Bruce Hoffman is actively engaged in an in-depth research project on these issues in California, Washington, and Oregon. His research and subsequent publications will tell the stories of the development of direct-entry midwifery in these key states (supplementing the work of Raymond DeVries [1996], who recounted the early history of the legislative efforts of the California midwives), and we urge our readers to watch for and read the results of his work. Suffice it to say that midwives' legislative success in these states benefited from all of the strategies mentioned above, and that the problems this success has generated are echoed and reflected in the descriptions of these same problems recorded in the chapters we do include in this book.

Part III, Core Issues in Mainstreaming Midwives

The four chapters in Part III of this book treat core issues in mainstreaming direct-entry midwives, from impediments to positive change. In chapter 10, midwife-sociologist Betty Anne Daviss describes the overarching tensions between midwifery as a social movement and its professionalizing enterprise, showing how social movement theory can both illuminate and inspire contemporary American midwives to engage in "social activist moments."

Some of the problems generated by legislative success are encapsulated in chapter 11, which deals with the issue of *renegade midwives*—those who occasionally or regularly reject state regulations or peer protocols to attend the births of women considered high risk. Renegade midwives, more dedicated to serving women's desires than to preserving midwifery as a viable profession, simultaneously preserve essential elements of midwifery knowledge, such as techniques for the home delivery of breeches and twins, and jeopardize the professional gains made by midwives in their states who are willing to abide by state regulations or peer protocols prohibiting such practices. Thus they constitute both assets and liabilities to contemporary American direct-entry midwives' struggle to enter the mainstream.

Chapter 12 describes the vagaries and successes of home-to-hospital transport, in which the very different worlds of homebirth midwifery and hospital obstetrics either collide or (temporarily) merge. Barbara and Robbie hoped, in writing this chapter, to offer a positive model to hospitals and homebirth midwives alike for the most effective forms of transport, which can constitute magical *mandorlas* (wholes created in small spaces by the merging of separate worlds).

The concluding chapter explains, fundamentally, "why midwives matter" through Christine's work on how midwives "care women into" a sense of autonomy and empowerment through pregnancy and birth. This chapter also addresses the primary barriers to a widely held dream—that midwives become the primary health care givers for the majority of childbearing women in the United States, while specialized obstetricians concentrate on the high-risk care they are trained to give. As Christine and Robbie delineate these barriers, they seek also to indicate the myriad strategies midwives and their many supporters are employing to overcome them.

Further information about the chapters in Parts I, II, and III can be found in the introductions to those parts.

The midwifery story we tell in this book is about politics, professionalization, and positive change; it is also deeply about identity. American midwives are still in the process of deciding and becoming who they want to be, both as professionals and as members of a social activist movement that seeks to change not only American birthways but also the cultural beliefs and values behind contemporary technocratic modes of birth. Collectively, midwives are still so marginal that their profession might vanish tomorrow if insurance companies, obstetricians, and health-care officials should decide to unite against them. Nevertheless, midwives do their best to provide women with birth options they would not otherwise enjoy and with lifetime health care based on notions of the normalcy of women's bodies and a sense of the importance of an ongoing relationship between the client and the practitioner. Legal or illegal, plain or professional, nurse- or direct-entry, American midwives remain dedicated to serving women and babies in woman-centered ways. We contend that in this endeavor they deserve the full support of the society whose need for childbirth alternatives generated, and continues to demand, their existence and their sociocultural, economic, and legal viability.

ACKNOWLEDGMENTS

We express our deep appreciation to the authors of the chapters in this book, who have worked long and hard to bring their original ethnographic studies to fruition in these pages, and to the following reviewers, whose careful attention to each chapter and helpful comments enabled us to ensure the accuracy of our statements and thus our accountability to the midwifery community, and to those who study and support it. These reviewers include Carol Nelson, Ida Darragh, Diane Holzer, Jo Anne Myers-Ciecko, Christa Craven, Susan Hodges, Katherine Camacho Carr, Deanne Williams, Judith Rooks, Raymond DeVries, and Barbara Katz Rothman. Special thanks to Deanne Williams for her challenging comments on this Introduction and to our Routledge editors, Michael Bickerstaff and Sarah Blackmon, for their excellent work and continuous support. Robbie Davis-Floyd also expresses appreciation to the Wenner-Gren Foundation for Anthropological Research for the grants (Nos. 6015 and 6247, extending from 1996 through 2000) that supported her research.

The title of this book was adapted from the theme of the 1998 Conference of the Midwives Alliance of North America in Traverse City, Michigan: "Midwifery in the Mainstream."

ENDNOTES

1. This original clarity has been blurred in recent years by the certification and licensure in New York of several CMs who graduated from MEAC-accredited programs, including the Seattle Midwifery School, as described in chapter 2.

2. Throughout this book we use female nouns and pronouns to refer to midwives. But it is important to remember that one percent of American midwives are male, and that many of these men have made important contributions to the development of American midwifery.

3. Indeed, a study conducted by nurse-midwifery researchers clearly demonstrated that higher education did not equal increased clinical competence (Rooks, Carr, and Sandvold 1991). But it does bring research skills, social credibility, and prestige.

4. Christine sought to obtain a representative sample of women who chose homebirth by contacting midwives, their clients, friends of homebirth organizations, and by using the snowball technique to increase the sample size. The sample reflects the profile of most women who choose homebirth—predominantly professional, white, and middle class. However, there is a significant minority of poor and working-class women who also consistently choose homebirth and are also included in the sample. To establish sufficient rapport for an authentic narrative account to emerge, each woman was interviewed using the in-depth, semi-structured interview technique. The interviews took from two to ten hours each, with the average interview running about four hours. To avoid the problems involved when collecting only retrospective data, Christine also located eleven women who were pregnant and were planning to give birth at home. Each of these eleven women was interviewed both before and after their birth experience. Every interview was transcribed in its entirety. Following this, recurring

themes and issues were identified in the resulting data, using a grounded theory approach. This technique is based on the generation of analytically-based categories through the *constant comparative method*, which validates the categories against the data in which they are grounded.

REFERENCES

American Medical Association. 1993. *Physician Characteristics and Distribution in the United States*. American Medical Association, Department of Data Services, Division of Survey Data Resources.

Benoit, Cecilia, Robbie Davis-Floyd, Edwin van Teijlingen, Sirpa Wrede, Jane Sandall, and Janneli Miller. 2001. "Designing Midwives: A Transnational Comparison of Educational Models." In *Birth by Design: Pregnancy, Maternity Care, and Midwifery in North America and Europe*, ed. Raymond DeVries, Edwin van Teijlingen, Sirpa Wrede, and Cecilia Benoit, 139–165. New York: Routledge.

Bourgeault, Ivy, Cecilia Benoit, and Robbie Davis-Floyd, eds. 2004. *Reconceiving Midwives: The New Canadian Model of Care*. Toronto: McGill-Queens University Press.

Davis-Floyd, Robbie E. 1990. "The Role of American Obstetrics in the Resolution of Cultural Anomaly." *Social Science and Medicine* 31(2):175–189.

———. 1992. "The Technocratic Body and the Organic Body: Cultural Models for Women's Birth Choices." In *The Anthropology of Science and Technology*, ed. David J. Hess and Linda L. Layne. Hartford, CT: JAI Press.

———. 1993. "The Technocratic Model of Birth." In *Feminist Theory in the Study of Folklore*, ed. Susan Tower Hollis, Linda Pershing, and M. J. Young, 297–326. Urbana: University of Illinois Press. (Updated and expanded revision of "The Technological Model of Birth," *Journal of American Folklore* 100(398):93–109, 1987.)

———. 1994a. "Mind over Body: The Pregnant Professional." In *Many Mirrors: Body Image and Social Relations in Anthropological Perspective*, ed. Nicole Sault. Brunswick, NJ: Rutgers University Press.

———. 1994b. "The Technocratic Body: American Childbirth as Cultural Expression," *Social Science and Medicine* 38(8):1125–40.

———. 1998a. "Autonomy in Midwifery: Definition, Education, Regulation." *Midwifery Today* 46 (Spring).

———. 1998b. "The Ups, Downs, and Interlinkages of Nurse- and Direct-Entry Midwifery: Status, Practice, and Education." In *Getting an Education: Paths to Becoming a Midwife*, 4th ed., ed. Jan Tritten and Joel Southern, 67–118. Eugene, OR: Midwifery Today.

———. 1998c. "Types of Midwifery Training: An Anthropological Overview." In *Getting an Education: Paths to Becoming a Midwife*, 4th ed., ed. Jan Tritten and Joel Southern, 119–133. Eugene, OR: Midwifery Today.

———. 1999. "Some Thoughts on Bridging the Gap between Nurse- and Direct-Entry Midwives." *Midwifery Today* (March).

———. 2000. "Mutual Accommodation or Biomedical Hegemony?: Anthropological Perspectives on Global Issues in Midwifery." *Midwifery Today* (March): 12–16, 68–69.

———. 2003a. "My Dream." *Midwifery Today* (January).

———. 2003b. "Home Birth Emergencies in the U.S. and Mexico: The Trouble with Transport." In "Reproduction Gone Awry," ed. Gwynne Jenkins and Marcia Inhorn. Special issue of *Social Science and Medicine* 56(9): 1913–1931.

———. 2004a. "Ways of Knowing: Open and Closed Systems." *Midwifery Today* 69 (Spring): 9–13.

———. 2004b. "Consuming Childbirth: The Qualified Commodification of Midwifery Care." In *Consuming Motherhood*, ed. Danielle Wozniak, Linda Layne, and Janelle Taylor. New Brunswick, NJ: Rutgers University Press.

———. 2004c. *Birth as an American Rite of Passage*, 2nd edition. Berkeley: University of California Press. (orig pub 1992.)

———. 2005 "Daughter of Time: The Postmodern Midwife." *MIDIRS Midwifery Digest.*

Davis-Floyd, Robbie, Sheila Cosminsky, and Stacy L. Pigg. 2001. "Introduction." *Daughters of Time: The Shifting Identities of Contemporary Midwives*. Special triple issue, *Medical Anthropology* 20: 2–3, 4.

Davis-Floyd, Robbie, and Elizabeth Davis. 1997. "Intuition as Authoritative Knowledge in Midwifery and Home Birth." In *Childbirth and Authoritative Knowledge: Cross-Cultural Perspectives*, pp. 315-349. ed. Robbie Davis-Floyd and Carolyn Sargent, University of California Press.

Davis-Floyd, Robbie, and Carolyn Sargent. 1997. "Introduction: The Anthropology of Childbirth." In *Childbirth and Authoritative Knowledge: Cross-Cultural Perspectives*, Berkeley: University of California Press.

Davis-Floyd, Robbie, and Carolyn Sargent, eds. 1997. *Childbirth and Authoritative Knowledge: Cross-Cultural Perspectives*, Berkeley: University of California Press.

DeVries, Raymond. 1996. *Making Midwives Legal: Childbirth, Medicine, and the Law*, 2nd ed. Columbus: Ohio State University Press.

Fraser, Gertrude. 1988. "Afro-American Midwives, Biomedicine, and the State: An Ethnohistorical Account of Birth and Its Transformation in Rural Virginia." Ph.D. diss, Dept. of Anthropology, Johns Hopkins University.

———. 1992. *Afro-American Midwives, Biomedicine, and the State*. Cambridge, MA: Harvard University Press.

Friedson, Eliot. 1983. "The Theory of Professions: State of the Art." In *The Sociology of the Professions: Lawyers, Doctors and Others*, ed. Robert Dingwall and Philip Lewis. New York: St. Martin's Press.

Hodges, Susan. 2004. "The Effects of Hospital Economics on Maternity Care." www.cfm.org.

Johnson, Christine Barbara. 1987. *Normalizing Birth*. Ph.D. diss., Boston University.

———. 2000. "The Public Face of Midwifery in Massachusetts." Paper presented at the May American Anthropological Association, San Francisco.

———. 2001. "The Ethic of Care and the Ethic of Autonomy." Paper presented at the May Pacific Sociological Association, San Francisco.

Johnson, Christine, and Priscilla Galvin. 2001. *Transforming the Health Care System with On-Line Technology*. United States National Library of Medicine Information Infrastructure Program, Contract N01-LM-6-3539.

Johnson, Kenneth, C. and Betty Anne Daviss. 2005. "Outcomes of Planned Home Births with Certified Professional Midwives: Large Prospective Study in North America." *British Medical Journal* 330(7505): 1416, June. www.bmj.com.

Jordan, Brigitte. 1986. *Brought to Bed: Childbearing in America 1750–1950*. New York: Oxford University Press.

———. 1989. "Cosmopolitical Obstetrics: Some Insights from the Training of Traditional Midwives." *Social Science and Medicine* 28(9):925–944.

———. 1993. *Birth in Four Cultures: A Cross-Cultural Investigation of Childbirth in Yucatan, Holland, Sweden and the United States*. Prospect Heights, Ohio: Waveland Press. (Orig. pub. 1978.)

Larson, M. 1979. "Professionalism: Rise and Fall," *International Journal of Health Services* 9

Leavitt, Judith Walzer. 1986. *Brought to Bed: Childbearing in America, 1750–1950*. NewYork: Oxford University Press.

Logan, Onnie Lee, as told to Katherine Clark. 1989. *Motherwit: An Alabama Midwife's Story*. New York: E.P. Dutton.

MacDonald, K. M. 1985. "Social Closure and Occupational Registration," *Sociology*, 19:541–56.

MacDorman, M., and G. Singh. 1998. "Midwifery Care, Social and Medical Risk Factors, and Birth Outcomes in the U.S.A." *Journal of Epidemiology and Community Health* 52:310–317.

Oakley, Ann. 1977. *Becoming a Mother*. New York: Schocken Books.

———. 1980. *Women Confined: Towards a Sociology of Childbirth*. New York: Schocken Books.

———. 1984. *The Captured Womb: A History of the Medical Care of Pregnant Women*. New York: Basil Blackwell.

Perkins, Barbara Bridgman. 2004. *The Medical Delivery Business: Health Reform, Childbirth, and the Economic Order*. New Brunswick, NJ: Rutgers University Press.

Reid, Margaret. 1989. "Sisterhood and Professionalization: A Case Study of the American Lay Midwife." In *Women as Healers: Cross-Cultural Perspectives*, ed. Carol McClain, 219–238. New Brunswick: Rutgers University Press.

Rooks, Judith. 1997. *Midwifery and Childbirth in America*. Philadephia: Temple University Press.

Rooks, Judith P., Katherine Camacho Carr, and Irene Sandvold. 1991. "The Importance of Non-Master's Degree Options in Nurse-Midwifery Education." *Journal of Nurse Midwifery* 36:124–130.

Rooks, Judith P., Norman L. Weatherby, Eunice K. M. Ernst, Susan Stapleton, David Rosen, and Allan Rosenfield. 1989. "Outcomes of Care in Birth Centers: The National Birth Center Study," *New England Journal of Medicine* 321:1804–1811.

Susie, Debra Ann. 1988. *In the Way of Our Grandmothers: A Cultural View of 20th-Century Midwifery in Florida*. Athens: University of Georgia.

Tew, Marjorie. 1982. "Obstetrics vs. Midwifery: The Verdict of the Statistics," *Journal of Maternal and Child Health*, May:193–201.

———. 1990. *Safer Childbirth: A Critical History of Maternity Care*. New York: Chapman and Hall.

Torstendahl, Rolf, and Michael Burrage. 1990. *The Formation of Professions: Knowledge, State and Strategy*. London, Newbury Park, New Delhi: Sage.

Witz, Anne. 1992. *Professions and Patriarchy*. London and New York: Routledge.

Part I

Developing Direct-Entry Midwifery in the United States

Chapter 1 ACNM and MANA: Divergent Histories and Convergent Trends

Chapter 2 Idealism and Pragmatism in the Creation of the Certified Midwife: The Development of Midwifery in New York and the New York Midwifery Practice Act of 1992

Chapter 3 Qualified Commodification: The Creation of the Certified Professional Midwife

These three chapters cumulatively paint a national picture of the development of nurse- and direct-entry midwifery in the United States in terms of history, politics, and national certification. In chapter 1, Robbie Davis-Floyd presents a comparative overview of ACNM and MANA through their divergent histories and contemporary convergent trends, analyzing the respective motivations of their members for creating two separate national direct-entry certifications, the CM and the CPM, at close to the same historical moment.

In chapter 2, Maureen May and Davis-Floyd describe the creation of the CM in the context of the history of nurse-midwifery in New York, which is intimately tied to the history of nurse-midwifery in the nation. They analyze the characteristics of the culture of pragmatism that developed among nurse-midwives and the ways in which this culture influenced their very practical reasons for conceptualizing and then working hard to create a new kind of midwife who would be both licensed in New York and certified by the ACNM Certification Council, without having to pass through nursing training. May and Davis-Floyd also describe the unsuccessful efforts of New York's homebirth direct-entry midwives to be included in the law that legalized the CM—the New York Midwifery Practice Act of 1992—and its effects on their practices and lives.

In chapter 3, Davis-Floyd analyzes the creation of the CPM by the North American Registry of Midwives, a daughter organization of MANA, using commodification theory to describe the alchemical process by which the requirements for this certification were developed as its creators struggled to "sell midwifery without selling midwifery out."

1

ACNM AND MANA: DIVERGENT HISTORIES AND CONVERGENT TRENDS

Robbie Davis-Floyd

• A Brief Social History of American Midwifery • Nurse-Midwifery's Shift to Hospital-Based Practice and the Founding of the ACNM • Lay and Direct-Entry Midwifery • The Founding of MANA and Its Work during the 1980s • The Carnegie Meetings of the Interorganizational Work Group • Apprenticeship in Canada and the United States • The Late 1990s: Convergent Trends • From Lay to Direct-Entry: The Development of the Certified Professional Midwife • ACNM, the Development of the Certified Midwife (CM), and MANA's Response • The Contemporary Status Quo • Conclusion: A Convergent Network of Options for American Women • Timeline of Events in the Comparative History of ACNM and MANA

The scene is the 1997 MANA conference in Seattle. The conference room is filling up with so many midwives that walls have to be moved to accommodate the crowd. I am on my way to the slide projector and I am so nervous that I drop my tray of slides, then have to work frantically to get them back in order before the panel—which I am facilitating—is supposed to start. Over the past ten years, I have given hundreds of public lectures and have chaired dozens of conference panels, so why am I trembling? Because this is the most politically charged topic I have ever taken on—a panel designed specifically to address the major issues that place MANA at loggerheads with ACNM.

The current president of ACNM is on this panel, along with the vice president and a past president. Representing MANA are its president, a board member of MANA's sister organization the North American Registry of Midwives (NARM),[1] and a well-known direct-entry midwifery educator. The title of the panel is "ACNM and MANA: A Direct-Entry Dialogue," and the burning question of the day is: What will be the relationship of the two new direct-entry certifications developed by MANA and the ACNM?

NARM began work on national direct-entry certification in the early 1990s and had its process up and running by 1994. A prime motivator for key members of the NARM board had been their belief that ACNM was going to stick to nurse-midwifery and leave direct-entry certification up to MANA and NARM. Thinking they had an open field, NARM board and committee members devoted thousands of volunteer hours to creating a new direct-entry credential, the Certified Professional Midwife (CPM).

But in 1994, after countless hours of deliberation on their own part, the ACNM passed a motion to develop its own direct-entry credential, which was later named the Certified Midwife (CM). From MANA's point of view, this was a massive infringement on the territory it had staked out—direct-entry or non-nurse midwifery. Making matters worse for MANA and NARM, ACNM had sent out a letter to legislators all over the country stating ACNM's support for its own CM credential and casting doubt on the validity of other certifications—an action many in MANA and NARM interpreted as a frontal attack.

Both organizations were facing battles to legalize these new direct-entry certifications in state legislatures across the country. What the 350 MANA midwives packed into the room wanted to know was, were they going to have to fight both the doctors and the ACNM to get their credential legalized, or could their sister midwives in the ACNM be convinced to support both certifications and work collaboratively with them to get both CPMs and CMs legalized and regulated in all 50 states?

So at one point, I asked the ACNM president to clarify whether she might support both certifications. Her response was that she could only stand by ACNM's standards and could not support the standards established by NARM.

Midwife after midwife, some speaking as members of MANA and some as members of ACNM, came to the mikes in dismay to plead for ACNM to take a more supportive position. And then Anessa Maize, the MANA representative from Canada, took the microphone in hand and said, "You know, in Canada, we have resolved these problems and we don't fight with each other like this. We believe we are creating systems that work, that are unifying and not divisive, and we invite you to come and take a look!"

In many areas of cultural life, Americans have prided themselves on establishing models of success that other countries try to emulate. But when the midwives of Canada initiated their worldwide search for the best models of midwifery education, legislation, and practice on which to base their "new midwifery" (Bourgeault, Benoit, and Davis-Floyd 2004), they did not look to the United States because they saw the American situation as something not to emulate but to avoid. Canadian midwives tend to view American midwifery as a fractured profession (Bourgeault and Fynes 1997), noting with dismay that the divisions between nurse- and direct-entry midwives have diverted their energies on multiple occasions into feuding with each other.

Since 1996 these struggles have constituted a focal point of my anthropological research—necessarily so, since my research project (described in the Introduction) has concentrated on the historical emergence at almost the same point in time of the two direct-entry certifications mentioned in the story above. These two new certifications encapsulate one significant agreement between the ACNM and MANA—that nursing should not be a mandatory part of midwifery education—and several significant disagreements over standards of education and practice.

Canadian midwives have both watched and participated as American midwives have tripped over pitfalls that the Canadians later worked hard to avoid. There were several attempts during the first part of the twentieth century, and again in the 1970s, to create American-style nurse-midwifery in Canada (Bourgeault and Fynes 1997:1056–1057), a number of American-trained nurse-midwives have long lived and practiced in Canada, MANA's second conference was held in Toronto (in 1984), and a number of Canadian midwives have been and are still members of MANA. Yet as midwives in Canada have worked to develop their new midwifery over the past two decades, the American story has served not as a model of inspiration, but rather as a *cautionary tale.*

In this chapter I will tell that tale, or at least the parts of it most relevant to our focus in this book on American midwives' efforts to mainstream themselves, in part through the development of direct-entry certification. I will occasionally refer to the Canadian perspective as a useful lens through which to view the American situation. An intracultural, U.S.-oriented telling would recount this story in its own terms, missing the important cross-cultural and transnational perspectives provided by taking an outsider's point of view. And indeed, the U.S. midwifery story has already been thoroughly recounted from an insider's point of view by Judith Rooks in her comprehensive book

Midwifery and Childbirth in America (1997; see also Donnison 1977, Donegan 1978, Leavitt 1986, Litoff 1978, Wertz and Wertz 1977).

In this chapter I seek to complement Rooks's work through an anthropological analysis that focuses directly on the relationships between nurse- and direct-entry midwives, and on points of time in which their interests either converged or diverged. I seek also to lay out the background information essential for understanding the transformations and divisions in contemporary American midwifery that are key to understanding the other chapters in this volume. Because these stem directly from historical developments, a portion of this chapter will recount that history to identify the evolutionary trajectories of nurse- and direct-entry midwifery that made today's clashes all but inevitable. I will identify some historical moments at which things could have unfolded differently, for therein lies the cautionary part of the cautionary tale: not to seize a moment that could lead to unity is, in effect, to accept and perpetuate the disadvantages of division. But that's not how the key players saw it at the time, and that's not how many of them see it even now. Division has its advantages too, and when midwives of good conscience see more to gain from staying separate than from joining together, those who seek to learn from their experience may wish to understand the reasons why.

A BRIEF SOCIAL HISTORY OF AMERICAN MIDWIFERY
The Development of Nurse-Midwifery

Well into the 1900s, in both Canada and the United States, midwives remained, as they always had been, the primary attendants at childbirth. Native American midwives continued to attend women in their tribal groups, as did colonial midwives among the white settlers, Hispanic midwives in their southwestern communities, immigrant midwives accompanying their ethnic groups, and black granny midwives in the American South. Nevertheless, Canada and the United States are the only two Western industrialized nations in which, by mid-century, midwifery was largely eradicated from the health care system. In the United States, three factors were primarily responsible:

Physician resistance. Starting in the early 1900s, physicians determined to take charge of childbirth, along with public health professionals and nurses, waged systematic and virulent propaganda campaigns against the thousands of immigrant midwives practicing in the northeastern cities, as they were seen to be the greatest threat to physician's attempts to take control of birth. These campaigns employed stereotypes of midwives as dirty, illiterate, ignorant, and irresponsible, in contrast to hospitals and physicians, which were portrayed as clean, educated, and the epitome of responsibility in health care. In *The Medical Delivery Business* (2004:31), Barbara Bridgman Perkins identifies "economic competition, professional and institutional needs to hospitalize birth [these include resident training], gender discrimination [specialization], and fear that midwife inclusion in the medical system would lead to more government regulation" as primary reasons for obstetric and academic rejection of midwifery.

Lack of professional organization by midwives. In Europe, midwifery developed as a profession with formal education and licensure requirements at a very early stage compared to the United States (DeVries et al. 2001). American midwives of the nineteenth and early twentieth centuries did not develop professional organizations to increase their political effectiveness and set standards and educational requirements. Cultural, socioeconomic, and language barrier contributed significantly; even professional immigrant midwives usually served only their own communities and were often not aware of the existence of other midwives serving other communities one neighborhood away. Other impediments to organization included legal and cultural prohibitions against women regarding public speaking, leadership, finances, and so forth, not to mention the non-existence of formal midwifery training programs in the United States, which resulted from all of the above-mentioned factors. So in spite of the high level of training many immigrant midwives obtained in professional European midwifery programs and their extensive experience, it was easy for the medical profession to portray them as untrained and ignorant, and impossible for them to combat these stereotypes in the wider cultural arena.

Cultural influences on women's choices. Fashion and assimilation played key roles here. As many of the ethnic communities within which midwives had flourished assimilated into the larger culture, they adopted its medical practices and values along with everything else. Minority women actively sought access to medical care in hospitals because the state touted it as the best care for their babies—but had also denied it to them for many years based on segregationist health care policies. Once these women finally gained access to hospitals, many began to perceive the use of midwives as "going backwards" (Holmes 1986:287; Brown and Toussaint 1998; Fraser 1998:103). The kind of culture that had supported midwives disappeared, and along with it the midwives (Borst 1988, 1989, 1995; DeVries 1996:179; Fraser 1995). In addition, from the late 1800s on in the United States, it increasingly became the fashion for middle-class women to employ male midwives and later, obstetricians, as the modern and progressive way to give birth. After all, male-developed technologies were bringing electricity, telephones, railways, cars, airplanes, vacuum cleaners, and a thousand other progressive and modern conveniences. Male, techno-logical attendance at birth seemed part and parcel of this process of modernization—a way up the social ladder of progress (Wilson 1995).

Throughout the 1800s, midwives attended the majority of births in the United States, but by the middle of the 1900s, marginalized and often practicing illegally, they attended only a tiny minority of births.

In reaction to the propaganda campaigns promulgated by obstetri-cians, public health officials, and some nurses, nurse-midwives (who were the first to create an organized and cohesive professional system of midwifery in the United States) took great care from the very beginning to act, and to portray themselves, as the opposite of the negative Sairy Gamp stereotype created by Charles Dickens of the fat, lower-class, gin-swilling midwife on her way to a birth carrying a bag of dirty instruments (including catheters to perform abortions). Their mechanism for the elevation of midwifery above this damning stereotype was the union of midwifery with public health nursing. This union was initiated in the United States in New York and in Kentucky in 1925 by Mary Breckenridge, who studied both mid-wifery and nursing and found the British combination of the two to be ideal to meet the needs of the rural Appalachian poor she had ded-icated her life to serve. The successful history of the Frontier Nursing Service (FNS) she founded in Hyden, Kentucky, has been recounted in detail elsewhere (Rooks 1997). Here, suffice it to say that the combi-nation of nursing and midwifery Breckenridge imported also seemed ideal for New York City (see chapter 2), where nurse-midwifery gained a toehold through the establishment (with Mary Breckenridge's help) in 1930 of the Lobenstine Clinic, the nation's second nurse-midwifery service, and in 1931 the site of the first American nurse-midwifery educational program, the Lobenstine Midwifery School (Rooks 1997:38). Both were affiliated with the Maternity Center Association (MCA, still extant today), which played a major role in their develop-ment, and both sent their midwives to practice in parts of New York City (Harlem, Hell's Kitchen, the Bronx) that had high rates of poverty and high rates of birth, maternal and infant death, and communicable diseases such as tuberculosis. As would be expected, given the ongoing medical campaign against midwives, the Lobenstine services did meet with opposition from physicians, but were able to overcome it because of their judicious combination of midwifery and public health nursing to meet the needs of a population that physicians had left severely under-served.

Thus, at its very beginning, three important elements of nurse-midwifery's evolutionary trajectory were set: First, nurse-midwives (albeit in very small numbers) overcame physicians' stereotypical thinking and got into the system by being educated as nurses and by serving populations (poor, black, inner city or rural) in dire need that physicians were not attending and did not wish to attend. Second, nurse-midwives managed to stay in the system by consistently demonstrating excellent results, right from the start. Mary Breckenridge's development of the Frontier Nursing Service (FNS) and the excellent care its horseback-riding nurse-midwives provided resulted in a dramatic drop in perinatal death rates in rural Leslie County, Kentucky (Rooks 1997:57). At a time when the national average for maternity mortality was 10.4 maternal deaths per 1,000 births, the maternal mortality rate for Lobenstine births was only 0.9 per 1,000, more than ten times lower (Roberts 1995). Excellent outcomes, often better than those demonstrated by physicians, have continued to characterize nurse-midwife-attended births ever since (see Rooks 1997, MacDorman and Singh 1998, Anderson and Murphy 1995, Murphy and Fullerton 1998, Davidson 2002). Third, as with all women's professions that manage to gain a place in a man's world, nurse-midwives benefited from the start from a small number of physicians who worked with them and supported their development. The nurse-midwives of both the FNS and the MCA collaborated with doctors from the beginning; one of Mary Breckenridge's first acts when she started the FNS was to hire a physician to serve as medical director. In both services the nurse-midwives had consultation available from one or more physicians on call twenty-four hours a day (Kitty Ernst, personal communication). Practicing autonomously, these early nurse-midwives and their supporting physicians developed collaborative models of care that still form an ideal for the CNMs of today.

For the next four decades, nurse-midwives opened a small number of other programs and steadily increased their numbers, albeit at a glacial pace. In 1955, the MCA reported that development was very slow, in part because of "connotations of untaught, non-professional midwifery" (Rooks 1997:39), and recommended greater efforts to overcome this stereotype through basing nurse-midwifery education in universities and standardizing educational curricula and admission requirements (Sharp 1983). MCA's recommendations led to the opening in 1956 of a program in maternal and infant health nursing in the graduate department of Yale's School of Nursing, which established a trend toward gearing midwifery education to the graduate level. By 1958 there were six nurse-midwifery programs in the United States; three awarded non-degree certificates and three offered master's degrees

(Roberts 1995). The graduates of these and other programs that formed served the rural and urban poor in the United States or joined missionary organizations and went to work in other countries; some were employed by the public health departments of various states. Many became leaders in public health and other fields, and the few who entered clinical practice were confined to rural areas where there were no doctors, or to urban areas where doctors did not choose to work (Rooks 1997: 40). From 1925 to 1955, those very few nurse-midwives who managed to work in clinical practice attended births in homes and maternity centers; the only hospital in which they could work as midwives was the Frontier Nursing Service's small hospital in Kentucky.

NURSE-MIDWIFERY'S SHIFT TO HOSPITAL-BASED PRACTICE AND THE FOUNDING OF THE ACNM

The FNS nurse-midwives were spread apart in small, isolated rural communities and were constantly available to the families they served. In 1929, sixteen FNS midwives formed an organization, which in 1941 became the American Association of Nurse-Midwives (AANM).[2] The focus of the early FNS nurse-midwives and their MCA colleagues, with whom they worked closely, was not on building nurse-midwifery as a profession, but rather on providing better maternity care for women and babies (Rooks 1997; Kitty Ernst, personal communication).

In 1944, the National Organization for Public Health Nursing (NOPHN) established a section for nurse-midwives; its members kept data on nurse-midwifery practitioners and educational programs and worked to popularize the concept of family-centered maternity care (Rooks 1997:41). The NOPHN dissolved in 1952 during the formation of two much larger nursing organizations: the American Nurses Association (ANA) and the National League for Nursing (NLN). Unable to create a niche for themselves in one of these new nursing organizations, in 1955 nurse-midwives formed the American College of Nurse-Midwifery (ACNM). ACNM's initial goals included developing educational standards and supporting the development of practices and educational programs, sponsoring research, and participating in the International Confederation of Midwives (Sharp 1983; Rooks 1997:42). In other words, with this organization's founding, nurse-midwives began active and sustained efforts to promote the profession of nurse-midwifery, which its members increasingly understood to be essential to eventual success in the larger cause of providing better maternity care to mothers and babies.

By 1955 when the ACNM was founded, the postwar baby boom had resulted in a dramatic increase in the number of U.S. births, overwhelming obstetric residency programs. A few large inner-city hospitals in New York and Baltimore sought relief by bringing nurse-midwives into their obstetric services. With the resultant shift to hospital-based practice, the nature of nurse-midwifery changed significantly over time: much was gained and much was lost. In these inner-city hospitals, nurse-midwives were able to serve far greater numbers of women than they had previously been able to reach, and to attend women with a wide range of complications, thereby expanding their knowledge base and their practice parameters and improving the care provided to poor women (the latter was their primary motivation). The increasing need for their services in hospitals fostered the development of new educational programs and helped to generate more employment opportunities in public charity hospitals, thereby raising their numbers.

These gains came at the price of the autonomy nurse-midwives had formerly enjoyed. In hospitals, nurse-midwives had to submit to some of the subordination that accompanies the nursing role in order to be accepted by doctors, to adapt to a far more interventive model of care, and to accept far greater medical influence over their educational programs and the loss of homebirth experience for their students (Rooks 1997:45). Nevertheless, the reality was that the hospital was where the vast majority of American women were going to give birth. So complete was nurse-midwifery's move into hospital-based practice that in 1973 the ACNM adopted a Statement on Homebirth, which named the hospital as "the preferred site for childbirth because of the distinct advantage to the physical welfare of mother and infant" (ACNM 1973, quoted in Rooks 1997:67).

From its original inception in 1955, the ACNM proved to be a formidable organizational force. ACNM members realized early on that the key to controlling the nature of their profession was to make sure that the ACNM would be the body to both certify nurse-midwives and accredit nurse-midwifery educational programs, so that it could control education and practice standards. By 1963, thirty-eight years after FNS was founded, there were only about forty nurse-midwives actually practicing midwifery in the United States. Most of the five hundred graduates of nurse-midwifery educational programs worked in nursing or public health, or as missionaries abroad (Judith Rooks, personal communication, 1999). Nevertheless, by 1965 ACNM had developed an accreditation process, and by 1970 was administering national certification and accreditation for all nurse-midwifery programs, a move that gave it enormous standard-setting power to define the boundaries and the nature of its profession.[3] The ACNM further ensured its control over nurse-midwifery education in 1978 by defining the *core competencies* of nurse-midwifery practice—the fundamental knowledge, skills, and behaviors that are the expected outcomes of nurse-midwifery education (ACNM Education Committee 1979).

At the end of the 1970s, after fifty years of hard work on the part of nurse-midwives to achieve cultural acceptance, set standards, and grow their profession, there were nineteen nurse-midwifery educational programs in operation and nurse-midwives were legal and practicing in forty-one states; all together, they attended only slightly more than one percent of American births (Rooks and Fishman 1980). It was in this context of extreme and continuing marginalization, in spite of their careful and rigorous professionalism, that the nurse-midwives of the late 1970s faced the challenge to the model of midwifery they had worked long and hard to create and solidify posed by the lay midwifery renaissance.

LAY AND DIRECT-ENTRY MIDWIFERY

Out of the cultural ferment of the 1960s and 1970s arose the countercultural and feminist movements, which became two powerful mainsprings of lay midwifery. A third generative force was women's reactions to the extreme overmedicalization of birth. In the 1950s thousands of women had begun to speak out in letters to magazines like *Redbook* and *Ladies Home Journal* about the horrors of hospital birth in the United States. From the 1930s to the 1970s, scopolamine was heavily employed. A psychedelic amnesiac that was supposed to take away memory, this drug often did not render women unconscious during birth, but rather made them wild. They were strapped down with lamb's wool bands (which did not leave marks on their arms) and often left alone to scream until the baby finally came; many women were subsequently haunted by spotty nightmarish memories. Technological interventions such as forceps and episiotomies became increasingly common as humanistic care for birthing women became increasingly rare.

Some women reacted by trying to change hospital birth. Consumer demand that hospitals change gave a strong boost to nurse-midwifery during the 1970s and 1980s. CNMs were instrumental in achieving the presence of partners, family, and friends in the delivery room, in the development of the labor-delivery-recovery room, in getting rid of restraints on the mother's arms and the sterile sheets that separated the mother from the baby, and in the growth of unmedicated births and of breastfeeding—so much so that hospitals began to market CNM services to attract patients (Deanne Williams, personal communication, 2005). Other women opted out of the hospital altogether. The choice to opt out was fostered by the countercultural movement, which offered that choice on multiple fronts, yet many women who made that choice were not countercultural at all. The homebirth mother of the late 1960s and 1970s was as likely to be a childbirth educator or a conservative preacher's wife reacting against a negative hospital experience as a feminist seeking self-empowerment through birth or a hippie rejecting the hegemony of the medical establishment. Then, as now, she was likely to be middle class, which meant in part that she was used to exercising her right to choose. Perceiving little room for choice in the standardized hospital births of the time, women across the country began to decide to give birth at home. Usually unable to find licensed practitioners to assist them, they asked their neighbors, their sisters, their friends. In 1970 the proportion of women giving birth in hospitals reached an all-time high of 99.4 percent, but between 1970 and 1977, the percentage of women giving birth at home more than doubled, from 0.6 percent in 1970 to 1.5 percent in 1977 (Institute of Medicine 1982).

Most of the lay midwives who responded to their call were mothers who had given birth themselves; some were childbirth educators, La Leche League leaders, or nurses who wanted to learn about nonmedicalized birth. Some were members of countercultural communes or intentional communities; some were Christians supporting members of Christian communities to give birth with God's help; some were entirely conventional in all other respects. Although a few of the early lay midwives were nurses who chose to opt out of the medical system, most were largely self-taught. They generally arrived at births with few preconceived notions, learning what they came to know from birth itself (see Gaskin 2003 for a fascinating recounting of this educational process as experienced by the midwives of the Farm in Tennessee). Because birth is a fundamentally successful natural process that turns out well the vast majority of the time, their early experiences of birth were mostly positive ones that generated in these incipient midwives a sense of trust in birth and belief in women's ability to give birth. Their positive experiences of birth were facilitated by the fact that they were attending a primarily middle-class population of women who enjoyed good nutrition and good health.

Understandably, lay midwives' grassroots emergence on the cultural scene horrified many of the nurse-midwives who had worked so hard to set educational standards and gain professional status. Here was the very stereotype they had tried so hard to overcome rearing its head again, this time activated by laywomen, most of whom, unlike those earlier generations of immigrant midwives, had no formal midwifery training. Occasional reports of the death of a mother or baby at home (despite the fact that babies also died in the hospital) fostered public perceptions that *all* such practitioners were practicing improperly, and nurse-midwives across the county began to take pains to distinguish themselves in the public eye from the lay midwives—an endeavor that usually proved fruitless because the American public did not then, and does not now, have a good understanding of who midwives are or what they do.

While nurse-midwives were concerned by what they perceived to be the lay midwives' lack of training, many were also in awe and sometimes jealous of the untrammeled beauty, naturalness, and woman-centeredness of the homebirths that lay midwives were attending (Rooks 1997:287). Here was midwifery in its pure, nonmedicalized form—women being with women as they gave birth. Photos and videos of radiant women pushing their babies out in the nurturing environment of their own homes, surrounded by family and friends, reminded nurse-midwives of what had been lost with their move into the hospital, and pointed up just how intensely medicalized hospital birth had become. The contrast made some nurse-midwives begin to question whether they were really offering midwifery care, and stimulated a debate over "who is a real midwife?" (Burst 1990).

The homebirth midwives were prolific and productive and quickly began to carve out a cultural space far greater than their small numbers would seem to warrant, in part because their generally countercultural philosophy was shocking, newsworthy, and ultimately critically important to the American cultural scene. The United States owes much of the expansion of its cultural range during the 1990s to the then-radical countercultural movement of the 1960s and 1970s, including the continued existence of homebirth.

Unlike nurse-midwifery, which arose from conscious efforts to develop a profession, lay midwifery was a grassroots movement. Throughout the 1970s, enclaves of lay midwives emerged all over the country, in Santa Cruz, California; in El Paso, Texas; in Boston; on the Farm in Summertown, Tennessee; at the Fremont Women's Clinic in Seattle, Washington; and in many other places. At first unknown to each other, through word of mouth, articles in newspapers and magazines, and eventually the publication of a number of books, they learned of each other's existence and realized they were part of a national movement. Raven Lang's *The Birth Book* came out in 1972 and started the cultural discussion of homebirth. Ina May Gaskin's *Spiritual Midwifery,* first published in 1975, became so popular that the printing presses on the

Farm (an intentional countercultural community that she and her husband Stephen helped found) were kept rolling twenty-four hours a day for four months straight to meet the national and global demand. In El Paso in 1977, Shari Daniels, who had started one of the first private midwifery schools, organized the first national gathering of lay midwives, called the First International Conference of Practicing Midwives. In Oregon, Arizona, California, and elsewhere, these new lay midwives began to get together and form statewide associations; meeting in groups at birth conferences, they began to generate a nationwide social movement.

Some of these early lay midwifery pioneers knew about nurse-midwives and consciously chose to avoid that route because they wanted to practice nonmedical midwifery outside of the hospital. Others practiced for years without even knowing that nurse-midwives existed. At the end of the 1970s, when nurse-midwives were attending around one percent of American births, lay midwives were also attending around one percent of American births. Both groups were very small in numbers, and in spite of nurse-midwifery's fifty-five-year history, both groups were about as culturally unknown and marginal as any group of health care practitioners can be.

Faced with a similar situation, in the early 1980s Canadian lay and nurse-midwives decided to join forces and establish common cause. The difference was that in Canada, neither group was legal and regulated: lay midwives practiced without regulation attending births at home; in hospitals nurse-midwives could only work as nurses (Bourgeault and Fynes 1997). So neither group had anything to lose from an alliance and much to gain, whereas the members of ACNM had already spent fifty years building a legal and regulated profession with a solid organizational base and long-established standards of education and practice in which they deeply believed. Thus many members of ACNM experienced the lay midwifery renaissance as a "gut-level threat" to all that they held dear.

THE FOUNDING OF MANA
AND ITS WORK DURING THE 1980s

In 1981, Sister Angela Murdaugh, the incoming president of ACNM, sat in an ACNM Open Forum meeting taking notes on a yellow pad. The topic on the floor was "lay midwifery." At the end of the heated discussion, during which some nurse-midwives expressed a desire to obliterate lay midwives and others took a more moderate stance, the overall message that Sister Angela (a woman of encompassing goodwill) wrote down was that the membership of the ACNM wanted to be "in dialogue with lay midwives." In response to that message, she invited a few well-known lay midwives, and some nurse-midwives who had started out as lay midwives, to meet at the ACNM headquarters in Washington, D.C. in late October of 1981. At that meeting she urged the lay midwives to organize themselves and create formal principles of practice. Some of them welcomed her suggestion while others were resistant, interpreting organization and standard setting as potential "sellouts to the patriarchy." Nevertheless, it was during that initial meeting called by Sister Angela that the idea leading to the creation of MANA was born. For her trouble, Sister Angela later took a great deal of criticism from various ACNM members, primarily those who identified nursing as the only viable route to professional midwifery. Some thought that she should not have given this kind of impetus to lay midwifery, while others insisted that instead of encouraging lay midwives to form their own organization, she should have urged them to obtain nurse-midwifery education and join ACNM.

Retrospectively, it is clear that decisions made by the ACNM in 1981 and 1982 were crucial to the events that later unfolded. For a brief moment in time, nurse-midwives very likely could have precluded the formation of MANA by opening the ACNM to non-nurse midwifery—a move they did make thirteen years later in 1994. We can imagine that had the leaders of the ACNM chosen to sit down with the lay midwives who came to that 1982 conference and ask them how ACNM might change to accommodate their values and needs, American midwifery today might be one unified profession, as Canadian midwifery has chosen to be. ACNM had already retracted its earlier position on homebirth, coming out in 1980 with a statement endorsing nurse-midwifery practice in all settings (hospital, freestanding birth centers, and homes) (Rooks 1997:182). A bachelor's degree was not a requirement at the time—many nurse-midwives graduated from certificate programs, so that would not have been an issue as it is today. Most of the midwives I interviewed who were practicing as lay midwives during this time have assured me that MANA quite likely would never have been formed if in 1981 ACNM had dropped the nursing requirement and addressed some of the lay midwives' philosophical concerns. Indeed, at that time there were some ACNM members who would have been happy to do so. In Ontario, by 1984 nurse- and direct-entry midwives were able to agree on goals and standards and to achieve unity (Bourgeault, Benoit, and Davis-Floyd 2004). But in the United States, that is not how history unfolded. The consensus among my ACNM interviewees is that ACNM would have been split in two by any such decision. Its current president, Katherine Camacho Carr, asks, "Did we want revolution or evolution? We chose evolution" (personal communication 2005).

So instead, during the 1982 ACNM convention in Lexington, Kentucky, a group of like-minded lay and nurse-midwives gathered in a hotel room to charter an organization that would give them and their "sisters" a sense of group identity and common cause. Some of them expected this to be an American organization; initial names they played around with included the "American Midwives Association" (AMA(!)) and the "National American Midwives Association" (NAMA—a bit too chant-like). The American midwives present at that meeting were keenly aware of the transnational nature of the grassroots movement they represented, and wanted to include the midwives they thought of as "their sisters" in Canada and Mexico, so the Midwives' Alliance of North America (MANA) was born. (This name was originally suggested by Fran Ventre, a former lay midwife who had become a CNM, and whose practice and ideology have ever since bridged the gap between the two. For more detail, see Schlinger 1992:14–27.)

Given the lack of consensus about change on ACNM's part, most of the midwives who created MANA could see no advantage to becoming nurse-midwives and joining ACNM because they believed that nursing training should not be a requirement for midwifery. In fact, they saw it as fundamentally detrimental to midwifery to require that midwives become nurses first, because they deeply believed in the value of a non-medicalized approach to birth. Past MANA vice president Anne Frye explains:

> As these original lay midwives became more sophisticated in their understanding of the details of medical training and practice, they saw quite clearly that what they were seeing at home-births often did not reflect what they were reading about and seeing in hospital birth. Understanding that they were developing a different knowledge system, over time they sought to develop educational methods and programs that would perpetuate that system, and to avoid incorporation into the more medicalized nurse-midwifery approach. (Personal communication 1998)

Throughout the 1980s, the women who started out in the late 1960s and early 1970s as lay midwives educated themselves, attended births, trained apprentices, and further developed a unique body of knowledge about out-of-hospital birth, eventually codifying it in books and articles (for examples, see Bruner et al. 1998; Frye 1996, 2005; Davis 1997, 2004; Gaskin 1990, 2003). They joined together to create core competencies and standards for practice, to lobby for workable legislation, and to create educational programs and state certification processes. In the mid-1980s they created an International Section of MANA consisting of midwives licensed in their states, which, despite ACNM's opposition, qualified for membership in the International Confederation of Midwives (which accepts as members only national groups whose members are government-recognized). They thrived in spite of the ill wishes and often-active persecution of the medical establishment and developed a powerful Statement of Values and Ethics that fully encapsulates the principle elements of their shared beliefs about birth.[4] As all this was being accomplished, MANA members, like the members of ACNM, gained a vested interest in preserving what they had worked so hard to create.

Over time, MANA became the spearhead of a movement powerful beyond its small numbers because of public support from the dedicated and numerous members of the alternative childbirth movement. In this effort, MANA has been continuously bolstered by support from many nurse-midwives: nurse-midwives participated in MANA's inception in that hotel room in Lexington, one-third of MANA's membership has always consisted of CNMs, and a number of CNMs have for many years trained direct-entry apprentices and taught in direct-entry programs and schools. Approximately 300 of ACNM's members belong to MANA, and a significant number of nurse-midwives were direct-entry midwives before they became CNMs; many of them retain an orientation to independent, out-of-hospital midwifery. The divisions between these organizations exist in spite of, and not because of, their multiple interlinkages and the extremely cooperative relationships of their members at the grassroots community level in some regions (Davis-Floyd 1998a).

The possible development of national certification was a subject for discussion at the annual MANA conventions as early as 1985. At the time, many MANA members were highly suspicious of such a potentially exclusionary move. From the start MANA defined itself as an inclusive organization, one that exists, ideally and ultimately, to represent all midwives. Unlike ACNM, which admits to voting into membership only midwives certified by the ACC (see note 1) and students enrolled in ACNM (DOA)-accredited programs, MANA then and now allows anyone who calls herself a midwife to become a voting member. Its inclusivity means that MANA cannot qualify as a professional organization in the usual sense; although its members developed core competencies, unlike ACNM, MANA could not enforce them as educational requirements. Nor could MANA ensure consistency or set national standards

for the many mentors training apprentices or for the educational programs its members developed, which tended to vary widely in scope and
quality. So although some state midwifery organizations did develop
rigorous credentialing programs, MANA members entered the 1990s
wide open to the accusation, often leveled at them by physicians and
nurse-midwives, that they had no national mechanism for protecting the
public: in most states anyone could "hang out a shingle and call herself a
midwife," regardless of her background or training. Compounding the
problem, the lack of such a mechanism was hindering midwives' fights
for legalization in many states.

THE CARNEGIE MEETINGS OF THE
INTERORGANIZATIONAL WORK GROUP

During this time of flux in MANA's development, the Carnegie Foundation for the Advancement of Teaching sponsored a series of meetings
between representatives from the ACNM and MANA; the meetings led
to the creation of an Interorganizational Work Group (IWG) charged
with trying to unify midwifery and thus to jumpstart its growth. During these meetings (1989 through 1994), the MANA and ACNM representatives compared their core competencies and deemed them to be
equivalent. This equivalence resulted in part from deliberate efforts on
the part of MANA members during the 1980s to model their core competencies on those of ACNM, in hopes of facilitating an eventual convergence. But by this time, the philosophical divides between the two
organizations were too deep. MANA had worked for a decade to
develop and to appreciate the value of its body of knowledge about
out-of-hospital birth, and one of its prime purposes had become the
preservation and perpetuation of that body of knowledge in unadulterated form. And MANA members had plenty of time to crystallize their
awareness of the value of apprenticeship training and the critical role it
plays in the preservation of homebirth midwifery knowledge.

The early, largely self-taught lay midwives soon began to train others
in the time-tested system of apprenticeship. Extensive interviews with
MANA midwives have led me to understand the importance they continue to attribute to apprenticeship. From their perspective, apprenticeship is more effective in fostering trust in the natural process of
birth and in women's ability to give birth than any other educational
system. Following a practicing midwife from home to home, the
apprentice experiences women in the fullness of their individuality,
rather than in the altered and often subjugated identities forced on
women in hospitals. The apprentice smells, touches, sees, hears, and

engages in birth at its most powerful and elemental, and for the most part witnesses woman after woman successfully giving birth with little or no technological intervention. She experiences the natural rhythms of birth, resonating with their ebbs and flows, and learns to avoid judgments about labor progress based on time charts, machines, and institutional routines. In such a context, her intuitive skills are honed. Reliance on intuition and trust in women's innate ability to give birth facilitate homebirth midwives' special ability to "normalize uniqueness" (Davis-Floyd and Davis 1997)—to make decisions based not on standardized measures but on what works for an individual woman at a given time and place. In short, everything important about the homebirth midwifery approach is most thoroughly and effectively transmitted through the intensely personal and committed relationship of mentor and apprentice. Thus apprenticeship remains far too important to MANA's essence and philosophy for its members to be willing to give it up as an educational pathway. The preservation of the choice to become a midwife through apprenticeship is as important to most MANA members as the choice to give birth at home, and so the MANA members of the IWG declared that it was impossible for them to compromise on this educational issue.

Given their long history of valuing university education, it was equally impossible for the ACNM members of the Carnegie group to accept pure apprenticeship. Leveling accusations of fostering illiteracy and ignorance among midwives at the MANA representatives, they decided that reaching effective agreements with them was also impossible. From the ACNM's point of view, it was disempowering to women to offer them a professional career that included study worthy of a university degree that did not result in that degree. Their focus was, as it had always been, a pragmatic one (see chapter 2): university degrees are what work in the wider society. From their perspective, apprenticeship, for all its sentimental value, implied the lack of a culturally valued education, as did the vocational schools that some MANA members had established. (For a comparison of apprenticeship, vocational, and university-based methods of educating midwives, see Davis-Floyd 1998b; Benoit et al. 2001.) Whereas the MANA midwives saw these private vocational programs as places where their brand of midwifery could be fully preserved, unadulterated by the hegemonic influences of university education, to the ACNM representatives, they were no more than "trade schools," an educational model they saw as hopelessly out of date. Ultimately the ACNM and MANA representatives to the Carnegie IWG settled on agreeing not to agree. They passed a statement acknowledging that there are different types of American midwives with overlapping scopes of practice, and ended the Carnegie dialogues in 1995. And so another chance for unity in American midwifery was lost.

APPRENTICESHIP IN CANADA
AND THE UNITED STATES

A bit of transnational comparison is in order here. Preserving apprenticeship was also a heartfelt desire of many of Ontario's lay midwives as they began to work for legalization in the early 1980s; they understood its value, as it was the manner in which most of them had been trained. In the end they adopted a pragmatic approach. They realized that neither the nurse-midwives, with whom they were in dialogue about alliance, nor the Ontario government, would accept anything less than university education as a bottom-line prerequisite for midwifery licensure. So they compromised, accepting university education but insisting that it be at the baccalaureate and not the postgraduate level, and that the community apprenticeship model form a major component of the baccalaureate program.[5] Today's Canadian midwifery students begin clinical training under a modified apprenticeship model from day one of their university education, following individual women through complete courses of care (see Kaufman and Soderstrom 2004; Bourgeault, Benoit, and Davis-Floyd 2004).

American nurse-midwives also value apprenticeship and have sought to incorporate it into their university programs in the form of clinical preceptorship. But unlike the Canadian model, university-based student nurse-midwives in the United States generally find their training split among the pre-, intra-, and postpartum periods, during which they often work in different sites under different preceptors. In contrast, this sort of split tends not to characterize the clinical training of American nurse-midwives enrolled in distance learning programs, which are university affiliated but allow students to remain at home studying didactics on computer, then spending a year in a preceptorship with a nurse-midwife who practices in the student's community.[6] This training is community based, allowing students to remain at home instead of having to leave their families to study in a university setting. It splits didactic and experiential learning, not only in place but also in time—students spend one year studying didactically at home before they enter their clinical preceptorship. Their clinical experience is gained almost entirely on an in-hospital basis, just as the training of direct-entry midwives (except CMs) takes place almost entirely out-of-hospital. In contrast, all Canadian midwives trained since passage of the new legislation in various provinces attend births in all settings throughout their training, and are then able, qualified, and supported by law and insurance to attend births in any setting. This is clearly a superior model for birthing women, as it allows them a full spectrum of choice and continuity of care along that spectrum, and for midwives, who are not limited by site of birth as they are in the United States. The practicality and success of this model is one of the reasons for the present rapid growth of midwifery in Canada (Bourgeault, Benoit, and Davis-Floyd 2004).

THE LATE 1990s: CONVERGENT TRENDS

The Carnegie IWG meetings, intended to generate dialogue and ideally to foster unity between MANA and the ACNM, ultimately deepened their divisions. I can imagine a different outcome only if these Carnegie meetings had taken place at a different time. Within a few years of their ending, certain unstoppable trends somewhat lessened the distance between lay and nurse-midwifery. These trends were visible at the time of the IWG meetings, but much less so than they were a few years later. In hindsight, one can see that a better understanding of these trends and their implications might have softened the Carnegie dialogues and opened up wider possibilities for collaboration. These convergent trends, which intensified throughout the 1990s and early 2000s, include:

1. A trend among MANA members toward the growth and improvement of formal direct-entry educational schools and programs. There were only a handful of such schools during the 1980s; today there are approximately twenty. These formal vocational schools combine a strong apprenticeship/preceptorship component with didactic classes, and are increasingly popular with a younger generation of direct-entry midwifery students most comfortable with formalized curricula, as long as what is taught is the out-of-hospital, holistic midwifery they seek. This trend was clearly visible during the Carnegie meetings, as by 1991, MANA educators had created the Midwifery Education and Accreditation Council (MEAC) (see note 1) to evaluate and accredit direct-entry educational programs. MEAC's stated mission was and is to improve the quality of direct-entry midwifery education, as well as to support innovative and diverse midwifery education programs, including apprenticeship. But at the time of the meetings, MEAC's work had barely begun. By 1999, MEAC had accredited ten of twenty existing programs, close to the number ACNM had accredited by the late 1960s (Davis-Floyd 1998b; Tritten and

Southern 1998, 2003; www.meacschools.org). In 2000, MEAC received federal government recognition as an accrediting agency for direct-entry midwifery schools from the U.S. Department of Education (DOE). ACNM's DOA had received DOE recognition as an accrediting agency for nurse-midwifery programs in 1982, and in 2001, the DOA was also recognized by the U.S. DOE as an accrediting agency for direct-entry (CM) programs. In other words, the United States government recognizes both MEAC and the DOA as being qualified to accredit direct-entry programs. This recognition entitles MEAC- and DOA-accredited programs to participate in the Title IV government funding program for student education, and ensures that graduates of such programs meet the international definition of a midwife, which requires graduation from a government-approved program. DOE recognition of both MEAC and the DOA has proved a powerful equalizer of the value and legitimacy of the education of both the CPM and the CM. In addition, as of January 2005, five of the twelve MEAC-accredited programs are degree-granting, further blurring the formerly distinct separation between ACNM's emphasis on university programs and MANA's lack of concern with them.[7]

2. A trend among MANA members toward the formalization of apprenticeship and its expansion as a learning system. In many cities, senior midwives take turns teaching weekly classes for all of their apprentices, adding a didactic element as part of the traditionally experiential apprenticeship. In addition, the Midwives College of Utah, the National Midwifery Institute, and the National College of Midwifery have developed modules that can be adapted for use by mentors and apprentices anywhere in the country. The modular form ensures that learning objectives can be formally set, and that what the apprentice learns can be tracked and evaluated; these became the first apprenticeship programs to receive MEAC accreditation. A charge often leveled against apprenticeship training is that it produces midwives who have very little experience with complications. This is less and less true: today most apprentice-trained midwives spend some months in a high-volume program where they can learn how to deal with multiple complications. Most apprentices study with at least two mentors, have completed relevant college-level courses, and participate in numerous continuing education programs given by nationally recognized experts (Jo Anne Myers-Ciecko, personal communication, 2005).

These two trends on the MANA side (the growth of formal direct-entry programs and the formalization of apprenticeship) are paralleled on the ACNM side by two equally significant developments:

1. ACNM's embrace in 1994 of the notion that one does not have to be a nurse before becoming a midwife, encapsulated in their creation of the CM (see chapter 2)—an idea that the lay midwives of the early 1980s tried to convey to nurse-midwives without success.

2. The massive expansion of ACNM's distance learning programs, which today graduate the majority of new nurse-midwives and are thus largely responsible for the rapid growth in the numbers of CNMs (see note 6). These programs are affiliated with a university and require a bachelor's degree for entry, but they do not require a move to a university campus. They allow the student to remain at home, studying didactic components on computer and in books, and learning clinical skills through one-on-one preceptorship with a practicing midwife in her community. Thus they foster a community-based approach to midwifery that has long been a MANA priority, and the educators who develop their curricula are freer than they might be on campus (where they are likely to be located inside of nursing or medical departments) to do so under a holistic, woman-centered midwifery philosophy. In addition to the benefit of being able to work with their preceptors in their geographical communities, students also report benefiting from the sense of community established through the periodic get-togethers of students and staff, and regular online communication. Nurse-midwives' development of these distance learning programs, which now graduate more students annually than resident university-based programs do, thus represents a trend toward convergence with more MANA-like educational philosophies and styles.

I will address further convergent trends, but let me mention one that is stylistic and very evident to the anthropological eye. The first MANA conferences I attended, beginning in 1991, were, in a word, flowing: time and schedules seemed not of the essence, sessions tended to be informal, openings and closings involved rituals, candles, poetry, and dance, many stories about beautiful births were told, and continuing education unit (CEU) forms were not much of an issue. In contrast, the first ACNM conferences I attended were far more formal, contained many more sessions about medicalized aspects of birth and women's health care, confined dancing to the Wednesday night party, and included rigorous requirements for the submission of CEUs. Since then, while MANA conferences continue to constitute "a dip in the holistic spring," many sessions are highly professional, schedules are more closely kept, and requirements for sessions have been standardized because licensed and certified homebirth midwives now also have ongoing CEU requirements to meet. ACNM conferences, while still very formal, now include storytelling sessions, sometimes dance and poetry at opening sessions, and more attention to the spiritual and intuitive aspects of birth. From what I can tell, these stylistic shifts within each organization stem, to some extent, from the influence of each on the other.

During the 1990s and early 2000s, MANA became a bit more like the ACNM, and the ACNM became a bit more like MANA. These convergent trends have not resulted in unification, as they did in Canada, because the ideological divisions between the groups over education are still deep, and in recent years have expanded to include differences in scope of practice. (The core competencies of both groups were declared equivalent during the Carnegie meetings, but subsequently, based on task analysis of what CNMs were actually doing, ACNM revised its core competencies to encompass gynecological practice and primary health care for women. MANA's core competencies remain focused on the childbearing year.) Nevertheless, these convergent trends represent increased possibilities for mutual respect, communication, and understanding across the ideological divides.

A fourth potential force for convergence has been a distinct trend among MANA members toward the professionalization of lay midwifery, including setting standards for the accreditation of educational programs and the professional certification of direct-entry midwives. During the Carnegie meetings, the dialogue was between one group of midwives who embraced professionalism in all its exclusivity and equated it with university training, and another group whose members were deeply ambivalent about calling themselves professionals and vehemently disagreed that to be a professional, one had to have a university degree. Some aspects of that situation have shifted, as the following section describes.

FROM LAY TO DIRECT-ENTRY: THE DEVELOPMENT OF THE CERTIFIED PROFESSIONAL MIDWIFE

By the early 1990s the word *professional* was a subject of much discussion in MANA, and the lack of consensus among MANA members on the appropriateness of its use was yet another source of tension in the Carnegie/IWG meetings. The nurse-midwives thought professionalism to be integral to the nature of midwifery, while the MANA midwives worried that calling themselves professionals would be too exclusive and hierarchical. But in spite of these doubts and the reluctance of the MANA IWG members to embrace the word, MANA midwives were increasingly feeling the need for a mechanism to prove the professional competency they had been developing. These midwives, whom the ACNM still characterized as *lay*, were feeling, acting, and running businesses like professionals. Their desire to rid themselves of the connotations of ignorance and lack of training encompassed by the word *lay* led them, during the early 1990s, to initiate efforts to drop that label in favor of the more professional term *direct-entry*. In Europe, this term had long been used to describe formal, government-recognized midwifery education that did not require nursing training as a prerequisite; MANA midwives, apparently beginning with MANA members in New York state (see chapter 2), adopted and transformed the term to mean simply that one enters any kind of midwifery education directly, without passing through nursing first.

During the Carnegie IWG meetings, the nurse-midwife participants repeatedly hammered on MANA's lack of educational requirements and general inability (beyond licensure in certain states) to evaluate the competence of its members. Their criticism came at a time when this call was being more loudly heard from MANA members themselves. Their transformation during the 1990s from lay to direct-entry midwives was paralleled by their increasing desire for a professional credential that would validate their knowledge of midwifery and help them interface with the medical system. (Those who had been the victims of medical persecution report being "forced" to this conclusion.) Problems generated by a few midwives who did practice without essential skills clarified the need for a common and established base of knowledge and skills, and for clear mechanisms for peer review and professional discipline (Pam Weaver, NARM board member, personal communication 1998).

The strong desire for such a credential on the part of many MANA members was paralleled by great concern that the uniqueness of the form of direct-entry midwifery they had been developing would become co-opted in the process of professionalization, which involved certain kinds of standardization. Concern about co-option led to the gradual step-by-step development of certification, as consensus had to be reached at each step.[8] After initial development of an examination and a national registry of those who had passed it, by 1994 MANA's daughter organization NARM had expanded into a full-fledged testing and certifying agency, designing, developing, and implementing the

Certified Professional Midwife (CPM) credential. (For more detail about this process, see chapter 3, this volume; see also Houghton and Windom 1996a, b; Rooks 1997: 248–252; and Davis-Floyd 1998a.)

CPM certification is competency based; *where* a midwife gains her knowledge, skills, and experience is not the issue—the fact that *she has them* is what counts. In keeping with MANA's values, NARM has been as inclusive as possible, honoring multiple routes of entry into midwifery, including self-study, apprenticeship, private midwifery schools, and university-affiliated programs, including those accredited by the ACNM. Thus the major criticism that ACNM educators level at NARM certification is that it does not require completion of a formal educational program. The NARM process has been streamlined for graduates from MEAC-accredited programs and from programs accredited by the ACNM's Division of Accreditation (DOA) (see note 1), but it is and will remain open to anyone trained by any method who can demonstrate that they meet NARM's entry-level requirements.

Here we find the crux of the philosophical differences involving educational issues that divide these two organizations. Although CPM certification can be obtained through formal educational programs, NARM board members do not accept the argument that formal, standardized education is essential for creating safe and competent practitioners. Citing recent trends in adult education in other fields, they stand behind competency-based education, and have designed a certification that can accommodate both midwives who graduate from formal programs and those who trained as apprentices. For the latter, CPM certification includes what is known in adult education as a *portfolio evaluation process* (nicknamed PEP). A portfolio is the formal documentation of a person's education through life experience. This documentation must be extensive and must demonstrate that the candidate meets NARM midwifery experience requirements: performance of seventy-five prenatal exams, attendance at twenty births as an active participant and twenty more as primary caregiver (a minimum of ten of these births must be on an out-of-hospital basis), and so forth, as listed in the NARM publication *How to Become a CPM* (available at www.narm.org). Knowledge is tested through the NARM written exam. The skills of apprentice-trained midwives are verified in two ways: the candidate's educational supervisor(s) or mentor(s) must attest that she has achieved proficiency in each area listed on the Skills, Knowledge, and Abilities Essential for Competent Practice Verification Form provided in the CPM application packet, and the candidate must take a hands-on skills exam.

In contrast, to be eligible for certification by the ACNM Certification Council (ACC), a student must graduate from a DOA-accredited educational program and pass the national ACC exam, which tests knowledge but not skills; these are attested to by the student's educational preceptors. While there is increasing variety among DOA-accredited programs, which now range from university- to community-based, all of them stress a system of knowledge based on in-hospital practice. Fewer than two percent of ACNM's members attend homebirths; most CNMs are prevented from doing so by state laws requiring physician supervision and/or the refusal of insurance companies to provide coverage for homebirth. Thus it is not surprising that MANA members feel so strongly that the preservation of the homebirth option is almost entirely up to them. They see their knowledge base as overlapping with that of the CNMs, but as fundamentally different, and they have designed their certification to preserve that knowledge base and their midwifery model of care[9]—a holistic approach to childbirth practiced by the first generation of midwives who founded MANA in 1982; in the same year, this midwifery model of care was, for the first time, fully described in writing by sociologist Barbara Katz Rothman in *In Labor: Women and Power in the Birthplace* (1982).

ACNM, THE DEVELOPMENT OF THE CERTIFIED MIDWIFE (CM), AND MANA'S RESPONSE

Of course, MANA midwives are not alone in laying claim to the midwifery model of care, as nurse-midwives also use this term to describe the woman-centered alternatives they offer in the hospital (Paine, Dower, and O'Neil 1999; Rooks 1999). And, as we noted above, MANA midwives are not alone in thinking that linking nursing with midwifery may at this point be causing more problems than it solves. Some influential members of the ACNM have been calling for its expansion into direct-entry education since the 1970s, believing that midwifery should be a unique, autonomous, and independent profession separate from nursing.

By the time of the Carnegie IWG meetings in the early 1990s, the dialogue within ACNM about the need for a direct-entry certification and new direct-entry educational programs was intensifying. The issue was brought to a head by events in New York state, where nurse-midwives in 1992 had achieved passage of the New York Midwifery Practice Act (see chapter 2). One of the conditions they had worked hardest to obtain was state acceptance of a new direct-entry certification. Now such a certification had to be developed, a void that ACNM could rush to fill or that could be left to New York state to develop on its own. Perceiving their window of opportunity, the proponents of direct-entry certification within the ACNM moved quickly to educate their membership about the reasoning behind a move into direct-entry certification.

Precedents for minimizing the role of nursing education in nurse-midwifery programs had been established in the 1970s with the development of a three-year masters' level program at Yale University (whose driver and visionary was Helen Varney Burst) that allowed a fast track through one year of nursing into two years of midwifery education. During the 1980s, several other such programs were developed. These programs stood in contrast to what had been the standard route: two to four years of nursing education, followed by several years of clinical practice as a labor and delivery nurse prior to applying to a nurse-midwifery education program. It was common in nursing programs to hear criticisms of midwifery students who did not practice labor and delivery nursing "long enough," as there still exists a belief among nurses that it takes years of practice to make one "a real nurse," and that extensive obstetrical nursing experience is a necessary precursor to midwifery training. Many within ACNM highly value their identity as both nurses and midwives and were vehemently opposed to creating a direct-entry route. Colloquially known as the "old guard" by direct-entry proponents, these nursing-oriented midwives resisted the development of the CM. But nurse-midwifery educators seeking more rapid growth for their profession realized that many students who wanted to become midwives did not want their lives "derailed" by a lengthy passage through nursing.

Other factors that influenced ACNM's move into direct-entry education and certification included the following: (1) the increasingly strong role identification felt by many CNMs with midwifery and not with nursing ("I am not a nurse, I am a midwife!" is a statement I have heard countless times during my interviews with CNMs; see also Scoggin 1996); (2) a desire for more autonomy coupled with resentment over regulation by state nursing boards, whose interests and priorities sometimes conflict with those of nurse-midwives; (3) the fact that physician assistants[10] with little obstetrical training had begun to attend births in some states (Burst 1995); these PAs needed to be able to obtain midwifery training but had already received all the basics of nursing training, which they should not be required to repeat; and (4) the realization that only specific aspects of nursing knowledge are relevant to providing quality midwifery care, and that this knowledge can be obtained outside of nursing education (Rooks 1998). In addition, although NARM was already in the process of creating a national direct-entry credential, many CNMs did not believe that NARM would set standards they could support. They believed that the midwives certified by NARM would be "substandard," and would endanger the midwifery profession with their "substandard practice." Thus they concluded that direct-entry certification should not be left to NARM, but should be taken on by the ACC.

In 1994, the year that NARM certified its first group of CPMs, ACNM members voted overwhelmingly for the ACC to create a direct-entry certification process and for the ACNM DOA to develop a process for accrediting direct-entry educational programs. In 1995 they chose Certified Midwife (CM) as the name of this new type of practitioner. In 1996, the first educational program leading to the CM (at State University of New York/Brooklyn in New York City) was preaccredited by the DOA; and in May 1997, when the first graduates of this program were anticipated to emerge, ACNM passed a resolution making this new CM a full-fledged voting member of the college. Only DOA-accredited university-based programs and university-affiliated distance learning programs lead to the CM credential.[11] CM entry-level requirements are based on entry-level CNM requirements; the exams taken by CMs and CNMs are exactly the same (Judith Fullerton, personal communication, 1998).

Eleven years after the 1994 ACNM vote to create the CM, SUNY Brooklyn (colloquially known as SUNY Downstate) is still the only DOA-accredited direct-entry program currently operating. It graduates approximately five students per year (approximately thirty-five students to date). (Other programs are under discussion, but lack of appropriate licensure and hospital privileges in all other states discourages their development).[12] CMs can presently be licensed as equivalent to CNMs in New York and New Jersey (except that in New Jersey they do not have prescriptive privileges as they do in New York). (To summarize the regulatory and practice variations in each of the states, the ACNM publishes *Direct Entry Midwifery: A Summary of State Laws and Regulations*, which is updated annually.) Nationally speaking, ACNM leaders and educators have not yet thrown their legislative support to this new CM certification, which has spoken strongly to issues in New York but has not seemed all that relevant to CNMs' concerns in other states (see chapter 2).

Many ACNM members felt that in accepting the CM, they were "opening up" their profession, generating the potential for easier ingress to all those who want to be midwives but don't want to be nurses. Thus some in ACNM felt more than justified in believing that ACNM should be the one and only national midwifery organization.

Insisting that having two national organizations only divides and weakens midwifery, they believed it would be best for midwifery if MANA members would rally around ACNM's new direct-entry standard.

In contrast, MANA members at the time did not see ACNM's move into direct-entry as an opening up but rather as a closing down, an exclusionary move to redefine direct-entry on ACNM's terms and shut out MANA-style (homebirth) direct-entry midwifery. As soon as ACNM's plans for creating the CM became known, those in MANA who equated direct-entry midwifery with out-of-hospital training and birth reacted with outrage to what they perceived as incursion into an area they had spent years developing and a co-option of the meaning of *direct-entry*, their chosen label. They believed that they were doing a very good job of defining direct-entry midwifery and of setting national standards for direct-entry education and practice. Anne Frye further explains:

> It seemed to us that nurse-midwives with no homebirth background teaching direct-entry students would be like direct-entry midwives suddenly deciding to open nurse-midwifery programs within hospitals. This would not only be ludicrous, but also a reinvention of the wheel. And the fact that the ACNM thought they could do this without so much as consulting any "real" direct-entry midwives was, in the minds of many MANA members, only proof positive that they did not have any understanding of the uniqueness of direct-entry midwifery as practiced by the members of MANA, NARM, and MEAC. To us it was clear that there are two distinct approaches to midwifery that both have value and which are similar in many ways but certainly not the same—a fact that calls for two different groups to oversee their ongoing development. (Personal communication, 1998)

In Frye's words we can see the effects of the semantic confusion generated by both organizations' use of the same term (direct-entry) to refer to these two very different models. Frye indicates the desire felt by many MANA members to maintain separation between the realms of nurse-midwifery and direct-entry midwifery, with the ACNM and its affiliates in charge of standard-setting and credentialing for the nurse-midwifery realm, and MANA and its affiliates in charge of standard-setting and credentialing for the direct-entry realm. The conceptual neatness of this distinction was blurred when ACNM established its own direct-entry certification process. Of course, ACNM never intended to create the same kind of direct-entry midwifery practiced by

MANA members, but rather is modeling its direct-entry educational programs on its existing nurse-midwifery programs.

In this chapter I have recounted several historical moments that could have led to increased unity in American midwifery but instead resulted in increased division. Another such pivotal moment occurred in Seattle in 1995. The Director of ACNM's Division of Accreditation (DOA) was paying a courtesy visit to the Seattle Midwifery School (SMS) shortly before the DOA was to meet to develop criteria for accrediting direct-entry programs. SMS was one of the first (vocational) direct-entry midwifery programs to be created in the United States, in 1978. The quality of its faculty and curriculum had earned it the respect of ACNM leaders, and much discussion had ensued around the possibility that the DOA would set accreditation criteria that SMS could meet. Then, the expectation went, SMS could arrange the requisite affiliation with a university and apply to the DOA for accreditation. DOA accreditation for SMS would mean that its graduates would be eligible to sit for the ACC exam and become certified as CMs. This development would have made SMS a major point of convergence between ACNM and MANA, would have increased student enrollment at SMS because education there would lead to either the CPM or the CM credential, and would have enabled SMS to establish relationships with hospitals and to offer hospital-based clinical training to its students along with their traditional out-of-hospital training. DOA accreditation for SMS would mean that direct-entry students with baccalaureate degrees could receive a holistic and feminist-oriented midwifery education, with out-of-hospital experience, in a private school with a strongly holistic midwifery model orientation.

Thus there was a great deal of excitement at SMS around the DOA director's visit. Things seemed to go pleasantly during her tour of the school, after which a small group settled down for tea. During that conversation, according to my interviews, the DOA director made a comment about MANA's choice (in October 1994) of the title Certified Professional Midwife—this was the name some had long thought would be used for ACNM's new direct-entry midwife, but by pure happenstance, MANA's Certification Task Force meeting to choose the name had occurred a few months before ACNM's meeting. The DOA director's comment was something to the effect that she wondered if this had been a challenge? The atmosphere was light, and SMS's director of education (jokingly, in her mind) responded, "Well I guess so!" A strong misunderstanding ensued, which seems to have affected the DOA's decisions to set standards for the accreditation of direct-entry programs that SMS could not meet. (These standards included the requirement that full-time faculty in such programs had to be either CNMs or CMs—something SMS could not achieve without changing its staff.) Feeling "betrayed" and "bitterly disappointed" by this DOA decision, the SMS staff turned the energies they would have devoted into convergence with ACNM toward MANA, NARM, the promotion of the CPM, and the development of MEAC. (Two SMS staff members became long-time members of MEAC's board and were instrumental in MEAC's achievement of DOE recognition.) And so, apparently because of a miscommunication resulting in ill feelings, another opportunity for increased midwifery unity was lost. Some ACNM leaders who had been hoping to choose CPM as the name of their new direct-entry credential felt that this choice by MANA was "a slap in the face" (it was not, as we shall clearly see in chapter 3). This example is but one of various miscommunications I could describe between ACNM and MANA members that illustrate how easily misunderstandings can result when ideological differences make every communication fraught.

In contrast to the feelings of many of MANA's direct-entry members, others, especially MANA's CNM members, welcomed ACNM's move into direct-entry education and certification, realizing that to some extent it *does* mean an opening of the college to new ways of thinking about and becoming a midwife. The existence of this entirely new kind of direct-entry midwife, the CM, represents fierce determination on the part of many committed CNMs to move their profession into a more autonomous position within the American health care system. The ACNM prime movers who created the CM faced down massive resistance from the nursing-oriented "old guard" members of the ACNM (and, in New York, from the nursing and medical professions) to bring the certification into existence. And they will have to face down opposition from state agencies, legislatures, and nursing and medical associations all over the country if they fight to obtain legal status for the CM in all fifty states.

ACNM has risked much and may risk more in the future to achieve its vision of an expanded and more autonomous midwifery profession. The mere existence of the CM has already had a profound conceptual effect. As soon as the CM was accepted as a full voting member of the college, Helen Varney Burst changed the name of her leading midwifery textbook from *Varney's Nurse-Midwifery* to *Varney's Midwifery;* the name of the ACNM journal was changed from the *Journal of Nurse-Midwifery* to the *Journal of Midwifery and Women's Health.* In addition, those most in support of letting go of the name *nurse-midwife* generated a serious movement within the college to change its name from the American College of Nurse-Midwives to the American College of

Midwifery. The proposal was put to a mail ballot in 1998. The fact that it did not pass seemed to indicate that the majority of the membership was not willing to let go of their identities as both nurses and midwives.

THE CONTEMPORARY STATUS QUO

Since the mid-1980s, nurse-midwives have been legal, licensed, regulated, and able to obtain insurance coverage from private companies and Medicaid in all fifty states and the District of Columbia. In February 2005 the total membership of the ACNM was around 7,000 and the voting membership was 5,411. Forty DOA-accredited nurse-midwifery (and one direct-entry) educational programs are currently in operation, graduating approximately 300 students each year (see www.acnm.org for the latest information). There are approximately 6,000 CNMs (about 25 percent of CNMs do not belong to the ACNM) and fifty CMs in active practice; exact figures are not available. Most CNMs stay in practice for an average of five years, earning salaries that average $65,000 per year. Most work in group practices that enable them to keep a reasonable work schedule and take time off for their families.

No one knows exactly how many non-ACNM direct-entry midwives are in practice across the United States; because many of them do not belong to MANA, they are difficult to count. My best estimate (based on informal surveys I have conducted) is that the number of state-licensed or nationally certified DEMs in the United States is around 2,000, while there are approximately 1,500 "plain" midwives who have neither state licensure nor national certification. MANA's total membership in February 2005 was 882 and its voting membership was approximately 750; 145 (around one-fifth) of these were CNMs and 287 were CPMs (most CPMs and many state-licensed midwives belong to their state organizations rather than MANA) (Nina McIndoe, MANA membership chair, personal communication 2005). Independent direct-entry midwives are legal, regulated, and licensed, registered, or certified in twenty-one states (over 700 DEMs practice in these states) and have varying status in the others (see www.narm.org for the latest information). Their services are covered by private insurance companies in most states where they are licensed, and by Medicaid (and sometimes managed care) in eight states. (In many other states licensed midwives are fighting for Medicaid and managed care coverage with varied results. In most states, homebirth attended by direct-entry midwives is still an out-of-pocket expense.) Most direct-entry midwives practice solo or in partnership with one other midwife; they are often constantly on call. Their annual incomes vary widely, according to the number of births they attend. Many make under $20,000 per year; a few make over $100,000.

In January of 1995, there were twenty-five CPMs. By June of 1998 there were approximately 400 CPMs; as of December 2005, there were 1,095—an average growth of 100 per year. (Today, one out of seven practicing midwives is a CPM.) All twenty-one states where direct-entry midwifery is "legal" use some or all of the CPM process as a requirement for licensure (www.narm.org). The CPM was conceived and created as an international certification. At present, there are forty-five CPMs in practice in Canada, four in Mexico, and one each in France, Ireland, South Africa, and Hungary. The CPM application process has been streamlined for United Kingdom midwives and may eventually become an option for midwives in the European Union who wish to practice in the United States or elsewhere, and who can document attendance at the requisite number of out-of-hospital births.

In the United States for the past two decades, ninety-nine percent of births have taken place in hospitals, with planned homebirths accounting for less than one percent of all births. Data from 2000 distributed by the National Center for Health Statistics show out-of-hospital births holding at .9 percent. That percentage is higher in Oregon (around six percent) and may rise in Florida, Washington, New Mexico, and other states where midwifery is legal and well integrated into the system, but on a national level it is still minuscule. While many decry this low figure, Ina May Gaskin, past president of MANA, points out that this low percentage of homebirths:

> can be seen as an accomplishment, given the highly financed, highly organized efforts that American physicians over the course of this century have made towards stamping out home-birth altogether. We have not only maintained that steady rate, but we have begun to experience what happens when a struggle such as this takes place over a generation. Given the opposition the medical profession has directed against midwifery, we in MANA believe that it has been an accomplishment for us to have survived at all! As more studies are carried out on the safety and efficacy of DEM practice, we believe that the percentage of homebirths will rise, not fall, during the years to come. We see the sixfold increase in homebirths in Oregon, where midwifery has long been legal, as significant. We are still in the stage of being a "best-kept secret" when it comes to mainstream culture. (Personal communication, 1998)

In fact, most of American midwifery is still a "best-kept secret." The medical monopoly in the United States remains firmly in control of birth: physicians attend around ninety percent of American births. Most American women think only of calling an obstetrician when they become pregnant; many people are unfamiliar with the benefits of midwifery practice and do not know that midwives are available in almost every city. The 8,000 or so practicing midwives, who cumulatively attend a mere nine percent of American births, [13] are still profoundly marginal in relation to the 35,000 or so obstetricians (and other doctors) who attend the rest. In this context, it might make sense for MANA and the ACNM to face the future battles they must fight for their continued existence by presenting a more unified front. After all, in various Canadian provinces nurse- and direct-entry midwives have come to agreement and unity by focusing on their shared values on woman-centered care and practice in all sites, a value that MANA and ACNM members also share.

In contrast to the Canadian situation, the divisions American midwives continue to face in part are created and defined by the philosophical divide between home- and hospital-based attendance at births. Although nurse-midwifery educators do make concerted efforts to stress the importance of minimizing interventions, hospital practice has had its effect: birth certificate data from 1997 showed that nurse-midwives use of technological interventions was rising at the same rates as obstetricians (Curtin 1999). This rise does not mean that nurse-midwifery care is not woman-centered: many American women expect and request interventions such as electronic monitoring and epidurals (Davis-Floyd 2004), and many nurse-midwives arrive at the realization that "woman-centered care" can mean meeting such requests.

Obviously, homebirth midwives are buffered from the medicalizing influences of such demands. Canadian midwives, who formerly practiced only at home, are finding themselves under increasing pressure to medicalize as they move more and more into hospital practice, serving a clientele that is less and less ideologically aligned with the spirit of the homebirth movement (Daviss 2001, Sharpe 2004). Ideally, Canadian midwives' continued presence at homebirths will effectively counteract the medicalizing pressures of hospital practice. Unfortunately, the mitigating influence of homebirth is not available to most American nurse-midwives, who are prevented from attending homebirths by various factors, including (1) their own lack of experience in (and sometimes fear of) homebirth; and (2) the conditions of their licensure in most states, which require them to have both insurance coverage and physician backup for homebirth, both of which are very difficult to obtain.

Largely confined to attending births in hospitals, like physicians many CNMs do become accustomed to routinely employing unnecessary interventions. In such cases, consumers point to the overmedicalization of CNM practice and training. On that panel discussion at the 1997 MANA conference in Seattle, ACNM President Joyce Roberts seemed to accept this criticism as a necessary price to pay for higher gain:

> You ask, what is the risk of this formalized education? You say it is overmedicalized. I would say it need not be, but I would also add that the risk of not having it is not being able to practice in all the domains that the World Health Organization [WHO] definition says midwives practice in. One has to weigh the risks of protecting themselves from overmedicalization and the realities of our health care system today, or take the consequences of limiting your practice to a very narrow domain.

Such limitation has indeed been the choice of many MANA midwives. They consider the degree of marginalization that results from out-of-hospital practice to be a worthy price to pay for maintaining autonomy, avoiding overmedicalization, and holding open a wide spectrum of care that the ACNM alone cannot preserve.

They are supported in this belief by the members of the Bridge Club, which was spontaneously formed at the 1997 MANA conference in Seattle the day after the Direct-Entry Dialogue panel (described at the beginning of this chapter) by a group of CNMs who are also members or supporters of MANA. Bridge Club members, who can belong to either or both organizations, now number over 100 and are trying to convince the ACNM Board to be more supportive of NARM certification, or at least to do nothing to undermine it. Supporting the CM, they also support the CPM, and advocate for the complementary coexistence of both. One result of their efforts was the establishment in 1999 of a liaison group consisting of three representatives each from ACNM and MANA, which at the very least constitutes a formal mechanism for dialogue between the two organizations.[14]

A very recent development is the creation by some members of MANA of the National Association of Certified Professional Midwives (NACPM). Its birth was sparked by events in Massachusetts: legislators there insisted that they could not accept the CPM unless it was backed by a professional organization that requires CPM certification for membership (which MANA does not) and sets national standards specifically for CPMs. The board members of NACPM, with the help of an advisory committee and with input from NARM, completed these standards in October 2004 (see chapter 3 for more detail, and www.nacpm.net).

NACPM's creation generated controversy within MANA, in part because some MANA members would have preferred such an organization be a section of MANA, and in part because of a fear that if all or most CPMs join NACPM (the professional organization) and leave MANA (the social movement organization), MANA's existence might be threatened in what could become a case of "matricide"—the daughter organization killing the mother organization. NACPM founders are making every effort to avoid such an event—the NACPM has no plans to hold its own national conferences, but rather will incorporate its meetings into MANA's annual conferences, and NACPM mailings have encouraged midwives to join both organizations. For the foreseeable future, it appears that MANA, to which hundreds of DEMs hold a 20-year allegiance, will continue to serve as the umbrella organization and the ideological catalyst that holds NARM, MEAC, the consumer organization Citizens for Midwifery, and the new NACPM in close alliance and cooperation.[15]

CONCLUSION: A CONVERGENT NETWORK OF OPTIONS FOR AMERICAN WOMEN

Thus ends my initial summary of the American midwifery story; far more detail is provided in the remainder of this volume. Two groups of midwives have so much in common that one came into existence at a conference held by the other, and some members of each belong to both. Yet they remain divided over seemingly irreconcilable differences in values and philosophy, most especially regarding educational routes (MANA values all routes, ACNM requires university degrees) and certification processes (MANA believes in the validity of CPM certification, which ACNM does not fully support). In the recent past, the members of these organizations have battled each other in state legislatures over whose direct-entry certification should prevail—a painful circumstance that often hinders the legislative efforts of both groups. The continued existence of these divisions means that every potential midwifery student, and many of the mothers seeking midwifery care, must examine these differences, consider their implications, and choose. A woman cannot at this point make a simple choice to use a midwife; rather, she must also choose which type, which educational philosophy, which knowledge system, which standards, and which site of care. Certainly, the existence of both ACNM and MANA in the United States creates a broader spectrum of choice for women than would exist if either organization and its members were to vanish, and the diversity these organizations represent gives women multiple options. But viewed in the Canadian context, where all midwives can practice at home or in hospital and can offer the full range from low- to high-tech birth, the home/hospital split that characterizes American midwifery can be seen to limit, not expand, women's spectrum of choice. And of course, it is these limitations which for Canadians, who have concentrated on unifying their profession, encompassing multiple knowledge bases, and developing systems that allow midwives to practice autonomously in all sites of care, have constituted the most cautionary part of this cautionary tale.

Happily, the American midwifery story does not end here. The most recent events in the evolution of MANA and the ACNM predict that a more positive, mutually accommodative part of the story will unfold. MANA members have largely accepted the existence of the CM and have come to see it as the step forward for midwifery that ACNM intended it to be. After initial rejection and scorn, increasing numbers of CNMs have gained respect for the CPM credential and the midwives who obtain it, especially because recent statistics on the outcomes of the births they attend have demonstrated the value and competence of their care.[16] Across the country there are hundreds of occurrences of interdependence between CNMs and DEMs. Sometimes, direct-entry midwives and nurse-midwives work together in private practices; often they create informal collaborative arrangements that benefit them both. CNMs sometimes mentor direct-entry apprentices and teach in direct-entry programs and schools.

Improved communication between ACNM and MANA members involved in national administration and in state legislation efforts has prevented a number of political battles that otherwise would have occurred. In some places the legislative efforts of nurse-midwives to expand their scope of practice, add prescriptive privileges, and so forth have benefited from long-established relationships between legislators and direct-entry midwifery state organizations, and the loyal support and social activism of homebirth midwifery clients often spills over to CNMs fired by hospitals or persecuted by physicians. Leaders of both national organizations have come to know and respect each other.[17] The two current presidents of ACNM and MANA, Kathy Camacho Carr and Diane Holzer, collaborate in many ways. They and other midwifery leaders participate mutually in national projects like the Safe Motherhood and the CIMS Mother-Friendly Initiative.[18] They meet at the conferences of MANA, the ACNM, Midwifery Today, and the International Confederation of Midwives (in which both organizations participate). As a result of careful epidemiological review of new data on CPM-attended homebirths (Johnson and Daviss 2005), ACNM leaders worked together with MANA leaders on a resolution passed by the American Public Health Association to increase access to out-of-hospital birth attended by direct-entry midwives (APHA 2002:453–455). The relationships they develop with each other in such arenas often lead to further dialogue and understanding. All these factors, combined with all midwives' intense devotion to women, babies, and their care will, over time, enhance the trends toward convergence I described above. While this convergence may take decades, or may never result in organizational unification, it is my hope that over time, the viable structures that members of both organizations are creating will form an increasingly strong network of options for American women and the ways they give birth.

TIMELINE OF EVENTS IN THE COMPARATIVE HISTORY OF ACNM AND MANA

This timeline is not a comprehensive history. It is based on the dates used in this chapter and provided to help the reader clarify the sequence of events discussed herein.

1925   Mary Breckenridge founds the Frontier Nursing Service in Hyden, Kentucky.

1929   Formation by FNS nurse-midwives of the American Association of Nurse-Midwives.

1930   Founding in New York of the Lobenstine Clinic.

1931   Founding of the Lobenstine Midwifery School.

1944   National Organization for Public Health Nursing establishes a section for nurse-midwives.

1955   Founding of the ACNM.

1956   Opening of Yale nurse-midwifery program.

1958   Six nurse-midwifery (NM) educational programs are operating in the United States.

1963   There are 500 graduates of these programs; only forty actually work as NMs in the United States.

1965   ACNM develops an educational accreditation process.

1970   ACNM begins administering national certification and accreditation for all NM programs.

1970   Hospital birth reaches an all-time high of 99.4 percent; homebirth at 0.6 percent.

1972   Publication of Raven Lang's *The Birth Book.*

1973 ACNM adopts a Statement on Homebirth naming the hospital as the "preferred site."

1975 Publication of Ina May Gaskin's *Spiritual Midwifery* and of Suzanne Arms's *Immaculate Deception.*

1976 Midwife Shari Daniels opens the Maternity Center, the first midwife-owned for-profit freestanding birth center, which she ran for ten years.

1977 Homebirth doubles to 1.5 percent as the grassroots lay midwifery movement grows.

1977 Shari Daniels opens the first professional direct-entry midwifery school, in El Paso, Texas.

1977 Shari Daniels organizes the First International Conference of Practicing Midwives, in El Paso, Texas.

1977 CNMs receive licensure in Massachusetts, one of the last states to grant it.

1979 Nine NM educational programs in operation.

1979 NMs attend one percent of births. Lay midwives also attend one percent of births.

1980 ACNM retracts its earlier position on homebirth, producing a statement endorsing NM practice in all settings (hospital, birth centers, homes).

1981 Sister Angela Murdaugh, president of ACNM, invites lay midwifery leaders to meet at ACNM headquarters in Washington, D.C.

1982 The midwifery model of care is fully described in writing by sociologist Barbara Katz Rothman in *In Labor: Woman and Power in the Birth Place.*

1982 ACNM's Division of Accreditation receives federal DOE recognition as an accrediting agency for nurse-midwifery programs.

1982 Founding of MANA.

1984 At the second MANA convention, held in Toronto, Ontario, Canadian nurse- and direct-entry midwives achieve organizational unity, creating the Ontario Association of Midwives (OAM).

1989 MANA establishes the Interim Registry Board to explore a national registry exam; the IRB later evolves into NARM.

1989–1995 Carnegie Inteorganizational Work Group (IWG).

1991 Creation of the Midwifery Education and Accreditation Council (MEAC).

1992 Passage of the New York Midwifery Practice Act legalizes the ACNM's new non-nurse-midwife.

1994 ACNM votes for the ACC to create a certification process and title for the new direct-entry midwife.

1994 NARM and the CTF choose Certified Professional Midwife as the name of the credential they are developing.

1994 Abby Kinne is the first to receive CPM certification, in October.

1995 ACC/ACNM choose Certified Midwife (CM) as the title for the new ACC-certified direct-entry midwife.

1995 NARM conducts a survey returned by 800 practicing midwives to determine entry-level requirements for the CPM, called the *1995 NARM Job Analysis.*

1995 ACNM/DOA sets criteria for the accreditation of direct-entry programs leading to the CM.

1996 The first educational program leading to the CM (at SUNY/Brooklyn in New York City) is preaccredited by the DOA.

1996 Linda Schutt CPM becomes the first CM in the United States.

1997 ACNM grants full voting membership to CMs.

1997 ACNM sends letter to state legislatures advocating recognition of only the CM. The Bridge Club forms.

1997 Helen Varney Burst changes the name of her leading midwifery textbook from *Varney's Nurse Midwifery* to *Varney's Midwifery.*

1997 The name of the ACNM journal is changed from the *Journal of Nurse-Midwifery* to the *Journal of Midwifery and Women's Health.*

1998 ACNM revises its core competencies to include lifetime gynecological, reproductive, and well-woman primary care, thus greatly enlarging its scope of practice. MANA's core competencies remain focused on the childbearing year, as mandated by NARM's Job Analysis (1995).

1998 A movement to change the name of the ACNM from the American College of Nurse-Midwives to the American College of Midwifery is put to a mail ballot but does not pass.

1999 MEAC has accredited ten of twenty existing direct-entry educational programs, close to the number of nurse-midwifery programs ACNM had accredited by the late 1960s.

2000 MEAC receives DOE recognition as a federally recognized accrediting body for direct-entry midwifery programs.

2001 The DOA receives DOE recognition as a federally recognized accrediting body for direct-entry midwifery programs.

2001 Formation of the NACPM at a MANA conference, and of a CPM section of MANA.

2005 Five of the twelve MEAC-accredited schools are degree-granting institutions.

2005 The total membership of the ACNM is around 7,000 and the voting membership is 5,411. There are forty-three ACNM/DOA-accredited programs.

2005 In January, NARM certifies its 1,000th CPM.

2005 Direct-entry midwifery legislation passes in Virginia and Utah, bringing the number of states in which non-ACC-certified DEMs are legal, regulated, and licensed, registered, or certified to 21.

ACKNOWLEDGMENTS

My thanks to Cecilia Benoit, Ivy Bourgeault, Joanne Myers-Ciecko, Judith Rooks, Anne Frye, Mary Anne Shah, Marcia Good Maust, Betty Cook, Christine Barbara Johnson, Mark Gridley, Ida Darragh, Diane Holzer, Christa Craven, Ray DeVries, Susan Hodges, Bruce Hoffman, Diane Holzer, Barbara Katz Rothman, and Deanne Williams for their helpful editorial comments, and to the Wenner-Gren Foundation for Anthropological Research for supporting the research on which this chapter is based.

ENDNOTES

1. The figure below shows the structural relationships between the organizations related to ACNM and MANA. In the United States, national legislation requires that certification and accreditation be carried out by separate bodies. The ACNM is a professional organization that requires certification as a certified nurse-midwife (CNM) or certified midwife (CM) by its affiliate, the ACNM Certification Council (ACC), for membership. All nurse-midwifery educational programs must be accredited by ACNM's Division of Accreditation (DOA). The DOA can accredit both intra-institutional programs and freestanding degree-granting institutions (Carrington and Dickerson 2004).

   MANA is not a professional organization in that it does not require certification for membership, but the North American Registry of Midwives (NARM) has created an optional certification, the Certified Professional Midwife (CPM), and a new professional organization, the National Association of Certified Professional Midwives, created in 2001, requires this certification for membership. MANA does not require program accreditation, but there is an accrediting body, the Midwifery Education Accreditation Council (MEAC), which has set rigorous standards and has accredited twelve direct-entry programs to date (www.meacschools.org). MEAC accredits both intra-institutional programs and freestanding degree-granting institutions.

These structural similarities mask important differences. The ACC and the DOA are true affiliates of ACNM, in the sense that they grew out of the ACNM and are fully philosophically and politically aligned with it. Likewise, NARM and MEAC grew out of MANA and share a strong ideological commitment to the midwifery movement and out-of-hospital birth. But MANA is inclusive and represents the midwifery movement. NARM's certification, while it has been made as accessible as possible is, by definition, exclusive. Thus NARM represents the professionalizing enterprise within direct-entry midwifery, as do MEAC and the new NACPM (National Association of Certified Professional Midwives, described more fully later in this chapter). So NARM, MEAC, and the NACPM are, strictly speaking, not affiliates of MANA, but rather sister or partner organizations with agendas that are related but distinct.

2. The American Association of Nurse-Midwives continued to exist until 1969; it consisted mostly of CNMs who had worked or did work at the Frontier Nursing Service. As roads were paved and the isolation of the FNS nurse-midwives decreased, there was no longer a need for the functions it had provided (Kitty Ernst, personal communication). And so in 1969 it merged with the ACNM, which at that point changed its name from the American College of Nurse-Midwifery to the American College of Nurse-Midwives, keeping the acronym (ACNM) the same.

3. In many other countries, the government sets midwifery educational standards, not the midwives themselves. This is common: governments of countries with national health services set the standards for medicine and nursing as well as for midwifery (Judith Rooks, personal communication). ACNM is one of the few national professional midwifery organizations in the world able to set standards for its own profession.

4. At the same time, factions of lay midwives around the country chose not to participate in any professionalizing efforts and to remain entirely outside the system. As I have done no research on these midwives, they are not considered in this chapter (but see chapter 5 by Mary Lay, and chapter 11 on "renegade" midwives). My estimate is that they number around 1,500.

5. In 1984, lay and nurse-midwives in Ontario merged into one organization, the Association of Ontario Midwives, which represented a union of the Ontario Nurse-Midwives Association and the Ontario Association of Midwives (see Bourgeault, Benoit, and Davis-Floyd 2004). Further illustrating the strong connections between midwives in Canada and the United States, this merger was accomplished at the 1984 MANA conference in Toronto, which carried the theme of "creating unity." The merger was fostered by (1) the congruence between the philosophies of both organizations, which focused on woman-centered care; and (2) a desire on the part of both to pursue integration into the public health care system (Bourgeault and Fynes 1997).

6. Distance learning is an important innovation in both nurse- and direct-entry midwifery. The program that graduates the largest number of nurse-midwifery students annually (approximately ninety-five) is a distance-learning program called the Community-based Nurse-midwifery Educational Program (CNEP)—an outgrowth of the Frontier Nursing Service, which is based in Hyden, Kentucky, at the original site of the FNS (www.midwives.org). Other major distance learning CNM programs include SUNY-Stonybrook in New York and the Institute of Midwifery and Women's Health (IMWHA) based in Philadelphia. In spite of the fact that most didactic instruction takes place over computer, these programs are characterized by a strong emphasis on the midwifery model and high degrees of teacher–student interaction (see Davis-Floyd 1998 a, b and Rooks 1997 for more detail.)

7. The five degree-granting institutions accredited by MEAC are:

   • Birthingway College of Midwifery (www.birthingway.org), which offers a Bachelor of Science in Midwifery;

- Midwives College of Utah (www.midwifery.edu), which offers Associate of Science in Midwifery, Bachelor of Science in Midwifery, and Master of Science in Midwifery degrees;
- National College of Midwifery (www.midwiferycollege.org), which offers the same three degrees plus a Doctorate of Science in Midwifery (Ph.D.);
- the Midwifery Program at Miami Dade Community College (www.mdc.edu/medical/Nursing/Programs/Midwifery_Prog/main.htm), which results in an Associate in Science Degree in Midwifery;
- the Midwifery Program at Bastyr University (www.bastyr.edu/academic/naturopath/midwifery/), which results in a Certificate of Naturopathic Midwifery in addition to the Naturopathic Doctor (N.D.) degree.

8. The ACNM makes major decisions by democratic vote of the membership; in contrast, MANA makes decisions based on consensus, which means that everyone has to agree. In both organizations, most decisions are made at the board level. The MANA board operates by consensus; in most cases, the ACNM board does as well.

9. Representatives of MANA, NARM, MEAC, and CfM developed the following definition of the Midwifery Model of Care, which was copyrighted in 1996 by the Midwifery Task Force (an already existing but inactive 501(c)3), which later also took on the task of maintaining the trademark registration of the logo developed to accompany the definition:

> The Midwifery Model of Care is based on the fact that pregnancy and birth are normal life events. The Midwifery Model of Care includes: monitoring the physical, psychological, and social well-being of the mother throughout the childbearing cycle; providing the mother with individualized education, counseling, and prenatal care, continuous hands-on assistance during labor and delivery, and postpartum support; minimizing technological interventions; identifying and referring women who require obstetrical attention. The application of this woman-centered model has been proven to reduce the incidence of birth injury, trauma, and cesarean section. (www.narm.org)

> In 2002, the name of this model as delineated above was changed to the Midwives Model of Care primarily because of the difficulty legislators and others have in pronouncing the word *midwifery.*

10. A physician's assistant (PA) receives extensive training in primary health care and is qualified in all fifty states for autonomous clinical practice.

11. Several direct-entry midwives who did not graduate from DOA-accredited programs have successfully challenged the licensure process in New York State and have been allowed to take the ACC exam; upon passing it, they qualified as CMs. (See chapter 2, note 10 for more detail.) As of 1999, like nurse-midwifery programs, all DOA-accredited direct-entry programs must either lead to a baccalaureate degree or require one for acceptance into the program. As noted previously, to date there are no pre-baccalaureate DOA-accredited direct-entry programs.

12. The nurse-midwifery program at Baystate Medical Center in Springfield, Massachusetts, developed a DOA-accredited direct-entry track for a particular student who had practiced as a lay midwife and is also a PA. She is now a CM and remains the only direct-entry graduate of this program, although other PAs could apply.

13. Although the percentage of births attended by midwives is still very small, it is steadily increasing. Between 1989 and 1997, it nearly doubled from 3.7 percent to 7 percent of total births (then rose very slowly to eight percent in 2002). Nearly all of this growth was due to increases in the number of in-hospital CNM-attended births; the percent of direct-entry midwife-attended births remained stable during that period, but may suffer from underreporting. In 2001, CNMs attended 305,606 births in the United States (*Quickening* 34(6):1, September/October 2003).

The U.S. Standard Certificate of Live Birth—source of data on the numbers and percentages of births attended by midwives—did not distinguish between any kinds of midwives until the 1989 revision, which distinguishes between CNMs and Other Midwives. The revisions made in 2003 distinguish between midwives certified by the ACNM or ACC—CNMs and CMs—and all other kinds of midwives.

Out-of-hospital births have accounted for less than one percent of all births in this country each year since 1989. CNMs attended fewer than 10,000 out-of-hospital births in 2002, of which the majority took place in freestanding birth centers (Martin et al., 2003). In 2002 the National Center for Health Statistics reported 5,689 births attended by CNMs in birth centers, and 2,726 births attended in birth centers by "other midwives" (Martin et al. 2003).

"Other midwives" attended almost 13,000 out-of-hospital births in 2002, the majority of which were homebirths. (Physicians attended almost 4,000 out-of-hospital births, including almost 2,000 in homes.) Someone other than a midwife or a physician signed the birth certificates of almost 9,000 babies born in out-of-hospital settings, including 7,500 that occurred in homes. Some of these were precipitous births with the baby caught by whomever was there. Some were planned homebirths with a family or church member attending, or midwife-attended homebirths in which the father signed the birth certificate. The latter is common in states where direct-entry midwifery is unregulated or illegal. Thus some of those births should also be attributed to "other midwives," raising the total of births attended by midwives who are not CNMs to somewhere between 13,000 and 20,000 per year. According to national vital statistics data from Centers for Disease Control (CDC), one out of twenty midwife-attended births is attended by midwives who are not CNMs (Martin et al. 2003, available at www.cdc.gov/nchs/data/nvsr/nvsr52/nvsr52_10.pdf).

14. The personal goals of members of this ACNM-MANA Liaison Group have at various times included developing appropriate language for a model state practice act that would encompass both new direct-entry certifications, and examining possibilities for making it easier for midwives credentialed by one organization to become certified by the other; these have not been realized. The group did develop a statement that endorsed all three national midwifery certifications (the CNM, CM, and CPM). This statement was accepted by the MANA Board but rejected by the ACNM Board of Directors. According to Rooks (2006): "The ACNM's budget was tight, and since the product of the group's work was inconsistent with ACNM positions, the ACNM ended its participation in the group in October 2001. In response to an outcry against this action by members attending the 2002 ACNM Convention, the ACNM [Board] re-instituted participation in the Liaison Group with guidelines regarding topics to be addressed by the group and the understanding that ACNM representatives would be self-funded. The group meets at both the MANA and ACNM annual meetings, although more of its members are usually present at the ACNM annual meeting." The ACNM Board of Directors and the MANA Board of Directors have agreed to three purposes for this group. They are: (1) to identify common areas of concern and mutual interest that may lead to joint ACNM/MANA initiatives; (2) to keep each organization informed on any state legislation that might impact the practice of the CPM and/or CNM/CM; and (3) to share with one another information related to the education and practice of CNMs, CMs, and CPMs.

15. Citizens for Midwifery is an independent consumer organization started by mothers who were interested in promoting and preserving the option of midwife-attended homebirth; thus its interests have always been in alignment with some of MANA's. President Susan Hodges (personal communication 2005) noted: "As CfM developed, the organization realized that our focus needed to be broader—that women really don't care what initials their midwife has or doesn't have after her name, they care

about the kind of care they get. Our mission/vision evolved and became: that the Midwives Model of Care should be the standard for maternity care and available to all women in all settings (regardless of provider)." CfM is also attempting to work with ACNM.

16. While nurse-midwives have a long-proven record of safety in attending both in- and out-of-hospital births (MacDorman and Singh 1998; Rooks 1997; 1999; Rooks et al. 1989), a constant criticism leveled at direct-entry homebirth midwives has been that they have no definitive statistics about the outcomes of their births. To combat this criticism, in the year 2000, all direct-entry midwives certified as CPMs were required to submit prospective data on all their clients, resulting in data on 7,000 courses of care (Johnson and Daviss 2005). I present the results of this study in chapter 3.

17. Examples of the increasing respect CNMs hold for CPMs include a 2000 article in *the Journal of Midwifery and Women's Health* in which Alyson Reed and Joyce Roberts suggested to CMs who need to find employment outside of the three states in which they are licensed that they obtain their CPM and practice out-of-hospital birth, and an initiative proposed by then-President of ACNM, Mary Ann Shah (2003), includes "explor[ing] ways of fast-tracking qualified CPMs . . . through ACNM-accredited education programs. Additionally, many of my more recent CNM interviewees express their appreciation for the CPM and the quality of practice for which it stands.

18. The Coalition for Improving Maternity Services (CIMS) was created through an alliance between various individuals and twenty-seven alternative birth organizations, including Lamaze International, ICEA, ACNM, MANA, AWHONN, DONA, La Leche League, and others. These groups realized that they had similar goals but were each working to achieve them on their own, and that they might have greater impact if they joined together. The common purpose all agreed on was the creation of a document called the Mother-Friendly Childbirth Initiative (MFCI) outlining "Ten Steps to Mother-Friendly Hospitals, Birth Centers, and Homebirth Services" and of a process of evaluation to achieve CIMS designation as "Mother-Friendly." The members of CIMS understand that many American women have little or no interest in natural childbirth; they are also keenly aware of the vast overuse of obstetrical interventions and the unnecessary damage to mothers and babies caused by this overuse. Their intention therefore is to work toward the goal that one day there will be a mother-friendly hospital in every community, so that women have access to all kinds of care, including care that is based on a natural childbirth/midwifery philosophy (see www.motherfriendly.org).

REFERENCES

ACNM Education Committee. 1979. "Core Competencies in Nurse-Midwifery: Expected Outcomes of Nurse-Midwifery Education." *Journal of Nurse-Midwifery* 24(1): 32–36.

American Public Health Association. 2002. "Increasing Access to Out-of-Hospital Maternity Care Services through State-Regulated and Nationally Certified Direct-Entry Midwives 2001–2003." *American Journal of Public Health* 92(3):453–455.

Anderson, R. E., and P. A. Murphy. 1995. "Outcomes of 11,788 Planned Homebirths Attended by Certified Nurse-Midwives. A Retrospective Descriptive Study." *Journal of Nurse Midwifery* 40(6):483–492.

Benoit, Cecilia, Robbie Davis-Floyd, Edwin van Teijlingen, Sirpa Wrede, and Janneli Miller. 2001. "Designing Midwives: A Transnational Comparison of Educational Models." In *Birth by Design: Pregnancy, Maternity Care, and Midwifery in North America and Europe*, ed. Raymond DeVries, Edwin van Teijlingen, Sirpa Wrede, and Cecilia Benoit, 139–165. New York: Routledge.

Borst, Charlotte. 1988. "The Training and Practice of Midwives: A Wisconsin Study." *Bulletin of the History of Medicine* 62:4 (606–627).

———. 1989. "Wisconsin's Midwives as Working Women: Immigrant Midwives and the Limits of a Traditional Occupation, 1870–1920." *Journal of American Ethnic History* 8(2):24–59.

———. 1995. *Catching Babies: The Professionalization of Childbirth, 1870–1920*. Cambridge, MA: Harvard University Press.

Bourgeault, Ivy, Cecilia Benoit, and Robbie Davis-Floyd, eds. 2004. *Reconceiving Midwives: The New Canadian Model of Care*. Toronto: McGill-Queens University Press.

Bourgeault, Ivy, and Mary Fynes. 1997. "Integrating Lay and Nurse-Midwifery into the United States and Canadian Health Care Systems." *Social Science and Medicine* 44, no.7: 1051–1063.

Brown, Dennis, and Pamela A. Toussaint. 1998. *Mama's Little Baby: The Black Woman's Guide to Pregnancy, Childbirth, and the Baby's First Year*. New York: Plume.

Bruner, Joseph P., Susan B. Drummond, Anna L. Meenan, and Ina May Gaskin. 1998. "All-Fours Maneuver for Reducing Shoulder Dystocia during Labor." *Journal of Reproductive Medicine* 43:439–443.

Burst, Helen Varney. 1990. "'Real' Midwifery." *Journal of Nurse-Midwifery* 35:189–191.

———. 1995. "An Update on the Credentialing of Midwives by the ACNM." *Journal of Nurse-Midwifery* 40(3): 290–296.

Carrington, Betty, and Nancy Dickerson. 2004. "Division of Accreditation (DOA) Marathon." *Quickening* (March/April). Available at http://www.midwife.org/edu/instaccred.cfm.

Curtin, Sally C. 1999. "Recent Changes in Birth Attendant, Place of Birth, and the Use of Obstetric Interventions." *Journal of Nurse-Midwifery* 44(4):349–354.

Davidson, Michele R. 2002. "Outcomes of High-Risk Women Cared for by Certified Nurse-Midwives." *Journal of Midwifery and Women's Health* 47(1):46–49.

Davis, Elizabeth. 1997. *Heart and Hands: A Midwife's Guide to Pregnancy and Birth*. 3d ed. Berkeley, CA: Celestial Arts.

———. 2004. *Heart and Hands: A Midwife's Guide to Pregnancy and Birth*, 4th ed. Berkley: Celetial Arts.

Davis-Floyd, Robbie E. 1998a. "The Ups, Downs, and Interlinkages of Nurse- and Direct-Entry Midwifery: Status, Practice, and Education." In *Getting an Education: Paths to Becoming a Midwife*. 4th ed., ed. Jan Tritten and Joel Southern, 67–118. Eugene, OR: Midwifery Today.

———. 1998b. "Types of Midwifery Training: An Anthropological Overview." In *Getting an Education: Paths to Becoming a Midwife*. 4th ed., ed. Jan Tritten and Joel Southern, 119–133. Eugene, OR: Midwifery Today.

Davis-Floyd, Robbie, and Elizabeth Davis. 1997. "Intuition as Authoritative Knowledge in Midwifery and Home Birth." In *Childbirth and Authoritative Knowledge: Cross-Cultural Perspectives*, pp. 315–349. ed. Robbie Davis-Floyd and Carolyn Sargent, University of California Press.

Daviss, Betty Anne. 2001a. "Reforming birth and (re)making midwifery in North America." In *Birth by Design: Pregnancy, Maternity Care, and Midwifery in North America and Europe*, ed. Raymond Devries, Cecilia Benoit, Edwin Teijingen, and Sirpa Wrede, 70–86. New York and London: Routledge.

DeVries, Raymond. 1996. *Making Midwives Legal: Childbirth, Medicine, and the Law*, 2nd ed. Columbus: Ohio State University Press.

DeVries, Raymond, Edwin van Teijlingen, Cecilia Benoit, and Sirpa Wrede. 2001. *Birth by Design: Midwives and Maternity Care in Europe and North America*. New York: Routledge.

Donegan, Jane B. 1978. *Women and Men Midwives: Medicine, Morality, and Misogyny in Early America*. Westport, CT: Greenwood Press.

Donnison, Jean 1977. *Midwives and Medical Men. A History of Inter-Professional Rivalries and Women's Rights.* New York: Schocken Books.

Fraser, Gertrude. 1995. "Modern Bodies, Modern Minds: Midwifery and Reproductive Change in an African American Community." In *Conceiving the New World Order: The Global Politics of Reproduction,* ed. Faye Ginsburg and Rayna Rapp, 42–58. Berkeley: University of California Press.

Fraser, Gertrude. 1998. *African American Midwifery in the South: Dialogues of Birth, Race, and Memory.* Cambridge: Harvard University Press.

Frye, Anne. 1995. *Holistic Midwifery: A Comprehensive Textbook for Midwives in Homebirth Practice,* Volume I, *Care during Pregnancy.* Portland, OR: Labyrs Press.

———. 2005. *Holistic Midwifery* Vol. II, *Care During Labor and Birth.* Portland, OR: Labyrs Press.

Fullerton, Judith. 1998. Personal communication. Judith Fullerton CNM is Professor of Nursing in the Department of Family Health Care, School of Nursing, University of Texas Health Sciences Center in San Antonio. A former test consultant to the ACNM Division of Competency Assessment and the ACNM Certification Council (ACC), she is the immediate past chair of the ACC Research Committee. She currently serves as a member of that committee.

Gaskin, Ina May. 1990. *Spiritual Midwifery.* 3d ed. Summertown, TN: The Book Publishing Company.

———. 1998. Personal communication. Ina May Gaskin, CPM is a direct-entry midwife on the Farm in Summertown, Tennessee, editor and publisher of the *Birth Gazette,* author of two books and numerous articles, and past-president of MANA. She is often referred to as "the most famous midwife in North America."

———. 2003. *Ina May's Guide to Childbirth.* New York: Bantam.

Haas, J. E., and Judith P. Rooks. 1986. National Survey of Factors Contributing to and Hindering the Successful Practice of Nurse-Midwifery: Summary of the American College of Nurse-Midwives Foundation Study. *Journal of Nurse-Midwifery* 32, no.5: 212–215.

Holmes, Linda Janet. 1986. "African American Midwives in the South." In *The American Way of Birth,* ed. Pamela Eakins, 273–291. Philadelphia, PA: Temple University Press.

Houghton, Pansy, and Kate Windom. 1996a. *1995 Job Analysis of the Role of Direct-Entry Midwives.* North American Registry of Midwives.

———. 1996b. *Executive Summary of the 1995 Job Analysis of the Role of Direct-Entry Midwives.* Copies can be obtained from the NARM Education and Advocacy Department (1-888-842-4784).

Institute of Medicine. 1982. *Research Issues in the Assessment of Birth Settings: Report of a Study.* Washington, D.C.: National Academy Press.

Johnson, Kenneth C. and Betty Anne Daviss. 2005. "Outcomes of Planned Home Births with Certified Professional Midwives: Large Prospective Study in North America." *British Medical Journal* 330:1416.

Kaufman, Karen and Bobbi Soderstrom. 2004. "Midwifery Education in Ontario: Its Origins, Operations, and Impact on the Profession." In *Reconceiving Midwives,* ed. Ivy Bourgeault, Cecilia Benoit, and Robbie Davis-Floyd, pp. 187–203. Toronto: McGuill-Queen's University Press.

Lang, Raven. 1972. *The Birth Book.* Palo Alto, CA: Genesis Press.

Langton, P. A. 1991. "Competing Occupational Ideologies, Identities, and the Practice of Nurse-Midwifery." *Research on Occupations and Professions* 6:149–177.

Litoff, Judy Barrett. 1978. *American Midwives. 1860 to the Present.* Westport, CT: Greenwood Press.

Leavitt, Judith Walzer. 1986. *Brought to Bed. Childbearing in America, 1750–1950.* Oxford: Oxford University Press.

MacDorman, M., and G. Singh. 1998. "Midwifery Care, Social and Medical Risk Factors, and Birth Outcomes in the U.S.A." *Journal of Epidemiology and Community Health* 52:310–317.

Martin, J. A., B. E. Hamilton, P. D. Sutton, S. J. Ventura, F. Menacker, and M. L. Munson. 2003. *Births: Final data for 2002.* National vital statistics reports, vol. 52, no.10. Hyattsville, MA: National Center for Health Statistics. http://www.cdc.gov/nchs/data/nvsr/nvsr52/nvsr52_10.pdf.

Murphy, P. A., and J. Fullerton. 1998c. "Outcomes of Intended Homebirths in Nurse-Midwifery Practice: A Prospective Descriptive Study." *Obstetrics and Gynecology* 92(3):461–470.

Myers-Ciecko, Joanne. 1999. "Evolution and Current Status of Direct-Entry Midwifery Education, Regulation, and Practice in the United States, with Examples from Washington State." *Journal of Nurse-Midwifery* 44(4):384–393.

Paine, Lisa L., Catherine M. Dower, and Edward O'Neil. 1999. "Midwifery in the 21st Century: Recommendations from the Pew Health Professions Commission/UCSF Center for the Health Professions 1998 Taskforce on Midwifery." *Journal of Nurse Midwifery* 44(4):341–348.

Perkins, Barbara Bridgman. 2004. *The Medical Delivery Business: Health Reform, Childbirth, and the Economic Order.* New Brunswick, NJ: Rutgers University Press.

Reed, Alyson, and Joyce E. Roberts. 2000. "State Regulation of Midwives: Issues and Options." *Journal of Midwifery and Women's Health* 45(2):130–149.

Roberts J. 1995. "The Role of Graduate Education in Midwifery in the USA." In *Issues in Midwifery,* Volume I, ed. T. Murphy-Black, 119–161. New York: Churchill Livingstone.

Roberts, Joyce E. 1991. "An Overview of Nurse-Midwifery Education and Accreditation." *Journal of Nurse-Midwifery* 36(6):373–376.

Rooks, Judith P. 1995. "The Role of Graduate Education in Midwifery in the USA." In *Issues in Midwifery,* ed. Patricia Murphy Black. Edinburgh: Churchill Livingstone.

———. 1997. *Midwifery and Childbirth in America.* Philadelphia, PA: Temple University Press.

———. 1998. "Unity in Midwifery? Realities and Alternatives." *Journal of Nurse-Midwifery,* 43:315–319.

———. 1999. "The Midwifery Model of Care." *Journal of Nurse-Midwifery* 44(4):370–374.

———. Forthcoming. "Relationships between ACNM-Certified Midwives and Other Midwives, Nurses, Physicians, and Doulas." In *Professional Issues in Midwifery,* ed. Lynette Ament. Sudbury, MA: Jones and Bartlett.

Rooks, Judith P., Norman L. Weatherby, Eunice K.M. Ernst, Susan Stapleton, David Rosen, and Allan Rosenfield. 1989. "Outcomes of Care in Birth Centers: The National Birth Centere Study," *New England Journal of Medicine* 321:1804–1811.

Rooks, Judith P., and S. H. Fishman. 1980. "American Nurse-Midwifery Practice in 1976–1977: Reflections on 50 Years of Growth and Development." *American Journal of Public Health* 70:990–996.

Rothman, Barbara Katz. 1982. *In Labor: Women and Power in the Birthplace.* New York: W.W. Norton.

Schlinger, Hillary. 1992. *Circle of Midwives.* Self-published.

Scoggin, Janet. 1996. "How Nurse-Midwives Define Themselves in Relation to Nursing, Medicine, and Midwifery." *Journal of Nurse-Midwifery* 41(1):36–42.

Shah, Mary Ann. 2003. "Midwifery Will Prevail." *Quickening* 34(5):3.

Sharp, E. S. 1983. "Nurse-Midwifery Education: Its Successes, Failures, and Future." *Journal of Nurse-Midwifery* 28(2):17–23.

Sharpe, Mary. 2004. "Exploring Legislated Midwifery: Texts and Rulings." In *Reconceiving Midwifery: The New Canadian Model of Care*, pp. ed. Ivy Bourgeault, Cecilia Benoit, and Robbie Davis-Floyd, 150–166. Montreal, Quebec: McGill-Queens University Press.

Tritten, Jan, and Joel Southern. 1998. *Getting an Education: Paths to Becoming a Midwife.* 4th ed. Eugene, OR: Midwifery Today.

Varney, Helen. 1997. *Varney's Midwifery.* 3d ed. Sudbury, MA: Jones and Bartlett.

Weaver, Pam. 1998. Personal communication. Pam Weaver CPM is a practicing direct-entry midwife in Alaska. She is co-author of the *Practical Skills Guide for Midwifery*, and served as the NARM board liaison to state legislatures and agencies.

Wertz, Richard W., and Dorothy C. Wertz. 1977. *Lying-In. A History of Childbirth in America.* New York: The Free Press.

Wilson, Adrian. 1995. *The Making of Man-Midwifery.* Cambridge, MA: Harvard University Press.

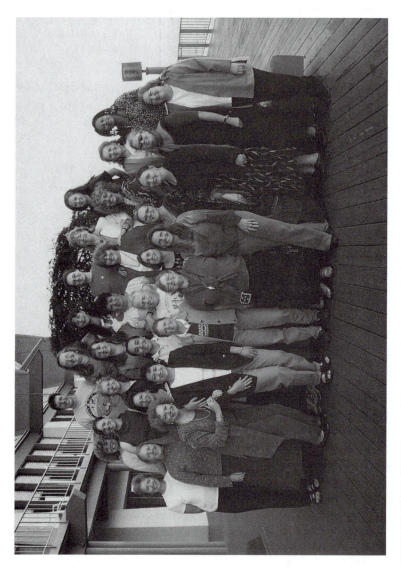

Fig. 1.1 Joint MANA/NARM/MEAC/NACPM Boards, October 2004. Photographer: Robbie Davis-Floyd

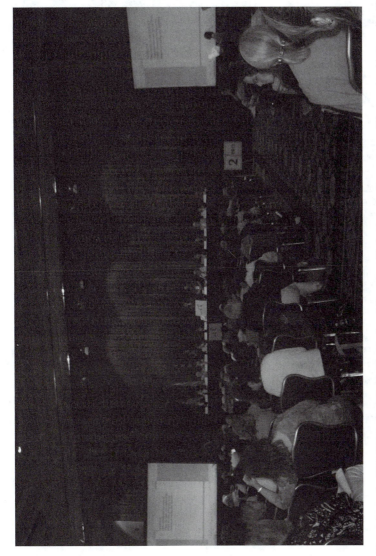

Fig. 1.2 "Floor Discussion at the 2005 ACNM convention in Washington, D.C. on June 13 about conducting a survey of the membership regarding their opinions about changing the name of the American College of Nurse-Midwives to the American College of Midwives. The resulting survey showed no clear majority opinion, so the name has not been changed."

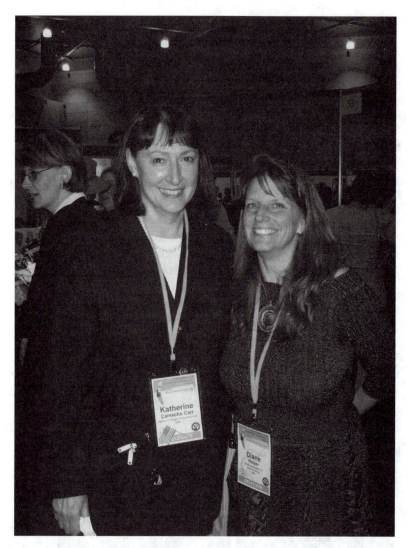

Fig. 1.3 Katherine Camacho Carr, ACNM President, and Diane Holzer, MANA President, at the triennial conference of the International Confederation of Midwives, Brisbane, Australia, 2005. Photographer: Robbie Davis-Floyd.

2

IDEALISM AND PRAGMATISM IN THE CREATION OF THE CERTIFIED MIDWIFE: THE DEVELOPMENT OF MIDWIFERY IN NEW YORK AND THE NEW YORK MIDWIFERY PRACTICE ACT OF 1992

Maureen May and Robbie Davis-Floyd

You don't get what you deserve, you get what you negotiate.

—**Dorothea Lang, New York CNM**

Historically, New York state has been a generative source for Certified Nurse-Midwives (CNMs) and for both of the two new types of direct-entry midwives—the Certified Midwife (CM) and the Certified Professional Midwife (CPM). Our focus in this chapter is on the creation of the CM through the enactment of a significant piece of legislation, the New York State Professional Midwifery Practice Act of 1992. The history we recount here provides background and context for the enactment of the legislation. This history opens a window into the development of the culture of nurse-midwifery, and seeks to describe how the ideological and political conflicts between nurse- and direct-entry midwives in New York have been primary catalysts for the conflicts, rivalries, and misunderstandings that still plague American midwifery in other states.

Until 1992, New York nurse-midwives were not licensed as midwives (the license they held was that of Registered Nurse) but were given permits to practice midwifery under an archaic 1907 statute in the state Sanitation Code while other professionals were licensed and regulated by the New York Education Department. Direct-entry, homebirth midwives practiced without licensure or legal status. Both groups of midwives worked for ten years on legislation that would grant them full and legal professional status. An additional desire of the New York CNMs was to create a new kind of direct-entry midwife (DEM) with the same training as the CNM but without the nursing requirement. The existing DEMs in New York thought that this new kind of midwife certification would and should include them and the training they valued—a training that focuses on homebirth and occurs either through apprenticeship or in one of the independent midwifery schools in the United States that exist outside of the university and medical center milieu (see chapter 1).

Those CNMs working for the legislation were certain that the New York state legislature would never pass a bill validating anything short of a university education for midwives. From their perspective, the legislation had absolutely nothing to do with the homebirth DEMs, but was about legitimizing CNMs and the new kind of DEM they envisioned. The eventual legislation, passed in 1992, did not give the CNMs everything they wanted but did achieve a number of their goals, and did lead directly to the creation of their new kind of midwife, later named the Certified Midwife (CM). It did not include the already existing unlicensed homebirth DEMs in any way except to turn the legal definition of their practice from misdemeanor to felony. This legal redefinition was not intended by the CNMs, but rather was put into the law by government staff because it is mandatory in any law creating and defining any licensed profession in New York.

While generating new opportunities and challenges for midwifery within New York state, the legislation has also had profound ramifications for midwifery throughout the country as the debate engendered by the creation of the CM has spilled over into political and legislative arenas in other states. In some states, efforts on the part of homebirth direct-entry midwives toward decriminalization and licensure have been actively opposed by some CNMs, with the unofficial support of the national ACNM leadership. In other states, CNMs have attempted to introduce legislation similar to that in New York, which would establish the ACNM-created Certified Midwife as the only legal direct-entry credential. In short, the New York situation set off a classic professional turf battle between midwives.

While to date there are only fifty CMs, what would appear to be something of little consequence is in fact a development of long-term consequence for American midwifery. The political, legislative battles over licensure, credentialing, education, and clinical preparation, as well as place of practice, are really about who has the right to legally practice and to claim the title *midwife*, which is, of course, ultimately all about identity—midwives' social, cultural, and historical identity.

METHODS AND FRAMEWORK

The research on which this chapter is based includes lengthy interviews conducted by the authors with fifty New York DEMs and CNMs, as well as with various government officials and consumer activists, between 1996 and 2000. Maureen May is a CNM with a Certificate of Midwifery from the Frontier School of Midwifery's Community-based Nurse-midwifery Educational Program (CNEP), and a Women's Health Nurse Practitioner with a Masters of Science in Nursing (MSN) from the University of Rochester. She is a homebirth midwife, a member of the ACNM who supports unity within the midwifery community, and is presently working on a PhD in social science with an emphasis on ethnography. Robbie Davis-Floyd is an anthropologist who has studied American midwifery since 1991 and supports both organizations and their philosophies of care (see Introduction, this volume). In addition to our interviews, we attended numerous professional and governmental meetings and investigated primary sources, including minutes from ACNM chapter meetings, the legislative jacket, and journal articles.

Ethnography is both a framework and a method of research. As a framework, ethnography holds as a core value the concept that there are real parts of the world and the human experience that cannot be quantified. Ethnographic research involves back-and-forth dialogue and close relationships between researchers and informants. Through this process, the ethnographer is able to access information unobtainable through other methodologies. Standard methods for data collection include interviews, observations, field notes, and the use of primary documents. We have utilized all of these in the process of our study. Ethnography recognizes that "facts" are not only contested, but are reflected in the richness and details of the informant's own words, and thus requires that the voices of the individuals under study be heard to the greatest extent possible. To that end, we have incorporated extensive quotes into our text from key interviewees on both sides, in order to offer our readers the feel and flavor of their experiences and thoughts. Consent has been obtained for all quotes from interviews. We name the quoted individuals when we have been given permission to do so; any quotes from unnamed individuals reflect their expressed desire to remain anonymous or the fact that the quoted words were repeated by various individuals.

At the onset, the goal of our research was to understand the development and ramifications of the New York midwifery legislation. During the coding of interviews, data on the professional culture of New York nurse-midwifery became so salient that we decided to include it in this chapter, in part because it breaks new ground in the anthropological study of midwifery, but primarily because it brightly illuminates the sociocultural context out of which New York CNMs created the law. For the same reasons, we highlight significant moments of time in the history of New York midwifery because this history is essential to a full understanding of how the culture of New York midwifery developed, why its members have always had a strong sense of specialness within American nurse-midwifery, and how their values came to include the licensing of midwives without nursing training.

Many discussions of present-day American midwifery drift into comparisons based on a binary framework. Analyzing American midwifery through professionalization or social movement theory leads to a focus on the structural and cultural changes (usually criticized by such theorists as negative or co-optive) that occur in a given group during its process of professionalization. Such analysis can easily result in labeling certain players *wrong* and others *right*. For example, if we view the CNM, the new CM, and ACNM as occupying an oppositional space in relationship to the direct-entry homebirth midwife, the Certified Professional Midwife (CPM), and MANA, we inevitably miss the reality, which is that in practice many midwives are occupying a space in between, both ideologically and in practice. Davis-Floyd (1998a; chapter 1 this volume) has documented the blurring of professional lines between these two types of midwives, demonstrating that within the grassroots of midwifery there is increasingly common ground. Our research has supported this analysis. Some nurse-midwives identify as professionals and as part of a social movement, and some direct-entry midwives continue both to embrace the social movement and engage in professionalization (as Betty Anne Daviss describes in further detail in chapter 12).

Concomitantly, we desired in this chapter to avoid a binary approach in an effort simply to tell, and to analyze, how the New York legislation came about—a story that in its full complexity has never before been written. But the core of this New York story revolves around professional rivalry between two groups of midwives. And so we found a binary approach impossible to avoid. There are two sides, and only two sides, to this New York midwifery story. During the writing process, we have often doubted our ability to tell both sides in a way that both groups will recognize as true. It has been a tremendous challenge to our ability as ethnographers to undertake this task. Early drafts of this chapter sent to midwives and others on both sides of this story for review resulted in responses that included desires to emphasize their parts of the story and discount the other side and accusations that we, the authors, were biased toward one side or the other. We have taken all comments into account in this final version, remaining determined to tell both sides of this New York story accurately and without bias. We have done our best to explain events, philosophies, and actions as both groups perceived and experienced them, and can only hope that in our final words both groups involved will find a fair and accurate portrayal of themselves and their versions of events.

Part of our writing challenge had to do with terminology. As anthropologists, it is our tradition to ascribe to subjects the name they claim, as a matter of respect and the right of people to self-definition. But it is precisely the contested claim to the term *direct-entry midwife* that constitutes the fulcrum around which this New York story revolves. Social scientists writing about midwifery had a much easier time when we could simply distinguish between *nurse-midwives* and *lay midwives*—the term used for themselves by many unlicensed homebirth midwives around the country throughout the 1970s, 1980s, and early 1990s. But then *lay* became politically incorrect as the professionalizing homebirth midwives rejected it for its pejorative connotations, and now is only properly used in a historical sense (a use we follow in this chapter). In the late 1980s, these midwives, especially in New York, began referring to themselves as *direct-entry*, a more professional term that they saw as more clearly describing their identity as it differs from nurse-midwifery. Concurrently, the New York nurse-midwifery leaders had been using the term direct-entry to describe the new kind of midwife they were trying to create, who would be trained not by any route but in specific, formal, university-based educational programs and would practice primarily in-hospital. So no easy distinctions have been possible in writing this chapter, as the term direct-entry properly includes both types of midwife without a nursing education.

In this chapter we wish to avoid confusion for the reader, while at the same time respecting all parties. So *direct-entry midwives* will, unless otherwise specified, refer to New York's independent, unlicensed homebirth midwives (some of whom formerly called themselves lay midwives). When referring to the new direct-entry midwife established after the 1992 legislation, we will use the full title Certified Midwife or the abbreviation CM.

Our goals in this chapter are threefold: (1) to write the history/her-story of the New York 1992 midwifery legislation from the points of view of both groups involved in trying to create it; (2) to present this history in the context of a sociological and anthropological (compara-tive) analysis of the motivations and ideologies of both groups; and (3) to extend this analysis to include the influence on both groups of their general marginalization in the American health care system and their subordination to the hegemony of obstetrics. Thus our analysis has been informed by James Scott's (1985, 1990) theory of domination and resistance in peasant societies. Scott's identification of "everyday acts of resistance" by subordinated classes against powerful dominating forces provides a useful framework for understanding the development of midwifery in New York. Our interviews revealed what Scott calls "hidden transcripts"—individual conversations taking place behind a group's public representations of itself.

In the United States, normal pregnancy falls within the professional purview of obstetrics. In most other developed countries, even where hospital birth is the norm, uncomplicated pregnancy falls within the professional province of an independent midwifery; obstetrics is con-sidered a medical specialty called upon to handle cases in which com-plications have developed. Both professions are recognized as having unique and distinct functions in the organization of maternity care. In contrast, American midwifery as a whole is a subjugated profession and the hidden transcripts that we have collected reflect differing beliefs and strategies on how to best position midwifery vis-à-vis the powerful dominating force of obstetrics.

THE DEVELOPMENT OF NURSE-MIDWIFERY
IN NEW YORK

Cultural beliefs regarding health and illness are not isolated from, but are always influenced by, a community's social history. The historical lens we provide here is critical for a full understanding of the significance that events in New York have held for the profession of nurse-midwifery from its early years to the present. In the following section, we touch on key aspects of this history that help explain recent events in New York.

New York nurse-midwives have long held strong influence within the ACNM, due both to their numbers and the quality of individual leaders who emerged early on from New York City midwifery schools and services, as well as to the early and continuing important role of nurse-midwifery in the city's health care system. This section will illustrate why New York nurse-midwives attach such importance and pride to their hospital-based midwifery services,[1] and how the history specific to New York midwifery has led to the sense of exceptionality and specialness held by many New York nurse-midwives—their strong feeling that what is good for New York must be good, and should provide the model for the rest of the country.

On the national level, contemporary nurse-midwives tend to strongly identify with a creation mythology that traces their historical roots from Mary Breckenridge and the Frontier Nursing Service. This creation mythology entails vivid imagery of bold, independent nurse-midwives riding horseback through rain and snow providing childbirth and primary health care to the households of the rural poor of Appalachia. While the Frontier Nursing Service is credited as the first "nurse-midwifery program" in the United States (Shoemaker 1947), its model of independent, rural, clinical practice is far from the reality of contemporary nurse-midwifery and is not the model for what ultimately evolved into the contemporary nurse-midwife. Nurse-midwives continue to practice in rural settings in many states (for example, CNMs now (2005) attend approximately thirty percent of births in New Mexico) and the percentage of births attended by CNMs in general is highest in rural states [National Center for Health Statistics, 1999]); but the type of nurse-midwifery that developed in urban New York also played a formative role in this profession's development in the rest of the nation.

New York City became a hot spot during the national campaign to eliminate the midwife in the early twentieth century. Forty percent of New York City deliveries were by midwives in 1905, all in the home (Harris, Daily, and Lang 1971). Many practicing immigrant midwives in New York City, referred to as "granny" midwives by public health reformers, were in fact professionally trained in government-approved midwifery programs in their countries of origin. One of the obstacles such immigrant midwives faced was the fact that there was "no provision in the law for examination" (Weisl 1964) of these midwives nor any equivalent type of educational facilities. As this brief history will show, the concept of nurse-midwifery was promoted in New York City by public health reformers who saw public health nurses trained as midwives and the movement of place of birth into the hospital as solutions to the public health crisis facing urban America, namely increasing infant and maternal mortality rates—a crisis associated with "the midwife problem" by a well-orchestrated public opinion campaign waged by organized medicine. Ironically, while traditional midwifery was systematically eliminated by this reform effort, many years passed before nurse-midwives were allowed to take the place of the midwives they had helped to eliminate and establish clinical practice in the hospital. And the professional independence held by midwives in other countries became lost and has yet to be reclaimed by American midwifery.

New York City became the first community to initiate reform aimed at reducing the infant mortality rate. A study of midwives was commissioned in 1906 by the Public Health Committee of the Association of Neighborhood Workers. In its report, Elisabeth Crowell, a nurse, produced a "scathing indictment of midwives which prompted the city to revise its laws pertaining to their regulation" describing the typical midwife as "foreigners of a low grade—ignorant, untrained women who find in the natural needs and life-long prejudice of the parturient woman a lucrative means of livelihood" (Litoff 1978:51). Prior to 1907, New York midwifery was loosely regulated by the state. Practicing midwives were required to register with the registrar of the city within which they provided service and present "certificates of character and expertise from two physicians. No supervision was maintained over their activities" (Weisl 1964:9). In 1907, state legislation gave the New York City Board of Health authority to regulate midwifery within its jurisdiction, placing regulation of New York City midwives within the Bureau of Child Hygiene. Section 196 of the Sanitary Code was enacted, establishing minimal regulations. In 1913, the Board of Health set up a Midwifery Division and the Bellevue School for Midwives was established along the lines of the European schools of midwifery (Weisl 1964). In 1914, as a further attempt to regulate and standardize the profession of midwifery, the New York City Health Code was altered so that permits to practice midwifery would be granted only to those midwives who had graduated from a recognized school of midwifery (Harris, Daily, and Lang 1971)—an effort fostered by those physicians who were supportive of the training and incorporation of midwives. But regulation of midwifery in New York City did not serve to strengthen the position of midwives within the health care system. By 1915, midwife-attended deliveries had dropped from forty percent (in 1905) to thirty percent (Corbin 1959; Harris, Daily, and Lang 1971). Hospital births at the time were also at thirty percent. (Regarding the other forty percent of births, it can only be assumed that doctors were taking over more of the home deliveries in New York City, that some mothers were delivering without official attendants, and that unlicensed midwives continued to attend births.)

Midwifery and homebirth were under increasing pressure from a variety of changing social patterns. Among these was the developing concept of prenatal care as an essential maternity service, a concept promoted through the work of the Federal Children's Bureau (established in 1912) and the Sheppard-Towner Maternity and Infancy Protection Act of 1921 (Corbin 1959; Rooks 1997). During this time a vision of nurse-midwifery began to take hold among public health reformers. The concept of midwifery as a clinical specialty of nursing was first discussed publicly in 1912, the same year as the influential and historic Federal Children's Bureau report. Clara Noyes, the Superintendent of Training Schools at Bellevue and Allied Hospitals in New York City, proposed in a speech to the International Congress of Hygiene and Demography that:

> if the midwife can gradually be replaced by the nurse who has, upon her general training super-imposed a course in practical midwifery, which has been clearly defined by obstetricians, it would seem a logical economic solution to the problem . . . we should be able to provide better teaching, better nursing and eventually better medical assistance to the less highly favored classes." (Quoted in Shoemaker 1947)

Two years later in 1914, at an annual meeting of the National Organization of Public Health Nurses, Dr. Fred Taussig endorsed the concept of establishing schools of midwifery limited to "graduate nurses" (Shoemaker 1947; Harris, Daily, and Lang 1971).

And so it was within the public health reform movement that today's nurse-midwifery was born. This movement's roots go back to the turn of the century and the Progressive Era—a time of public health reform and the urban settlement house movement with its mission to serve the underserved in large urban communities. Key reforms of the Progressive Era involved the establishment of a public health system serving the growing urban population. This is where nurse-midwives gained their initial toehold—in the public health clinics of the urban centers, in the northeast and New York City in particular (Dye 1987; Harris, Daily and Lang 1971; Howard 1994; Kobrin 1966; Litoff 1978; Reagan 1995).[2]

In 1917, the Women's City Club of New York City, an organization of 2,000 influential women, citing its concern for the extreme maternal and infant mortality rates evident in New York City and the United States, established the Maternity Protection Committee to take on a special project, a maternity center, which would provide both clinical and social service to mothers lacking adequate maternity care (*Bulletin of the Women's City Club of New York,* 1(6) October 1917). The goal of the maternity center was to "give adequate medical and nursing care to every woman" and to provide "thorough coordination of all the work of all the agencies" in the community (Stevens 1918). Within a year the center achieved success beyond hopes and expectations, with over 2,300 women asking for assistance, far more than the 1,000 women they initially hoped to reach (Women's City Club of New York. February 1919. *Summary of the First Year's Work. Preliminary Report to Club Members on the Maternity Center. From Its Opening September 15, 1917 to October 1, 1918).* After little more than two years, the Maternity Center Project could claim the following gains in a pamphlet entitled *Our Hopes Justified.*

> Results of Pre-natal Work carried on for more than two years show: 1. Where three babies die in the entire city only one dies when under our care. 2. When ten are still-born, we have but three. 3. Where five mothers die under ordinary conditions, only two die when under our supervision. Is this not worthwhile? (Women's City Club of New York, *Our Hopes Justified*)

In May 1920, the center project was turned over to the Maternity Center Association (MCA). Formed in 1918, MCA held as a primary goal the establishment of maternity centers throughout New York City. Its mission was to facilitate pregnant women's access to health care so that "every pregnant mother in the City of New York" could be "brought under medical and nursing supervision" (Stevens 1919). This goal was to be accomplished by training "a limited number of selected public health nurses who can find a place to use their training in the new order; not to work as private practitioners or midwives, but as instructors and supervisors for the untrained midwives and for nurses with only an elementary, deficient training in obstetric nursing" (Hemschemeyer 1962:7). This developing vision of a new type of midwife "contained essential differences from the system of midwifery practice in some countries in Europe and Great Britain and [provided] the guidelines for establishing an American system of nurse-midwifery" (Hemschemeyer 1962:7). A clear—and pragmatically necessary—acquiescence to physicians was evident. These early activities of the MCA, while not directly aimed at the elimination of the midwife, encouraged women to avail themselves of medical care and discouraged the use of midwives in childbirth. Eventually, however, these negative attitudes toward midwives were changed by the excellent results of the Frontier Nursing Service in Hyden, Kentucky (see chapter 1). Its highly successful and well-documented outcomes were noted in New York, to such an extent that by 1931 the MCA had established an educational school of nurse-midwifery,[3] "appropriately so since recognition of the concept of midwifery and the responsibility for its standardization had early precedence here" (Harris, Daily, and Lang 1971:65).

Shoemaker (1947) documents the Manhattan Midwifery School, associated with the Manhattan Maternity and Dispensary and existing from 1928 to 1932, as the first U.S. school of nurse-midwifery. However, the founding in 1931 of the Lobenstine Clinic and School of Midwifery, affiliated with the MCA, was of greater significance (Shoemaker 1947, Lang 1977). According to Rooks (1997), the establishment of this school was an organized effort by individuals within the MCA and Mary Breckenridge.

> In 1921, MCA decided to concentrate on a single demonstration center that could provide complete maternity care. In 1923, MCA tried to arrange for the Bellevue School for Midwives [in New York City] to instruct its public health nurses in midwifery. The plan was rejected by a city commissioner. In 1930, a group of MCA board members and others, including Mary Breckinridge, incorporated themselves as the Association for the Promotion and Standardization of Midwifery. After much work, the two affiliated organizations opened the Lobenstine Clinic, the nation's second nurse-midwifery service and, in 1931, the Lobenstine Midwifery School, the first nurse-midwifery educational program, in New York City. (Rooks 1997:38)

The decision by MCA to establish a midwifery training program and a clinic was controversial, extending beyond its original mission: "It violated a principle to which it had long subscribed; namely, that antepartum and postpartum clinics should be part of an obstetric service in a general hospital. MCA acted because of the immediate, urgent need for public health nurses, equipped not only with theoretical knowledge of obstetrics but with actual clinical knowledge. Midwifery, like any art, can only be learned by doing" (Corbin 1959:22). The objectives of the Lobenstine School and clinic were substantially different from the type of midwifery practiced by European midwives and the nurse-midwives at the Frontier School of Midwifery in Kentucky.

> First, the nurse-midwife trained at the Lobenstine School would accept the responsibility of maternity care of normal patients delegated to her by the obstetrician after a complete physical examination had been given. And secondly, the nurse-midwife would not be a private practitioner as was the principle of work in Kentucky. These differences made it necessary that nurse-midwives be employed only where medical care and medical consultation services are available. Their principle work would be in the field of supervision and instruction. (Shoemaker 1947:30)

The willingness to compromise professional independence in order to gain that primary toehold within the mainstream maternity care system is seen early on in this New York experience.

Rose McNaught, a nurse-midwife from FNS, was sent by Mary Breckenridge to lead the clinic. McNaught, Hattie Hemschemeyer (a public health nurse), and a physician were the initial staff (Shoemaker 1947). The first class of six student nurse-midwives "gave priority to public health nurses from states with high infant mortality and many untrained granny midwives" (Rooks 1997:38). These nurse-midwifery students at MCA, the first of whom graduated in 1934, attended births in women's homes during training. Upon graduation most went to work within the public health system, taught in nursing schools, or did mission work abroad. "Wherever they worked, the level of maternity care improved . . . The demand for their services outran the supply" (Corbin 1959:188). Yet growth in numbers was slight and job opportunities in active clinical midwifery practice were not forthcoming. The effort to eliminate the traditional midwife was very successful. As the number of traditional midwives with practice permits dwindled, nurse-midwives did not take their places.

The following table is from Bernard Weisl's 1964 article "The Nurse-Midwife and the New York City Health Code," published in the *Bulletin of the American College of Nurse-Midwifery* (forerunner of the *Journal of Nurse-Midwifery*, later renamed the *Journal of Midwifery and Women's Health*, see references). It illustrates an efficient and thorough elimination of the traditional midwife through the efforts of physicians, public health reformers, and New York nurses and nurse-midwives. Many years passed before the nurse-midwife would be allowed to take the place of the traditional and immigrant professional midwives these groups worked to eliminate.

As the table shows, in 1934, "granny midwives" held 1,997 permits to practice in New York City while nurse-midwives held six. Five years later in 1939, granny midwives held only 270 permits to practice and in

Table 2.1 Permits in Force, New York City, December 31, Annually

Year	Total Midwife Permits	" Granny Midwives"	Maternity Center Midwives
1934	1203	1997	6
1939	276	270	6
1940	235	229	6
1942	170	162	8
1943	151	142	9
1944	129	119	10
1945	113	97	16
1946	47	31	16
1947	36	7	29
1948	26	6	20
1950	24	9	15
1951	21	6	15
1952	21	6	15
1953	22	6	16
1954	18	5	13
1955	19	4	15
1956	19	4	15
1957	13	2	11
1958	17	2	15
1959	13	2	11
1960	25	2	23
1961	2	2	0
1962	1	1	0

	Nurse-Midwife Permits		
	Total	**Original**	**Renewal**
1960	5	5	0
1961	15	10	5
1962	21	8	13

1940 had declined further to 229 permits. In 1941, citing a lack of granny midwives to regulate, New York City's Midwifery Board eliminated itself and midwifery became regulated under what became the Bureau of Child Health. By 1957 there were only thirteen midwifery permits in New York City, eleven of which were held by staff of the MCA. By 1962, New York City nurse-midwives held twenty-one permits to practice (Weisl 1964). All were educators or new graduating midwife interns (Dorothea Lang, personal communication 2005).

Professional recognition for nurse-midwives was nonexistent for decades, and clinical positions were scarce. Many graduate nurse-midwives left the United States to work in international settings where they could practice full scope clinical nurse-midwifery (Lang 1977:94–95). This small profession sought out ways to meet the needs of women. "Much of the credit for the pioneering work toward prepared childbirth education and family-centered care goes to these CNMs" (Lang 1977:94–95). However, as hospital birth rapidly replaced homebirth, the doors to providing midwifery care in the hospital remained closed to nurse-midwives. In 1963, a national study of nurse-midwives carried out by the United States Children's Bureau under the Department of Health, Education, and Welfare (HEW) documented that only thirty certified nurse-midwives out of 535 residing in the United States at the time were providing the scope of care for which they were trained (Lang 1977:97).

The Hospital-Based Nurse-Midwife in New York City

New York City cannot lay claim to the first urban nurse-midwifery deliveries. That honor goes to Johns Hopkins Hospital where a nurse-midwife was invited in 1953 to deliver on an experimental basis, followed by a similar experiment at Columbia /Presbyterian Hospital in New York City (Lang 1977). In subsequent years, CNMs began gaining entrance to the New York City hospital system, although not yet at the clinical level. In 1956, Columbia University Teachers College established the first masters-level program available to nurse-midwives, a Masters of Nursing Education. The City of New York Health Code was amended in 1959 making both RN licensure and nurse-midwifery certification a requirement for a midwife permit (Weisl 1964). New York City was the second locale to grant legal status to CNMs. (New Mexico granted state licensure to CNMs in 1945.) Following this Health Code modification, in 1960 five nurse-midwives were given a permit to practice in New York City and by 1968 a total of sixty-seven permits to practice had been obtained by CNMs (Harris, Daily, and Lang 1971).

In 1958, obstetrician Louis Hellman asked the MCA school of Nurse-Midwifery to come to Kings County Hospital in Brooklyn, where the first hospital-based nurse-midwifery class began. In 1961, New York City made a commitment to nurse-midwifery services by making nurse-midwifery educator salaries a budget line in the Department of Hospitals (Hellman 1971:75). In 1963, as an experiment, Cumberland Hospital and Harlem Hospital offered employment to CNMs (Cumberland Hospital, three CNMs; Harlem Hospital, two CNMs) serving mothers in the hospital labor and delivery unit (personal communication, Dorothea Lang, 2005).

In 1962, the Panel on Mental Retardation created the opening nurse-midwives had been waiting for by drawing a connection between inadequate maternity care and prematurity and brain damage. "The report led to legislation which authorized the Maternity and Infant Care Projects under Title V of the Social Security Act beginning in 1963" (Lesser 1972:111). Fifty-six projects were quickly funded through this legislation, two of which hired nurse-midwives, resulting in a new source of employment for graduates. The Maternal and Infant Care (MIC) Project of New York City, responsible for community-based maternity and infant care clinics throughout the city, came out of this federal effort and played an important role in propagating midwifery services throughout the city's hospital system.

In 1970, the MIC project established the first hospital-based nurse-midwifery service in New York at Delafield Hospital's Obstetrics and Family Practice Center, with permission to attend births at Columbia/Presbyterian Hospital. At the same time, the MIC published a guide for the development of nurse-midwifery services for twelve hospitals affiliated with the MIC project. A unique relationship developed between the MIC project and the twelve affiliated hospitals. Nurse-midwives hired by MIC for each hospital provided both community and hospital-based services; half of their time in intrapartum care and the other half in pre- and postnatal care at the community-based clinics. Nurse-midwives expanded their scope of practice as they began to staff family planning clinics (Hellman 1971). By 1971, 100 nurse-midwives at eighteen hospitals had attended the births of 3,650 babies in New York City (Lesser 1972).

Under this unique organizational scheme, New York midwifery services grew in number and flourished. By 1981, CNMs were providing care and managing labor and delivery services at five hospitals and nine prenatal clinics. Although initially a pioneering strategy allowing for a degree of independence for nurse-midwives, this unusual organizational framework with its multiple lines of institutional accountability and corresponding responsibility to multiple authorities became increasingly unworkable for nurse-midwives. The confusion this framework created and its limitations for long-term practice and identity led directly to the push to separate midwifery from nursing at the clinical level, an underlying motivation for nurse-midwifery to have its own legislation in New York state.

In 1981, nurse-midwives attended four percent of deliveries in New York state, most of which took place in hospitals. Six midwives—five CNMs and one lay midwife—attended homebirths in New York City. One freestanding birth center existed—the MCA Childbearing Center in Manhattan (Wolfe 1982). This was the first urban birth center in the United States, becoming a prestigious role model for independent midwifery and seen by its leaders, at its creation, as an alternative to homebirths attended by lay midwives (Judith Rooks, personal communication, 2004). It also became "an alternative to nurse-midwife-attended hospital births where strict regulation of practice and lack of family-centered care prevailed" (Katherine Carr, personal communication, 2005). The number of hospital deliveries attended by CNMs steadily increased to eight percent by 1994 (New York State Department of Health and New York State Education Department, 1997).

PRAGMATISM, IDEOLOGY, AND
EVERYDAY ACTS OF RESISTANCE

In order to be able to function as best we can in whatever system we're in, we find ourselves in the constant, and tiring, position of having to negotiate, balance, and compromise; be skilled politically and in interpersonal relations; and take put-down with a smile, coolness of response, and outward negation of pride... .

Maternity care is a political issue and our purpose [is] one of identifying recommendations, which would address the redistribution of power pertaining to maternity care. . . . Now I, like most of you, am for progress and against impotence; but I do not believe in annihilation. There must be a way. When I was a student nurse I frequently heard a great deal of pride given to an attribute, which was presented as characteristic of nurses. This attribute was ingenuity, i.e., figuring out how to create necessary items out of materials not before considered for that purpose. As we are *nurse-midwives* [italics in original] I call upon us, individually and collectively, to create the modes of practice that will take us out of our binds and conflicts without destroying ourselves in the process.

—Helen Varney Burst, Presidential address to the ACNM 23rd Annual
Meeting, 1978

Pragmatism has been of high value and is a fundamental cultural characteristic within nurse-midwifery (May 1999). The nurse-midwives in New York state had a practical vision and a long-term strategic plan that culminated in the Professional Midwifery Act of 1992. They had a "dream," as do many pragmatists, but the tactics and strategies they use to achieve their goals are influenced by the pragmatic nature of their thinking. As opposed to the idealist, the pragmatist is more likely to settle for less in the short run in order to stay "in the game."

From its inception, nurse-midwifery has occupied a position on the margins between midwifery and medicine, having to balance these two traditions. Since the 1960s, its focus has been on: (1) hospital-based midwifery; (2) education within universities; and (3) the carving out of a sustainable niche within the medical system, the culture of which is often hostile to the midwifery model of care. These early sustainable niches were often in areas where few, if any, physicians were available or willing to provide care to those women who were underserved.

Many nurse-midwives describe their practice as occupying a space along a continuum of care, with ideal midwifery care on one end and obstetrical (interventive) birth at the other. As nurse-midwives began positioning themselves in hospitals and operating along this continuum of care, survival depended on the ability to negotiate care processes filled with tension and dichotomy. Flexibility, the ability to compromise, a comfort with ambiguity, and a distrust of extreme viewpoints are key values within the nurse-midwifery profession. Such flexibility has proven so helpful that the nurse-midwife is often loath to adjust her pragmatism for idealism. From her standpoint, the ability to survive within a hostile environment depends on these cultural characteristics, which empower her to serve a far greater number of women than would otherwise be possible, as well as to bring humanistic care to disadvantaged women.

One nurse-midwife, who no longer delivers babies but instead cares for women with AIDS, calls herself "a poverty worker." This commitment to serving women comes through in the words of another New York City nurse-midwife, Ronnie Lichtman (personal communication, 2005):

> The decision to practice as a midwife in a hospital, particularly in the inner city, can be seen as both an ideological and an idealistic choice. It isn't merely that this is where we are hired, or where we have a regular salary—those issues, of course, are real. Nor is it merely because of the numbers of women who birth in hospitals—which is, of course, most American women. It is because of

the "who" we wish to serve and our desire to make the midwifery model of care available to underserved, undereducated, oppressed women—who do not have the wherewithal, for whatever reasons, to even consider a homebirth, let alone carry it out. It is to make midwifery available to these often-disenfranchised women that we choose to work in hospitals. Sometimes, the best we can do is offer a kinder approach—despite the hospital's policy of routine use of technology. We can, at the very least, provide physical and emotional support that otherwise would not necessarily be available to the woman in our care. Moving along the continuum of midwifery practice, we can frequently avoid some of the interventions that would make the woman high risk or lead her down the slippery slope to complications and cesarean birth. At the most positive end of the continuum, we can influence practice and make substantial change . . . .

[T]he discussion is not only about higher or lower skills, or whether a given salary is worth the sacrifice of the midwifery model of care. I'm trying to point out that the reasons (for some of us at least) behind the choices we make are for equally idealistic reasons—only different ones—as the reasons to become a homebirth midwife.

Lichtman's words provide us with a deeper understanding of the value placed on altruism and the care of women by nurse-midwives. These values are the context for the pragmatic nature of nurse-midwifery's survival strategies.

Scoggin (1996) documents the growing professional identity of nurse-midwives as unique and separate from both nursing and medicine. She also identifies five fundamental concepts and core values of nurse-midwifery: (1) advocacy—supporting and protecting clients, (2) normalcy of the birth process, (3) a high regard for competence, (4) authority—the ability to command respect, and (5) autonomy—the ability to practice independently within the CNM's area of expertise. As the obstetrical technocracy spirals out of control in the United States, holding true to these values while continuing to negotiate the midwifery–obstetrical continuum both strains and renders more essential the coping values of CNMs—patience, flexibility, negotiation, and comfort—with ambiguity. We find evidence of all these values in the voices of our informants.

The ingenuity—the ability to create "necessary items out of materials not before considered for that purpose"—referred to above by Varney is a form of nurse-midwifery resistance to the overwhelming presence of the technocratic model of childbirth within which nurse-midwives, against great odds, daily find themselves working. Within the unavoidable (in the hospital) constraints on the midwifery model of care, nurse-midwives look for small and subtle means of subversion to bring midwifery care to mothers and babies. This daily resistance runs as a thread in the voices of the New York nurse-midwives we interviewed during our research.

For example, one nurse-midwife who has been in practice in New York for several decades described how she used carefully worded "informed consent" (a legal and ethical responsibility of all health care professionals) as a means of subverting the actions of an aggressive on-site anesthesiologist who wanted to give as many epidurals as possible to laboring women. It became well known that when she was on the schedule, the anesthesiologist could expect to be called for fewer epidurals because she made sure that her clients understood the role that epidurals play in the cascade of events that can ultimately lead to an unnecessary cesarean. In her hands, informed consent also became a form of everyday resistance. "I didn't buck the system," she said. "I just did what clients asked me to do. If they wanted that epidural then I made sure that they understood benefits, risks and alternatives to it and I wasn't going to dissuade them in any way. But if they wanted that natural childbirth, they got it. I never went out of my way to provide epidural service to people because I viewed birth as normal." It mattered not a bit to this nurse-midwife that at Christmastime, the anesthesiologist let it be known that she was the only staff member who would not be receiving a gift from him. Laughing, she said, "The anesthesiologist was passing out the bottles of wine to the staff and he said, 'You don't get one.' And he smiled and laughed. And I said, 'Why's that?' He goes, 'Because your patients never have epidurals.'" This CNM went on to describe her impact on her labor and delivery unit: "Here's a statistic for you. . . . [when] I went out on a leave . . . he told me that the epidural rate on evenings . . . I was a permanent evening shift . . . went up by ninety-five percent while my foot was broken."

Time and again nurse-midwives describe how they employ the skills of patience, negotiation, and subtle manipulation of the technocratic obstetrical model to bring the midwifery model of care to the many women who give birth in a hospital. One nurse-midwife described her relationship with "my guy," her term for the obstetrician for whom she worked. At first their relationship was difficult for her because he "micromanaged my care. But over time he came to trust my judgment, and I now can do pretty much what I want without his interference. When I want to do something that I think he might not go along with,

I know how to handle my guy. I can call him and talk him into going along with just about whatever I think is best."

This strategy (establishing a relationship with an obstetrician who then backs off enough to allow the midwife room to practice her model of care) is repeatedly expressed by nurse-midwives as key to survival in the hospital setting. The danger they note is that the instinct of flexibility and compromise, so intrinsic to nurse-midwifery, can turn into its opposite—hesitancy and a fear of rocking the boat. Another nurse-midwife, in a late 1990s interview, described her frustration with her CNM colleagues who were unwilling to support her attempts to confront what she felt was a sexualized work environment because of their fear that it would jeopardize the arrangements that had been worked out over the years.

> It's an issue of power and control. As long as we're good little girls . . . [To be told] "Oh you just don't know how to deal with these people." What [I'm really being told is] "You're not willing to play the nurse game." Because that's what we were taught as nurses . . . play the nurse game, how to manipulate the doctors to get what we wanted. [There were] twelve OBs in the group that we worked with. . . . And I had issue probably with eight of them who would think that they could either touch you or talk to you in an inappropriate way. Like, "sweetheart, honey, dear, darlin'" . . . hug, kiss or touch me in any way inappropriate. And when I'd say to my other midwife colleagues, "I want to bring this issue up at the next staff meeting with the OBs," [none] were supportive. "We understand what you're saying. We don't like it either. But we're going to pick our battles and this is not key or important."
>
> If the way we conduct ourselves with each other is not key or important to us moving things forward, I don't know what the hell is. I don't know what else would be more important than communicating to these physicians that we were not an object that they could slap on the ass when they felt like it. . . . [But] I was told I should cut them a little slack because they're in their fifties and sixties and seventies and of a generation when that was appropriate. I don't buy that line either. A lot of [my CNM colleagues said] "Tolerate it because after all, we're not going to change them." But do you know what I found out personally? Probably all but one of these eight that I eventually had opportunity to interact with and confront on my own, I felt I had better relationships with them when I stood up to them. Most of

them understood because . . . I turned it around. I said, "It isn't appropriate for *me* to call *you* 'honey,' or 'sweetheart,' or 'dear,' or to come up and start touching you." And [when they stopped] I would comment to them, "I appreciate you respecting that I don't want you to touch me, that I don't want you to call me these certain names."

By the way, these other midwives—I was by far younger than all of them. These are midwives who are in their fifties, who have been practicing for years . . . and [it was] like, "You're a little neophyte about this but you'll learn too that this is something to tolerate." I'm not ignorant about male-female relationships. But I'm establishing myself and midwifery.

Of course, such issues and struggles are not unique to nurse-midwifery practice; they are the same issues confronting women in many other professional arenas dominated by men, and also by new professions trying to make inroads into established hierarchies. This CNM did eventually tactfully and successfully negotiate nonsexualized professional relationships with the obstetricians, yet lost her job when she encountered an issue unique to hospital-based midwifery. She participated, on her own time, in a homebirth that was entirely legal and for which she had a written medical agreement. Her participation in this birth was known by only a small number of people. Nonetheless, she was fired by her midwifery service director, a CNM. When asked if she believed that liability was at issue in the firing, she responded:

That was the fear but they didn't use that word. They used philosophy. "There is a difference in philosophy and we do not want to discuss it." There was so much damage to my self-esteem to be fired. I felt so alone. [Those midwives I felt were my colleagues—not one] talked to me for three months. Not a phone call, not a card, not one word, because they'd go down too for the association with me. . . . But they knew what kind of a midwife I was.

From the mid-1960s until the early 1990s, nurse-midwives gained their first experiences in the labor and delivery room milieu. (For many years, nurse-midwifery programs required labor and delivery experience as a prerequisite for application.) There they learned what nurses viewed as the necessary survival skills of negotiation, compromise, and flexibility—skills that can also take the form of manipulation, evasion and passive resistance. Significantly, this New York CNM entered nurse-midwifery school without labor and delivery nursing experience. The culture of pragmatism often does not come easily to those newer CNMs, who unlike their veteran colleagues, do not have the years of labor and delivery nursing once thought essential to becoming a nurse-midwife. This CNM has now found her place in a successful homebirth practice—she is one of approximately twenty CNMs who legally practice homebirth in New York State and who are consciously blurring the line between home and hospital birth midwifery.

The relationship between survival and change remains a central theme in the discourse of CNMs. Veteran nurse-midwives defend their culture in terms of surviving in order to bring about change. Their words echo throughout our interviews. In order to bring about change one has to still "be here, and being here involves shifting and survival." Future midwives need to be prepared for the "reality that they must be better than" and that reality involves having a clear view of "what one has rather than acting like you have what you don't."

NURSES OR MIDWIVES?
AN IDENTITY CRISIS WITHIN NURSE-MIDWIFERY

In keeping with its beginnings as a clinical specialty of nursing and an alternative to traditional midwifery, nurse-midwives made a point of emphasizing their distinctness from traditional midwifery. A 1987 ACNM brochure entitled *What Is a Nurse-Midwife?* stated, "For centuries, women who assist at births have been called midwives. But other than a shared tradition of caring for mothers and infants, today's certified nurse-midwives have little in common with their historical counterparts."

In contemporary nurse-midwifery we witness a growing identification with a model of independent practice unlike that of American nursing and akin to that of some European professional midwives. This identity crisis has been fueled in part by the evolution of homebirth midwifery (see chapter 1) whose practitioners held as a central philosophical tenet a radical critique of nurse-midwifery as being dominated by, identified with, and subordinated to the obstetrical profession. Central to this critique has been the viewpoint that nursing education is not only unnecessary for midwifery training, but has tied American midwifery to a highly technocratic model of childbirth. The identity crisis within nurse-midwifery has also been fueled by the growing power of the technocratic obstetrical model (bringing with it increased control over both women and midwives) along with a growing discomfort among nurse-midwives with their identity as advanced practice nurses.

Throughout the 1980s, the relationship of nurse-midwifery to the profession of nursing became a point of intense debate among CNMs, even as they began to grow in numbers and make inroads into hospital practice across the country. Arguments for separation from nursing have originated from two different standpoints, one ideological and one pragmatic: (1) nurse-midwifery's position within nursing has led the profession to turn away from the midwifery model of non-interventive birth; and (2) in the interests of autonomy and establishing itself as a recognized and identifiable profession, nurse-midwifery should separate from nursing to avoid being regulated under evolving state legislative initiatives as advanced nursing practice.

During the decade or more of debate on the professional identity of nurse-midwifery, growing numbers of women identifying with this alternative vision of midwifery entered nursing school for the sole purpose of jumping through the necessary hoops to gain admittance to nurse-midwifery school. These new nurse-midwives held little loyalty to the nursing profession and shared a common sense of purpose with direct-entry midwives. Many held (and still hold) dual loyalty to both the ACNM and MANA (see Davis-Floyd 1998a and chapter 1, this volume). And so the critique of nurse-midwifery's relationship to nursing became internal as well as external to the profession.

The influence of these internal and external debates was summed up well in 1978 by Helen Varney Burst in her President's Address to the ACNM's 23rd Annual Meeting in Phoenix, Arizona. "In many very real ways," she states, "we are beset upon from all sides, pressured simultaneously by medicine, lay midwifery, the alternative childbirth movement, and nursing" (1978:11). Burst's warnings regarding nursing did not involve rejection of nursing education as a prerequisite for midwifery, but rather expressed many nurse-midwives' fears of being subsumed organizationally and structurally by nursing. With regard to physicians, Burst noted, "On one side we have some physicians whom we threaten either economically or professionally or both. They fear our entry into private practice and attempt to restrain our practice to the indigent and/or rural underserved as well as to restrict us to always be in the role of an employee." Additionally, Burst noted, physicians feared being relegated to the role of high-risk obstetrical specialists as midwives laid claim to normal childbirth. Nurse-midwifery has always believed in "the philosophy of a team relationship" but "in self-defense will have to get competitive vis-à-vis the obstetrical profession—exactly what they don't want" (1978:11).

"Lay midwifery," Burst continued, "threatens us and in other instances scares us." While admitting that some lay midwives "are serving the consumer well," she stated that nurse-midwives are "frightened for the consumer" by those lay midwives who are "unprepared, unread, inexperienced, unsupervised. . . ." At the same time, nurse-midwives are threatened by lay midwifery "because they claim a population we thought we were serving: the consumer population. . . . We may also be jealous of the lay midwife because of her freedom from the professional restraints which sometimes frustrate us" (1978:11).

Early lay midwives and the alternative childbirth movement critiqued the merging of nursing and midwifery, asserting that this encouraged the medicalization of midwifery. They also questioned whether nursing education was necessary for training competent midwives. A growing number of nurse-midwives shared this critique. In contrast, the earlier questioning by ACNM leadership of its relationship to nursing had focused not on this radical critique but on awareness of the danger of becoming subsumed, absorbed, and controlled by nursing.

One of the earliest calls for separation of nurse-midwifery from nursing was articulated in a 1973 editorial in the *Journal of Nurse-Midwifery*, "Cut the Cord," by Dolores Fiedler, MD, a New York City physician associated with MIC (Maternal and Infant Care Project of New York City). To foster its attempt to demarcate itself from traditional midwifery, nurse-midwifery had needed the status, the image of competence, and the public respectability of nursing. But now, Fiedler argued, separation from nursing was in the interest of nurse-midwifery; her arguments were clinically and structurally based. First of all, nurse-midwifery faced limitation of its growth as only one profession among the variety of midlevel health care professions emerging at the time (which included physician assistants and nurse-practitioners in addition to nurse-anesthetists and paramedics). "The delegation of granting licensure of midwives to the nursing discipline will hamper and stagnate the profession of midwifery. . . . With the advent of the nurse-clinician, nurse obstetrician, paramedic, obstetrical technician, etc. the distinctive role and the unique potential of the midwife will become diminished, diluted, and devitalized . . ." (Fiedler 1973:3). Nurse-midwifery had outgrown its need for nursing; Fiedler notes:

Midwifery has enough status to be considered and regulated as an independent and distinct profession. . . . Simply stated the question is: Are midwives content to be an extension and expansion of the nursing role, or is it the desire of midwives to become completely unique professionals, capable of delivering services to women by a discipline of education and training exclusively developed for a new profession? (3)

Louis H. Hellman(obstetrician, Director of the Ob/GYN department at Kings County Hospital/SUNY [State University of New York] Downstate Medical Center, and leading academic and health care policy spokesperson) was a strong supporter of the developing New York City nurse-midwifery services and the expansion of their scope of practice beyond nursing. In an editorial in the *Bulletin of the American College of Nurse-Midwives* (1971) and again at a 1972 speech given to the International Confederation of Midwives, Hellman critiqued the institutional position of New York City's nurse-midwifery services, which were subject to several lines of authority. Warning that nurse-midwifery's position was untenable, he stated, "I do not believe that the organization of maternity care under a triumvirate of nurse-midwives, nurses, and obstetricians is beneficial or viable" (Hellman 1971:21). He continued, "the organizational system under which nurse-midwifery answered to several lines of authority presents too many interfaces and too much fragmentation of responsibility; academic progression is cumbersome and funding may be impossible to achieve" (78). Insisting that nurse-midwifery should establish a separate place for itself, he stated, "Nurse-midwifery could survive as part of the medical cadre, but it would never achieve its full stature, and achieving academic status for its staff might present difficulties. American nursing has been rigid and inflexible for at least a generation" (78). His proposed solution for resolving institutional conflict with nursing was to make nurse-midwifery clearly responsible for all maternity care; all maternity nurses would be nurse-midwives and all activities and academic positions having to do with maternity nurses would be filled by nurse-midwives.

In New York state, many nurse-midwives work in private medical services. But New York City has been unique because of its large, city-run maternity care program in which nurse-midwives played a major role. Throughout the next decades, the debate over their relationship to nursing persisted among New York nurse-midwives and continued to focus on the need to separate structurally from nursing (e.g., Cuddihy 1984). This discussion was primarily based in New York City; its subsequent legislative efforts culminated in the New York State Professional Midwifery Practice Act of 1992, which we address in the following sections.

THE NEW YORK PROFESSIONAL MIDWIFERY ACT OF 1992: HISTORY AND PERSONAL MOTIVATIONS

Legislative Efforts of the CNMs

In the early 1980s, New York CNMs embarked on a process of strategizing and lobbying to create state legislation legitimizing nurse-midwifery as a viable health care profession. Their legal status was ambiguous. The only statute regulating midwifery was the State Department of Health Sanitation Code, under which nurse-midwives received a permit to practice through the Department of Health. The permit required a physician signature to show "medical direction" and so was usually time-limited, tied to each individual nurse-midwife's employment. A legal midwife in New York was required to hold a nursing license and therefore came under the jurisdiction of the Board of Nursing within the Department of Education, yet as nurse-midwives they were also regulated by the Department of Health.

Throughout the 1970s and 1980s, nurse-midwives around the country, along with nurse practitioners, promoted legislation defining and regulating midwifery as advanced practice nursing. The result has been that in most states today, nurse-midwifery is defined under legislative statute as advanced practice nursing, so that nurse-midwives, nurse-anesthetists, and a wide variety of nurse-practitioners work under the jurisdiction of the State Board of Nursing, which also regulates Registered Nurses (RNs) and Licensed Practical Nurses (LPNs). In New York, at the same time that nurse-midwives were pushing the Midwifery Practice Act, nurse-practitioners were lobbying for advanced practice nursing legislation. Their legislation passed several years before the midwifery legislation also successfully passed. It gave legal recognition to advanced nursing practice, granted licensure to nurse practitioners, established regulations for their practice, and allowed them prescriptive privileges.[4] New York nurse-midwives rejected the opportunity to be included in the New York advanced nursing practice legislation, opting to write and promote their own bill. Unlike their colleagues in other states, the New York CNMs made a decision that not only did they need legislation clarifying the legal status of midwifery, they wanted to be a profession separate and distinct from nursing. Separation from nursing was *the* bottom-line issue on which they would not compromise (Redman 1997). There would be "one type of midwife; one level of midwifery" that would not require a nursing education. The intent of the promoters of this new legislation was to create an "open door" for foreign-trained and other midwives who wished to pursue a career in licensed midwifery practice without first attending nursing school (Dorothea Lang, personal communication, 2005).

By all accounts, the New York midwifery legislation, while certainly an idea whose time had come and had from its conception included the idea of separation from nursing, was the brainchild of Dorothea Lang, past president of the ACNM and longtime Director of the Maternal and Infant Care Project (MIC) of New York City from 1968 until her recent retirement. During her many years of active practice and administration, Dorothea dreamed of freeing the profession of midwifery from the constraints of nursing. Her own birth in Japan in the 1940s was attended by professional midwives, whose persistent presence at the majority of Japanese births (though they became nurse-midwives after World War II) helped to give that country one of the lowest perinatal mortality rates in the world. A return visit to Japan in 1962 and again during the 1970s further convinced Dorothea of the viability of an independent midwifery.

Another major factor motivating Dorothea's support for direct-entry midwifery was her understanding of the circuitous nature of the nursing route:

> I remember in the early days when I interviewed almost every new graduate [in New York City], I always used to ask them, "Would you have come into midwifery without nursing if there would have been a route?" And ninety percentof my applicants used to say, "Yes! . . . I would not have wasted six to eight years of my life coming before you now as my first job potential. If I had another route I would have been in midwifery four years ago, two years ago, three years ago. It was costly. It was agonizing. It took many years for me to finally be a midwife."

With Dorothea's dream in mind, a committed group of CNMs began to envision and later lobby for a bill that would establish New York midwifery as a licensed, independent profession governed by its own Board of Midwifery (as opposed to the Board of Nursing), prescriptive privileges (which are essential to autonomous practice), and the freedom as independent practitioners to practice without a written physician agreement. Registered nurse licensure and a degree in nursing would not be necessary to practice as a midwife. Embracing direct-entry midwifery became an essential, fundamental piece of their rationale that midwifery in New York state should be separate from nursing, with its own licensing mechanism and its own separate lines of authority at both the regulatory and clinical levels. "This new New York legislation was a confirmation that New York recognized midwifery as an identifiable profession. . . . This now enables midwives to help guide/control the practice of midwifery and the licensed professional midwife" (personal communication, Dorothea Lang, 2005).

When New York nurse-midwives laid claim to direct-entry midwifery, it was with a different meaning than that of the homebirth direct-entry midwives who had been practicing in New York since the early 1980s. For New York CNMs, "direct-entry" did not mean apprenticeship learning and homebirth practice. Rather, it meant escape from the institutional and structural dominance of nursing—for example, having budget lines separate from nursing in hospitals with midwifery services. Midwifery Service Directors would no longer be answerable to a Director of Nursing, and midwifery staff would no longer be claimed by the Nursing Department. Midwifery salaries and benefits would no longer have to correlate with those of advanced practice nurses. Perhaps most importantly, midwives could lay claim to clinical activities as being distinctly midwifery, which would help protect those activities from encroachment by other professionals (such as the Physician Assistants and Women's Health Nurse Practitioners who were beginning to attend labor and delivery patients in New York under the auspices of employer obstetricians). Direct-entry midwifery education was a fundamental piece of the overall rationale for institutional separation from nursing. It was as much a means to an end as it was a dream.

In 1983, the initial draft of what was to become the Professional Midwifery Act of 1992 was supported through the Legislative Committee of the New York City chapter of ACNM Region II. Funds from the legislative committee were used to hire a lobbyist. Meeting in the lobbyist's office, four nurse-midwives wrote the initial draft—Nancy Cuddihy, a nurse-midwife at the state Health Department in Albany, Sue Piening from SUNY Downstate, Beth Cooper from Rochester, and Elaine Mielcarski from Syracuse (personal communication, Elaine Mielcarski, 2004). The legislation was promoted strongly by the New York City ACNM chapter's Legislative Committee. The Midwifery Council, representing midwifery service directors in New York City, became actively involved behind the scenes after its formation in 1984. Richard Gottfried, a Democratic State Representative from Manhattan, chair of the New York State Assembly Committee on Health, and a powerful player within the Democrat-controlled New York Assembly, became the House sponsor of the Midwifery Practice Act, ultimately known as the Gottfried-Lomardi Act; once enacted, it became the Professional Midwifery Practice Act of 1992.

   Through the persistent lobbying efforts of Elaine Mielcarski, State
Senator Tarky Lombardi of Syracuse became convinced to take over
sponsorship of the midwifery legislation in the New York State Senate.
Lombardi, at the time, was a powerful Republican in the Republican
dominated state Senate serving as Chair of the Senate Committee on
Finance, Health and Public Authorities, and Chair of the Governor's
Council on Health Care Financing. His sponsorship and personal
support of the bill became instrumental in its eventual successful passage.
With two powerful sponsors combined with the massive efforts of
nurse-midwives Dorothea Lang, Pixie Ellsberry, Nancy Cuddihy, and
others, Elaine's ten-year lobbying effort, and as we shall see, the support of the direct-entry midwives who believed that they would be
legalized, resulted in legislation establishing a Board of Midwifery
within the State Education Department that would license and regulate
midwives in New York state. CNMs in upstate New York, fewer in
number and more widely dispersed geographically, were nevertheless
heavily involved in the early stages of developing and supporting the
legislation. Elaine Mielcarski was an early key proponent of the legislation and one of its primary drivers. Already certified as a nurse-practitioner, Elaine had been inspired to become a midwife by Dorothea
Lang. She felt that the training she received at the Medical University of
South Carolina with a poor, high-risk population well equipped her to
practice in New York. But on her return to New York, she faced the
realization that the midwifery statute was outdated and that the
circumstances for nurse-practitioners were changing.

> When I came back to New York state and looked at the original
> [1907] statute and the Sanitary Codes governing midwifery
> practice, I realized that it was a very old, archaic law. It said that
> we had to have "clean nails, clean aprons, clean minds" and we
> delivered babies, but there was nothing there that spoke to how
> we did it and what types of—It didn't codify our practice at all.

She went on to explain:

> Nursing became very upset when the nurse-practitioners tried
> to break away and become licensed as nurse-practitioners and
> not just under the Nurse Practice Act in New York state. . . . The
> Board of Nursing sent around a memo to the hospitals, to nurs-
> ing services, and told them that nurses could not take orders
> from nurse-practitioners anymore. And they were legally right
> in doing that because there was nothing in the statute that

allowed them to write on an order sheet and give them [nurses] orders [without a physician signature]. So therefore there was nothing legally supporting nurses who took those orders. . . .

And when they sent that memo around . . . the labor and delivery nurses were standing at the counter, where I was also standing. And they said, "We can take orders from nurse-midwives. Why can't we take orders from nurse-practitioners? Elaine, we can take orders from you, can't we?" Well, I wanted to sink right onto the floor because I knew there wasn't anything in our statute either that we could prescribe medication. . . . An anesthesiologist, who was very anti-midwife, happened to be in the utility room and overheard the conversation. He went to the administration of the hospital and told them that there were no legal grounds for my practice, that I could not write orders on the order sheet or could not give phone orders. I could not admit patients to the hospital. And he was smart enough before he did this to look up the act and he was absolutely right.

This was in 1982 when my hospital privileges were suspended by the hospital. I had been practicing since 1979 at PHP [an early HMO in the Syracuse area with its own clinics] in Baldwinsville. It was a tremendous blow to our patients. It was a tremendous blow to the center in which I practiced. Not to even mention that I had moved with three children to another state and had worked two jobs to earn the money to do that prior to becoming a student, and then took out loans at thirteen percent interest to pay for my education.

Elaine saw New York City as more insulated from this threat: since 1907 the Sanitary Code had legalized the practice of midwifery in New York City, midwives there were providing thirty-five percent of prenatal care and attending twenty-five percent of births for the Health and Hospital Corporation, so that "New York City could not just wipe out midwifery without major catastrophes." But the larger threat was that "as the competition between midwives and obstetricians became more keen, the existing law would be enforced throughout the state." Elaine called Dorothea to alert the New York City midwives:

that we had to band together to begin legislation to codify the practice of midwifery. And Dorothea asked me to come down to the next chapter meeting in New York City, which I did. And that was in December of 1982. I went down and . . . started a lobbying fund. . . . And so we hired a lobbyist through the dues that the upstate chapters of the American College of Nurse-Midwives had put together. We each went to our chapters and asked for lobbying funds.

It was entirely clear to the New York CNMs that if they had not been so committed to creating their version of direct-entry midwifery, they could have either joined the nurse-practitioners, or passed their own bill legitimizing their profession, granting them prescriptive privileges, and giving them autonomy from physicians, at least five years before they actually achieved passage of the 1992 bill. Why did they fight so hard for that five extra years to create a new kind of midwife who would then have to struggle for legislation and licensure in the other forty-nine states?

Elaine: Initially we wanted to codify the practice of *nurse*-midwifery. [The initial language of the bill] talked about the American College of *Nurse*-Midwives. I always was in favor of being totally separate from nursing and developing a profession, a professional language, and licensure in our own right as midwives.

Robbie: Why? I mean here you were trained as a nurse and a nurse-practitioner. Why would you, of all people, want to separate from nursing?

Elaine: Because midwifery is not nursing. Nor has it ever been promoted as nursing in the College. When I became a nurse-midwife, if you looked at the language in the documents from the American College of Nurse-Midwives, and you looked at the definition, it said that nurse-midwives are trained in the two disciplines of nursing and midwifery.

Robbie: Which implies that midwifery is a separate . . .

Elaine: A separate profession. And if you look in the documents that further expand and explain that, they talked about midwifery not being nursing. That we're colleagues and it's an interdisciplinary teamwork approach. . . . But that midwives do not do nursing. That's how I was educated. My knowledge of midwifery at that point purely came from the American College of Nurse-Midwives. The ACNM did not ever consider themselves to be practicing nursing.

And as nursing saw the positive legislation that midwifery was getting all over the country and the positive laws for midwifery and the number of dollars that legislators were setting aside for midwifery education . . . the feeling by nursing of being an underappreciated and demeaned profession. . . . I think that they looked at this golden egg as something that they wanted to hitch their star to. . . . I saw at the Medical University of South Carolina totally separate units. I saw the nursing division try to put more and more tentacles into nurse-midwifery.

And if Dorothea and I didn't have the brainstorm that we actually pushed until all nurse-midwives accepted it in New York state. . . . remember that we had a hard sell, not just to the legislators, but we had a hard sell to nurse-midwives, to open . . . to expand the law beyond nurse-midwifery, to expand the language in the legislation. Because nurse-midwives knew the safety of nurse-midwifery practice and they had strong feelings about the value of nurse-midwifery education.

And those feelings were good. I mean nurse-midwifery education has proven to be a good educational process to become a midwife. Not the only one, but it's proved to be a good avenue to do it. We had to convince . . . I was chapter chair for four years. Prior to that, as being legislative chair, we had to convince nurse-midwives in both of our regions—Carol Bronte and Dorothea Lang downstate and myself upstate—that you could have the same educational process that is most valued in midwifery education without becoming a nurse first.

Like Dorothea, Elaine was spurred on by the international context:

Robbie: So why is direct-entry so important that you were willing work for five extra years to achieve it?
Elaine: Because it's honest. It's honest. It's dishonest to say that...nursing is a prerequisite, is the only way of producing a competent midwife. Look at the Netherlands. Look at their outcomes.

Midwifery was never eliminated in Europe as it was in the United States and Canada; rather, European midwives professionalized, creating national organizations in every European country and incorporating their education and practices into the formal health care systems. Midwives still attend the majority of European births, as they always have. In particular, the Netherlands is widely regarded as having one of the best midwifery systems in the world (DeVries et al. 2001; DeVries 2005). The Dutch midwifery educational system has never been involved with nursing; midwives attend a four-year vocational program in midwifery. Elaine had spent time in the Netherlands studying the Dutch system, its autonomous midwives, and its excellent outcomes, and had concluded that even without nursing, the courses necessary for midwives were "all there—microbiology, anatomy, physiology, social and health care sciences."

Elaine further explained her incentive for separating from nursing:

Nurses have to take orders from midwives, not the other way around, and putting a midwife under nursing is a serious conflict of interest. I was outspoken about this when I entered the

Medical University of South Carolina [MUSC] in '78 and told the faculty that midwifery was the goose laying the golden egg and nursing was robbing the hen house. I don't know why they didn't kick me out. The reality was at that time that nursing had no way of generating income, that legislators awarded money for midwifery that entered the coffers of the colleges of nursing and that a minuscule amount if any filtered into the departments of midwifery. Midwifery faculty at MUSC had to exist with old beat-up desks, cracked linoleum floors, and offices that looked like they belonged in third-world countries. . . . Guess what the nursing administration and faculty's floor and offices looked like?! Carpeted, decorated and well supplied with textbooks etc.

Many of the faculty I had were originally missionary nuns or missionary midwives. All of them only saw the needs of women and babies. They saw infant and maternal mortality and morbidity that could be decreased . . . .[At MUSC] we had a high-risk, black teen patient population, with a high incidence of preeclampsia. Yet I came out of that program revering the beauty of holistic birth, an attitude that I already had but gained the confidence to pursue at all cost. One of the OB residents told me that the mortality rate was very high before the midwifery department was formed at MUSC. The midwives decreased those statistics significantly. They also supervised "granny" education.

Elaine's desire to separate American midwifery from nursing was tempered by reality. In order for the legislation to be passed, two major opponents had to be neutralized: the New York State Medical Association and the New York State Nurses Association (NYSNA). Both groups strongly opposed licensure of midwives without a nursing education. During last-minute negotiations, the Medical Association agreed to drop its opposition to this new direct-entry midwife in return for the requirement that all CNMs and CMs would be required to have a "written practice agreement" with an obstetrician, a family physician with obstetrical privileges, or a hospital obstetrical service, without which they could not practice legally. So in effect the CNMs traded the autonomy from physicians they had hoped to achieve for the right to incorporate direct-entry midwifery as a legal health profession in New York state. The New York State Nursing Association, while officially opposed to the new legislation, softened its opposition because the CNMs agreed to insert the wording that this new direct-entry midwife would have to obtain "nursing equivalency" in her midwifery educational process. Members of NYSNA understood that few direct-entry midwives would meet the requirement for "nursing equivalency," and therefore nursing education would remain the entrée to midwifery for the vast majority of midwives in New York. These last minute negotiations occurred without the presence of direct-entry midwives and resulted in a redrafted bill in the House that was very different from the original draft legislation (personal communication, Sharon Wells, 2005). The determination of what constitutes "nursing equivalency" comes under the jurisdiction of the Office of Comparative Education within the New York State Education Department. Its function is to compare and evaluate curricula to determine which educational programs are equivalent to those of New York state. Additionally, the Office of Comparative Education evaluates the educational credentials of professional immigrants—doctors, nurses, engineers, etc. About this term, Dorothea said:

> We got "equivalent" in there. That was our goal. We knew we didn't want the future midwives to be any less than the nurse-midwives. We wanted her to possibly be more. . . .That's a step for midwifery. Because if you get people from all walks of life coming into one profession, you get a much broader base of professional colleagues. You get the people who write well, who sing well . . . the physical therapist knows the whole pelvic muscles far better than the nurse would ever know it. And they will then take over the leadership in midwifery. And the nurses will then sit back and say, "Hey, I never thought of that." And all of us, [five] thousand midwives all come from nursing. And we only are . . . all brainwashed only in one chain of thinking. And now this new thinking is coming in. This is a threat to the midwifery community. And I say, "It's a wonderful threat. Let's have it." Because I'm sick and tired of people stuck in the mud. We have to think futuristic!

Elaine explained further:

Robbie: Why does the law read "nursing education or the equivalent?"
Elaine: Well what happened was that we had the Medical Society and New York nursing absolutely opposed to this legislation. Big numbers. Big money. We could have passed the legislation years and years and years sooner had it just been nurse-midwifery. . . . There's no question

about it. We could have passed it without a written agreement in it. That was a last-minute compromise to keep [direct-entry].

And so in the final few days of the legislation, there was a major skirmish, and roundtable discussions, and hours of hammering out with the chairs of some of the committees, and with [our] key legislative proponents, [who] absolutely agreed that there could be a professional midwife. Because I had given the curriculum of the Netherlands to them years before and the United Kingdom's curriculum. They absolutely agreed that this was a professional midwife who had a sound academic and clinical program and all the components that were necessary. You didn't need geriatrics. You didn't need all the nursing courses to be a midwife. And it wasn't the practice of nursing anyway.

Elaine drove from Syracuse to Albany almost every week for ten years to work for this legislation. Like Elaine, all of the nurse-midwives responsible for creating and giving birth to this legislation were quite aware of the role they were playing in nurse-midwifery's struggle to redefine itself, and were certain that they were leading the way for the profession. "It is in New York where midwifery in the U.S. primarily evolved," said Dorothea Lang, "and the New York vision is leading the College right now. New midwives are receiving the benefits of all the efforts of the pioneering midwives in New York" (Chapter Minutes; ACNM Region II, Chapter 1; June 22, 1998).

RELATIONSHIPS BETWEEN NURSE- AND LAY-MIDWIVES IN NEW YORK: FAILED POTENTIALS
New York City: A Positive Beginning

The involvement of the New York lay/direct-entry midwives in the New York legislation must be understood in the context of the history of their relationships with New York nurse-midwives. We will chronicle both the positive and the negative sides of this "herstory," for the purposes of our analysis of both groups as subordinated and to indicate that this mutual subordination could have resulted in productive alliances, as indeed it has in other states. The first instance we know of their interactions was a mutually supportive relationship that developed in the late 1970s between Carol Nelson, an apprentice-trained midwife from the Farm in Tennessee, who later became a leader of the development of direct-entry midwifery in the United States, and Therese Dondero, the founder of the North Central Bronx Nurse-Midwifery Service and a leader in the development of nurse-midwifery in New York. As an RN, Carol Nelson had worked labor and delivery in Illinois in the late 1960s and early 1970s.

Her disillusionment with hospital maternity care was one factor that led her in 1973 to the Farm—a mecca for midwives involved in innovative birth practices (Gaskin 1978, 2003). During this era, hundreds of women traveled to the Farm from throughout the country in order to have an out-of-hospital birth. At the Farm, despite her years of labor and delivery experience, Carol assisted in over 100 births as an apprentice before she became a primary midwife attending births on her own.

Members of the Farm, which is variously known as a "hippie commune," a "social experiment," and an "intentional community," although poor themselves by American middle-class standards, in 1977 created an affiliated nonprofit health care collective, PLENTY, to carry out relief projects in Guatemala, South Africa, and the Caribbean. Their goodwill efforts also took them to the South Bronx in New York when they learned that this poverty-stricken area suffered from a lack of accessible ambulance service, which PLENTY realized it could provide.

Sharon Wells, who later became a major player in the political drama that unfolded around the midwifery legislation, was a member of PLENTY. Although not yet a midwife, she was an EMT and was involved in the efforts to establish the ambulance service. She also provided labor support for pregnant women and volunteered at North Central Bronx in the labor and delivery unit, the ER, and the NICU. Later, as the major lobbyist for the direct-entry midwives during the efforts to pass midwifery legislation, she was to encounter nurse-midwives from the North Central Bronx that she had once considered friends and colleagues.

At one of PLENTY's numerous meetings with the New York City Health Department and various hospital department heads, Therese Dondero was present to represent North Central Bronx midwives, although the North Central Bronx midwifery service did not exist separately from labor and delivery. According to Carol, Therese "honed right in, asking me 'are you doing homebirths?' And I said, 'I wouldn't consider doing births without an adequate backup system.' And she said, 'We're it!' She really encouraged me." And so the Farm in Tennessee began referring women in the Northeast who desired out-of-hospital birth to their PLENTY affiliate in the South Bronx.

While waiting for city permission to run the ambulance service, members of the PLENTY cadre in New York, including Carol, volunteered at emergency rooms in the South Bronx. Carol said, "A couple of us were CPR instructors and we started giving CPR classes, which at that time was a pretty new thing. A lot of the doctors and nurses didn't even have it at that point. I gave classes for the doctors and nurses at North Central Bronx Hospital, and for people at Montifiore Hospital, Lincoln Hospital, along with our volunteer work in the emergency rooms." At Therese Dondero's invitation, Carol also began volunteering in labor and delivery at North Central Bronx, serving as what today we would call a doula. Carol and Therese met on a regular basis and Carol attended rounds occasionally, on invitation from Therese. What ensued was an open and supportive relationship between these two midwives who represented very different cultures and traditions, which turned into a "learning exchange" between Carol and the North Central Bronx midwives. Carol describes an example of this learning exchange:

> One night there was a lady . . . it wasn't her first baby but this baby was posterior so the labor was taking a while and it was real hard on the mother. Therese asked me, "What would you do in a situation like that?" So I told her that I would get the mother up and change positions and do some exercises, maybe pushing a bit on the baby with her hand to try to change the position, and then also some herbs to get the labor a little stronger. . . . This all seemed new to them because they didn't consider getting people out of bed once you were there and you were getting along in labor. . . . They might have her up walking the halls occasionally maybe early but changing positions so much was kind of a new concept. This was over time. . . . We did some labor coaching techniques. . . . I would do something and then the nurse-midwife would be right there doing it also, breathing with the woman.

So for a two-year period in the late 1970s, Carol Nelson attended homebirths in New York City with informal backup by the nurse-midwives at North Central Bronx and by Therese Dondero's future husband, North Central Bronx obstetrician Dr. Samuel ("Sandy") Oberlander. Carol notes that there also existed at that time a tiny network of direct-entry midwives in New York City who met together to study and discuss cases, whose meetings she attended. These home-birth midwives were "very underground." This situation ended abruptly when PLENTY was informed, off the record, that the City of New York Health Department was aware that Carol was delivering babies and that PLENTY would not receive its license to provide ambulance service as long as she continued to do so. So she left New York to continue midwifery practice on the Farm. The ambulance service became licensed to operate and did so very successfully until it was eventually absorbed by the city in 1984.

The open and mutually supportive relationship between Therese and Carol in part had to do with the 1970s, an era characterized by openness to new ideas. Physicians and nurse-midwives were not as protocol-driven as they are today, and malpractice, shared liability, and insurance issues had not yet become barriers to innovation. Although the ACNM clearly differentiated itself from MANA, as a result of the growing grassroots homebirth movement and the midwives who developed from it, Therese Dondero recognized an opportunity for collaboration that would benefit women. Sadly, Therese died at the young age of forty in 1986. Carol said:

> Therese was such a powerful person, so strong in who she was and such a strong midwife and such a big influence on midwifery in New York that I think [the legislation] probably would have come down differently had she remained alive. I know that things changed at North Central Bronx when Therese was no longer alive. She made me feel welcome. . . . She gave me her home phone number. She said, "If you have to transport somebody, if you ever have any trouble, if the residents are giving you any trouble, you call me up and let me know." So it was a safe space. It was a sacred space. And she gave me the confidence that I knew I had a good backup system, which is such a vital issue, such a key issue with out-of-hospital birth and direct-entry midwives.

The relationship between Therese and Carol had the potential to create a positive model for other relationships between nurse- and direct-entry homebirth midwives in New York state. As the following section shows, this potential was not realized in the relationships that developed between these two types of midwives during the 1980s and 1990s.

UPSTATE NEW YORK: DISPARATE IDEOLOGIES AND UNWORKABLE RELATIONSHIPS

Outside the greater New York City area, following the elimination of the traditional midwife, midwifery had little presence until the 1970s when the new homebirth midwives (some of whom were licensed in other states, and now call themselves direct-entry) began practicing. During the 1980s and early 1990s, while less than a handful of unlicensed midwives were practicing in New York City (Wolfe 1982), approximately fifty were attending births in upstate communities. Unlicensed midwives began providing homebirth services in Albany in the mid-1970s—a time when CNMs were not yet practicing there. They came from a variety of educational settings. Linda Schutt of Ithaca, having graduated from a formal, accredited school of midwifery in England, provided homebirth services without a license as her education was not recognized as legitimate in New York state. Hilary Schlinger and Anne Frye had attended independent schools of midwifery in El Paso, Texas. After leaving New York City, Sharon Wells (who holds a master's in education) attended the North Florida School of Midwifery, a three-year program approved by the Florida Department of Education, and then practiced as a licensed midwife in the state of Florida. She returned to New York and was attending homebirths on Long Island when she became involved in the legislative efforts surrounding the proposed midwifery legislation. Others were apprenticeship-trained, studying in groups led by the more experienced midwives and working with a primary midwife in an apprenticeship relationship. These unlicensed midwives took their education seriously, delivering many babies under the supervision of a primary midwife before establishing their own independent homebirth practices. The ACNM standard in nurse-midwifery schools was twenty supervised deliveries as primary attendant prior to graduation. Most of the new unlicensed homebirth midwives had many more supervised deliveries than new CNMs. For example, Linda Schutt was required to attend fifty births as primary midwife in her British midwifery education. Hilary Schlinger, in obtaining her New Mexico licensure, also delivered approximately fifty babies as primary midwife. Their education did not match the "see one, do one" stereotype used as a pejorative characterization by some nurse-midwifery leaders. Over time these homebirth midwives came to be highly regarded and relied upon by the women in their communities.

In Syracuse throughout the 1970s, unlicensed homebirth midwives served an active alternative childbirth community outside the parameters of the medical establishment. These midwives practiced in an extremely cautious manner, with potential clients carefully screened about their commitment to having a homebirth by a group of supporters known as Advocates for Choices in Childbirth, a grassroots childbirth activist organization. This underground situation changed in the early 1980s when midwives who are now nationally known (Anne Frye, Dev Kirn Khalsa and later, Hilary Schlinger) moved to Syracuse and, although unlicensed in New York, began to openly practice homebirth midwifery. Their arrival roughly coincided with that of the first nurse-midwife in Syracuse, Elaine Mielcarski. In the beginning, the presence in Syracuse of one hospital-based nurse-midwife and three unlicensed homebirth midwives offered the hope of collaboration, and so on a few occasions these homebirth midwives brought women they were concerned about to Elaine for evaluation. Elaine's initial willingness to work with them stemmed from a shared participation in an incipient national midwifery movement and a shared ethos of woman-centered care. But this potentially collaborative effort foundered. From the homebirth midwives' point of view, they were appropriately asking Elaine for advice on conditions about which another opinion would be helpful. They believed that they were referring in a responsible manner and that this reflected sound clinical judgment. But Elaine found herself "shocked" at what she perceived as their "lack of knowledge," and began to view them as "insufficiently educated" and "incompetent." Her opinions, once formed, remained frozen in time. Although the unlicensed homebirth midwives considered themselves to be experienced and well-educated, and continued to evolve as such, Elaine, no longer involved with them, did not experience this evolution. She did not believe that they should have a place in the nurse-midwifery legislation because she did not think their training was sufficient; rather, she hoped they would go on through further education to achieve the new kind of direct-entry certification she was trying to create.

By the late 1980s to early 1990s, approximately six direct-entry midwives attended homebirths in the area surrounding Syracuse and about the same number of CNMs attended hospital birth. As also happened in other upstate areas, CNMs newly employed by hospitals or physician practices encountered homebirth direct-entry midwives already in clinical practice. Differences in ideologies, styles of practice, and educational routes often generated conflict. The more pragmatic CNMs integrated themselves into the biomedical health care system and came to see homebirth midwives as uneducated, unsafe, and a threat to their public credibility. The more idealistic homebirth midwives were vocal in their criticism of nurse-midwives as being overly medical and not "real midwives." Among the homebirth midwives there also existed the feelings that come with marginalization by others—anger, bitterness, resentment. Communication and understanding between these two types of midwives, which ran smoothly in some states, became increasingly hard to achieve in New York.

Upstate New York has often been in the center of social movements of the day. The religious revivalism of the 1800s, the religious alternative community movements of which Oneida was but one example, the abolitionist movement, the women's suffrage movement, the labor movement, the antiwar movement, and the alternative childbirth movement—all have been a significant part of the history of upstate New York. (For example, the Cesarean Prevention Movement, now known as the International Cesarean Awareness Network, was founded and headquartered in Syracuse.) The unlicensed homebirth midwives in Syracuse were surrounded and protected by a strong social movement of women who desired alternatives in childbirth—a factor that may have contributed to the divisions between homebirth midwives and the first CNMs in Syracuse.

Although some of the dialogue between midwives takes place in the public arena, more takes place outside of the power relations of the dominating class, in this case biomedicine. Such dialogues exemplify what Scott (1985, 1990) calls the "hidden transcripts" of subordinates. For example, the public critique of direct-entry midwifery by nurse-midwives focuses on issues of clinical competence and consumer safety. Privately, many nurse-midwives today recognize that direct-entry midwives are safe, competent practitioners. Their fundamental private critique has to do with image—the lack of a university-based credential, which has become a powerful symbol for competence in our health care system and accepted by nurse-midwives as necessary to establish credibility in a credentialed society. A representation of these hidden transcripts looks like this:

Nurse-Midwife: "You have copped out."
Direct-Entry Midwife: "No I haven't. I've opted out."

Direct-Entry Midwife: "You have sold out."
Nurse-Midwife: "No I haven't. I'm holding out."

Actual quotations from our interviewees flesh out these differing philosophies.

> Direct-entry midwife: [Nurse-midwives] don't understand the difference in the models of care. They think they are preserving midwifery. They cry in meetings because of the care they have to give, but they don't see that they could support us to keep giving the kind of care they wish they could give. They are oppressed by an oppressive system that puts them on report for the slightest thing, so they will be more cautious next time. They have been co-opted by the oppressor.

> Nurse-midwife: Lay midwives are selling themselves, women in general, and the profession of midwifery short by accepting an education that society regards as inferior. They make all of us look bad. No obstetrician would practice without degrees! Why should women accept anything less?

When asked, "But why can't both groups coexist?" one New York nurse-midwifery leader consistently responds, "In order to be strong there must be one midwife—one type of midwife, one standard of care. Otherwise everyone is confused—the consumer, the insurance companies. The physicians knew this. That's why there is only one type of doctor." Of course she is referring to the historic contest between the *regular* physicians and the so-called *irregulars* at the turn of this century, in which the irregular physicians were regulated out of existence, interestingly enough roughly at the same time as the traditional midwife was being regulated out of existence. This historical parallel is very provocative because today there is not only one type of publicly recognized and accepted doctor, there are two—the Medical Doctor (MD) and the Doctor of Osteopathy (DO), whose historical evolutions and underlying philosophies for a while differed profoundly and are beginning to do so again, as DOs increasingly reclaim their original holistic orientation (Davis-Floyd and St. John 1998). (In addition, chiropractors and naturopaths claim the title "doctor." After decades of work, chiropractors succeeded in their legislative efforts in all fifty states, while naturopathic doctors [NDs] are legal and licensed in only seven states; their battle continues.) The DOs won acceptance and legitimacy by moving to university-based education equivalent to that of MDs, while many homebirth, direct-entry midwives held, and still hold, to their beliefs that university education entails a sellout to the medical model (as do thousands of naturopaths around the country who are also apprentice-trained). For the direct-entry midwife, opting out of hospital birth is a less pragmatic and more idealistic strategy to provide the freedom to define midwifery independently from medicine and to protect childbirth in the face of growing technocratic interference. In contrast, the pragmatic strategy of nurse-midwives for holding out a space within the medical system serves to reach greater numbers of women, particularly disadvantaged women, often in the face of intense opposition.

THE LEGISLATIVE EFFORTS OF THE DEMS
AND THE CNMS' RESPONSE

In 1987 the unlicensed homebirth midwives of upstate New York became aware of the midwifery legislation in the New York legislature initiated by New York nurse-midwives. Hilary Schlinger, an unlicensed homebirth midwife in Syracuse at the time, remembers her reaction as "Why *haven't* we been included in the discussions and formulating of the bill?" Realizing that the midwifery legislation would inevitably impact them (their homebirth practices, while not legal, had been carried out without official interference), the unlicensed homebirth midwives of upstate New York decided to act.

Their first action was to contact several of the nurse-midwives leading the legislative effort to "ask for a seat at the table." After being "rebuffed," says Hilary Schlinger, "Alice Sammon and I quickly got ourselves—I would say pushed ourselves—into the discussion [by introducing our own bill.] We did so not because we thought that our bill had a chance of succeeding but because it was the only way we could see of stopping the momentum of the Gottfried bill, of getting a voice in the negotiations . . . and not be like flies that were swatted away. We were advised that the legislature would not act if there were two competing bills, and would press both parties to work out a compromise form."

Hilary holds a bachelor's degree from Cornell University, attended a direct-entry midwifery program in Texas, became a licensed midwife in New Mexico in 1982, and by her own account, "had a thriving home-birth practice in New York from 1982 to 1996." Alice Sammon, an RN and mother of five with two of her own children born at home, undertook a two-year apprenticeship and practiced as a homebirth midwife in Warwick from the early 1980s to the late 1990s. Their idea that the unlicensed direct-entry midwives should proceed with their own legislation in order to gain licensure and certification had not been a popular one with some unlicensed, homebirth midwives who remained suspicious of any kind of professionalization effort that might limit their autonomy, but Hilary and Alice were able to convince most DEMs in New York of the need for legislative action. So the unlicensed homebirth midwives (who had by this time formed an organization, the Midwives Alliance of New York [MANY]) introduced the Saunders Bill into the New York Legislature as an alternative to the Gottfried Act. With two competing bills before them, the New York Assembly Committee on Higher Education put aside both, requiring "the two groups get together and come back with one piece of legislation." MANY believed this accomplished what they had intended—the nurse-midwifery bill was stalled and they now had a place as stakeholders at the table. From the CNMs' point of view, the DEMs were unwelcome players and spoilers.

Rather than reintroduce their own legislation or work with nursing to kill the nurse-midwives' bill (which for a while appeared to be an option), the DEMs threw their legislative support behind the nurse-midwives' bill. Alice Sammon described her hopes and motivations in so doing:

> We were called to do what we do [homebirth] not for ourselves but out of necessity. Women wanted choices and options in birth and that included homebirth. That's what we were committed to—maintaining the option of homebirth that was safe

and where we could also depend on a reliable and consistent means of transport to the hospital when needed. We wanted homebirth to be open; we wanted to be able to collaborate and be an integral part of the health care community. . . .

[It was clear to us that] the nurse-midwives would own the title of midwife unless we did something. . . . We were fighting for our right to practice, to exist, for the right of diversity of educational opportunities within midwifery, to maintain apprenticeship education. We were looking for a mechanism where those of us who were already trained under an apprenticeship model and had years of experience could be granted licensure.

A shared ethos of serving the childbearing woman is reflected in both Alice's words and those we heard previously from nurse-midwives.

"It's not that we conceded" in supporting the Gottfried-Lombardi bill, Hilary states. "In reality, we were duped."

We were promised a seat at the table. I sat in on legislative meetings (most memorable to me being one in Tarky Lombardi's office) and negotiated wording on the bill. At that meeting, we were told (by his aide) that both the consumer seat on the board and the educator seat would go to direct-entry midwives [a term that the homebirth, unlicensed midwives at the time believed referred to themselves], so that we would have a voice in the board even if we couldn't hold midwifery seats on the first board incarnation. This never occurred.

We were later told that our educations would be considered for equivalency. As you know, all were rejected outright. We even had a meeting with the Board of Regents College to discuss the feasibility of them being the agency, which would validate our "independent education," much as they do for LPNs becoming RNs. We also met with a representative from Empire State College looking for a similar way to validate our educations.

Sharon Wells was the major lobbyist for the New York direct-entry midwives' legislative process. While in Florida, she had worked on successful midwifery legislation there (see chapter 4). She moved to New York in 1990 and opened a homebirth practice on Shelter Island. Even before her arrival in New York, Sharon had become involved in the New York process through meeting Dorothea Lang at the 1989 MANA conference in New Orleans and hearing Dorothea describe her legislative work in New York, which Sharon thought was a "great idea." Sharon said, "Dorothea told me that she wanted to combine midwifery under one law and to make nurse-midwifery and direct-entry midwifery equal. At that point I said, 'Well, that would work. I'll help you do that.' We had a long dialogue about this." In Sharon's words above, we again see the confusion generated by the disparate meanings given to the term *direct-entry* by nurse- and direct-entry midwives in New York. As we saw in the Introduction and chapter 1, this designation was commonly used in Europe to distinguish midwives professionally trained in government-approved programs designed for midwives who entered midwifery training without first having nursing education. To recap, this term was adopted and adapted from the European usage by the fifty or so unlicensed homebirth midwives of New York, most of whom by the early 1990s had at least ten years or more of practice under their belts and had developed considerable professional expertise. Thus they rejected the term *lay* in favor of direct-entry, a more professional title, which they believed best reflected their point of demarcation from nurse-midwifery and their beliefs that neither university education nor nursing training should be a prerequisite for training as a midwife. Direct-entry, as the formerly lay midwives adapted it, means entry directly into diverse educational settings, including apprenticeship, and does not necessarily require a college degree; direct-entry, as the nurse-midwives were using it, means entry into a formal university-based program that does not require nursing as a prerequisite.

Schlinger emphasizes now that the stance of the unlicensed homebirth midwives was not at the time "anti-university."

> Again, the issue is not place, or that we reject higher education, but who controls the content. We saw such programs as "nurse-midwifery minus the nursing" and with no seat at the table for those of us who had long been practicing direct-entry midwifery and even designing direct-entry programs. What a different outcome could have occurred had we been given an equal voice in the process! Imagine educators from both the nurse-midwifery and direct-entry realms sitting down as equals together to design educational programs drawing from the best of both worlds! Instead, we were pushed out again and again.
>
> We did not reject university training in and of itself but as the only route into the profession. As evidenced by meetings with such institutions as Regents College and Empire State College, we were looking for ways to validate experiential learning. We were also working nationally to form NARM and MEAC (both Alice and

I were on the MANA board), with the national Department of Education, with such entities as the National College of Midwifery and the Seattle Midwifery School, etc. to find ways to validate direct-entry education. Furthermore, we believed that apprenticeship should be retained as a vital part of training, and should not be abandoned in favor of only a classroom-based model. Our call was for multiple routes of entry, not anti-university.

In contrast, the New York CNMs were determined that the new direct-entry midwife they were seeking to create would emerge from midwifery programs within credentialed institutions of higher education recognized by the New York State Education Department. While some New York midwives, both direct-entry and nurse-midwives, thought the new legislation would lead the way toward legalization of the already established direct-entry homebirth midwives (as happened in Ontario in 1993), the key nurse-midwifery players behind the legislation were clear from the beginning that it would not do so unless the homebirth DEMs undertook higher education or were able to establish "equivalent" education. The ACNM legislative leaders hoped and expected that the university-based direct-entry programs they wished to establish would provide an accelerated route to this higher education—an open door through which the formerly lay midwives could pass. Elaine Mielcarski, in particular, had pinpointed funding opportunities she hoped to use to create direct-entry programs around the state, and Dorothea Lang provided written proposals that demonstrated specific plans for creating streamlined pathways for practicing midwives to enter such programs. But like Hilary, Alice Sammon regrets that "we [direct-entry midwives] were never consulted or included in the development of the equivalency process. We had practicing midwives, educated but educated differently, and the CNM leadership felt that they could decide what we needed to do. We should have been included in the developmental process. Our input would have been valuable" (personal communication 2005).

While Elaine's early contacts with direct-entry midwives had been largely negative from her perspective, Dorothea had attended MANA conferences for many years, despairing that the ACNM would ever develop and accredit direct-entry midwifery educational programs. Once it became clear that she could achieve her dream of direct-entry professional midwifery education through ACNM after all, Dorothea used her knowledge about the educational processes of direct-entry midwives to develop specific charts and tables for making ANCM-style direct-entry education as simple and straightforward as possible for them to achieve.

By the mid-1980s, all New York state–approved nurse-midwifery programs were affiliated with a university; admission prerequisites included being an RN with upper level credit in the health and social sciences toward a baccalaureate degree. Between 1984 and 1992, advice from legislators and discussions with the Health and Education Department made it crystal clear to Dorothea and the other CNM legislative leaders that "the potential for developing a new licensure mechanism for professional midwives would be viable *only* if the new law continued to require similar or higher academic degree preparations, knowledge, and skills." Dorothea explains:

> The upstate and downstate leaders of the NYS [New York state] chapter of the ACNM strategized ways to achieve this kind of higher education for non-nurse-midwives. . . . These could culminate in the required university-affiliated midwifery education core curriculum and clinical practice requirements. Sets of these documents and graphic charts were circulated to legislators, their education and health committees, the Education and Health Departments, the Board of Regents, other key decision-making leaders in New York state, as well as to SUNY and Empire College, which specializes in adult education. (Dorothea Lang, personal communication, 2005)

The New York DEMs we interviewed report that over ten years of lobbying effort, they had spent approximately $20,000 to pay their own lobbyist and had acquired support from various legislators, but in the end they were faced with two alternatives: to support the nurse-midwives' bill, or to work with nursing to kill it. The latter option existed because they had been approached by representatives of NYSNA proposing a bargain: help NYSNA kill the Gottfreid-Lombardi Bill, thereby keeping nurse-midwifery under the jurisdiction of the Board of Nursing, and NYSNA in turn would help the DEMs pass a bill of their own. Having grown out of the alternative birth movement of the 1960s and 1970s, these homebirth midwives held a jaundiced and distrustful view of the nursing profession. They saw entering into a political "you scratch my back, I'll scratch yours" agreement with NYSNA as an ethical sellout that went against their idealism and desire for a united midwifery profession (see chapter 1). A third alternative—to withdraw from the process altogether—did not seem possible because they knew that inevitably they would be affected by any midwifery bill. Alice said, "If they got a bill passed that said 'midwifery,' and we were not identified and included in it, we would be excluded, which is exactly what happened."

So despite their status as unwelcome participants, the New York DEMs continued to support and attempted to influence the wording of the nurse-midwives' bill. As far as they understood at the time, the bill did not contain statements about "nursing equivalency" or "physician supervision" or "written practice agreements" and gave more leeway to educational diversity. During their negotiations with the CNMs, they came to believe that they would come away with a seat on the new Board of Midwifery and would have input into the creation of direct-entry educational programs. In addition, they expected that their participation in the process would result in a law providing them with a means towards licensure and recognition. They participated in what Alice called "this tremendous lobbying wheel that had been created that we were a part of. We had our whole network across the state in place lobbying for this bill for a full year [1991–1992]. Letters, phone calls, the whole thing."

Sharon Wells said,

> I practically lived in Albany that year. . . . Visiting senators. Visiting all the legislators. Taking in packets. Being available to comment on the floor. It's a never-ending process to lobby because as soon as you get through all of them, you need to go back and start over with new information. . . . If you look at the bill jacket, it had twenty sponsors from each house on it. That's all my work. All the sponsors that I went out and gathered for it. Without my help they couldn't have gotten this bill through.
>
> We fought for every word. We wrote a section that actually was intended for me, a board position, of a midwifery educator. I was led to believe from the beginning that this was a position they were writing for me, so that direct-entry midwives could be included. It was the only way to get direct-entry midwives included. So we put that into the bill as one of the board positions—the only board position that was available to us at that point.
>
> I think we had one meeting [with the nurse-midwifery leaders, and we had some major disagreements] and after that they would never sit down with us. People would not return my phone calls. They wouldn't dialogue with us.
>
> And then lobbying . . . Hilary, Alice, and I would run into them in Albany. We were working on the same bill, really, and they would have to deal with us at times, and they always said it included us. But they were rude and not nice.

Subculture and personality clashes intensified this difficulty in communication. CNM legislative leaders saw the DEM legislative leaders as "contentious, tactless, and unprofessionally dressed." DEM leaders saw the CNMs as "sneaky, closed-mouthed, and conspiratorial." The DEMs insist that their defensiveness and contentiousness arose from their growing conviction that the CNM leaders really did not want to work with them. Later they realized that their desire to reach unity of legislative intent with the nurse-midwives set them off on a kind of parallel lobbying path that left them out of any real decision making between the legislators and the nurse-midwives.

Alice Sammon's perceptions of these events are very different from those of the nurse-midwives directly involved.

Alice: ACOG [American College of Obstetrics and Gynecology] had been invited into the process for a full year and had refused to sit at a negotiating table with the direct-entry midwives and the nurse-midwives. In the meantime we met but we never agreed. There were always arguments. Always [they would tell us] we had to let X happen and "don't worry, you would be gotten in."

           So two weeks before the bill went to the floor of the Senate and the assembly . . . in a closed-door meeting that we did not find out about until after . . . it was ACOG and the certified nurse-midwives and different representatives from the state legislature and state education department. We to this day do not know exactly what went down at that meeting. But deals were made. And we were cut out. Totally cut out.

Robbie: But [a state official] told me that the Midwifery Practice Act never had anything to do with you. That he had no idea why you thought it ever had anything to do with you. That he had spent years telling you guys that it had nothing to do with you. And he wondered, "Where on earth did you get the illusion that it had something to do with you?"

Alice: Well, in his mind it never had, even though for years we were trying to get the bill written so it would clearly deal with us. Even though we had been lobbying for years, even though we . . . would be placated. We were always hearing about meetings just before they happened . . . always pushing our way in . . . always trying to have our voice represented. But never seen as key players, as anything that needed to be listened to. Because of the bill's implications, we felt we needed to have input into it. That input was never accepted. . . . And in fact the bill *does* clearly deal with us—it clearly makes us illegal and does not provide a mechanism for us to be legal. . . . So we need to be now chastised for not complying with the law. We realize *now* that from the beginning the bill was never going to be about us.

From a factual point of view, parts of the stories of the DEMs and the CNMs are irreconcilable. The DEMs involved in the legislative efforts bitterly insist to this day that "we were promised a voice in the bill," while CNMs say they were not. Hilary Schlinger sums up the DEMs' beliefs: "At every turn there was deception. [They would say] 'Of course we're working with you' when in fact they were working against us." Sharon Wells told us that she realized only after all was over that the bottom line for the New York midwives was separation from nursing and that they would, in Sharon's words, "compromise anything to accomplish that." She didn't understand at the time that her conception of direct-entry and that of the New York CNMs were so fundamentally different:

> The bill was so horrendous. It was like night and day. It went from being an autonomous practice act to being under the control of the doctors. And as far as I could see, the nurse-midwives were in no better shape. In fact, they had given up freedom to have this bill . . . their main focus was to get out from under nursing. It was an obsession. That's all they cared about. They sold us out to get out from under nursing.
>
> Donald Ross, our lobbyist, and I tried to salvage anything we possibly could in the proposed law. We went through it word by word and tried to make it so it wasn't as bad by taking a word out here, or putting a word in there. Just altering it so that it didn't come out that the doctor had complete control. That it didn't come out that it had to be signed protocols. It doesn't say signed protocols. It says written protocols.
>
> There were certain little things that I could do—the education. I thought I had preserved the education. We thought we had one board position, like I said. Then when it all got played out and the law . . . became a law . . . and we started actually going for interviews as people who wanted to be on the board, I was turned down.
>
> We had lost everything. I knew we had lost everything. We lost autonomous practice. That was number one. The nurse-midwives lost any ground that they had.
>
> After they passed the law, it was such a bad law, I was so devastated that I came to the Farm. I went to Ina May's house. It took me a week before I could even hardly talk. That's how bad a shape I was in. So Ina May put me down at the computer and had me start writing "The New York Sell Out" (Wells 1992).

That was when I wrote that, when it was right fresh from coming from that.
    To me it looks like they went from the frying pan into the fire.
I still believe that.

Few of the nurse-midwifery leaders we interviewed respond directly
to the accusations of the direct-entry midwives in this story, repeating,
"It wasn't about them. It was never about them." In other words, the
motivation behind the legislation had nothing to do with homebirth or
the direct-entry midwives providing homebirth services. From their
viewpoint, it was first and foremost about autonomy from nursing.
Secondly, they perceived the legislation as a means of guaranteeing the
competence and safety of midwives without nursing education. "It's
not about homebirth, it's about education," stated a prominent New
York City nurse-midwife. (Hilary Schlinger disagrees: "No, it's about
ownership of the word midwife!")
    The educational issue was key. Elaine Mielcarski (personal communi-
cation, 2004) stated:

> Right from the start, I gave articles to the governmental and leg-
> islative people showing the Netherlands statistics and the Neth-
> erlands curriculum full of basic sciences, health sciences, etc.
> Remember that the midwives graduating from the Netherlands
> program who chose to go on could be accepted right into the
> Ph.D. program of the University of Amsterdam. Their under-
> graduate education, which entailed many more academic weeks
> per year, times four years, probably was the equivalent of our
> master degree programs. Unfortunately for them, the lay mid-
> wives also spoke of the Netherlands outcomes and homebirth,
> then submitted a bill fashioned after ours but requiring only
> apprentice education. They were able to get a sponsor in only
> one house with no other signatures on that bill. Their effort
> failed on its own merits. It blew me away. I never conceived that
> they would not be willing to expand their education. To be fair,
> some were.

The firm belief of the nurse-midwives was that any legislation that did
not include nursing equivalency for direct-entry education would be
doomed to fail. Dorothea said, "To get out of nursing, this [nursing
equivalency] was absolutely necessary or else only nursing education
would be allowed as a prerequisite into midwifery. Some lay midwives

still do not understand all of the intricate New York state educational, licensure, and practice requirements. The Saunders Bill, or any bill, if passed would have needed similar New York state requirements in order to become legally enacted" (personal communication 2005).

Although the CNMs insist that there was no sellout, negotiations did take place prior to the passage of the legislation around what nursing equivalency would entail. According to Dorothea, these negotiations took place with the following concepts in mind:

1. If the basic academic core prerequisites and the health and social sciences for entrance into nurse-midwifery education (traditionally acquired during the academic years for a bachelors degree nursing credential) could also be acquired in a similar/equivalent academic baccalaureate-level science pathway, then the equivalent prerequisites for entering a midwifery education program could be met.
2. Once admitted into a NYS-approved university-affiliated midwifery education program, both applicant groups (the post-nurse applicant and the post-health science applicant) would be required to master the identical academic, clinical, and practical components of the midwifery education program.
3. Upon successful completion and graduation, all must pass the New York State Board of Midwifery–approved midwifery examination.
4. Any midwife who meets all prerequisites and who successfully passes this examination and pays the fee is eligible for New York state licensure to fully practice professional midwifery (CNMs and CMs).
5. As was required prior to the new legislation, all private and public midwifery education programs have to seek approval via the NYS Education Department to educate midwives for practice in New York state.

To this day, the original New York DEMs continue to wonder what would have happened if they had entered into a political alliance with the NYSNA nurses to prevent the CNMs from creating their new type of direct-entry midwife and to get a law of their own. They refused such an alliance because of their commitment to midwifery and reluctance to associate with nursing, and because they did not want to impede the CNMs' legislation; they just wanted to be included in it. At the same time, the CNMs are certain that no matter what the home-birth direct-entry midwives had tried, they would not have succeeded without incorporating university education into their training because of New York's strong and long-standing emphasis on higher education for all professions. Dorothea continues to emphasize the importance of university-based credentials—her vision included "multiple pathways giving university credit for a variety of prior education and would include extra courses in pharmacology, well-woman care—whatever would help the DEMs meet CM or CNM requirements." But Hilary Schlinger, who went on to become a CNM, stated, "What we needed was not *more* education, but a way to validate our education. From my perspective now, having become a CNM, my education at the time was more adequate than that of many CNMs I have met." She continues:

> University-based education is not the issue. The issue is who gets to define what this education looks like. A university education based on Anne Frye's *Holistic Midwifery* looks very different from one based on *Varney's Midwifery*. To us it was about direct-entry midwives being able to define midwifery education. What we saw was a model of (medicalized) direct-entry midwifery education being offered up that looked like (medicalized) nurse-midwifery minus the nursing. Again, it was a fundamental issue of who got to define the word "midwife," starting with who got to define the parameters of midwifery education. It [the proposed direct-entry education] didn't incorporate the midwifery *I* know. (Personal communication, 2005)

Anthropologically speaking, Hilary is correct: education and identity are intimately linked. The way a midwife is educated and thus socialized into midwifery does indeed have a profound effect on the kind of midwife she is likely to become (see Benoit et al. 2001). Fundamental disagreements about identity will lead to fundamental fights about education, as happened among the midwives of New York.

THE CREATION OF THE CERTIFIED MIDWIFE

The New York State Professional Midwifery Practice Act was passed in 1992, and in 1994 the New York State Education Department established a Board of Midwifery to provide regulatory governance over the profession of midwifery separate from nursing and medicine—a situation unique in the United States for nurse-midwives.[5] Thus the New York CNMs were the first to create a new classification of hospital-based midwife for whom licensure as a Registered Nurse (RN) would no longer be a requirement.

At first there was a great deal of resistance to the idea of direct-entry on the part of ACNM members who were deeply committed to both their nursing and midwifery identities and wanted to keep an unbreakable link between the two, but ultimately most New York CNMs came to support the legislation. This large-scale membership support was in many ways a direct result of strategic efforts by a strong, informal, national coalition of midwifery leaders who had been meeting and strategizing how to convince ACNM members that direct-entry midwifery should be embraced by the ACNM. The members of this informal national coalition included Dorothea Lang, Elaine Mielcarski, Helen Varney Burst (then Director of the Nurse-Midwifery Program at Yale and of the ACNM's Division of Accreditation [DOA]), Joyce Roberts (then President of ACNM), Katherine Camacho Carr (then Vice President of ACNM, elected President in 2005), Richard Jennings (then Director of Midwifery at Pennsylvania Hospital and Chapter Chair for the ACNM in Pennsylvania), and nationally known researcher and midwifery proponent Doris Haire. The articles they wrote and their informational and lobbying efforts within ACNM generated agreement among most of the membership that the time had come to open the ACNM to direct-entry education. Many CNMs began referring to the opponents of direct-entry as "the old guard" who were "stuck" in their commitment to nursing.

One of the agendas of this informal coalition of ACNM leaders was to stave off the crisis that would result if New York midwives established their own credentialing exam. If necessary, the New York CNMs were prepared to "go it alone," meaning that the New York Department of Education would create its own testing for licensure. But from the standpoint of New York's CNMs, it made much more sense for the ACNM Certification Council (ACC) to be the testing agency for all New York midwives—both nurse-midwives and the new direct-entry midwife. This would allow for the immediate licensure of nurse-midwives under the new Board of Midwifery. New York CNMs also believed that using the ACC exam would provide increased legitimacy for this new direct-entry midwife.

In the end, the ACNM, ACC, and DOA leaders endorsed the concept rather than have New York create its own licensing mechanism.[6] Joyce Roberts, then President of ACNM, worked with the DOA to carry out a Delphi Study to identify "the nursing knowledge, skills, and competencies that are essential for midwifery." The DOA reached "consensus" on these items and then developed "a mechanism for accrediting non-nurse midwifery education programs" based on criteria "developed for accreditation of basic midwifery educational programs" (Roberts 1996:1–2). The ACC subsequently adapted its national certifying exam to test both nurse- and direct-entry midwives for ACC certification, which would then qualify them for state licensure in New York as a Certified Midwife (CM). This series of events made it possible for the nurse-midwifery program at the SUNY Health Science Center at Brooklyn (informally referred to as SUNY Downstate) to expand its program to encompass direct-entry students and develop a means of teaching this identified set of skills to direct-entry students (those without a nursing degree). Over 100 potential students and others attended SUNY Downstate's first presentation of the new direct-entry program to the public. Six students were accepted into the first class, which began in 1996. Originally desiring to make the process so streamlined that the educational program would take only one year, the downstate educators, with feedback from students, realized that the learning curve was too steep, and so in 1999 expanded the program to two years and offered a Masters of Science in Midwifery degree at completion. A student with a baccalaureate degree in any field can take any of the thirteen basic science prerequisites she has not already had (which for liberal arts students may take one year), and enter the SUNY Downstate program and graduate as a midwife two years later.[7]

For years, CNM leaders debated the question of what to name this new kind of midwife. In articles calling for her creation, Helen Varney Burst had tentatively titled her a Certified Professional Midwife (CPM). Some ACNM members favored this term, while others felt that to call her a professional might imply that nurses were not professionals. The issue became moot when MANA members met in October 1994 to choose the name of their own new kind of certified direct-entry midwife. In an ironic twist of history, their meeting took place a few months before the meeting in which the ACNM was to pick its name for its own new kind of certified direct-entry midwife. Because they felt a strong need to identify themselves as professionals in order to rid themselves of the "lay" appellation, the members of MANA's Certification Task Force chose Certified Professional Midwife, CPM (see chapter 3), as the title for their new certification, leaving the ACNM with little choice but Certified Midwife (CM). At first some ACNM leaders felt deep resentment about this "preemption" of their designation, but later came to embrace the term, as "Certified Midwife" satisfied their deep desire to be midwives.[8]

EFFECTS OF THE NEW YORK
MIDWIFERY PRACTICE ACT
ON DIRECT-ENTRY HOMEBIRTH
MIDWIVES IN NEW YORK

The new law has resulted in both winners and losers in New York state. The winners, whose dream turned into reality, have been nurse-midwives, the new certified midwives (CMs), and consumers seeking a hospital birth assisted by a recognized professional midwife. The losers, whose experience turned into a nightmare, have been homebirth consumers, especially in upstate New York, and the unlicensed homebirth midwives who served them. While not legal under the previous statutes, these midwives had nevertheless practiced openly, providing homebirth services mostly in upstate communities. The new law resulted in redefinition: practicing midwifery without a license, formerly a misdemeanor, became a felony. Dorothea Lang (personal communication, 2005) reemphasizes the point that "*any* professional midwifery act would have had the same result."

The effects of this redefinition were not immediate. It took until 1994 for New York state to form the New York Board of Midwifery. The first elected chairman was Elaine Mielcarski. Licenses to practice midwifery were issued to approximately 450 nurse-midwives who had held permits to practice under the old law. Some months later, New York's practicing direct-entry midwives were invited by the Board of Midwifery to apply for licensure; approximately thirteen did so. This invitation appeared sincere: some board members hoped that at least some of the practicing DEMs would meet the criteria for state licensure, which would entail evaluation of their education and passing the ACC exam. Following ten months without a response, all applicants received a letter of denial from the board, dated December 8, 1995, with the recommendation that they "attend a registered midwifery program, to work towards a certificate of midwifery" (Linda Schutt, personal communication, 2004). The fact that the educations of Linda's direct-entry homebirth colleagues were not deemed by the New York State Office of Comparative Education to meet the standards for nursing equivalency became the basis for the state's rejection of their license applications.

Again, from the perspective of nurse-midwives, this was not intentional on the part of board members. As described above, they had hoped to create many "open doors" to the requisite higher education for the practicing homebirth midwives. But the funding they hoped to put behind this effort never came through, and to date (2005), thirteen years after passage of the New York law, the SUNY Downstate program is still (effectively) the only one of its kind in the nation—an

ACNM/DOA-accredited midwifery educational program in which students can become an ACC-credentialed midwife without also obtaining a nursing degree.

Hilary Schlinger expresses a common feeling among New York's DEMs: "I believe, but have no proof, that the information given in our original applications was then used in prosecuting us—perhaps passed on to investigators within the department. I do know that cease-and-desist orders quickly followed." On December 13, 1995, five days after receiving her letter of rejection from the Board of Midwifery, DEM Roberta Devers-Scott of Syracuse was arrested in her home, taken away in handcuffs, and charged with the felony of practicing midwifery without a license. Within days, ten or so homebirth midwives received cease-and-desist orders from the state of New York. (Hilary received her cease-and-desist order in January 1996.) Three were arrested and/or prosecuted, and some homebirth clients were investigated and harassed. These actions were carried out by the Office of Professional Discipline, the enforcement office within the Office of the Professions of the State Education Department. Members of the Board of Midwifery denied that they had anything to do with these events, and nurse-midwives central to the statutory process insisted that the inclusion of a felony count was not initially part of the wording of the bill. It was placed into the bill at the end by legislative staff because in New York, it is a felony to practice *any* profession without a license. (It is important to remember that nurse-midwifery in New York was not a licensed profession until the passage of this bill. Nurse-midwives were licensed only as nurses. As midwives, they received a "permit" to practice under the 1907 Sanitation Code.) Several nurse-midwifery leaders stated, "We didn't know that was going to happen. We just didn't know." Pat Burkhart, director of the nurse-midwifery educational program at New York University, who became a member of the New York Midwifery Board, expressed their feelings:

> We nurse-midwives in New York state who were working desperately to obtain passage of the bill were focused on fighting off the state medical and nursing societies and did not stop to consider the ultimate consequences of legalizing ACNM-certified direct-entry midwives. Once the law passed and was being implemented, most of us were shocked to realize that the practice of unlicensed midwifery had been transformed into a felony. When the members of the new Board of Midwifery became aware that the state attorney's office had begun prosecuting unlicensed midwives, we were appalled and we did not understand

why they were doing so. We were told that complaints from consumers were what led to the prosecutions, but our further investigations did not completely verify that statement. We talked
with the state attorney's office, asking them to back off and
insisting that unless there was clear indication of a need to investigate a particular midwife, there was no reason to enforce a law
just to enforce a law.

Nevertheless, the history of negative political interactions with
nurse-midwives ensured that the New York DEMs would be quick to
assume that the criminalization of their practices was intentional
on the part of the CNMs who had promoted the bill. They met the
denials of intent with skepticism, and accusations were made that
a "witch hunt" was underway. Their sense of injustice, and that
of their consumer supporters, were expressed in various public demonstrations in favor of the homebirth midwives who had been
harassed.

Justified or not, the feelings of betrayal, anger, and grief on the part of
New York direct-entry midwives have been and remain profound.
Sharon Wells went for an interview to try to achieve a place on the
board but was turned down. She received a cease-and-desist order from
the state telling her to stop practicing, but after an expensive legal battle
was never actually charged. Disillusioned and emotionally wounded,
Sharon moved back to the Farm in Tennessee, where she continued to
work with the North American Registry of Midwives to develop its
own national certification for direct-entry midwives, the CPM (see
chapter 3). Roberta Devers-Scott eventually plea-bargained her case and
moved to Vermont, where she became licensed and opened a homebirth
practice. Defeated and newly terrified of arrest and prosecution, most
homebirth direct-entry midwives also left the state, moving to New
Hampshire or Vermont, where they can practice legally. Alice Sammon
moved to Maine, where she continues to work as a homebirth midwife
and as adjunct faculty at Birthwise Midwifery School in Maine (a
MEAC-accredited program). Hilary Schlinger moved to Albuquerque,
set up a homebirth practice, and proceeded to work toward meeting the
legislative requirements for New York licensure. She did finally gain
licensure as a CNM after receiving an RN degree through New York
state's distance learning program, the Regents College. Moving back to
New York to open a homebirth practice, she was unable to obtain the
requisite written physician agreement and has recently returned to
Albuquerque. The few unlicensed direct-entry homebirth midwives
who remain have to practice as invisibly as possible. The end result has

been to make access to homebirth very difficult in upstate communities where few CNMs or CMs provide homebirths.

The small number of CNMs and CMs licensed under the new law in New York who offer homebirth services find themselves traveling longer distances to serve consumer demand for homebirth and/or suffering from a lack of physician backup. These legal homebirth midwives also find themselves overcome by illegitimate complaints from hospitals, doctors, and labor and delivery room nurses who do not understand homebirth. The Disciplinary Committee within the Department of Health takes up these complaints and has been particularly aggressive in pursing complaints against homebirth midwives, legal and illegal, creating financial as well as emotional distress for these few legal homebirth midwives. As a result, there has been a further marginalization of, and lack of access to, homebirth in communities previously served by unlicensed direct-entry midwives.

Alice Sammon's and Sharon Well's New York "nightmare" did not diminish their commitment to homebirth midwifery. Asked how she felt about devoting ten years of hard work to the New York legislative process, Alice responded with a resigned smile, "some good had come out of it after all." She and Sharon both noted that had they been included in any way in the New York legislation, they would have thrown all of their prodigious energy into working together with the CNMs for the future of midwifery in New York. Rejected and excluded, they turned their attention to the national level and were instrumental in realizing the wider dream of generating a national certification designed to support and preserve the apprenticeship training and the midwifery model of care they value so highly (see chapter 3). In 1995, both Alice and Sharon became CPMs. Their critical involvement in this national process—a direct result of being "shut out" in New York—is yet another example of how formative the events in New York have been for American midwifery as a whole.

Like the massive ripples created by dropping a large boulder into a small pond, what happened in New York has affected legislative efforts in other states and has had a hugely negative impact nationwide on relationships between CNMs and homebirth direct-entry midwives.[9] Local nurse-midwifery leaders in a few states have attempted to introduce legislation similar to New York that would establish the Certified Midwife as the only legal direct-entry midwifery credential, and have attempted to block legislative efforts to legalize CPMs. Perhaps most sadly, because of the suspicion engendered by events in New York, even when local ACNM leadership proffers no opposition to direct-entry licensure, DEMs in various states have assumed that such opposition exists. Their distrust has led them to reject real opportunities to work with nurse-midwives on various types of legislation, engendering the same lack of trust on the other side. For the most part, this lack of trust comes from DEMs' felt sense that even if they collaborate with CNMs on legislation, the CNMs could "sell them out" at the last minute by making agreements with physicians that the legislation will not include them after all. DEMs think this is what happened in New York—that the nurse-midwives sold them out to the doctors at the end. In contrast, the nurse-midwives think they did no such thing; they insist that their last-minute agreement with the doctors to accept written practice agreements had nothing to do with the unlicensed homebirth midwives of New York: "It was never about them." But perception is powerful, and the perception among DEMs around the country of a "New York sellout" has been a major impediment to establishing trust between these groups.

After both the positive and negative effects of the passage of the New York Midwifery Practice Act of 1992 became clear, many New York CNMs came to deeply regret its results for the practicing DEMs, and to wish for means for them to achieve licensure in New York. Linda Schutt, the British-trained midwife who practiced (illegally) for years as an independent, unlicensed, homebirth midwife in upstate New York, was one of the original thirteen unlicensed homebirth midwives to apply for licensure (her application was initially denied). Her direct-entry training in England met the New York educational standard for midwifery education, but she had to meet the nursing equivalency requirement by taking courses at SUNY's Regents College. Eventually allowed to sit for the ACC exam, which she passed, she became the first midwife to obtain CM certification in New York state (and thus in the nation). Her example made it clear that the New York midwifery legislation can work for foreign-trained midwives, who previously would have had to complete an American nurse-midwifery program in order to be licensed. Linda Schutt is now (2005) the chair of the New York Board of Midwifery—a fact that New York nurse-midwives point to with pride and view as proof that the legislation is ultimately leading to the end result they intended.

Julia Lange-Kessler, a longtime homebirth midwife practicing in Orange County, New York, who became a CPM in 1995, did walk through ACNM's open door. Receiving twenty-two hours of credit for her CPM certification from SUNY Downstate and taking basic science courses, she entered SUNY Downstate's direct-entry program, graduated, and is now both a CPM and a licensed CM providing hospital birth services in her community.

When we asked other New York direct-entry homebirth midwives why they did not, like Julia, choose to walk through ACNM's open door by becoming CMs, they were passionate in their responses, emphasizing the "offensiveness" of the compromises that would be entailed. For example, Alice Sammon, already an RN with a college degree who probably would have had easy ingress into the new direct-entry (CM) program, exclaimed:

> It's because direct-entry midwives were not included in the creation of that program. That is a *nurse*-midwifery program that they are *saying* is a direct-entry midwifery program. You want to be a midwife, and you don't want to be a nurse, and you start out with these high ideals, and then you comply and compromise in your educational program, saying, "Oh, I'll just go through these hoops because then, when I get out, I can work the way I want to and I can make it change. Then because you have to pay back loans, or you need a steady salary, you take a job. Now you're dependent on that job. Your vision of working for women and changing the system fades as you do what you have to do to keep your job.
>
> The job situation for CNMs in New York has been very challenging. I have listened to them over and over again complain about how they cannot do midwifery care. They are required to provide a medical model of prenatal and birthing services. The more you are criticized or your position is jeopardized, the more you attempt to conform, do it right, achieve higher educational standards, because now we will be accepted and now we will be able to give midwifery care. Well, acceptance has come at the price of compromising the model of care. Increasingly CNM services and birth centers have been closed. The compromises are not providing a diversity of services.
>
> I think that we hold truths that keep a balance. There needs to be a mechanism for me, and women like me, to be legal. Creating a program based on ACNM standards, and telling me I have to go through that, is not providing a mechanism for me to be licensed, acknowledging who I am and the skills I hold, and the whole system that we have created that is equally as valid. I could see them for political reasons deciding they have to survive but to ignore the truth makes them part of the same thing that they think they're fighting against.

Another original direct-entry homebirth midwife still questions the right of the CNM legislative proponents to define direct-entry midwifery, noting that women are taken care of in the neighboring states of New Hampshire and Vermont by state-licensed homebirth DEMs who are competent practitioners but whose training is not recognized in New York. And Hilary Schlinger noted sadly that

> whereas once central New York was a hotbed of birth activism, the place where the Cesarean Prevention Movement arose, where there were vital consumer organizations like Syracuse's Advocates for Choices in Childbirth, where we had an ongoing midwifery study group for more than a decade, where midwives from diverse communities (I mean diverse—Mennonite, Native American, Lesbian, Fundamentalist Christian, among others) unitd to work on a common cause, there is now a void—no consumer groups, no homebirth midwives, seemingly little demand for homebirth. If the intent of the nurse-midwives, in laying claim to the title of "midwife," had been to destroy any vestige of the fact that other midwives had ever existed, then they succeeded. (Personal communication, 2005)

ANALYSIS: PLACE OF BIRTH AS A STRUCTURAL FACTOR

While education and identity are core issues in this New York midwifery struggle, place of birth is the underlying determinant of the differences in approach to these issues. Nationwide, ninety-seven percent of CNMs attend births only in hospitals, while ninety-seven percent of DEMs attend only births at home. The ACNM states that standards of care are the same regardless of place of birth. But the place of birth inevitably affects the nature of the birth experience for both mother and midwife. In hospitals the childbirth milieu reflects the competing care models of midwifery and obstetrics, and everyday decision-making by nurse-midwives involves negotiation and compromise between these models. Homebirth midwives do not wish to make such compromises: they tend to see their integrity as midwives as part and parcel of their autonomous homebirth practice under a holistic model of birth that honors the woman's individual rhythms, not hospital protocols and routines. (Freestanding birth centers, in which both CNMs and CPMs attend births, account for fewer births than at home. Many are forced to close because of malpractice costs and reimbursement problems.)

The educational traditions of each group reflect this division in place of birth. The intimate and complex nature of apprenticeship training is particularly fitting for a focused, specialized training in homebirths, which are intimate, complex, and unique. University training, combined with clinical experience in a hospital and community-based public health setting, is more appropriate to the exigencies of hospital practice and to the full-scope primary care for women of all ages that CNMs now provide.

Throughout the process of working for the Midwifery Practice Act, the call by New York nurse-midwives for "one type of midwife, one standard of care" became a mantra encoding the political and philosophical rationale for the development of direct-entry midwifery by nurse-midwives. Many CNMs see the knowledge base of nurse-midwifery and hospital care as more complex and superior to that of homebirth midwifery, insisting that if a midwife is experienced as a hospital midwife, she is capable of doing homebirths, and that midwives must first become proficient at attending births in hospital. (The reality is that New York midwifery students in ACNM/DOA-accredited university programs who desire exposure to homebirth are rarely able to achieve it because these programs are not allowed by malpractice carriers to incorporate homebirth.) In contrast, DEMs see homebirth as primary:

> The direct-entry view of midwifery education holds that we first learn birth from women, from observing un-interfered-with normal birth that can best be seen at home. All other knowledge builds from this base. It holds that the physical realm emphasized by institutionalized, medical-model practice and education leaves out the many other dimensions of the birthing process. It holds that midwives cannot truly understand birth by learning in a system that provides fragmented care. It holds that the emphasis on classroom learning often occurs at the expense of actual experience, that it is experience with birth that dissipates fear of birth. It holds that fear of birth motivates interference, while knowledge of, and respect for, the process make such high rates of intervention unconscionable. (Hilary Schlinger, personal communication, 2005)

Alice Sammon expands upon Hilary's point, again illustrating the primacy of place of birth:

> Rather than the emphasis on learning care of the women as a totality and as a whole unit, the education is fragmented. You're taught to give fragmented care, and you're not taught to see the

person as a whole system. They're seen in pieces. And your education supports that because you're taught in pieces. A true apprenticeship program . . . you learn as the situation comes up to you. So if you, in a clinical setting, are confronted with postpartum hemorrhage, or shoulder dystocia, or whatever, then you build your didactic learning for that week or month . . . on what you've just seen.

The approach is backwards in an institutionalized educational system. It's Thursday, so on Thursday we are studying pre-eclampsia. Well it doesn't matter that yesterday you just saw a postpartum hemorrhage. This is Thursday and you're studying pre-eclampsia. Or this semester we're doing microbiology . . . you know . . . or whatever else.

Rather than expanding, this kind of education funnels midwives' thought processes. It creates a mentality that's dependent on a system to provide you answers rather than building inherent knowledge and an intuition base so that the midwife learns to trust that whatever she needs at that time is available to her. You're taught to depend on only what you can see in books . . . only what you can call down to the doctor for . . . I'm a firm believer that there needs to be very strong didactic education. But this other component is missing in institutionalized education. And I think that is the heart and soul of midwifery.

The lack of concern regarding the impact of the New York legislation on access to homebirth service and independent practice throughout the state has been justified by the idea, stated by several nurse-midwifery leaders, that "first we must be strong in the hospital, then we can push outwards to include homebirth"—a strategy often heard from those same midwives who call for "one type of midwife, one standard of care." Implicit in this strategy is the notion that the homebirth DEM is less than the nurse-midwife, more on a par with the traditional birth attendant—someone who needs to be "brought up" to the level of the ACC-certified midwife.

New York's original DEMs argue that this viewpoint belies the reality of diversity within American midwifery in both place of birth and educational tradition, and reflects a hierarchical philosophy of knowledge. Many DEMs around the country believe that homebirth constitutes a fundamentally different kind of midwifery with a distinct if overlapping knowledge base. Homebirth may appear simple to the uninitiated because of its standard of avoiding unnecessary intervention. Yet the pieces that make up a successful homebirth are as complex as those comprising a hospital birth. The homebirth midwife dances a fine tango with the birthing mother and family. The ability to refrain from inserting oneself into the birthing situation while at the same time keeping the ability to observe, draw conclusions, and carry out a safe birth are skills not easily honed in the hospital. Also, the hospital-based midwife easily becomes accustomed to the support of nursing staff, on-call physicians, etc. Homebirth midwives become used to independence and the reality that the buck stops with them. They must be able to manage the entire range of prenatal care, labor and delivery, postpartum care, observation of the neonate, education on breastfeeding, and support for the family in the home during the first few days and weeks after birth. Additionally, as they are almost always self-employed practitioners, they develop an entrepreneurial spirit and the skills necessary for managing a small health-care practice.

In spite of these differences, a growing trend within the grassroots of midwifery recognizes that home and hospital midwifery, nurse- and direct-entry midwifery, share a knowledge base and skills even as each holds unique characteristics. This trend is reflected in the growing respect among many nurse-midwives for the knowledge base of the CPM as evaluated and validated by NARM. One result is that in New York, some CNM leaders are now working to create streamlined routes for CPMs who hold baccalaureates and graduate from MEAC-accredited programs to become CMs in New York, despite their lack of hospital experience (Mary Ann Shah, personal communication, 2004). Already, several midwives who graduated from MEAC-accredited direct-entry midwifery programs in other states (including the Seattle Midwifery School and the National College of Midwifery) have had their education deemed to meet nurse-midwifery equivalency, have taken and passed the ACC exam, and have been licensed in New York.[10]

In December 2003, NARM presented its certification process and exam to the New York Board of Midwifery and the New York State Education department, which had long stated that it would consider the NARM exam as a possible route to licensure for midwives in New York state. The committee that reviewed the exam found it "to have matured and improved significantly over the years," but "still lacking in well-woman and primary care as well as pharmacology, all necessary for the NYS scope of practice" (Linda Schutt, personal communication, 2005). Having committed itself to the ACC (ACNM) exam, New York state is loath to incorporate a second exam into its licensure process.

Sharon Wells describes an irony in this story that cannot be lost. The numbers of CPMs nationwide have far outpaced the numbers of CMs over the past ten years.

The CM and the CPM were created basically at the same time. Now there are about fifty CMs and over 1,000 CPMs. As of September 2005, the CPM process is used as part of the regulatory process in twenty-one states. The number of CMs is quite small compared to this growing number of CPMs. In fact, I do not see how an institution of higher education can continue to support a degree that produces so few graduates. On the other hand, the CPM is steadily increasing and now with the recently published Johnson-Daviss [2005] journal article documenting homebirth outcomes, out-of-hospital birth with a CPM has been shown to be a safe option. (Sharon Wells, personal communication, 2005)

THE SITUATION IN NEW YORK TODAY

The health care system in New York City continues to hold national significance. In the 2002–2003 academic year, 14.8 percent of our nation's medical residents and 14.3 percent of the obstetrical residents nationwide were trained in New York state, the majority within the New York City hospital system, even though New York state represents only six percent of the population nationwide. This large concentration of medical residents is a major source of health-care dollars from the federal government, which helps keep the New York City hospital system afloat (Physician Workforce Studies Unit, Center for Health Workforce Studies, SUNY Albany, personal communication, 2004).

New York City in particular depends on medical residents to provide care to the underserved. There is a financial incentive for the hospitals to have as many residents as possible; for example, in downstate New York, hospitals are given a $150,000 premium for each obstetrical resident. This situation is complicated by recent changes in state regulations limiting the number of hours a resident may work. The midwifery services within the city's hospital system, some at large teaching hospitals, have been players in health-care politics and compete toe to toe with obstetrical residents for space, money, and clients, as well as with nursing for funding. "Where once there were no residents, now residents compete with midwives for the deliveries. Throughout the system in New York City midwives are asked to work longer hours, for less pay and with less support," stated a nurse-midwife who works at a long-established midwifery service.

Over 1,000 CNMs/CMs (in 2005) hold a New York state midwifery license. Foreign-trained and other midwives can apply for licensure and furnish their academic credentials to the New York State Education Department Office of Comparable Education to be screened for equivalency.

Despite a growing trend among nurse-midwives toward employment with physician groups, in 1997, thirty-two percent of New York state licensed midwives (all of whom are CNMs or CMs) were employed by hospitals. Nineteen percent reported working in a midwifery group practice, and three percent in a freestanding birth center (New York State Department of Health and the New York State Education Department 1997).[11] Throughout the state, the number of births attended by midwives has grown at a steady pace, from seven percent in 1998 to 10.66 percent in 2002 (National Center of Health Statistics 1999). But in New York City, midwifery births have declined. In 1997 nurse-midwives accounted for 12.2 percent of Big Apple births, falling to 9.7 percent in 2002 (Perez-Pena 2004). Causes for this decline include: the closing of long-standing midwifery services, reimbursement issues, changes in birth certificate information (e.g., physician signing birth certificates for midwife deliveries), hospital reorganizations, a growing liability insurance crisis involving all childbirth professionals, the competition between midwives and OB residents over normal deliveries, and high transfer rates out of midwifery services due to restrictive protocols. These collectively constitute a threat to midwives' share of normal deliveries. Recent economic pressures on city-owned hospitals and the Health and Hospital Corporation of New York (previously the Department of Hospitals) have placed some midwifery services at risk.

The Elizabeth Seton Childbearing Center, a freestanding birthing center associated with St. Vincent Catholic Medical Center (previously known as the Maternity Center Association Childbearing Center) has shut down. This leaves only two freestanding birth centers operating in New York City—Morris Heights Childbearing Center in the Bronx and the Brooklyn Birth Center. In nearby New Jersey, the only three independent birthing centers run by midwives have also closed. In all cases, drastic rises in malpractice insurance have been cited as the reason for the closings. The popular September Hill Birth Center near Ithaca, New York, also closed, leaving upstate New York without a freestanding birth center. Midwife Lonnie Morris, who attended more than 7,000 births in twenty years, shut Englewood New Jersey Birth Center after her malpractice rates jumped from $30,000 to $300,000 a year. She simply stated, "I couldn't pay my bills" (personal communication, 2004). The Columbia/Presbyterian Midwifery team at the Allen Pavilion Hospital, considered a mainstay of New York City midwifery services along with North Central Bronx, has become greatly restricted in its labor and delivery service, presently doing very few births. This development has been a sore point for New York City midwives, as the midwifery service at Columbia/Presbyterian Hospital in New York City was the first New York hospital to permit a nurse-midwifery delivery (in 1955 on an experimental basis).

As elsewhere, rising professional liability insurance rates, low payment rates, and the difficulty of being included in managed care panels have become major obstacles in carrying out the dream of an independent midwifery in New York state. When Medical Liability Mutual Insurance Company (MLMIC), the primary insurance carrier for obstetricians and nurse-midwives in New York, was denied a sixty-one percent policy rate increase and was offered only a ten percent increase for Licensed Midwives by the New York Insurance Department, MLMIC informed New York Licensed Midwives that new applications for coverage would be denied and that existing policies would not be renewed. MLMIC will continue to provide policies to hospitals that employ midwives, but not to private physicians who employ midwives (personal communication from New York Friends of Midwives 2004). TIG Insurance Company, underwriter for ACNM's malpractice insurance, announced that it would no longer accept new applications and would not renew policies after June 30, 2003 (letter from Kathleen McMahon CNM to Gregory Serio, New York State Insurance Department). The new malpractice carrier for ACNM, Contemporary Insurance Services, is placing high prices on individual midwives, with yearly policies starting at $16,000 and annually rising incrementally to $25,000 in the fourth year.

In New York state the trend toward group practice and shared liability is particularly strong. The parameters of clinical decision-making and practice guidelines have become the purview of the physician group, as opposed to the individual clinician. As a result, the rise in group practice has made the tradition-bound profession of medicine all the more conservative. Solo practitioners, particularly those with untraditional, innovative practices (the very practitioners most likely to support homebirth) are increasingly the targets of state investigations in New York.

The statutory requirement of a written practice agreement with a physician (the compromise made by nurse-midwives with the New York Medical Association in order to achieve the right to create licensed direct-entry midwifery in New York) presents a powerful barrier to independent practice, including homebirth, by licensed midwives in New York, as well as in other states. (Unlicensed direct-entry homebirth midwives practiced without formal practice agreements in New York, although most had informal arrangements with physicians.) Few physicians are willing to enter into formal practice agreements involving homebirths or independent midwifery practice, and even those few who are privately supportive find themselves hindered by the realities of professional politics and economics, including ACOG's anti-home-birth stance, which makes professional marginalization a likely end for any physician who enters into a practice agreement with a midwife who practices independently and/or delivers in the home—legal or illegal. Family practice physicians who practice obstetrics risk losing referral arrangements with obstetricians if they enter into such arrangements. Thus, although many New York CNMs have expressed to us that they would prefer to practice independently and attend births at home, by 2005 only about twenty licensed midwives (out of 1000+) have been able to obtain the requisite agreements with physicians.

Just as New York midwives find it difficult to attend homebirths, so women who wish to birth at home find it difficult to find a midwife since passage of the midwifery legislation. Carolyn Keefe, a childbirth activist representing New York Friends of Midwives (NYFOM), reports that "consumers and midwives who move into most of New York state are pretty stunned at how hard it can be to find homebirth services and at the ways the law impedes access to those services" (personal communication, 2004). Keefe goes on to state:

> Midwifery in New York state remains at the mercy of the medical profession. In most cases, it is the doctor who decides the midwife's scope of practice. Midwives are dependent on the individual doctor's recognition of midwifery's value—whether medical, philosophical, or economic. . . . As long as the written practice agreement is in place that will continue to be the case. It makes midwives reluctant to challenge the obstetrical community and organization.
>
> It's also important to note that a concentrated effort by medical and obstetric organizations to eliminate midwifery in New York state would be frighteningly easy. By putting pressure on physicians and hospitals, most, if not all, of the written practice agreements could easily be pulled and access to midwifery in New York state all but eliminated. This state regulated midwives nearly out of existence once and could do so all too easily again, this time using liability insurance as an excuse. That's one of my fears as a consumer advocate, and I fear that the lack of consciousness about this risk allows midwives to remain divided.

Nurse-midwives nationwide share the barriers to practice described above. However, in New York it is significant that the unique legislation granting the profession its own board and its own professional oversight has not served to insulate nurse-midwives from these barriers. The legislation has not provided any special protection or power, nor has it improved the ability of New York licensed midwives to establish independent practices. Additionally, the large midwifery services within the New York City hospital system, long a source of great pride for New York midwives, have become particularly vulnerable to the systemic shake-up occurring at this time within the American health care system. New York licensed midwives have organized a statewide association to begin to take on these barriers to practice and to initiate reform initiatives—the New York State Association of Licensed Midwives (NYSALM) (www.nysalm.org).

CONCLUSION: "WE'RE ALL *MIDWIVES* NOW"

Nurse-midwifery as we know it today, particularly in New York state, has its roots in the intersection of significant historical trends that culminated in the shift from home to hospital birth and the elimination of the traditional midwife. As we have seen, the profession grounded its beginning in the rise of the modern health care system and has developed a professional culture characterized by pragmatism, flexibility, and resilience, all of which have allowed it to survive within a medical model of care often at odds with the midwifery model. Our analysis of this culture has been informed by James Scott's (1985, 1990) analysis of "everyday acts of resistance" by subordinated classes against powerful dominating forces. It is both too easy and inaccurate to view the seeming acquiescence and daily conformity of the CNM to obstetrical domination of childbirth as representing "false consciousness" (identification with one's dominator). The goal of the profession nationwide is to practice midwifery to the greatest extent possible under obstetrical and nursing regulatory authority. Symbolic conformity to some obstetrical norms, what Scott (1985) would call a "mask of compliance," often shapes a strategy for resistance. Core values of the profession—avoidance of open confrontation, patience, flexibility, and negotiation—characterize this mask of compliance with its everyday acts of resistance. Although the New York CNMs did not gain everything they had hoped for with the passage of their legislation, it can be understood from their standpoint as a pragmatic series of giant steps toward survival and a still-hoped-for clinical independence from obstetrics.

The legislative success of New York state CNMs in achieving their goals through pragmatism, strategy, and negotiation, along with the failure of the homebirth direct-entry midwives to be included in the law, is the essence of the story we have told in this chapter. In temporal terms, this discussion is moot: ACNM-certified midwives (CNMs and CMs) are solidly established in New York state and other kinds of midwives are not. The licensed midwives practicing in New York are now regulated by their own Board of Midwifery and they have created a new kind of culture around their inclusion of the CM, dropping the term nurse-midwife in most circumstances and insisting that in New York, "we're all *midwives* now." The gains that have been made, the uniqueness of the midwifery services within the city's hospital system, and the numerous women in many walks of life that are served by the city's midwives, constitute a source of deep pride among nurse-midwives.

New York's direct-entry homebirth midwives, proud of their entrepreneurial spirit and independence from the obstetrical profession, turned their defeat in New York and their idealism, now tempered by a hard-learned pragmatism, into a new national certification. The giant steps they have recently taken toward achieving legitimacy while remaining autonomous are described in chapter 3.

TIMELINE OF EVENTS IN NEW YORK MIDWIFERY

1906   New York City midwives are studied by the Public Health Commission of the Association of Neighborhood Workers. Its report paints a negative picture of New York City's traditional midwives.

1907   New York state changes the state Sanitation Code to establish regulations for midwives under the State Health Department. New York City midwives are regulated and given permits to practice by the City's Health Department.

1912   The concept of nurse-midwifery is publicly articulated for the first time by Clara Noyes, a New York nurse educator, at the International Congress of Hygiene and Demography.

1914   Dr. Fred Taussig, at the annual meeting of the National Organization of Public Health Nurses, endorses the concept of establishing schools of midwifery limited to "graduate nurses."

1917   The Women's City Club of New York City establishes the Maternity Center Project, providing prenatal care to 2,400 women in its first year of operation.

1918   The Maternity Center Association is established, its goal to set up neighborhood clinics bringing "every pregnant mother . . . under medical and nursing supervision." In 1921, the Maternity Center Project is turned over to the MCA.

1931 A nurse-midwifery educational program, the Lobenstine Clinic and School of Midwifery (affiliated with MCA) opens its doors.

1941 New York City's Midwifery Board eliminates itself, citing a lack of granny midwives to regulate. In 1934, granny midwives held 1,997 permits. Within five years, they held only 270 permits and their numbers continued to dwindle. The number of nurse-midwives did not make up for the losses. For decades, professional recognition and clinical positions remain almost nonexistent. In 1962, only twenty-one nurse-midwives hold a permit to practice in New York City.

1958 MCA's School of Nurse-Midwifery moves to Kings County Hospital in Brooklyn (precursor to SUNY Downstate) becoming the first hospital-based nurse-midwifery educational program.

1959 New York City's Health Code is amended, making both RN licensure and nurse-midwifery certification requirements for obtaining a midwife permit.

1970 The Maternal and Infant Care Project of New York City (part of the federal public health campaign aimed at improving infant mortality rates, arising out of Social Security Act of 1963) establishes the first hospital-based nurse-midwifery service in New York at Delafield Hospital's Obstetrics and Family Practice Center with permission to attend births at Columbia/Presbyterian Hospital.

1975 The first urban freestanding birth center is opened in New York City by the Maternity Center Association (MCA).

1982 Legislative campaign begins to pass what ultimately becomes the Midwifery Practice Act.

1992 The Professional Midwifery Practice Act passes the New York House and Senate and becomes law.

1994 The New York Board of Midwifery is formed. Licenses to practice midwifery issued to 450 CNMs who held permits under the old law. Nurse-midwifery-attended births are at eight percent in New York state, having increased from four percent in 1981. Twelve DEMs apply for state licensure and are denied ten months later.

1995 ACC/ACNM choose Certified Midwife as the title for the new ACC-certified direct-entry midwife. Thirteen DEMs apply for state licensure and are denied. Cease-and-desist orders sent to approximately ten unlicensed homebirth DEMs.

1996 SUNY Downstate's direct-entry educational program initiated. Linda Schutt CPM becomes the first CM.

1997 ACNM gives full voting privileges to CMs.

2000 The New York State Association of Licensed Midwives (NYSALM) is formed. (www.nysalm.org)

2003 NARM process and exam evaluated by New York State Education Department, but not accepted for New York.

2005 Over 1,000 CNMs and around fifty CMs hold New York state midwifery licenses.

ACKNOWLEDGMENTS

First and foremost, we thank our New York interviewees for the time they spent with us, patiently answering our questions and forthrightly explaining their actions and points of view. We also express deep appreciation for their comments and helpful edits on this chapter to Anne Frye, Kathy Carr, Carolyn Keefe, Dorothea Lang, Ronnie Lichtman, Elaine Mielcarski, Carol Nelson, Judith Rooks, Barbara Katz Rothman, Hilary Schlinger, Linda Schutt, Nancy Villa, Richard Waldman, Deanne Williams, and Raymond DeVries.

Maureen's personal acknowledgment: I dedicate this work to my two men (my husband and son). They put up with me these seven years while I, together with Robbie, gave birth to this postdates baby—the New York chapter.

ENDNOTES

1. When we speak of hospital-based midwifery services, we are referring to midwifery services that are distinct from traditional labor and delivery services, administered by a Midwifery Service Director and where nurse-midwives are salaried by the hospital or by the Ob/gyn department faculty practice, to work in its midwifery service. In New York state these midwifery services are mainly found in New York City. Outside of New York City there are only several such services in New York state. Most New York-licensed midwives are employed by an Ob/gyn physician group and attend hospital births in this capacity.

2. Lilian Wald, an RN, public health nurse and personal friend to some of the earliest nurse-midwives, was one of the movers and shakers in the settlement house movement, establishing the Henry St. Settlement House in New York City.

3. During the 1930s and 1940s, several other nurse-midwifery schools and services were established in other states. In 1939, the Frontier Nursing Service established the Frontier Graduate School of Nurse-Midwifery in Hyden, Kentucky. In 1941, the Alabama Department of Health established a nurse-midwifery educational program at Tuskegee College as well as a homebirth service demonstration project. The Tuskegee project closed after only five years, but its demonstration of the ability of trained midwives to significantly decrease maternal infant mortality rates in rural Alabama within

a short period of time made its mark on the history of nurse-midwifery. In 1943, the Medical Mission Sisters established a nurse-midwifery service in Santa Fe, New Mexico, and in 1944 a nurse-midwifery educational program, the Catholic Maternity Institute, began at this service. Through its affiliation with the Catholic University of America, the Catholic Maternity Institute in Santa Fe became the first nurse-midwifery school to grant a university degree (Corbin 1959).

4. By statute, nurse-practitioners in New York state are licensed as nurses and also receive an additional license to practice their advanced nursing specialty (i.e., Adult Nurse Practitioner, Pediatric Nurse Practitioner, Family Health Nurse-Practitioners, Women's Health Nurse-Practitioner, Ob-Gyn Nurse Practitioner, etc.). The Board of Nursing within the New York State Education Department governs them.

5. Other models for regulatory governance of nurse-midwifery are as follows: Utah has a Board of Nurse-Midwifery but has no means for incorporating direct-entry midwifery under its jurisdiction. New Jersey has incorporated the ACC-credentialed Certified Midwife under its Board of Nursing but has not granted the CM prescriptive authority. CNMs in Rhode Island, New Mexico, Connecticut, and American Samoa are licensed under their Boards of Health. Illinois has an Advanced Practice Nursing Board with jurisdiction over all advanced practice nursing, including nurse-midwifery. CNMs in the remaining states practice within the purview of a combination of models—Boards of Nursing, Boards of Medicine, Joint Boards of Medicine and Nursing, Boards of Public Health. In a direct effort to avoid the turf battles in New York, midwives in Massachusetts are proposing legislation that would also establish a Board of Midwifery, this time including CNMs, CMs, and CPMs (see chapter 9).

6. It is not difficult to understand why the possibility of a separate licensing process in New York state would present a threat to the ACNM. Nationwide credentialing has provided a stabilizing effect on the profession and aided its growth. Another example lies in nursing. Nationwide reciprocity for RNs has existed only since 1978 with establishment of the NCSBN (National Council of State Boards of Nursing), which then instituted a national nursing exam, the National Council Licensure Examination (NCLEX), and became recognized as the national testing agency for the nursing profession. In the 1980s, a move by the California Board of Registered Nursing to establish its own licensing exam was taken seriously as a threat to the entire nursing profession and was prevented.

7. Graduations of direct-entry students from SUNY Downstate by year are as follows: 1997, four; 1998, four; 2000, four; 2001, four; 2002, two; 2003, five; 2004, six; 2005, four. Total: thirty-three graduates (an average of four per year), all of whom have been certified as CMs. (Ronnie Lichtman, personal communication, 2005)

8. Nurse-midwifery in New Hampshire, as in most states, comes under the jurisdiction of the Board of Nursing. The apprenticeship-trained midwives practiced without legal recognition until the early 1980s, when New Hampshire passed legislation providing voluntary certification for direct-entry, homebirth midwives. The statute established requirements for certification and a process for certification through a state exam. The statute gave the title of Certified Midwife to those midwives who became certified by the state through this process. In 1990, two years prior to the 1992 New York midwifery legislation, the New Hampshire Midwives Association (NHMA) registered (state trademarked) the title of Certified Midwife with New Hampshire's Secretary of State as "owned by the New Hampshire Midwives Association (NHMA)."

Following the passage of the New York midwifery legislation and the change of ACNM bylaws recognizing the ACC-certified CM as eligible for membership in the ACNM, the ACNM federally trademarked the title Certified Midwife. Mary Ann

Shah, then President of ACNM, sent a cease-and-desist letter to the New Hampshire Midwives Association warning them to stop using the title or face legal action. New Hampshire's Attorney General ruled that the federal trademark of the CM title held no legal validity in New Hampshire. In order to differentiate themselves, the New Hampshire direct-entry midwives began calling themselves New Hampshire Certified Midwives (NHCM). In 1999 a second midwifery statute passed the New Hampshire legislature further regulating direct-entry midwifery. This second statute mandated CM licensure for direct-entry, homebirth midwives. It established a Board of Midwifery, which would oversee the practice of state-licensed Certified Midwives. Further, the statue makes the NARM exam the certification exam for New Hampshire Certified Midwives. Despite the threats of the ACNM, the statute did not change the title of Certified Midwife. One midwifery leader in New Hampshire stated, "We could have chosen to change the title from Certified Midwife to Certified Professional Midwife at that time . . . but we had been practicing under the title Certified Midwife since 1980 and we didn't want to give it up. We wanted the historical continuity that the title gives us here in New Hampshire. It's what we have been called, and called ourselves, for so many years."

In an extreme irony, an ACC-certified CM from New York applied for licensure in New Hampshire. New Hampshire's Attorney General has ruled that any ACC credentialed CM, in order to obtain a license to practice midwifery in New Hampshire, must first take the CPM exam and then apply to the Board of Midwifery as a CPM for CM state licensure.

9. As an example, in Texas a law beneficial to DEMs was defeated by CNMs because of failed communications between the two groups resulting directly from the mistrust engendered by the New York situation. In Ohio, a bill revising nurse-midwifery regulation, which would have made direct-entry midwifery illegal, was changed only through the efforts of direct-entry midwives. In Utah and Tennessee, legislative efforts by DEMs to become legal were fought by local CNMs. Nevertheless, DEM legislation was successfully passed in both states.

10. As of February 2005, there were forty-eight CMs: twenty-nine graduates of SUNY Downstate, two graduates of other DOA-accredited programs, and twenty graduates of programs not accredited by the ACNM (some of these are foreign-trained and some are graduates of MEAC-accredited schools). The breakdown of the CMs who did not graduate from SUNY Downstate is as follows. One CM, who had previously practiced as an unlicensed direct-entry midwife and a PA, graduated from a DOA-accredited direct-entry track created especially for her by the nurse-midwifery program at the Baystate Medical Center in Springfield, Massachusetts. She remains the only direct-entry graduate of this program, although other PAs could apply. Another CM graduated from the now-defunct EPA program in California. Of the twenty CMs who graduated from midwifery schools not accredited by the ACNM, two were educated in the United Kingdom, and one each in the Netherlands, Peru, Chile, and Iran. At least five graduated from MEAC-accredited programs: one from Seattle Midwifery School; three from the National College of Midwifery; and one from the naturopathic midwifery program at Bastyr University. One is a PA in Washington state. On the other seven, we could find no information. (Our thanks to Ronnie Lichtman, Director of the SUNY Downstate program, for much of this information.)

11. These figures represent midwives throughout the state and are not broken down by regions. Because there are few hospital-based midwifery services outside of New York City, the percentage of New York City midwives who work within one of the city's midwifery services is most likely greater than shown by these numbers.

REFERENCES

American College of Nurse-Midwives. 1987. *What Is A Nurse-Midwife?* (Brochure). Washington, D.C.: American College of Nurse-Midwives.

American College of Nurse-Midwives. Chapter Minutes; ACNM Region II, Chapter 1 (June 22, 1998):22.

Benoit, Cecilia, Robbie Davis-Floyd, Edwin van Teijlingen, Sirpa Wrede, Jane Sandall, and Janneli Miller. 2001. "Designing Midwives: A Transnational Comparison of Educational Models." In *Birth by Design: Pregnancy, Maternity Care, and Midwifery in North America and Europe*, ed. Raymond DeVries, Edwin van Teijlingen, Sirpa Wrede, and Cecilia Benoit, 139–165. New York: Routledge.

Burst, Helen V. 1978. "Our Three-Ring Circus." *Journal of Nurse-Midwifery* XXIII(fall):11–14.

Corbin, Hazel. 1959. "Historical Development of Nurse-Midwifery in this Country and Present Trends." *Bulletin of the American College of Nurse-Midwifery* 4(1):13–26.

Cuddihy, Nancy R. 1984. "On Nurse-Midwifery Legislation." *Journal of Nurse-Midwifery* 29(2): 55–56.

Davis-Floyd, Robbie. 1998. "The Ups, Downs and Interlinkages of Nurse- and Direct-Entry Midwifery: Status, Practice and Education." In *Paths to Becoming a Midwife: Getting an Education*, ed. Jan Tritten and Joel Southern. Eugene, OR: Midwifery Today, Inc.

Davis-Floyd, Robbie, and Gloria St. John. 1998. *From Doctor to Healer: The Transformative Journey*. New Brunswick, NJ: Rutgers University Press.

DeVries, Raymond. 2005. "A Pleasing Birth." In *Dutch Maternity Care and the Cultured Science of Obstetrics*. Philadelphia, PA: Temple University Press.

DeVries, Raymond, Edwin van Teijlingen, Sirpa Wrede, and Cecilia Benoit, eds. 2001. *Birth by Design: Pregnancy, Maternity Care, and Midwifery in North America and Europe*. New York: Routledge Press.

Dye, Nancy Schrom. 1987. "Modern Obstetrics and Working-Class Women: The New York Midwife Dispensary, 1890–1920." *Journal of Social History*, 20 (spring 1987):549–564.

Fiedler, Dolores E. 1971. "Cut the Cord." *Journal of Nurse-Midwifery* 18(3):3.

Harris, David, Edwin F. Daily, and Dorothea M. Lang. 1971. "Nurse-Midwifery in New York City." *American Journal of Public Health* 61(1): 64–77.

Hellman, Louis H. 1967. "Nurse-Midwifery in the United States." *Obstetrics and Gynecology* 30(6):883–888.

———. 1971. "Nurse-Midwifery: Fifteen Years." *Bulletin of the American College of Nurse-Midwives* XXI(3):71–79.

———. 1972. "Challenges for Nurse-Midwifery in the Seventies." In *New Horizons in Midwifery*. Proceedings of the Sixteenth Triennial Congress of the International Confederation of Midwives, October 28–November 3, 1972, Washington, D.C., ed. Alice M. Forman, Susan H. Fischman, and Lucille Woodville. London: The International Confederation of Midwives.

Hemschemeyer, Hattie. 1962. "Our 30th Anniversary—A Tribute." *Bulletin of the American College of Nurse-Midwifery* VII(1):5–14.

Howard, Esme J. 1994. *Navigating the Stormy Sea: The Maternity Center Association and the Development of Prenatal Care 1900–1930*. Master's thesis, Yale University School of Nursing.

Gaskin, Ina May. 1978. *Spiritual Midwifery*. Summertown, TN: The Book Publishing Company.

———. 2003. *Ina May's Guide to Childbirth*. New York: Bantam.

Johnson, Kenneth C. and Betty Anne Daviss. 2005."Outcomes of Planned Home Births with Certified Professional Midwives: Large Prospective Study in North America.." *British Medical Journal* 330(7505): 1416, June. www.bmj.com.

Kobrin, Frances E. 1966. "The American Midwife Controversy: A Crisis of Professionalization." *The Bulletin of the History of Medicine* 40(4):350–363.

Lang, Dorothea. 1977. "The American College of Nurse-Midwives; What Is the future for Certified Nurse-Midwives in Hospitals? Childbearing Centers? Homebirths?" In *21st Century Obstetrics Now*. Vol. 1. published by the National Association of Parents and Professionals for Safe Alternatives in Childbirth.

Lesser, Arthur J. 1972. "Issues in Planning for Better Maternity Services in the United States." In *New Horizons in Midwifery*. Proceedings of the Sixteenth Triennial Congress of the International Confederation of Midwives October 28–November 3, 1972, Washington, D.C., ed. Alice M. Forman, Susan H. Fischman, and Lucille Woodville. London: The International Confederation of Midwives.

Litoff, Judy Barrett. 1978. *American Midwives. 1860 to the Present*. Westport, CT: Greenwood Press.

May, Maureen. 1999. "Midwifery in New York State: Identity, Power and Politics." Paper presented at the Annual Meetings of the American Anthropological Association, Chicago, Illinois, in the session "Daughters of Time: The Shifting Identities of Postmodern Midwives," organized by Robbie Davis-Floyd and Sheila Cosminsky.

National Center for Health Statistics. 1999. *National Vital Statistics Reports*. Volume 47, Number 27 (December 2).

New York State Department of Health and the New York State Education Department. 1997. *Professional Midwifery Preparation and Practice in New York State* (July).

Perez-Pena, Richard. 2004. "Use of Midwives, a Childbirth Phenomenon, Fades in City." *New York Times*. March 15, 2004.

Pew Health Professions Commission. 1995. *Pew Commission Report on Reform of the Health Professions*. San Francisco: UCSF Center for the Health Professions.

———. 1999. *Charting a Course for the 21st Century. The Future of Midwifery*. San Francisco: UCSF Center for the Health Professions.

Reagan, Leslie J. 1995. "Linking Midwives and Abortion in the Progressive Era." *The Bulletin of the History of Medicine* 69:569–598.

Redman, Annie. 1997. "Professional Midwifery Practice Act of New York, 1992: A Case Study of Nurse-Midwifery Politics." Master's thesis, Yale University School of Nursing.

Roberts, Joyce Roberts. 1996. "The Certification of Non-nurse-midwives by the American College of Nurse-Midwives." *Journal of Nurse-Midwifery* 41(1):1–2.

Rooks, Judith. 1997. *Midwifery and Childbirth in America*. Philadelphia, PA: Temple University Press.

Rosenthal, Elisabeth. 1997. "To Pay New York Hospitals Not to Train Doctors, Easing Glut." *New York Times*. February 1, 1997.

Scoggin, Janet C. 1996. "How Nurse-Midwives Define Themselves in Relation to Nursing, Medicine, and Midwifery." *Journal of Nurse-Midwifery* 41(1): 36–42.

Scott, James C. 1985. *Weapons of the Weak. Everyday Forms of Peasant Resistance*. New Haven, CT: Yale University Press.

———. 1990. *Domination and the Arts of Resistance: Hidden Transcripts*. New Haven, CT: Yale University Press.

Shoemaker, M. Theophane, Sr. 1947. *History of Nurse-Midwifery in the United States*. Washington, D.C.: Catholic University Press.

Stevens, Anne A. 1918. "An Experiment in Maternity Protection: Report of the Work of the Maternity Center of the Women's City Club of New York City." Unpublished paper Presented at the Biannual Meeting of the National Nurses Association. Cleveland, Ohio, May 1918. WCCNY microfilm, reel 20, frames 205–207.

———. 1918. "The Work of the Maternity Center Association." Transactions, 10th Annual Meeting, American Child Hygiene Association, November 11–13, 1919, Asheville, NC (WCCNY microfilm reel 20, frames 209–231).

Weisl, Bernard A.G. 1964. "The Nurse-Midwife and the New York City Health Code." *Bulletin of the American College of Nurse-Midwifery* IX(1):8–14.

Wells, Sharon. 1992. "The New York Legislative Sellout." *Birth Gazette* 8(4):32–33.

Wolfe, Leanna. 1982. *Giving Birth in New York City. A Guide to Childbirth Options.* New York: New York Public Interest Research Group, Inc. (NYPIRG).

Women's City Club of New York. 1917. Bulletin published by the Women's City Club of New York, vol. 1, no. 6 (October).

———. 1919. *Summary of the First Year's Work. Preliminary report to Club Members on the Maternity Center. From its opening September 15, 1917 to October 1, 1918.* New York: Women's City Club of New York, February.

———. 1920. *Our Hopes Justified.* New York: Women's City Club of New York.

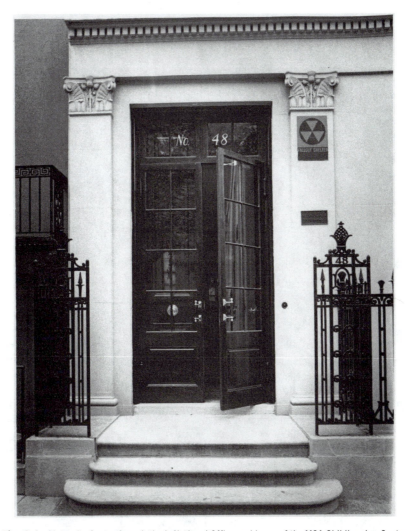

Fig. 2.1 Maternity Center Association's National Office and home of the MCA Childbearing Center from 1952 to 1996. Photo from the MCA archives.

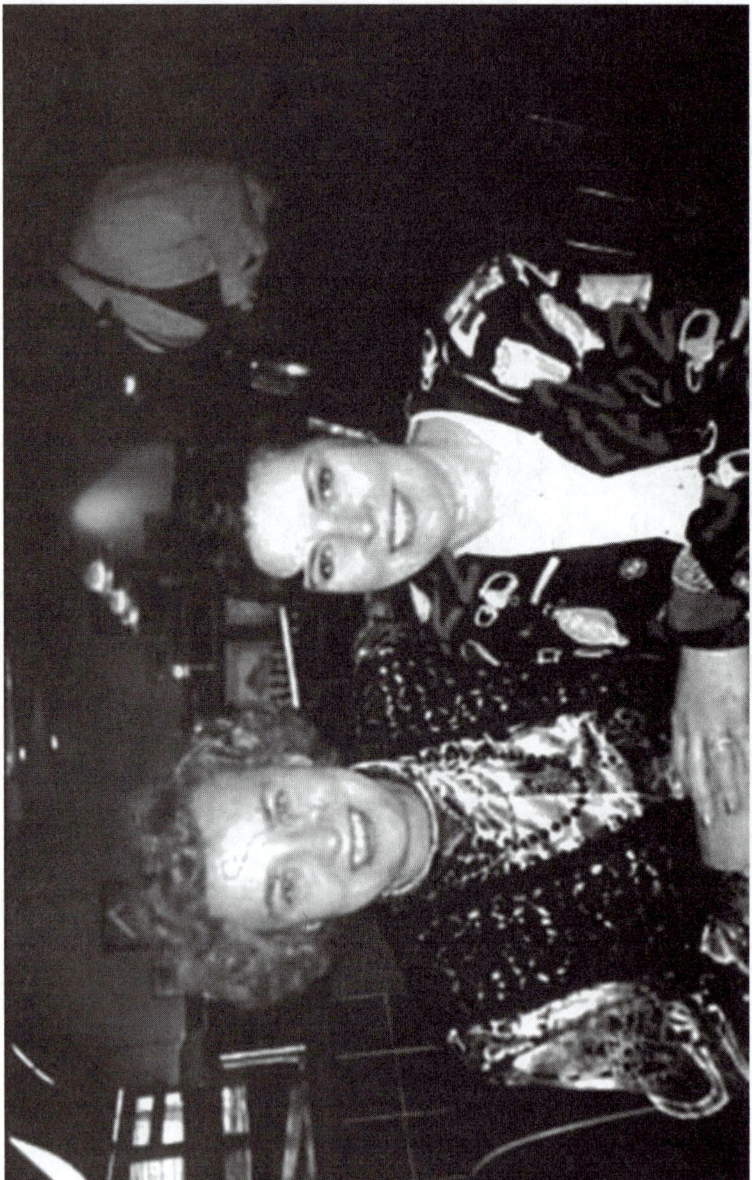

Fig. 2.2 Dorothea Lang and Elaine Mielcarski, 1997. Photographer: Robbie Davis-Floyd

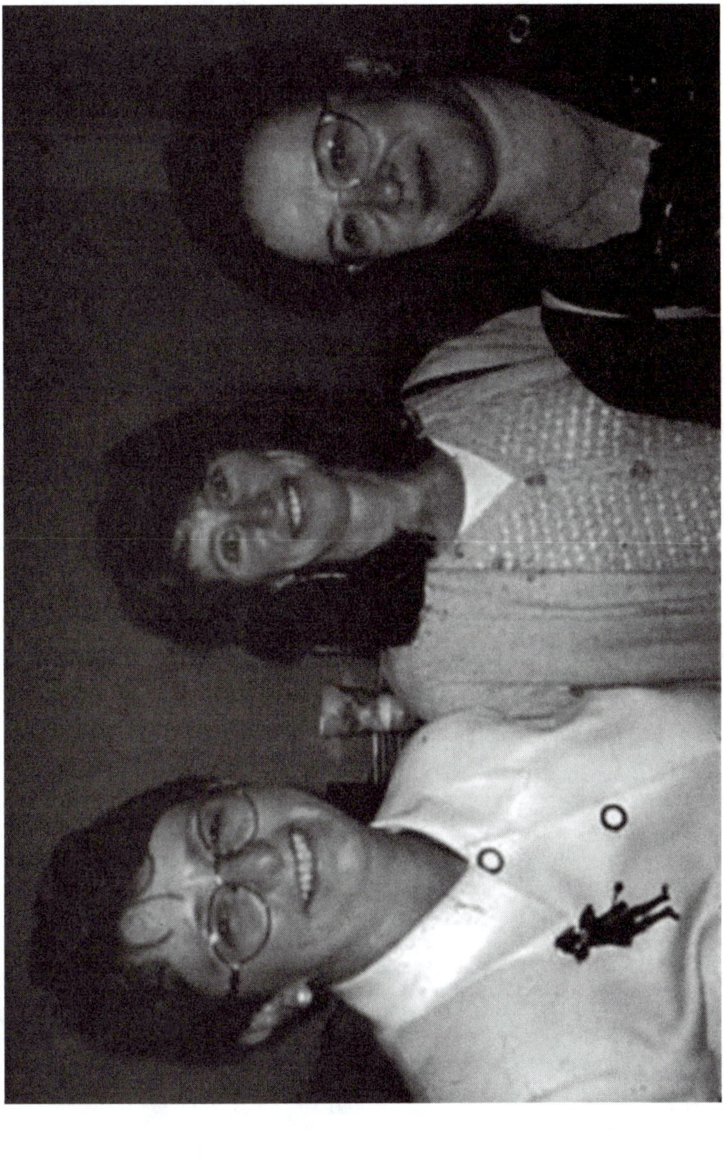

Fig. 2.3 Linda Schutt, the first CM, flanked left to right by ACNM Chief Executive Officer Deanne Williams and President Joyce Roberts, 1997. Photographer: Robbie Davis-Floyd

3

QUALIFIED COMMODIFICATION:
THE CREATION OF THE
CERTIFIED PROFESSIONAL MIDWIFE[1]

Robbie Davis-Floyd

• **The Midwifery Appropriation of Commodification Strategies** • **The Politics of Representing Midwives** • **Qualified Commodification: Mainstreaming Midwives** • **Characteristics of Commodification and How CPMs Fit** • **Conclusion: Maintaining a Tireless Vigilance**

> **commodity** 1. Something useful that can be turned to commercial or other advantage. 2. An article of trade or commerce.
>
> —**dictionary.com 2005**

This chapter incorporates a rather extreme change in theoretical tone from the preceding chapters, to which I must ask our readers to adjust. I originally wrote it for an anthropological book called *Consuming Motherhood* (Taylor, Wozniak, and Layne, 2004), which utilizes various kinds of theories of commodification and consumption to analyze multiple aspects of motherhood in the contemporary United States, and have adapted it for this book (with permission) because I found that analyzing the creation of the CPM in terms of commodification theory sheds a great deal of light on the richness and complexity of the process the midwives who created the CPM went through, and on its ultimate results. While homebirth midwives may not immediately appreciate thinking of themselves as commodities, in the introduction to *Consuming Motherhood*, Janelle Taylor writes,

> Scholars of consumption have argued persuasively that we must understand consumption itself as a site of cultural creativity and political agency, and also . . . of subversion and resistance. Consumers are neither passive nor without agency, but rather appropriate mass-produced goods to their own projects and purposes, producing selves and making worlds in the process. (2004:11–12)

These are notions to which I think midwives can easily relate. In fact, contemporary homebirth midwives are engaged in precisely the enterprise Taylor identifies: by appropriating certain aspects of mass production to their own projects and purposes, they are using consumption as a site of subversion and resistance to create new selves and alternative worlds. Starting out at the margins of a consumer society they view with a jaundiced and critical eye, these midwives came to realize over time that their survival as viable practitioners required participation in the technocracy's core processes of commodification and consumption. Their own views of these processes, while initially negative and derogatory, have subsequently expanded to encompass the ambiguity inherent in commodification.

In other words, these midwives came to see that processes of commodification can be not only agents of co-option into standardized mass markets, but also forms of cultural creativity and political agency, and indeed also of subversion and resistance to mass standardization. The selves/identities such midwives make as they commodify in order to occupy a wider terrain in the consumer market, and the alternative realities they explored through the process of commodification as they created the CPM, are the subject of this chapter. I will illustrate their appropriation of the language and strategies of the kinds of consumption and marketing that they themselves originally perceived as negative, in what I identify as a process of *qualified commodification*. Webster's New World Dictionary (2000) gives as the fourth and fifth definitions of the word *qualify*: "to modify, restrict, limit [to qualify one's approval]; to moderate, soften [to qualify a punishment]." Thus, with this term I seek to name the alchemical process through which direct-entry homebirth midwives appropriated the rhetoric and core cultural characteristics of mass forms of commodification in order to move themselves into the mainstream through creation of the CPM, but modified and moderated those characteristics in an effort to simultaneously remain true to the countercultural ideals and values they have long called their own. Are you with me?

THE MIDWIFERY APPROPRIATION OF COMMODIFICATION STRATEGIES

The intense commodification of reproduction has had some interesting consequences for American midwives, who are managing in some rather creative ways to appropriate it to their own ends. Effectively shut out of birth during the modern industrial era, in the postmodern technocracy American midwives have been fighting their way back (Davis-Floyd, Cosminsky, and Pigg 2001). Their numbers are growing, as is their political and legislative presence in the birth arena. Increasingly unwilling to accept their cultural marginalization, both nurse- and direct-entry midwives are actively starting to think of themselves, and to present themselves to the public, as valuable health-care commodities. Appropriating the notion of women as agentic consumers of maternity care (an image they helped to create), midwives have added themselves to the list of birth care options from which women can now choose. Marketing has become a keystone of their strategies for success in the twenty-first century: in recent years midwives have produced advertisements, brochures, leaflets, videos, and books touting the benefits of midwifery care. They have also become master politicians, successfully selling midwifery to state legislators, nursing and medical societies, and regulatory boards. In some states their search is for greater representation on the boards that govern them and more beneficial rules and regulations; in others, the fight is for so basic a thing as the right to practice legally and to be licensed by the state.

Within these parameters of the commodification of American midwifery, as we saw in chapter 1, two models and philosophies of midwifery education and practice coexist and sometimes compete for legal status and cultural recognition: the nurse-midwifery and the lay/direct-entry midwifery models. In particular, direct-entry midwives' efforts at professionalization and commodification contrast in fascinating ways with the ongoing value they place on their relationships with their clients and their grassroots social movement fervor. As we have seen, nurse-midwives have worked hard to create a professional image and reputation in keeping with that of other health-care professionals—an image that was seriously threatened by the relatively sudden advent of the lay midwife. In chapter 1, I noted that these new lay midwives came from a wide diversity of backgrounds; they included hippies, feminists, members of various religious groups, and conservative Midwestern housewives. Yet their most visible public face was countercultural: long hair, long flowy skirts, and Birkenstocks constituted the visual representation they came to conjure up, along with a hippie ethos, a countercultural lifestyle and values, and a laid-back attitude. This public image often had nothing to do with the individual characteristics of particular lay midwives, yet it developed as a stereotype and has tended to remain. This image was a major threat, both stylistically and professionally, to the short-haired, stockinged, and white-jacketed image of mainstream professionalism and competence that nurse-midwives had worked hard to build.

THE POLITICS OF REPRESENTING MIDWIVES

As every anthropologist knows, ethnography is all about representation. As an ethnographer, I first became aware of how concerned direct-entry midwives were becoming with revamping their public image when I began work on a chapter for a book (Davis-Floyd 1998a) being put together by *Midwifery Today* (a magazine and company dedicated to the preservation and promotion of midwifery) called *Paths to Becoming a Midwife: Getting an Education* (Tritten and Southern 1998). For that book, I had been asked to write a comparative description of "the ups and downs of nurse- and direct-entry midwifery" in nine pages or less—a task I should have known would be impossible. Yet I had been conducting fieldwork among nurse- and direct-entry midwives for four years at that point, in an attempt to understand their similarities, differences, and political motivations vis-à-vis each other. I (foolishly) thought that the interviews I had conducted with these midwives, and the dozens of midwifery conferences I had attended, would make it easy to describe them in simple, generalized terms. In the first draft of that chapter, which I wrote in a few days, I noted that direct-entry midwives are more culturally marginalized, work longer hours, and make far less money than nurse-midwives. The direct-entry midwives who saw that first draft reacted with outrage, telling me that I made them sound like "marginalized losers" and the hospital-based nurse-midwives, who make a great deal more money and have more reasonable working hours, like winners. Aware that this *Midwifery Today* book would be read by students trying to make a decision as to whether to become a direct-entry midwife (DEM) or a certified nurse-midwife (CNM), the DEMs wanted me to represent them in the most positive light possible. I asked for suggestions for alternative wording that would be as true as what I originally had said but that would make them look better; putting our heads together, we came up with the following:

> Direct-entry midwives often work alone or in practices with one or two primary midwives, and are almost always on call. For some, burnout is the result of this constant availability; others find this a viable way of life.... Many direct-entry midwives appreciate the flexibility they enjoy as independent practitioners: should they desire more time off, they can cut down on the number of clients they take on. In areas where interest in homebirth is steady or growing, they can choose to accept more clients until they build their practice to the level they desire. Thus their incomes vary widely: those who attend only a few births a year may make only a few thousand dollars, while some direct-entry midwives make upwards of $60,000 per year. . . .
>
> In short, DEMs face the challenges and reap the benefits of being self-employed entrepreneurs. Like some MDs, they run independent practices; their earning ability is not constrained by salaries but rather depends on their level of energy and their ability to attract clients (which itself is constrained by cultural attitudes toward homebirth). In states where they are licensed and regulated, they often serve as the sole proprietors of thriving businesses (at a time when many MDs are being forced to trade in their economically advantageous positions as independent practitioners for the rigid payment schedules of HMOs). Many DEMs make a good living, many do not, but all of them love their work. Most DEMs would not trade the challenges, tribulations, and rewards of their entrepreneurial practices for the constraints of working in a hospital setting. (Davis-Floyd 1998a:75)

Although I had some qualms about being made into an active agent of their marketing strategies, I felt responsible to them to describe them the way they tend to see themselves, so I was happy to find this alternative wording. But the battle was not over; they took me severely to task once again when I tried, in that same article, to describe the damaging stereotypes hospital practitioners tend to create and disseminate about direct-entry midwives. What I said in that first draft was:

> Many medical practitioners, and some nurse-midwives, have serious concerns about the safety of direct-entry practice; they point to the fact that there are some DEMs in practice with truly

inadequate training. Thus when a DEM makes a mistake, no matter what her individual knowledge and skills, most people in the medical community are only too ready to assume that she is "ignorant" and "incompetent," and go on to assume that incompetence and lack of education characterize all midwives of her ilk.

Immediately I received irate phone calls from a midwife and a midwifery advocate, both of whom asked me "how dare I call direct-entry midwives 'ignorant' and 'incompetent'?" Of course I had not done so—I had simply tried to describe the stereotypes other people held. Painful and irrational as this accusation was, it pointed out to me the extreme level of concern today's DEMs bring to public representations of their image. Fighting generations of such stereotypes applied to them by the medical profession, today's professionalizing homebirth midwives react strongly to any such negative associations. They and their clients sometimes suffer in extreme ways from the effects of such stereotypes, as the home-to-hospital transport stories recounted in chapter 10 describe in detail. The negative reactions midwives encounter when they transport a client to the hospital (not to mention those they also encounter in state legislatures) vivify the problematic nature of the interface between midwives and medical practitioners and the consequent deep need midwives feel for cultural legitimacy. It is one thing to proudly hold a countercultural space in which women can make alternative choices, and another to watch your clients suffer the effects of the negative stereotyping of midwives. Thus, although many direct-entry midwives remain countercultural to the core, they are keenly aware of the need to make themselves more viable in the technocracy, not only to keep themselves out of jail, but also to protect their clients from being medically mistreated because they chose a homebirth midwife. One obvious route to cultural viability would have been nurse-midwifery, but that would have meant losing the kind of independent midwifery they had worked so hard to create. How could they sell themselves without selling themselves out?

QUALIFIED COMMODIFICATION:
MAINSTREAMING MIDWIVES

A Certified Professional Midwife (CPM) is a knowledgeable, skilled, and professional independent midwifery practitioner who has met the standards for certification set by the North American Registry of Midwives (NARM) and is qualified to provide the Midwifery Model of Care. The CPM is the only international credential that requires knowledge about and experience in out-of-hospital settings.

—NARM, *How to Become a Certified Professional Midwife*

For the first three decades of their existence, several factors handicapped direct-entry midwives in their efforts to gain a toehold in the technocracy. These included: (1) some degree of public awareness of their lack of credentials and their illegal status in various states; (2) the vast variances in their educational processes, which range from pure apprenticeship to private three-year schools; (3) the negative publicity generated around occasional bad outcomes at homebirths, some of which were attended by insufficiently trained practitioners (a publicity rarely applied to negative hospital outcomes); (4) the negative stereotyping of midwives in general as less competent than physicians. As I described in chapter 1, they created a national organization, MANA, in 1982 and developed national practice standards and identified core competencies during the 1980s. But full voting membership in MANA was open to anyone who called herself a midwife, and there was no obligation to abide by the standards that MANA had set. Increasingly aware that only a standardized national certification process could convince the public, including politicians, legislators, and the courts that they were safe and savvy practitioners, compensate for the variations in their educational processes, help them avoid arrest and legal persecution, and minimize the possibility of inadequately trained midwives out there doing births, the members of MANA were at the same time concerned that any kind of nationally standardized certification would compromise their ability to meet women's unique needs and requirements in out-of-hospital settings.

No one was more aware of this danger than the members of the organization created by MANA to develop an exam and later a full-fledged certification process—the North American Registry of Midwives (NARM). Desiring to design a psychometrically valid testing and certification process in line with the standards set by the National Organization of Certifying Agencies (NOCA), NARM board members also, and just as ardently, desired not to co-opt themselves and their sisters or compromise their practices in the process. Since 1994, in my dual roles as ethnographer and member of the NARM Board, I have watched them struggle with the tensions generated by the often conflicting pulls to (1) enhance their public image to better market themselves to the public through creating a rigorous certification process; (2) preserve their ability to practice according to their own individual values and beliefs and those of their clients, which they believe constitutes the essence of out-of-hospital midwifery; and (3) establish certification requirements that work with the logistical realities of their day-to-day practices, educational processes, and the legislation in various states.

Karl Marx asserted that commodification is a transformative process, but he viewed it in negative terms. Since then, anthropological theories about commodification have come to encompass its many variables and its often-creative qualities (Hebbdige 1979, McRobbie 1988). MANA midwives not familiar with such writings maintain deep suspicions about commodification and tend to see it in more culturally negative terms. Their view of commodification resonates more with those of social scientists like Adorno and Horkheimer (1999), Bourdieu (1984), Baudrillard (1988), and others. In what follows I will utilize a list of the characteristics I have noted that midwives seem to associate with commodities and commodification, combining those characteristics with some thoughts of my own.

For wide success, a commodity must, among other things, be:

1. produced in a standardized way.
2. subject to mechanisms of quality control.
3. quantifiable, measurable, and legally accessible.
4. purchasable and user-friendly.
5. able to tap or to create a market niche and to be marketed successfully through advertisements or other means to reach that market niche.
6. designed and redesigned in ways responsive to consumer desires and cultural trends.
7. have a brand name that gives it a unique identity (the most successful commodities, from Coca-Cola to the iMac, have a brand name that maintains consumer demand for that particular product, even in the face of clones and competitors).
8. reflect market conditions and fluctuations (inevitably, commodities are embedded in the local/global political economy—their price, availability, and symbolic worth reflect market fluctuations, competitive pressures, government priorities, political realities and tensions, and *glocal* [local and global] cultural biases and beliefs).

Most of the above characteristics of commodification are antithetical to the ethos and the values that characterized lay midwives in the early days of their development (Reid 1989, DeVries 1996). They started out in resistance to the standardization of hospital birth, experienced a non-quantifiable spiritual calling to midwifery, often attended women who could not pay, and would not have dreamed of marketing themselves too visibly, as they were illegal or alegal in most states.[2] But in the early 1980s they gained legalization and licensure in Washington state, Florida, New Mexico, Arizona, and Texas, created their national association (MANA) in 1982, started to formalize and codify their knowledge base in books, articles, and formal vocational curricula, and by the mid-1980s began to exhibit many of the characteristics of incipient professionalization, including developing various state certifications. By the early 1990s many of them were moving into full-scale participation in the technocracy.

From their beginnings as a grassroots social movement, they had created a unique style of midwifery that they wanted to preserve, so their challenge in the 1990s became how to professionalize and commodify themselves without losing the essence of who they are and what, uniquely, they have to contribute. In the rest of this chapter, I will utilize the above list of characteristics to shed light on their commodifying strategies and to analyze their degree of success in achieving their primary goal: preserving the autonomous, woman-centered, and holistic style of midwifery they had created by making it viable in the technocracy, primarily through the development of CPM certification.

CHARACTERISTICS OF COMMODIFICATION AND HOW CPMS FIT
Standardized Production

The Certified Professional Midwife (CPM) has been educated through a variety of routes, including programs accredited by the Midwifery Education Accreditation Council (MEAC), the American College of Nurse-Midwives Division of Accreditation (ACNM-DOA), apprenticeship education, and self-study.

—NARM, *How to Become a Certified Professional Midwife*

As this quotation indicates, direct-entry midwifery education takes many forms and shapes; it cannot be considered standardized. Rather, DEM training ranges along a spectrum, from the most hands-on and the least didactic (self-study and apprenticeship) at one end, to highly didactic formal programs at the other. This lack of standardization has been the source of many of its public relations problems. For many years, ACNM's rigorous educational standards (see chapter 1) contrasted sharply with the lack of such standards for DEMs. Some DEMs responded to this situation by creating rigorous licensure processes in a few states, and/or by opening formal vocational programs, usually of three years' duration. Within these formal programs, students are evaluated according to standards set by the faculty of each program. By the mid-1990s, these programs themselves could apply for evaluation by the Midwifery Education and Accreditation Council (MEAC). In an effort to maintain clarity and consistency for midwifery students, MEAC kept its educational requirements in line with those established by NARM; often, details were worked out jointly by both groups.

But how do you evaluate in a publicly convincing way the knowledge, skills, and experience obtained through self-study or apprenticeship with a practicing midwife? How do you standardize the unstandardizable learning process called apprenticeship? How, in other words, do you commodify an anti-commodity? This was one of the most daunting challenges of developing NARM certification. Midwifery apprenticeship is a thoroughly individualized process whose shape and nature depends on the personalities and abilities of the apprentice and the mentor(s), and most especially on the relationship that develops between them. When it is successful, the apprentice/mentor relationship provides a supportive and nurturing educational context within which the apprentice can learn about pregnancy and birth through the immediacy of touch and experience, and can supplement that embodied knowledge with reading and long discussion with her mentor and others. Apprentices accompany their mentors to homebirths, witnessing woman after woman give birth successfully on her own, and developing comprehension of the normal birth process. Where hospital training tends to focus on pathology and generate a fear-based approach to birth, homebirth apprentice training generates trust. Midwives who fundamentally trust birth are more likely to be able to create an atmosphere within which women can find their own power and trust themselves to give birth. Thus, preserving apprenticeship has been and remains essential to the ethos and ethics of MANA members' philosophy and practice (Davis-Floyd 1998a, 1998b; Benoit et al. 2001).

NARM's response to the challenge apprenticeship presented was to standardize its educational *requirements* without trying to standardize direct-entry educational *processes*. NARM certification is open to midwives educated through all possible routes, including apprenticeship, self-study, formal vocational programs, university training, and all combinations thereof. NARM certification is competency based: where or how you gained your knowledge, skills, and experience is not the issue; that you have them is what counts. In other words, it is what you know and can do that matters, not how you learned it or what degrees you obtained.

Thus the decisions the members of the NARM board had to make as they developed CPM certification came to center around the issue of what criteria to use for standardizing their educational requirements. The discussion quickly crystallized around three ingredients—knowledge, skills, and experience. What knowledge base did an entry-level applicant have to master; what skills did she have to learn; how much experience was enough? In establishing answers to these questions, the eight members of the NARM board[3] faced the difficult task of balancing the competent and professional public image they desired for the new CPM against the pragmatic realities of her training and practice. Urged by the MANA membership not to undertake this task alone, the NARM board held five Certification Task Force (CTF) meetings around the country to seek input from the American midwifery community. Any midwife of any kind was welcome to participate in these meetings, as were consumers and advocates; approximately 150 did so, including some CNM members of MANA (Alice Sammon, personal communication, 2003). All NARM and CTF decisions were consensus-based, meaning that everyone present had to agree to every major decision. Strict adherence to the consensus process carried its own set of challenges, but ultimately ensured that the outcome of the process was supported by all of its creators, as it continues to be.

One of the early issues the members of the NARM board and the CTF faced was the number of births to require that CPM candidates must have attended. They knew it would "look better" to the outside world if CPM candidates had to attend more births as primary caregivers than the twenty births required of student nurse-midwives, but resisted that temptation because requiring more births would, among other reasons, make achieving certification too difficult for midwives practicing in rural areas where the births can be few and far between. Likewise, they knew it would look better, more "midwifery-like," to require that CPM candidates give large numbers of courses of continuity of care to their clients (caring for the same woman throughout the childbearing cycle), but resisted that temptation because some of the most important midwifery training centers, such as Maternidad La Luz in El Paso, primarily serve poor Hispanic women from northern Mexico, many of whom do not show up for any kind of prenatal care nor return for postpartum visits, making continuity of care extremely difficult for many students to achieve. (Wanting to require ten or more courses of continuity of care, they ultimately settled on three.)

They also knew it would "look better" to require the ability to insert IVs as an entry-level skill required of all CPM candidates—in the extensive discussion of this issue during a CTF meeting, one of the arguments repeatedly used in favor of requiring this skill was that homebirth midwives "look really good" to hospital personnel when they transport a woman who is hemorrhaging with the IV already in place. Another was that this skill is essential to safe homebirth practice. It was here, in this heated debate over whether or not to require IV insertion as an entry-level skill, that the depth of their commitment to preserving midwifery (as it is understood and practiced by homebirth midwives) through this new certification was put to its greatest test.

It was January of 1995. The members of the CTF, including myself,[4] were in a hotel on Captiva Island in Florida. These members of MANA knew that this was about creating the future of their brand of midwifery, so a full forty of them showed up at their own expense. The sun was shining and the beach was calling on that warm and breezy day. Nevertheless, we sat in a meeting while everyone in turn spoke their mind on the important issue of which skills should be required for entry-level practice. Written on the board were IV insertion, catheter insertion, and pitocin administration for hemorrhage as the skills in immediate question. Many participants saw these as high-tech and highly medical skills, yet, as I listened with astonishment, midwife after midwife spoke in favor of requiring all of these skills for entry-level midwives.

Halfway into the process I raised my hand and asked for a quick sense of the room—how many of the midwives present favored requiring all these skills? When thirty-six out of the forty sets of hands went up, I was amazed to realize that I was bearing direct witness to the professionalization of lay midwifery. Even Ina May Gaskin, an irrepressible and eternal hippie and internationally known point person for "spiritual midwifery," argued for the IV requirement. She noted that after many years of holistic midwifery practice, she realized she had been relying on EMT technicians on the Farm to insert IVs in those rare cases of severe postpartum hemorrhage, and had finally taken responsibility for learning the skill herself. She felt that it was now an invaluable part of her midwifery repertoire, and she stressed not only its lifesaving potential, but also its positive value in terms of the public image of midwives, saying, "When we have a hemorrhage and we transport the woman with an IV already in place, we really look good to the hospital personnel who receive our clients. It helps them to trust us as practitioners."

Only four of the midwives there were in active opposition. Their primary spokesperson was Sandra MorningStar, a midwife from Missouri who had been sent to the meeting with a mandate from her state midwifery association not to allow IVs to be required as an entry-level skill for CPM certification. (In the consensus process used by members of MANA, one person can block a proposal even if everyone else supports it.) As midwife after midwife tried to get her to change her mind, Sandi held fast, insisting that requiring IV insertion sent the wrong message to student midwives. She said that IV insertion was "an advanced, not an entry-level skill," because the proper first courses of action in case of a hemorrhage were, in this order: (1) to speak to the mother, commanding her to stop bleeding (an intervention that midwife/anthropologist Janelli Miller calls "magical speech"), (2) to administer the herb shepherd's purse, (3) to utilize bimanual compression of the uterus, (4) to give a pitocin injection, and only after all that had been tried, (5) to insert an IV and transport. Sandi herself had learned IV skills a decade before, but she didn't want student midwives thinking that they should jump straight to the IV without learning all the other techniques that homebirth midwives had "rediscovered" for dealing with hemorrhage, because usually those less interventionist techniques were all that is needed. The midwives in her state, who were practicing illegally, did not want to be required to carry IV equipment, as this would open them to the serious charge of practicing medicine without a license. So steadfast was Sandi in her insistence on blocking the IV requirement that, after four hours of trying to get her to change her mind, the others gave up, put the matter in the hands of the steering committee, of which Sandi was a member, and took a break before dinner.

At dinner I was curious to see how Sandi would be treated by those who had opposed her so vehemently only an hour before. (She had been in tears at one point, openly questioning whether she should even become a CPM.) Ina May got to the dining room first, rushed over to Sandi, gave her a big hug, and thanked her for "speaking her truth" and "holding her space." Ina May said that when one midwife holds her space, it always works out better for everyone than if she had given in against her will and compromised her principles. And so the dinner went, with everyone hugging Sandi and expressing their appreciation. They still disagreed with her, but their trust in the consensus process was deep—experience had taught them that somehow it would work out.

By the time the steering committee met, everyone on it was exhausted. We sprawled around the room and tentatively started the discussion. Sandi still wouldn't budge until someone said, "Well, Sandi, if you knew that most of the midwives in the United States wanted IVs to be required, would you still hold this position?" Sandi answered, "Of course not! I'm not here to tell the majority of midwives what they *should* do! It's just that I don't think the forty women at this meeting [all of whom were midwifery leaders or directors of private midwifery schools] really represent the majority of practicing midwives—I'm trying to speak out for the ones who are not here, who don't think as you do." At that point, with dawning amazement, the group began to realize that they had just been handed a golden key. It occurred to all of us simultaneously that none of us could really say *what* the majority of practicing midwives thought about which skills should be required for entry-level practice, and it wasn't long before the steering committee was actively and excitedly planning what later turned out to be the largest survey of practicing midwives ever conducted in the United States, the *NARM 1995 Job Analysis.*

Some months later, after hundreds of volunteer hours of work, 3,000 surveys were mailed, and although they were so detailed they took over twelve hours to fill out, 800 of them were returned in usable form (Houghton and Windom 1996 a, 1996b).[5] As a result, the NARM process is based on midwifery as actually practiced by these 800 out-of-hospital midwives, not just by the forty who had been present on Captiva Island that day. These grassroots midwives themselves set the standards by which they were to be judged, and thereby avoided two of what they saw as the primary potential downsides of commodification—the many being co-opted by the rule-making few, and quality and individualized design and service giving way to mass standardization. They ultimately did standardize the production of CPMs, but the criteria they used were not arbitrarily established by an elite governing group, but rather were consensually chosen by a majority of practicing DEMs. In other words, they qualified (modified, moderated) the ways in which they commodified according to the internal standards of the larger, and still countercultural, group.

Quality Control

The education, skills, and experience necessary for entry into the profession of direct-entry midwifery were mandated by the Midwives' Alliance of North America (MANA) Core Competencies and the Certification Task Force; were authenticated by NARM's current Job Analysis; and are outlined in NARM's *Candidate Information Bulletin* and the *How to Become a Certified Professional Midwife (CPM)* booklet.

—How to Become a Certified Professional Midwife

As these midwives perceived it, a commodity must be subject to mechanisms of quality control. Part of the professionalizing enterprise is the inclusion of those who meet established criteria for education and practice—in other words, for quality—and the exclusion of those who do not. This simple fact was the subject of intense debate among MANA midwives during the 1980s and early 1990s. At that time, the social movement was (and remains) MANA's dominant ethos, and inclusiveness its dominant ethic. MANA's nonprofessional inclusiveness was in deliberate and direct contrast to the ACNM's professional exclusiveness.

Voting membership in ACNM entailed ACC (ACNM Certification Council) certification as a CNM (or later, as a CM) (see chapters 1 and 2). Membership in MANA entailed the simple statement that one was a midwife. At the first MANA conference I attended in El Paso in 1991, some MANA midwives were refusing even to utter the word "professional" because of its exclusionary connotations. Nevertheless, it was clear that they were evolving into professional midwives with a codified and cohesive body of knowledge and skills. Their creation of NARM certification was a strong expression of this evolving sense of professionalism.

Their motivations for seeking a more secure cultural status included not only their desire to protect mothers and babies from the mistreatment that results from medical stereotyping of midwives, but also to protect them from mistreatment by midwives who are insufficiently educated. Although DEMs do not like to talk about it, it is a fact that in the early days of lay midwifery, when everyone was on a learning curve, occasional bad outcomes in out-of-hospital births resulted from a midwife's lack of knowledge or skill. Today, DEMs have a named category for the *renegade midwife* (see chapter 11) who practices outside the protocols and parameters of her peers in her local midwifery community. Thus, a means of testing midwives to ensure that they have the necessary knowledge, skills, and experience became increasingly desirable to DEMs themselves, and NARM certification became the mechanism of quality control they chose.

It is a given that any certification process will include those who meet all requirements and exclude those who do not. This process of exclusion starts with requirements for candidacy. The DEMs' desire to minimize the exclusiveness of their certifying process led NARM board members, in consensus with the Certification Task Force, to establish four educational categories through which student midwives can apply for NARM certification as a CPM. Applicants in all four categories must meet NARM's General Education Requirements, which include attendance at forty births, twenty as primary attendant under supervision; three courses of continuity of care; seventy-five prenatal exams; twenty newborn exams; forty postpartum exams; CPR (adult and neonatal) certification; and other criteria (see www.narm.org for more details), but how an applicant must demonstrate that these requirements have been met varies by the educational category through which she applies.

The first category listed in *NARM's How to Become a CPM* booklet is graduation from a formal program accredited by the Midwifery Education and Accreditation Council (MEAC). Because the education of these students has already been evaluated by the faculty of the school, in general, upon completion of their program, they have only to pass the NARM written exam.

The second category is "certification by the ACNM Certification Council (ACC)." Inclusion of this category was not without effort. As we saw in chapter 2, Sharon Wells and Alice Sammon had been prime movers in the DEMs' effort to be included in the CNM bill. Defeated in New York, they had turned their prodigious energies to the national level, and had become two of the most influential and visionary members of the NARM board, along with Carol Nelson, who had also practiced midwifery in New York. Thus, and understandably, the initial debate among the members of the NARM board over whether or not to allow ACNM-certified midwives (CNMs and CMs) to apply for CPM certification was tinged with intense bitterness and exclusionary desires.

But in the end, MANA's core ethics of inclusiveness and sisterhood once again prevailed, and the NARM board consensually decided to keep its certification open to all midwives, including CNMs and CMs. While NARM was aware that most nurse-midwives would not want or need NARM certification, its members were also aware that some CNMs would want to become NARM-certified out of a philosophical commitment to MANA and to homebirth and midwifery as social movements, while others might need to become CPMs so that they could practice autonomously outside of hospitals, which in some states their CNM or CM certification might not allow them to do. To date, four CNMs have chosen to also become NARM-certified, and as we shall see later on, NARM certification may come to have particular significance to ACNM's new CMs.

Once NARM decided that CPM certification should be open to ACNM/ACC-certified midwives, there was much discussion among board members as to whether additional requirements should be established for candidates in this educational category. This discussion led to a general philosophical agreement among NARM board members and the CTF that in-hospital experience, which is all that ACNM-accredited programs require, is not sufficient preparation for out-of-hospital practice. So it was decided that CNMs and CMs who apply for NARM certification must document attendance as primary midwife at a minimum of ten out-of-hospital births and three courses of continuity of care, and must pass the NARM written examination. (This exam tests knowledge about birth outside the hospital, where as one NARM member put it, "there is no button to push to call for backup and a midwife must know how to handle sudden emergencies herself.")

With these requirements, NARM both kept its certification process open to and inclusive of nurse-midwives, and held its own conceptual space as an organization dedicated to establishing and evaluating the knowledge, skills, and experience required to attend out-of-hospital births.

NARM's third educational category is legal recognition in states previously evaluated for educational equivalency. This category recognizes the equivalency between some pre-existing state certification or licensure processes and NARM certification. Candidates from these states can, with some exceptions, simply submit a copy of their state license and take the NARM written exam.

The fourth category, and the most innovative and complex, is completion of NARM's portfolio evaluation process, also known as PEP—the route established by NARM to evaluate the education, skills, and experience of midwives trained through apprenticeship and self-study. PEP applicants are divided into two categories: "entry-level" and "special circumstances."[6] Entry-level candidates must document their fulfillment of NARM's General Education Requirements; provide written verification from their preceptor(s) that they have achieved proficiency in the numerous skills listed on NARM's Skills, Knowledge, and Abilities Essential for Competent Practice Verification Form; provide a written affidavit from their preceptor(s) that the applicant meets various other requirements; provide three professional letters of reference; and pass the NARM Skills Assessment (a hands-on exam conducted on a pregnant volunteer and an infant). Because an apprentice-trained midwife may have only one or two preceptors during her entire training (individuals who may be her friends), NARM and the CTF felt a need to establish a mechanism for testing her actual skills. Ideally, such an exam would evaluate the skills demonstrated by the student midwife at a birth, but that would have required the exam administrator, called a NARM Qualified Evaluator, to travel to wherever the midwife lived and wait there until her client went into labor. Cost, logistical, and liability difficulties make this impossible. So instead, NARM board members utilized the list of required skills that stemmed from 1995 *Job Analysis* (Houghton and Windom 1996a), emphasizing the skills that can be demonstrated on a pregnant volunteer and an infant. For each exam, the skills that will actually be tested are randomly chosen from this list by a computer. The Qualified Evaluator asks the applicant to demonstrate each skill and grades her performance. This skills exam has formed an essential part of NARM's success in establishing the CPM as a valid credential, as it helps to resolve the issue of how apprentice-trained midwives can prove that they have obtained the skills that were identified as necessary for entry-level practice, thus ensuring the requisite degree of uniformity in quality among CPMs.

Within a profession, another major aspect of quality control is what mechanisms exist for taking disciplinary action against members who are accused of malpractice. The creation of an effective peer review process has been a major challenge for the NARM board, as it requires them to sit in judgment of their own, a painful position for midwives operating under an ethos of sisterhood and inclusivity. Due to space limitations, I will not discuss the complexities of this process here, as to date there have been very few cases in which the peer review process has had to be activated (three CPM certifications have been revoked). More important for the issue of quality control is birth outcome, which for midwives is the ultimate litmus test of quality control.

Quantification, Legality, and Midwifery's Market Niche

Quantification   A commodity must be quantifiable and measurable. How many are produced, how many are sold, how many are used, how well do they work? And a commodity must be able to tap into an existing market niche or, like the personal computer, create one where none previously existed. Lay midwifery in the United States arose in response to the desires of some women to avoid hospital birth. In other words, the market niche existed and lay midwifery rose to fill it. But as long as midwifery remained primarily a social movement, the numbers of women utilizing lay midwives' services remained miniscule. In the United States, as we saw in chapter 1, out-of-hospital births still account for less than one percent of all births.

Direct-entry midwives have long contended that more women want homebirth than are able to achieve it because of the limitations on their accessibility, imposed by lack of legalization, licensure, and/or insurance reimbursement. Where DEM practice is illegal, it is accessed only by the tiny minority of women so committed to the philosophy and spirit of the homebirth movement that they are willing to go outside the law to achieve it. Where DEMs are legal but not reimbursable under insurance, they are accessed only by women who can pay out of pocket for their services. Where they are legal, licensed, and insurance reimbursed, their accessibility to a much wider clientele is reflected in the higher homebirth rates in Oregon, which are paralleled by rising homebirth rates in Florida, New Mexico, Arizona, Vermont (where the homebirth rate doubled in the two years after licensure was achieved), and Washington state. In certain areas of Seattle, for example, where licensed midwives are easily accessible to large numbers of women and are fully covered under insurance, homebirth rates have risen to eight percent or more, reinforcing the point Ina May Gaskin made in chapter 1 that the "one percent barrier," as it used to be known, was a reflection not of women's lack of interest in homebirth, but rather of its culturally imposed inaccessibility.

Over the past decade, this inaccessibility, which was nearly universal in the United States in the 1960s, has given way to wild variation in the legal status of (and thus consumer access to) DEMs from state to state (see chapter 1). For midwives, issues of quantification, measurability, and marketability in terms of their public image center primarily on outcome. Over time, MANA had accumulated a database of the outcomes of 14,000 births, but this data was not considered epidemiologically valid because it was voluntarily and retrospectively submitted, leaving the results open to the charge that midwives had simply not sent in any bad outcomes they may have had. In 1999 the NARM board decided to address this problem by requiring that every CPM submit a prospective form for every client she accepted in the year 2000, and then account for the outcome of each of those births. Participation in this endeavor, which became known as the CPM2000 Statistics Project, was made mandatory for recertification as a CPM (which must be done every three years). The outcome forms had to be verified by the client whose birth they describe. In this way, the members of the NARM board and the MANA statistics committee intended to generate outcome data for CPMs that meets epidemiological standards for validity. In a sense, they "bet the company" that the outcomes would be good; if they were not, the public image of the CPM and her value as a health care commodity would suffer accordingly.

Preliminary results of the CPM2000 project were presented at the 2001 and 2002 meetings of the American Public Health Association (Johnson and Daviss 2001) and the 2001 and 2003 MANA conventions, and in 2005 were published in the *British Medical Journal* (Johnson and Daviss 2005). Three hundred fifty CPMs sent in data on over 7,000 courses of care. The transport rates from homes (or birth centers) to a hospital were 12.1 percent, meaning that out of every 100 women who started out intending to give birth at home, eighty-eight did so successfully and twelve were transported. Half of the transfers were for failure to progress, pain relief, or maternal exhaustion, and the midwife considered the transfer urgent in only 3.6 percent of intended homebirths. (When a homebirth mother lives thirty minutes from a hospital, the time from start of transport to cesarean is that same thirty minutes. Inside the hospital, the time from "decision to incision" is also about thirty minutes.) The cesarean rate was 3.7 percent, and the perinatal mortality rate (PNMR), which is the most critically scrutinized figure, was two in 1,000 (1.7 in 1,000 without breeches), equivalent to what it is for nurse-midwives attending homebirths and for physicians attending low-risk births in hospitals. This study shows that planned homebirth attended by a CPM is as safe as hospital birth for low-risk women, and a good deal less interventive. These good outcomes, which demonstrate safe and effective care, will now be included in every legislative package and will become a major marketing tool.

As I have tracked the evolution of the CPM, I have wondered with fascination at what point, if ever, MANA would evolve into a professional organization requiring CPM certification for voting membership. Conversations about creating a separate organization representing CPMs began around 1997, but were usually squelched with the argument that such an organization would generate a further fracturing of an already over-fractured midwifery community. With only 882 members, MANA could hardly afford to lose one-third or more of them to a separate organization. In 1999, yet another problem became visible. While ACNM's membership was growing by 500 or more a year, as new students graduating from the forty-five existing nurse-midwifery programs became full voting members, MANA's membership had hovered at between 700 and 1,000 for years. Part of the problem, it turned out, was that only about one-half of the new CPMs belonged to MANA. All the members of the NARM board are longtime members of MANA and were concerned by this trend. So the NARM board decided to run an ad in the spring 2000 edition of the CPM News; here is how it read:

Numbers Matter!

MANA is the only national organization that is open to all midwives.
The ACNM's membership has surpassed 8000 while MANA's membership has held steady at around 1000 for nine years. In order to continue to provide an effective counterbalance to the medicalization of midwifery, and to promote the Midwifery Model of Care and the CPM, MANA must grow! Only half of all CPMs currently belong to MANA.
JOIN MANA, SO THAT WE CAN STAND TOGETHER AND BE COUNTED!
Benefits of membership include:
The MANA News—a primary source of information about political issues affecting CPMs.
Ensuring that MANA represents the interests of CPMs.
Being part of the Sisterhood of Midwives.

Fostering midwifery as a social movement.
Helping to preserve out-of-hospital birth.
Being counted in the national tally of direct-entry midwives.
ASK NOT WHAT MANA CAN DO FOR YOU—
ASK WHAT YOU CAN DO FOR MIDWIFERY BY JOINING MANA!!

It is an ironic twist that its concern with numbers has placed MANA, whose members created CPM certification, in the position of having to market itself to CPMs. Querying those CPMS who hesitated to join MANA, I found that many of them preferred to pay membership dues to their state associations, which represented them as regulated professionals or were lobbying to make them so; they did not perceive membership in MANA as relevant to their concerns as professionals. This situation represents a further transformation in American direct-entry midwifery, demonstrating that a significant portion of CPMs are more committed to the professionalizing enterprise than to the social movement (see Daviss 2001, and chapter 12 of this volume) and/or to local political struggles over national issues (Christa Craven, personal communication, 2005).

Potential need for a separate organization for CPMs became manifest during the attempt that nurse- and direct-entry midwives are currently making for legislation in Massachusetts (see chapter 9), a move intended to heal the breach created in New York by regulating both types of midwives under the same state midwifery board. Legislators understand professional organizations and the official standards they set. The Massachusetts CNMs could point to national practice standards set by ACNM, but CPMs could not because although MANA had set practice standards similar to those of ACNM, MANA is not a professional organization that requires certification for membership. So the direct-entry midwives of Massachusetts felt the need to create a national organization requiring CPM certification for membership that could set specific standards for CPMs. (Not only are such standards reassuring to legislators, but they also help midwives themselves retain control over their profession—a better situation than having standards set for them by regulatory groups with non-midwife members.) A new CTF meeting was held at MANA 2001 in Albuquerque, New Mexico; the discussion revolved around whether the new CPM organization should be independent or should be a section of MANA, albeit with its own independent governing board. At the time, consensus crystallized around the latter option. The thirty or so midwives at the task force meeting wanted to honor the need of CPMs for their own organization and representation without fracturing MANA. But many interested parties were not present at that meeting (it occurred shortly after 9/11), so the discussion continued, ultimately resulting in the creation of a CPM section within MANA *and* an independent organization, the National Association of Certified Professional Midwives (NACPM).[7] Their strong and inclusive consensus tradition led MANA members to form both, and then see which one would receive the most grassroots support. This interesting development reflects the identity struggles of the new CPMs—are they primarily invested in the professionalizing/commodifying processes of certification and licensure that the NACPM represents or in the social movement of midwifery and its inclusivity that MANA represents? Or will they accomplish and support both simultaneously? As of the date of this writing (May 2005), the NACPM had only about 100 members, but its board, with the help of an advisory committee, has completed national standards of practice for CPMs (www.nacpm.net), which have already been of help in successful legislation in Utah and Virginia and proposed legislation in Wisconsin, as well as in Massachusetts. The CPM section of MANA appears to have few members; time will tell if it will continue to exist.

Legality, Illegality, and the Price of Licensure   The multibillion-dollar international drug trade makes it clear that it is not absolutely necessary for a commodity to be legal to be successful in creating and reaching its market niche. Where consumer demand exists, entrepreneurs will try to fill that demand even if it means breaking the law and risking jail. In most such cases, there is nothing noble about this enterprise; it's simply about money and power. In contrast, the early "lay" midwives and contemporary "direct-entry" midwives (many of whom are the same people) flouted the law and continue to do so in some states, not out of a quest for money and power, but out of the moral imperative they feel to keep the homebirth option open to the women in their communities. Members of social movements regularly break the law in the name of their cause; part of the point is to get the laws changed to reflect the realities the social movement is trying to generate. Commodification forms a major part of the strategy midwives and their consumer allies employ to obtain legality.

In many such states, groups of midwifery supporters, often called Friends of Midwives (as in Massachusetts Friends of Midwives), work to help direct-entry midwives gain legal status. At the national level, a consumer group called Citizens for Midwifery (CfM) has generated a number of helpful publications, from brochures on the Midwives Model of Care (MMOC) to information on lobbying and working with media (www.cfmidwifery.org). CfM focuses on networking, sharing information and resources, promoting the MMOC, encouraging public education efforts, and helping state organizations with legislative initiatives. CfM's stated vision is "to see that the Midwives Model of Care is recognized as the optimal model of care in all settings and available to all women" (Susan Hodges, personal communication, 2003). Through such consumer support groups, direct-entry midwifery's market niche loudly proclaims its existence in highly public ways. For example, when DEMs are arrested or persecuted, or are actively promoting legislation or trying to change an unfavorable bill, they are often helped to win their cases by the public demonstrations consumer groups sponsor and the press coverage they generate.

When lay practitioners become professionals and obtain the benefits of legalization and licensure (which include not only insurance reimbursement, but also not having to worry about being arrested), there is usually a price to be paid. Licensure means regulation, and regulation means restrictions on one's decision-making power and thus on one's autonomy. When DEMs practiced illegally, they did pretty much everything they wanted to do—it was all illegal, so what was the difference? Thus their practices often included attending women choosing homebirth who would be classified in the hospital as high risk, most especially women with babies in the breech position and women giving birth to twins. While most entry-level DEMs would themselves consider these to be high-risk conditions meriting transport, some highly experienced DEMs have gained special expertise in attending such births and are often more skilled at it than most physicians. (Increasingly, vaginal birth after cesarean (VBAC) is considered high-risk in hospitals; some DEMs do not consider them so and continue to attend them at home.)

Nevertheless, getting state legislatures to legalize DEMs and state boards to regulate them in ways that actually allow them to continue to practice almost always requires certain compromises; most often it is these three kinds of births (VBACs, breeches, and twins) that midwives must give up the right to attend out-of-hospital. Before regulation, attendance at such births was a matter of a midwife's individual choice; after regulation, they would be breaking the law to do so, and in danger of losing their license. So midwives seeking commodification have had to decide which is more important: full autonomy or being able to sleep at night instead of lying awake in fear of a knock on the door.[8] Most of the time they compromise and accept these sorts of restrictions in return for the benefits of licensure; in other words, most of the time they are willing to pay the price of commodification.

Some midwives, however, refuse to pay that price. In Pennsylvania and other states, such midwives call themselves "plain midwives," to differentiate themselves from the professionalizing direct-entry mid-wives. Few such midwives belong to MANA. Often they are members of religious groups; in general, they just want to serve their communities according to their particular customs and beliefs, preferring to remain completely outside of the system. Although they run the risk of being arrested for practicing medicine without a license, in actuality they are so few in number and so adept at avoiding publicity that they are usually left alone; to them that seems better than the closer scrutiny that comes with legalization and regulation. In other words, content to remain in the cultural margins, the plain midwives reject both professionalization and commodification, while their direct-entry colleagues actively seek, through both of these strategies, to enter the mainstream. After sometimes bitter rhetorical battles with plain midwives in their states, DEMs often decide to accept or actively generate a fissioning of their social movement by clearly differentiating themselves from midwives who do not want any kind of licensure or regulation. Mary Lay has documented this process in detail for Minnesota, a state in which the professionalizing DEMs formed a midwifery guild and eventually won state licensure based on NARM certification. One of the rhetorical strategies they employed was actively distancing themselves from their nonprofessionalized colleagues. Lay (2000:78) notes that during the legislative hearings:

> the Minnesota direct-entry midwives made clear that the midwifery community was divided, and to some extent took advantage of that division. As those involved in the hearings struggled to define the "good midwife," they did so by acknowledging an "other" midwife who seemed not to rely on medical knowledge to screen her homebirth clients and who was in essence silenced in the hearings.

Such silencing is not atypical of the results of successful commodification processes. Midwives who succeed in professionalizing and obtaining licensure often find it both ironic and intensely distressing that their mainstream status results in the establishment of exclusionary hierarchies in a community where before, there were none. In Washington state, for example, in the early 1980s DEMs succeeded in gaining legalization and licensure via an old law on the books that allowed for midwives to be licensed if they graduated from a formal vocational school. The Seattle Midwifery School (SMS) thus became the first, and is by now the best-known three-year DEM vocational program. Its founders were countercultural self-help feminists who thought they were going to end up in jail for practicing midwifery, but ended up founding a school instead. The downside was that no DEM could become legal and licensed in Washington without graduating from this school, which takes three years and costs over $25,000 in tuition. The result has been the hierarchization of non-nurse midwifery in the state: SMS graduates, who call themselves direct-entry midwives, are legal, licensed, regulated, and insurance-reimbursed. The "other midwife" thus created is called a *lay midwife*; she can practice legally only if she does not accept any money in payment for her services. Thus the victory of some has been the defeat of others. Because this result was never their intention, the directors and staff of SMS have been trying for years (and have recently succeeded) to get the legislature to open other routes to licensure in Washington state. In one sense, opening such routes is like shooting themselves in the foot, as it may limit the number of applicants they receive, but their commitment to the spirit and inclusive ethos of the social movement remains strong, and they would prefer to qualify, even compromise, the success of their commodification rather than continue to live with the exclusions and hierarchies it has created.

This respect for and appreciation of nonprofessionalizing lay or plain midwives is one of the primary reasons MANA members voted at their Florida convention in 2000 to keep their membership open to all midwives. Licensed midwives responsible to the state often find themselves torn between parents' wishes and regulatory protocols. They stand to lose their licenses if they accept out-of-protocol home-birth clients (e.g., VBACs, breeches, or twins). Sometimes licensed midwives take such cases anyway; other times they refer such clients to the unlicensed, illegal, or alegal "lay" midwives nearby (if they respect those midwives' skills), who are often termed "renegade midwives" because they do not follow peer group protocols, but rather consider the wishes of the parents to be primary (see chapter 11). The professionalizing members of MANA, who used to have the same priorities, regard these lay midwives with an odd combination of distrust and wistfulness, but they would never want to exclude such midwives from membership in MANA. Having to turn away certain clients one has the skills to attend is the price many pay for licensure, and there is a great deal of respect within MANA for skilled and responsible unlicensed midwives who are unwilling to pay that price and so will serve the clients licensed midwives are supposed to refuse.

Purchasability, Marketing, and Brand Name Recognition

Certified Professional Midwives (CPMs) are skilled professionals qualified to provide the Midwives Model of Care, which is appropriate for the majority of births.

—NARM brochure, *The Certified Professional Midwife*

Commodities are sold and bought. This kind of purchasability came after the fact to many lay midwifery pioneers who began their work out of an ethic of service to women. Over time and across the country, these early pioneers evolved into seasoned professionals with set fees, bookkeeping systems, and a desire for insurance reimbursement. But to be bought, commodities must be readily available. In states where direct-entry midwifery remains illegal, their practice is very much underground and they can be extremely hard to find. In contrast, in states where they are fully legal, licensed, and regulated, midwives' advertisements often appear in bold letters in the yellow pages. For example, an ad for the Austin Area Birthing Center in Austin, Texas, reads as follows:

Create an Ideal Birth for You and Your Baby:
With Gentleness and Individual Care in a beautiful, warm, homelike environment!

  • Staffed with Certified Professional Midwives and Licensed Nurses
  • Medical backup
  • Covered by most insurance
  • Spacious birthing rooms with fire place & waterbirth tub
  • Complete care from prenatal through birth
  • Over 1800 successful births since 1981

Childbirth the Way It Should Be!

Fees for midwifery services vary widely from rural to urban areas. For a quick example, in Austin, direct-entry midwives charge $3,000 for one entire course of care, including prenatal care, labor and delivery, and postpartum follow-up. Although their fees are markedly lower in most areas than those charged by obstetricians and CNMs, DEMs remain at a disadvantage because in most states their fees must be paid out of pocket, a fact that often limits their client base to the middle class. Lack of insurance reimbursement has in some places been a powerful motivator for midwives to obtain NARM certification and to drive for legislation recognizing the CPM as a legitimate health care provider. In this endeavor, cost-effectiveness is one of their major supporting points. Because DEMs employ few technological interventions and practice out of hospital, from a governmental perspective they are a cost-effective alternative to highly expensive obstetrical care. But the costs of state testing and licensure are high, so the expenses of the boards that must regulate licensed midwives can be prohibitive. Thus one of NARM's most effective marketing strategies has been pointing out to state agencies how much money they can save if they let NARM do the testing and credentialing instead of the state. A fact sheet developed by NARM, dated August 12, 1999, reads as follows:

HOW CAN THE CERTIFIED PROFESSIONAL MIDWIFE (CPM) CREDENTIAL SAVE GOVERNMENT AGENCIES MONEY ?

When the CPM is used as the state credential for midwives practicing in out-of-hospital settings, government agencies can:

1. Avoid expending valuable staff time to validate the education of direct-entry midwives who practice in primarily out-of-hospital settings;
2. Avoid test construction and maintenance costs associated with the creation of a licensure examination;
3. Save the costs of test administration;
4. Save the costs of continuing education monitoring for re-licensure.

IT'S A GOOD DEAL FOR THE MIDWIVES! IT'S A $$ SAVER FOR THE STATE!

Through such promotional literature, NARM seeks to demonstrate not just its cost-effectiveness, but also its user-friendliness to state agencies, whose beleagured workers are often delighted to be relieved of some of their administrative burdens.

Of course, user-friendliness has become a buzzword for accessibility in technology; likewise, brand name recognition is often an essential ingredient of a commodity's success. User-friendliness has been a central distinguishing feature of midwives' practices from the beginning, one that they have long branded *woman-centered care* in order to contrast their approach to that of physicians, who often place their own needs or the requirements of the institution above those of the mother. Another identifying phrase, a sort of generic label adopted by all American midwives, has been "the midwifery model of care." These two phrases are universally used by both nurse- and direct-entry midwives. But as NARM crystallized its certification, its members and many others worked for months to develop and copyright their own "brand name," which turned out to be a definition of what they originally called the Midwifery Model of Care (adding the capitalization to distinguish its wording as uniquely theirs).

This focus on the model of care rather than the midwife was a contribution from consumers, as Susan Hodges, president of the national consumer group Citizens for Midwifery, recounts:

When representatives of MANA, MEAC, and NARM began having regular phone calls (spring of 1996), one of the first things that came up was the need for some way to succinctly describe what we were all working for. The idea was to come up with a definition of *midwife*. It was Citizens for Midwifery that suggested a definition of a kind of care rather than of a midwife. As consumers, we were very aware that the kind of care you get is much more important than the letters after someone's name. [We knew] that there was tremendous variation among midwives in terms of how they practice. So it was the consumers who strongly suggested a definition of the model of care, which has turned out to be much more useful than a definition of midwife. (Personal communication, 2003)

As MANA, NARM, MEAC, and CfM began to organize their marketing strategies around this model, they were increasingly disconcerted by the fact that the word "midwifery" was not user-friendly: many people, including legislators, had a problem pronouncing it, which often resulted in embarrassment and a general turnoff on the legislator's part. On the advice of a professional marketing organization they had hired to help them revamp their public image, they changed the name to "Midwives Model of Care," trademarking the label and the brief description of that model on which they had all agreed:

The Midwives Model of Care is based on the fact that pregnancy and
    birth are normal life events.
The Midwives Model of Care includes:
  • monitoring the physical, psychological, and social well-being of
    the mother throughout the childbearing cycle;
  • providing the mother with individualized education, counsel-
    ing, and prenatal care, continuous hands-on assistance during
    labor and delivery, and postpartum support;
  • minimizing technological interventions;
  • identifying and referring women who require obstetrical atten-
    tion.
The application of this woman-centered model has been proven to
    reduce the incidence of birth injury, trauma, and cesarean
    section. (NARM, *How To Become a CPM*, 2002:2).

This description was originally copyrighted in May 1996 by the Midwifery Task Force (a nonprofit corporation), under the title "Midwifery Model of Care." It was recopyrighted in 2000 with the new title

"Midwives Model of Care." This brief description of the MMOC appears in all NARM literature, including its consumer brochures and legislative lobbying packets. A much more detailed description of what a woman should expect from a practitioner promising this kind of care is published in CfM brochures. Many thousands of copies have been distributed in the United States and around the world. As the brochure points out, any practitioner, including physicians, can provide this model of care. This focus on a user-friendly and consumer-oriented brand name—the Midwives Model of Care—instead of on the midwives themselves, is an intentional strategy suggested by consumers and agreed on by midwives. This consensus arose to focus more attention on the pregnant woman as the deserving recipient of a certain kind of care, and less on the self-promotion of midwives who seek to provide that kind of care (even though the ultimate effect may be the same). Through this brand name choice, CPMs remind themselves, even through their self-marketing, that their primary mission is to mothers.

Design and Redesign: Commodities as Responsive to Consumer Demands and Market Trends

> The term "midwifery consumer" . . . implies a certain agency and choice on the part of women having midwifery care that has always been important to midwifery. Indeed, the consumer-based campaign for choices in childbirth was a key factor that fueled midwifery as a social movement over the last several decades. The idea of the midwifery consumer, however, is not simply a result of the self-conscious feminist agenda of woman-centred care and the critique of biomedicine. It also speaks to the political economy of reproduction . . . in the context of late capitalism and demographic transition, specifically, the trend towards having fewer children later in life and the trend towards treating pregnancy and childbirth as valuable experiences.
>
> —Margaret MacDonald, "The Role of Midwifery Clients in the New Midwifery in Canada: Postmodern Negotiations with Medical Technology"

Successful commodities in today's market frequently shape-shift in response to technological advances, consumer trends, and market demands. Computers were beige and boxy until the iMac set new standards for attractiveness in computer design, reshaping consumer expectations for how computers should look. The ugly but functional toaster from Target is elegantly redesigned; the software upgraded; the dishwasher computerized. The "redesign" of direct-entry midwives in response to consumer trends has, to date, been most obvious in Ontario, where the legalization of midwifery in 1993 was accomplished through an alliance of nurse- and lay midwives who united behind a model of midwifery practice based on the principle that "the midwife follows the mother." In other words, women select their site of birth—home, birth center, or hospital—and the midwife will attend them there. As a result, Ontario's former lay midwives, who practiced only outside of the hospital for two decades when midwifery was a social movement and not yet a profession, have had to familiarize themselves with hospital protocols and technologies. And, as documented by MacDonald (2001), Sharpe (2004), and Daviss (2001), Ontario midwives' client base has shifted from homebirthers dedicated to the holistic principles of the midwifery and homebirth movements to consumers who have had no involvement in these movements and may simply want more personalized care.

In particular, Margaret MacDonald (2001) points to the agentic role midwifery consumers are playing in reshaping the nature of Ontario midwifery. North American consumers display increasing familiarity with and respect for information obtained through high technology; when they choose midwifery care, they add to this familiarity the midwifery principle of fully informed choice. The result is that even when midwives themselves recommend against certain technologies, such as repeat ultrasounds or certain kinds of genetic testing (e.g., the triple screen), consumers often choose them anyway, and midwives find themselves the go-betweens in a game they are very uncomfortable playing. As Canadian midwife and social scientist Mary Sharpe (2001) expressed it:

> Midwives felt that the requirement to offer testing shifted their care towards a focus of verifying rather than assuming that pregnancy is normal, and were concerned that midwives themselves might be moving away from a wellness model towards a pathology-oriented model, relying on ultrasounds and an increased use of the system and spending less time on woman-generated discussions relating to the woman's feelings, questions, and circumstances.

In addition to the shape shifting they are undergoing in response to consumer demands, Ontario midwives find themselves changing even more as they attend more births in hospitals. In other words, the market for midwives to attend hospital births, which is larger than the market for midwives to attend homebirths, is slowly but inexorably reshaping the nature of Ontario midwifery. Sharpe describes their experiences at the beginning of their entry into the hospital.

[M]idwives. . . . were on a steep learning curve with respect to orientation to hospital procedures, protocols, equipment and paperwork, as well as client admission and discharge. While attending their first hospital births as primary caregivers following legislation, it would take two midwives up to four hours following the birth to accomplish the usual postpartum care and the new paperwork. . . . Comments from midwives expressed how they felt their practices were ruled by these new procedures.

> "The hospital is the most disturbing situation to me because I'm finding it difficult to feel like I'm both fulfilling my expected role as a health care professional in the hierarchy of the system in the hospital as well as just being with someone which is what I feel my primary role is." (Anna)

Some midwives felt closely monitored and scrutinized in hospital, and that the hospital staff was testing them, waiting to assess their level of competence. There was great pressure to be very careful about what they did. . . . In exchange for hospital privileges, some midwives felt compromised, now required to comply with certain hospital rules with which they didn't agree. Some midwives implied that they had to "behave like good girls" and "move into line" in order to get what they wanted for their clients in the hospital setting and to maintain their credibility. . . . The definition of being a good midwife in the hospital had changed for one midwife: before the legislation it had to do with her labour supporting skills, now, with her clinical care and charting. Another noted that experiences in the hospital were influencing how she worked at homebirths in that she didn't have as much hands on caring for the woman in either setting. . . . The client of one midwife who previously appreciated the spiritual aspect of her work, hired a "spiritual midwife." She wondered if she was now the "clinical midwife."

Decades of hospital practice have also clearly had their effect on American nurse-midwives; an examination of birth certificate data shows that CNMs' use of some technological interventions, such as electronic fetal monitoring, has been rising at the same rates as that of physicians (Curtin 1999). My interview data indicate that nurse-midwives' use of hospital technologies is influenced by the degree to which they are taught to rely on such technologies during their midwifery education, by pressures placed on them by other hospital personnel to utilize high technologies, and by the choices and demands of their clients, many of whom feel reassured by the application of high technologies to their births and actively choose their use (see Davis-Floyd 2003). This brief glance at the influence of hospital practice on Canadian midwives and American nurse-midwives clearly illustrates how the market and its consumers can reshape the nature of the commodity.

Predictably, American DEMs are often heard to suggest that CNMs have sold out to or been co-opted by the medical system, noting that while out-of-hospital practice certainly limits DEMs' accessibility as a health care commodity, it also significantly limits the extent to which they can be co-opted into overmedicalization. While they have done some shape-shifting themselves in response to market trends and consumer demands, as long as they remain outside of hospitals, DEMs may be able to successfully limit the degree of change they undergo as they professionalize and commodify.

Commodities as Embedded in the Global Political Economy

American DEMs respect Ontario's former lay midwives for their success at achieving full integration into the Canadian health-care system and American nurse-midwives for being there for women who choose hospital birth, but DEMs are simultaneously aware that their purely out-of-hospital independent midwifery system is unique. Recently I coauthored, with a group of international scholars, a chapter comparing midwifery education in the United States, Canada, and Europe (Benoit et al 2001), which we organized around the three basic models of midwifery education: apprenticeship, vocational training, and university education. As I worked on the sections on the United States, I was fascinated to note that because of the American DEMs, the United States is the only Euro-American country in which all three basic models of midwifery training are alive and flourishing. All over the developed world, I have heard American direct-entry midwives extolled as examples of "holistic midwifery," "pure midwifery," and "real midwifery." Many long-professionalized midwives in the United Kingdom, Italy, Australia, and other Western countries consider American direct-entry midwives to represent the heart or essence of what midwifery should be, and engage in long discussions about how they might try to recapture some of the spirituality and woman-centeredness that they feel they have lost in their professionalism. Thus American midwives feel a special responsibility not only to themselves but also to the world to preserve what they have created. Their sense of the value of their independent midwifery system and out-of-hospital knowledge base, in relation to midwives everywhere, has led the members of the NARM board to make the CPM an international certification, available to midwives in any country who might choose to adopt it. Some beginnings have been made: the Canadian province of Manitoba recognizes NARM certification, and at present there are forty-five CPMs in practice in Canada. Four midwives in Mexico have become CPMs (Naoli Vinaver, Alison Bastien, Marian Tudela, and Laura Cao Romero; see Davis-Floyd 2001). One CPM per country is in practice in France, Ireland, South Africa, Namibia, and Hungary. While there is no government recognition of the CPM in these countries, the fact that it is an American-created credential gives it some authoritative status. In addition, as I mentioned in chapter 1, NARM has created a streamlined route for British midwives to be able to obtain CPM certification (which includes documenting attendance at the requisite ten out-of-hospital births and passing the NARM exam). If this process continues, the CPM may become an option for all European Union midwives who wish to practice in the United States attending out-of-hospital births.

CONCLUSION: MAINTAINING A TIRELESS VIGILANCE

> With legislation, midwives are learning new texts and engaging in new rulings. Are these rulings slowing us down, fixing us gradually and inexorably into new relationships and new ways of acting and being? Or do these rulings provide structure and support and free us? . . . The bottom line for midwives is: can legislation enhance creativity and expand possibilities for women and midwifery or limit them? . . . We need continuously to hold our behaviour in question. . . . We require a tireless vigilance to maintain what some would say are midwifery's gains, and others would call our compromises. And we must continue to examine our practices in order to recognize how we, for better or for worse, are implicated in the rulings of our profession.
>
> **—Mary Sharpe, "Exploring Legislated Ontario Midwifery"**

I have often heard members of NARM and MANA echo Sharpe's words as they work to maintain a tireless vigilance over the gains they achieve and the losses they suffer in their professionalizing and commodifying enterprises. What I have observed over and over is that every time these midwives face a choice between enhancing their public image as health-care commodities and compromising their values, their practices, or their training programs, they let go of image and concentrate on what works and what, in their eyes, preserves the essence of who they are. Speaking for all those who participated in the development of CPM certification (during a 1997 panel discussion), direct-entry midwives Pam Weaver, Elizabeth Davis, and Alice Sammon exclaimed, "We did it! We actually managed to develop a certification that encompasses everything we hold dear!"

To be sure, many midwives who have struggled to fill out NARM's detailed forms, to come up with the required documentation, or to pay NARM's fees, have done their share of complaining about the number and complexity of the hoops they are asked to jump through, as have those who failed the NARM exam on their first and even second attempts and had to take it again. But I have watched this process long enough to be awed by the lack of controversy now surrounding it among MANA members, who have moved from initial deep suspicion of any standardizing moves to acceptance of the CPM as a credential that supports them far more than it gets in their way. As longtime homebirth midwife Sharon Wells put it, "the CPM is the only ground we have to stand on." Even the thirty direct-entry students I have inter-viewed, instead of complaining about NARM requirements, were happy to have specific goals to work toward. Several of them noted to me that apprentice-trained midwives are often not sure at what point during their training they can actually start to call themselves midwives instead of students. The arrival of their CPM certificate in the mail has become a concrete marker for them that they have earned the right to say, "I am a midwife."

Nevertheless, debates continue in various states between midwives willing and unwilling to compromise in order to gain a toehold in the technocracy, with one group accusing the other of selling out to get in. Many midwives mourn some of their lost freedoms to serve their clients as they saw best (see chapter 11) while they rejoice in their legal status and the many new clients who are seeking them out because they are legal and insurance-reimbursed.

When I focus on the big picture, what I see, all things considered, is that American direct-entry midwives, even as they professionalize and commodify, are simultaneously striving to maintain themselves as the woman-centered, family-serving, intuition-honoring, birth-trusting, and system-flouting guides and guardians of birth that they have always been. Clearly, commodification can be more than a means of selling out to capitalism. When qualified according to the values of a particular group newly perceiving itself as a commodity, it can also be a creative way of generating needed services that offer consumers a rich array of alternatives, precluding homogenization and facilitating the heterogenization of individual choice.

ENDNOTES

1. This chapter is a revised version of a chapter that appears in *Consuming Motherhood*, eds. Janelle Taylor, Danielle Wozniak, and Linda Layne (2004). I wish to thank anthro-pologists Linda Layne, Janelle Taylor, and Danielle Wozniak, CPMs Shannon Anton, Elizabeth Davis, Abby Kinne, Carol Nelson, Holly Scholles, and Alice Sammon; con-sumer advocates Susan Hodges and Jo Anne Myers-Ciecko; and sociologists Christine Barbara Johnson and Betty Anne Daviss (who is also a midwife) for their helpful com-ments and suggestions.

2. As Margaret Reid put it in "Sisterhood and Professionalization: A Case Study of the American Lay Midwife" (1989:229), "The first transformation to occur was often an internal one, a change in self-perception or self-image. . . . It was always a significant change, as one midwife's comments illustrate: 'it took me a long time [to realize]—I want some money for this. I'm spending maybe sixty hours a week, I'm away from my family . . . and I want to be compensated.' And with that grew the birth of a professional."

3. At that time, the members of the NARM board, who held primary responsibility for developing CPM certification, included Sondra Abdullah-Zaimah, Shannon Anton, Robbie Davis-Floyd (since 1994, I have served as the consumer representative on the NARM board; my role has been largely advisory), Alice Sammon, Suzanne Suarez, Ruth Walsh, Pam Weaver, and Sharon Wells. Key committee heads included Ann Cairns, Susan Hodges, Debbie Pulley, Abby Kinne, and Sandra MorningStar.

4. I was invited to become a member of the NARM board in 1994, in the position of consumer representative. Before I accepted the invitation, I made it clear that if I accepted, I would want to be studying NARM's work even as I participated in it, a request that was approved by the board members at the time. The members of the NARM board and the Certification Task Force have always been tolerant of, and helpful with, my dual roles as participant and observer, and I would like to express my appreciation to them for accepting me in both capacities.

5. Regarding the IV question, a large majority of survey respondents indicated that IV insertion should not be required for entry-level practice, and so it was not. Another fascinating result of the survey was in the category of Well-Woman Care. Respondents indicated that they did not wish the category as a whole to be required; however, they did wish all the skills listed under it to be required. At first puzzled by this response, the NARM board eventually ascertained that this meant that practicing midwives wanted entry-level midwives to be able to perform all these skills, but not to be required to offer general well-woman (gynecological) care.

6. NARM's inclusivity is perhaps best demonstrated by the Special Circumstances category, which is designed to allow midwives trained in other countries, *grand midwives* who began practice before 1965, or midwives trained through other unusual circumstances to apply. Special Circumstances applicants must document attendance at a minimum of seventy-five births in the last ten years (ten of which must have occurred in the preceding two years) and fulfill an extensive set of further requirements; they are individually evaluated by a special NARM committee. In addition, for the first two years of CPM certification, NARM held open an Experienced Midwife category as a mechanism to quickly evaluate and certify experienced practicing midwives. Qualification for the Experienced Midwife category required being in practice for more than five years and attending a minimum of seventy-five births as primary. Although this move was criticized by some members of ACNM and others as an easy way of granting certification to the "members of the club," it proved to be a critical and viable transition strategy for creating a base of qualified midwives who could then mentor student midwives through their certification process.

7. CPMs are not required to belong to MANA (or the NACPM). CNMs and CMs are not required to belong to the ACNM, but they are intensively socialized during their educational processes to think of ACNM as their professional organization, and the vast majority (approximately seventy-five percent) of them do. In contrast, MANA remains aprofessional, trying to meet the needs of both professionally licensed or certified midwives and those who are not, an increasingly difficult task.

8. Ohio midwife Abby J. Kinne CPM points to another crucial issue regarding midwifery autonomy even where state regulations do not exist. (In Ohio, direct-entry midwifery is not legally defined, but not prohibited.)

It is not just fear of the knock on the door—for many of us, it is the trade-off for making the midwifery model of care more accessible to the homebirth community at large. Although Ohio has yet to institute regulations (which are quite likely, in the end, to restrict our ability to attend VBACs, twins, and breeches) some of us already are limited in such special circumstances in order to maintain good relations with supportive backup physicians. You can choose to help these moms and risk losing good backup, or you can make a concession to your backup doc so that you can continue to provide good backup to the vast majority of our clients who do not face these rare circumstances. It is a major dilemma for us. (Personal communication, 2003.)

REFERENCES

Adorno, T., and M. Horkheimer. 1999 [1972]. *Dialectic of Enlightenment*. New York: Continuum.

Appadurai, Arjun, ed. 1986. *The Social Life of Things: Commodities in Cultural Perspective*. Cambridge: Cambridge University Press.

Arms, Suzanne. 1975. *Immaculate Deception*. New York: Houghton Mifflin.

Baudrillard, J., ed. 1988. *Selected Writings*. Stanford, CA: Stanford University Press.

Benoit, Cecilia, Robbie Davis-Floyd, Edwin van Teijlingen, Sirpa Wrede, Jane Sandall, and Janneli Miller. 2001. "Designing Midwives: A Transnational Comparison of Educational Models." In *Birth by Design: The Social Shaping of Maternity Care in Euro-America*, ed. Raymond DeVries, Edwin van Teijlingen, Sirpa Wrede, and Cecilia Benoit. New York: Routledge.

Bourdieu, Pierre. 1984. *Distinction: A Social Critique of the Judgment of Tastes*. Cambridge, MA: Harvard University Press.

Bourgeault, Ivy, Cecilia Benoit, and Robbie Davis-Floyd, eds. 2004. *Reconceiving Midwifery: The New Canadian Model of Care*. Toronto: McGill-Queens University Press.

Bourgeault, Ivy, and Mary Fynes. 1997. "Integrating Lay and Nurse-Midwifery into the U.S. and Canadian Health Care Systems." *Social Science and Medicine* 44(7):1051–1063.

Bruner, Joseph P., Susan B. Drummond, Anna L. Meenan, and Ina May Gaskin. 1998. "All-Fours Maneuver for Reducing Shoulder Dystocia During Labor." *Journal of Reproductive Medicine* 43:439–443.

Cartwright, Elizabeth. 1998. "The Logic of Heartbeats: Electronic Fetal Monitoring and Biomedically Constructed Birth." In *Cyborg Babies: From Techno-Sex to Techno-Tots*, ed. Robbie Davis-Floyd and Joseph Dumit, 240–254. New York: Routledge.

Casper, Monica J. 1998. *The Making of the Unborn Patient: A Social Anatomy of Fetal Surgery*. New Brunswick, NJ: Rutgers University Press.

Curtin, Sally C. 1999. "Recent Changes in Birth Attendant, Place of Birth, and the Use of Obstetric Interventions." *Journal of Nurse-Midwifery* 44(4):349–354.

Davis, Elizabeth. 1997 [1983]. *Heart and Hands: A Midwife's Guide to Pregnancy and Birth*, 3rd edition. Berkeley, CA: Celestial Arts.

Davis-Floyd, Robbie E. 1987. "Obstetric Training as a Rite of Passage." *Medical Anthropology Quarterly* 1(3):288–318.

———. 1992. *Birth as an American Rite of Passage*. Berkeley: University of California Press.

———. 1998a. "The Ups, Downs, and Interlinkages of Nurse- and Direct-Entry Midwifery: Status, Practice, and Education." In *Getting an Education: Paths to Becoming a Midwife*, 4th ed., ed. Jan Tritten and Joel Southern, 67–118. Eugene, OR: Midwifery Today. Also available at www.davis-floyd.com.

———. 1998b. "Types of Midwifery Training: An Anthropological Overview." In *Getting an Education: Paths to Becoming a Midwife*, 4th ed., ed. Jan Tritten and Joel Southern, 119–133. Eugene, OR: Midwifery Today. Also available at www.davis-floyd.com.

———. 1999. "Some Thoughts on Bridging the Gap between Nurse- and Direct-Entry Midwives." *Midwifery Today*, March.

———. 2001. "*La Partera Profesional*: Articulating Identity and Cultural Space for a New Kind of Midwife in Mexico." In "Daughters of Time: The Shifting Identities of Contemporary Midwives," ed. Robbie Davis-Floyd, Sheila Cosminsky, and Stacy Leigh Pigg. Special issue of *Medical Anthropology* 20(2–3):185–243.

———. 2002. "The Technocratic, Humanistic, and Holistic Models of Birth." *International Journal of Gynecology & Obstetrics* 75, Supplement no. 1, S5–S23. Also available at www.davis-floyd.com.

———. 2003. "Homebirth Emergencies in the United States and Mexico: The Trouble with Transport." In "Reproduction Gone Awry," ed. Gywnne Jenkins and Marcia Inhorn. Special issue of *Social Science and Medicine* 56(9):1913–1991.

Davis-Floyd, Robbie, Sheila Cosminsky, and Stacy Leigh Pigg, eds. 2001. "Daughters of Time: The Shifting Identities of Contemporary Midwives." Special triple issue of *Medical Anthropology*, nos. 2–3/4.

Davis-Floyd, Robbie, and Joseph Dumit, eds. 1998. *Cyborg Babies: From Techno-Sex to Techno-Tots*. New York: Routledge.

Davis-Floyd, Robbie, and Carolyn Sargent, eds. 1997.*Childbirth and Authoritative Knowledge: Cross-cultural Perspectives*. Berkeley: University of California Press.

Daviss, Betty Anne. 2001. "Reforming Birth and (Re)making Midwifery in North America." In *Birth by Design: Pregnancy, Maternity Care and Midwifery in North America and Europe*, ed. Raymond DeVries, Edwin van Teijlingen, Sirpa Wrede, and Cecilia Benoit, 15–168. New York: Routledge.

De Certeau, Michelle. 1984. *The Practice of Everyday Life*. Berkeley: University of California Press.

DeVries, Raymond. 1996. *Making Midwives Legal: Childbirth, Medicine, and the Law*, 2nd ed. Columbus: Ohio State University Press.

Fiedler, Deborah Cordero, and Robbie Davis-Floyd. 2001. Entry on "Midwifery as a Reproductive Right." In the *Historical and Multicultural Encyclopedia of Female Reproductive Rights in the United States*, ed. Judith A. Baer. Westport, CT: Greenwood Press.

Frye, Anne. 1995. *Holistic Midwifery: A Comprehensive Textbook for Midwives in Homebirth Practice*, Vol. I, *Care During Pregnancy*. Portland, OR: Labyrs Press.

Gaskin, Ina May. 1990. *Spiritual Midwifery*, 3rd ed. Summertown, TN: The Book Publishing Company.

———. 1998. Personal communication. Ina May Gaskin CPM is a direct-entry midwife on the Farm in Summertown, Tennessee, editor and publisher of the *Birth Gazette*, author of two books and numerous articles, and former president of MANA. She is often referred to as "the most famous midwife in North America."

Hartouni, Valerie. 1997. *Cultural Conceptions: On Reproductive Technologies and the Remaking of Life*. Minneapolis: University of Minnesota Press.

Hazzell, Lester Dessez. 1976 [1969]. *Commonsense Childbirth*. New York: Berkeley Medallion Books.

Hebbidge, Dick. 1979. *The Meaning of Style*. London: Melthuen.

Hodges, Susan. 2003. Personal communication. Susan Hodges is a longtime consumer advocate for preserving the homebirth option for women and for the Midwives Model of Care. She is president of Citizens for Midwifery.

Houghton, Pansy, and Kate Windom. 1996a. *1995 Job Analysis of the Role of Direct-Entry Midwives*. Marlton, NJ: North American Registry of Midwives.

———. 1996b. *Executive Summary of the 1995 Job Analysis of the Role of Direct-Entry Midwives*. Copies can be obtained from the NARM Education and Advocacy Department (1-888-842-4784) or see http://www.mana.org/narm.

Johnson, Kenneth. 1997. "Randomized Controlled Trials as Authoritative Knowledge: Keeping an Ally from Becoming a Threat to North American Midwifery Practice." In *Childbirth and Authoritative Knowledge: Cross-Cultural Perspectives*, ed. Robbie Davis-Floyd and Carolyn F. Sargent, 350–365. Berkeley: University of California Press.

Johnson, Kenneth C., and Betty Anne Daviss. 2001 (October). "Results of the CPM Statistics Project 2000: A Prospective Study of Births by Certified Professional Midwives in North America." Abstract presented at the annual meeting of the American Public Health Association, Atlanta, GA.

———. "Outcomes of Planned Home Births with Certified Professional Midwives: Large Prospective Study in North America." *British Medical Journal* 330(7505): 1416, June. www.bmj.com.

Kinne, Abby. 2003. Personal communication. Abby Kinne was one of the earliest homebirth midwives in Ohio and has long been a midwifery pioneer and activist in promoting Ohio legislation for direct-entry midwives. She was the first to receive CPM certification (in November 1994). She is currently working on opening a direct-entry midwifery school near Columbus.

Kunisch, Jill 1989. "Electronic Fetal Monitors: Marketing Forces and the Resulting Controversy." In *Healing Technology: Feminist Perspectives*, ed. Kathryn Strother Ratcliff, 41–60. Ann Arbor: University of Michigan Press.

Lang, Raven. 1972. *The Birth Book*. Palo Alto, CA: Genesis Press.

Lay, Mary. 2000. *The Rhetoric of Midwifery: Gender, Knowledge, and Power*. New Brunswick, NJ: Rutgers University Press.

Layne, Linda. 2000a. "'He was a real baby with real baby things': A Material Culture Analysis of Personhood and Pregnancy Loss." *Journal of Material Culture* 5(3):321–345.

———. 2000b. "The Cultural Fix: An Anthropological Contribution to Science and Technology Studies." *Science, Technology and Human Values* 25(4):355–77.

———2000c. "Baby Things as Fetishes? Memorial Goods, Simulacra, and the 'Realness' Problem of Pregnancy Loss." In *Ideologies and Technologies of Motherhood*, ed. Helena Ragone and F. Twine, 111–138. New York: Routledge.

———. ed. 2000. *Transformative Motherhood: On Giving and Getting in a Consumer Culture*. New York: New York University Press.

MacDonald, Margaret. 2001. "The Role of Midwifery Clients in the New Midwifery in Canada: Postmodern Negotiations with Medical Technology." In *Daughters of Time: The Shifting Identities of Postmodern Midwives*, ed. Robbie Davis-Floyd and Sheila Cominsky. Special issue of *Medical Anthropology* 20(2–3):245–276.

MacDorman, M., and G. Singh. 1998. "Midwifery Care, Social and Medical Risk Factors, and Birth Outcomes in the U.S.A." *Journal of Epidemiology and Community Health* 52:310–317.

Martin, Emily. 1987. *The Woman in the Body*. Boston, MA: Beacon Press.

Marx, Karl. 1978. "The Fetishism of Commodities and the Secret Thereof" [from Capital, Vol.1]. In *The Marx-Engels Reader*, 2nd ed., ed. R. Tucker, 319–329. New York: W.W. Norton and Company.

McRobbie, Angela. 1988. *Zoot Suits and Second Hand Dresses: An Anthology of Fashion and Music*. Boston, MA: Unwin and Hyman.

Miller, Janneli. 2002. "Midwives' Magical Speech." Unpublished ms.

Morgan, Lynn M., and Meredith W. Michaels, eds. 1999. *Fetal Subjects, Feminist Positions*. Philadelphia: University of Pennsylvania Press.

Myers-Ciecko, Joanne. 1999. "Evolution and Current Status of Direct-Entry Midwifery Education, Regulation, and Practice in the United States, with examples from Washington State." *Journal of Nurse-Midwifery* 44(4):384–393.

North American Registry of Midwives (NARM). *How to Become a CPM*. www.narm.org.

Paine, Lisa L., Catherine M. Dower, and Edward O'Neil. 1999. "Midwifery in the 21st Century: Recommendations from the Pew Health Professions Commission/UCSF Center for the Health Professions 1998 Taskforce on Midwifery." *Journal of Nurse Midwifery* 44(4):341–348.

Reed, Alyson, and Joyce E. Roberts. 2000. "State Regulation of Midwives: Issues and Options." *Journal of Midwifery and Women's Health* 45(2):130–149.

Reid, Margaret. 1989. "Sisterhood and Professionalization: A Case Study of the American Lay Midwife." In *Women as Healers: Cross-Cultural Perspectives*, ed. Carol McClain, 219–238. New Brunswick, NJ: Rutgers University Press.

Rooks, Judith P. 1997. *Midwifery and Childbirth in America*. Philadelphia, PA: Temple University Press.

Rooks, Judith P., and S. H. Fishman. 1980. "American Nurse-Midwifery Practice in 1976–1977: Reflections on 50 Years of Growth and Development." *American Journal of Public Health* 70:990–996.

Rothman, Barbara Katz. 1982. *In Labor: Women and Power in the Birthplace*. New York: W.W. Norton.

Sammon, Alice. 2003. Personal communication. Alice Sammon practiced homebirth midwifery in New York state for twenty-five years (see chapter 2, this volume) and was one of the original members of the NARM board. She was instrumental in creating CPM certification, and currently resides and practices midwifery in Maine.

Schlinger, Hillary. 1992. *Circle of Midwives*. Self-published.

Schor, Julius, and Douglas Hope, eds. 2000. *The Consumer Society Reader*. New York: New Press.

Scoggin, Janet. 1996. "How Nurse-Midwives Define Themselves in Relation to Nursing, Medicine, and Midwifery." *Journal of Nurse-Midwifery* 41(1):36–42.

Sharpe, Mary. 2004. "Exploring Legislated Ontario Midwifery: Texts, Ruling Relations, and Ideological Practices." In *Reconceiving Midwifery: The New Canadian Model of Care*, ed. Ivy Bourgeault, Cecilia Benoit, and Robbie Davis-Floyd. Toronto: McGill-Queens University Press.

Taylor, Janelle, Danielle Wozniak, and Linda Layne, eds. 2004. *Consuming Motherhood*. New Brunswick, NJ: Rutgers University Press.

Tritten, Jan, and Joel Southern, 1998. *Paths to Becoming a Midwife: Getting an Education*, 4th ed., Eugene, OR: Midwifery Today.

Varney, Helen. 1997. *Varney's Midwifery*, 3rd ed, Sudbury, MA: Jones and Bartlett Publishers.

Weaver, Pam. 1998. Personal communication. Pam Weaver CPM is a practicing direct-entry midwife in Alaska. She is coauthor of the *Practical Skills Guide for Midwifery*, and currently serves as the NARM board liaison to state legislatures and agencies.

Weaver, Pam, and Sharon Evans. 2001. *Practical Skills Guide for Midwifery*, 3rd ed. Chugiak, Alaska: MorningStar Publishing.

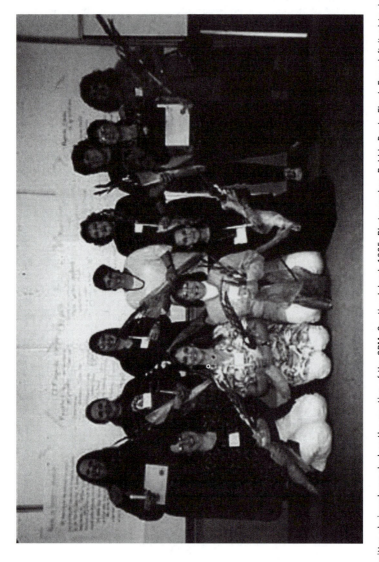

Fig. 3.1 Committee chairs who worked on the creation of the CPM, Captiva Island, 1995. Photographer: Robbie Davis-Floyd. From left (top) to right: Sharon Wells, Carol Nelson, Ann Cairns, Alice Sammon, Susan Hodges, Pam Weaver, Ruth Walsh, Justine Clegg. From left (bottom) to right: Jo Anne Myers-Ciecko, Marimikel Penn, Abby Kinne, Sandra MorningStar.

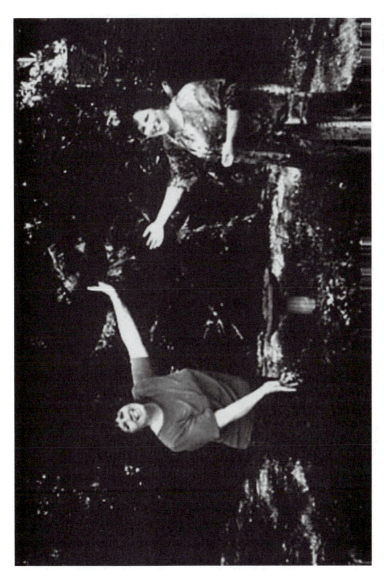

Fig. 3.2 Midwives Pam Weaver and Alice Sammon expressing their vision of the CPM as the gateway to the future for direct-entry midwifery, 1996. Photographer: Robbie Davis-Floyd

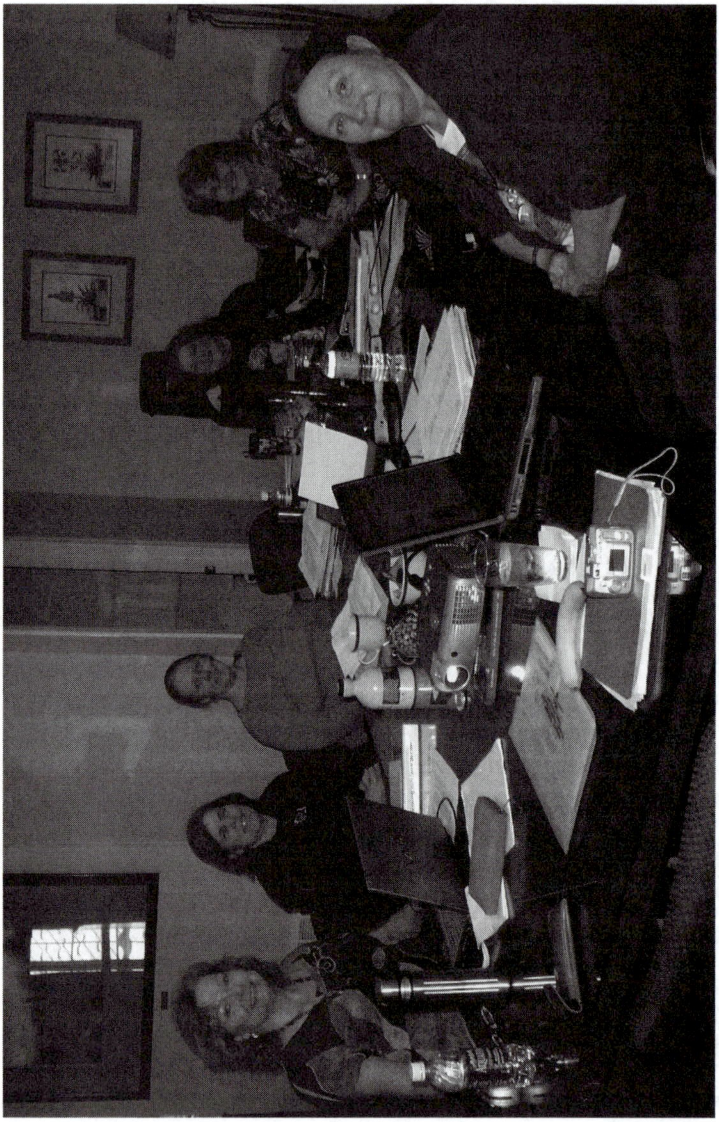

Fig. 3.3 The NARM Board, March 2005. From left to right around table: Robbie Davis-Floyd, Joanne Gottschall, Shannon Anton, Ida Darragh, Debbie Pulley, and Carol Nelson. Photographer: Robbie Davis-Floyd

Part II

State-Based Studies in the Legislation of Direct-Entry Midwifery

These six chapters constitute case studies of efforts, successful in the first four states and unsuccessful as of yet in the latter two, to achieve legalization and licensure for direct-entry midwives. The social scientists and midwives who write about these processes have both studied and participated in them. Cumulatively their case studies provide the full spectrum of the legal struggles and situations of homebirth direct-entry midwives in the contemporary United States. Thus these chapters offer profound lessons about what works and what does not in attempts to legalize direct-entry midwifery. Salient successful strategies that emerge from these chapters and from consultation with other midwives include:

- The formation of state direct-entry midwifery and consumer organizations.
- The formulation and presentation to state legislatures of a united front among these groups, which must agree on key aspects of legalization and regulation instead of fighting over them in public forums. Ultimate agreement between midwives who do not wish for licensure and those who do can be achieved by making the licensure voluntary or by creating ways for unlicensed midwives to practice without sanctions.
- Judicious use of the NARM/CPM certification process and national NACPM practice standards.
- Consultation with midwives and consumers in other states experienced in legislative processes, especially members of the MANA Legislative Committee, which offers conference calls for that purpose, and with NARM, which has published a Planning for Legislation Handbook (2005) (info@narm.org).
- Careful reading of all laws legalizing direct-entry midwives already passed in twenty-one states; the full text of these laws is available at www.mana.org.
- Advance consultation with nurse-midwives on proposed laws to make sure these laws will not interfere with CNM rights or practice, in order to avoid CNM opposition to these laws.
- Compilation of a database of members, organized by legislative district, allowing organizers to target key legislators by mobilizing constituents to contact their local representatives.
- Effective communication of the legislative agendas of these groups and of the reasons why these agendas matter to the public.
- Savvy lobbying of legislators and public officials through multiple means.
- Presentation of midwives and midwifery advocates as regular citizens asking for their rights for birth options.
- Cultivation of particular officials and supportive physicians.
- Education of consumers and legislators through the distribution of clear information and judicious communication with the media.
- Ongoing collaborative efforts among midwives and related groups.
- Effective consumer support as demonstrated by consumer communication with politicians, public rallies, and other means.

- Taking advantage of particular points in time during which opposition groups are focused on other issues.
- Creating midwives' own protocols for dealing with complications (or using national standards) and referring to these in the legislation, rather than letting the legislation itself restrict or prohibit dealing with specific complications or attendance at certain kinds of births (like vaginal birth after caesarean [VBACs] and breeches).
- Stressing midwives' abilities to screen out high-risk clients and their willingness to collaborate with, but not be supervised by, physicians.
- Including birth in homes and birth centers as legitimate sites of midwifery practice.
- Including rights to carry and utilize necessary pharmaceuticals and equipment.
- Avoiding written practice agreements with physicians through assurances of voluntary collaboration when needed (this involves convincing legislators of midwives' good judgment).
- Seeking to include state-mandated third-party reimbursement in the legislation.
- Ensuring the presence of direct-entry midwives themselves, and midwifery consumers, on governing boards or advisory councils.
- Perseverance over many years, especially on the part of midwives and consumers who become well-schooled in the political process.
- Entry of new advocates who can bring fresh energy when the longtime advocates become weary and "burned out."
- Occasional serendipitous doses of luck that must be noticed and utilized to full advantage.

The foundational basis of the success of all of these strategies is the midwives' documentation of, and the consumers' testaments to, the excellent, evidence-based, and woman-centered care they provide.

In addition to these larger conclusions, each chapter offers unique perspectives and insights. In both Florida and Virginia, black granny midwives were deliberately phased out by the medical and public health systems by the 1960s; the process of their demise in some places coincided with the advent of the new white middle-class lay midwife. While in Florida the story Melissa Denmark tells is primarily one of white middle-class activism, in Virginia, Christa Craven points to what she calls "cross-class political mobilization" for midwifery as primary in the very recent success of the Virginia legislative effort.

In Florida, direct-entry midwives chose formal education in three-year vocational programs as the only acceptable route to licensure; indeed, some of the original DEMs practicing there themselves developed such schools and went through their programs in order to achieve legitimacy to further their legalization efforts. Apprenticeship connected to CPM certification (or at least passing the NARM exam) remains a viable route in Minnesota, Colorado, and Virginia. Preserving apprenticeship is still a part of midwives' legislative plans in Iowa. In Massachusetts, in a historic move, CPMs and CNMs are working together for joint legislation creating a board that would govern all three types of nationally certified midwives (CNMs, CPMs, and CMs). To the Massachusetts CPMs, it seems clear that formal MEAC-accredited schools (like the distance learning program created by the Seattle Midwifery School) will serve this cause best. Part of the overall goal of the Massachusetts midwives is to end the legacy of distrust created during the 1990s in New York.

In the first four states discussed in this section, DEMs had already agreed that legalization and licensure were essential both to protect the public and for their own professional safety; those chapters focus most on their process of achieving it. But in many of the states in which direct-entry midwifery is still alegal or illegal, midwives are still debating the virtues and the pitfalls of licensure. Carrie Hough's chapter on Iowa, where direct-entry midwifery is still alegal, lets us in on the complexities of this debate among midwives like Eliza, who at present attends VBACs, but is concerned that she would "sell out" and refuse VBAC clients in order to preserve her legal and regulated status (were that to be achieved), and Lydia, who notes that "every single other profession out there, from chef to cutting hair to doing fingernails requires licensing" and debates with *herself* over whether midwifery should be different. Across the nation, midwives are increasingly resolving these debates in favor of the step toward professionalization that licensure represents, yet their concerns about biomedical and bureaucratic cooptation also increase as they watch these processes happen in states where licensure has been achieved.

In Colorado, DEMs have been licensed for over ten years, yet they have been forced to return to the legislature three times, twice for formal sunset reviews of their law. Compared to other states where homebirth midwifery is regulated, Colorado homebirth midwives have the greatest restriction on the scope of care they can legally provide (e.g., medications, suturing, IV fluids). And the legal wrangling the legislative fight entailed, as Susan Erickson and Amy Colo note, "has resulted in a fractious homebirth midwifery community and a decidedly more obstetrically-oriented practice of midwifery." The authors do not suggest that Colorado midwives would be better off without legal status and the degree of professionalization they have achieved, but show that the process of legalization served as a catalyst for certain changes within Colorado midwifery culture, including the "strategic removal from public view" of some aspects of the midwifery arts.

In contrast, Minnesota midwives now enjoy one of the most liberal licensing laws in the nation, one that safeguards their midwifery knowledge system. Mary Lay and Kerry Dixon's chapter summarizes this law, the process by which it was achieved, and the impetus it received from Minnesota's exploration of the new NARM/CPM certification process. Lay and Dixon stress that ultimately, the most effective strategy the Minnesota midwives developed was unified agreement among them that allowed them to present a united public front. Massachusetts midwives have reached such agreement, and have received support for their legislative process from all three branches of the state government—judicial, legislative, and administrative. The major impediment to their success is now economic—the potential costs of the new midwifery board they hope to create seem to remain the only barrier to the successful passage of their proposed legislation. The same costs are also at issue in states such as Oregon and Florida, where such costs render the maintenance of midwifery boards increasingly tenuous and thus jeopardize midwives' gains and impede state acceptance of the CM, who cannot be regulated by nursing boards.

4

"THE GOVERNOR'S FULL SUPPORT": LEGALIZING DIRECT-ENTRY MIDWIFERY IN FLORIDA

Melissa Denmark

• A History in Context • Woman with Woman and
the Days of the "Old Law" • Flushed Out of the Underground
• Snipped Off at the Bud • The Long Road to Legality, Again
• Developing a Profession: The Privileges and Prices of Swimming in
the Mainstream • Conclusion: The Value of History • Timeline:
A Brief History of Licensed Midwifery in Florida

There are a lot of crosscurrents of issues that have come together in the
20th century regarding midwifery in Florida. . . . You have to see it in the
context of Southern history, rural history, women's history, matters of
race, matters of struggle within the profession for who controls health
care, and consumer resurgence. . . . What we have in midwifery today is
just the confluence of all of those various forces and it's moving rapidly
and it still has the potential to be very, very different as other forces come
to play, like managed care and epidurals.

—Joan McTigue, Florida midwife

Florida has a particularly interesting history in regard to midwifery:
from a legal standpoint, reading and writing this history is like riding a

roller coaster, from up to down and up again, with multiple twists and turns along the way. A Southern state with many rural, impoverished areas, Florida was one of the last domains of the African-American "granny" midwife who attended the births of predominantly minority women up until the mid-1970s, and whose history is documented in Debra Susie's *In the Way of Our Grandmothers* (1988). Thus I only briefly touch on that history here. Around the time the granny midwife was almost completely eliminated from the Florida landscape, a resurgence of midwifery energy awakened in a different group of women. They were white, middle-class, and educated, attending births for a demographically similar population whose members consciously wanted an alternative to the standard obstetric hospital birth. These new midwives were few in number but were deeply committed to their ideological stance on childbirth. They stood up for their beliefs and organized themselves socially and later politically to revolutionize state law. Their battle was fought against larger, more powerful, and well-funded opponents, but through personal dedication, networking, and political efforts, their goals were realized. Their efforts and the medical community's resistance to them are the primary subjects of this chapter.

During my first semester of graduate studies in medical anthropology at the University of Florida, I discovered midwifery after listening to a lecture by Ina May Gaskin, one of midwifery's heroines. In order to learn more, I chose to write most of my assigned papers on women's reproductive health and birth. The idea for my master's research project was inspired by Robbie Davis-Floyd. She suggested to me that Florida has had a long and fascinating midwifery history, but no one had yet documented the most recent changes. I took on the challenge. This chapter is an abbreviated version of one of the chapters in my master's thesis (Denmark 2002). In this chapter, I historically reconstruct direct-entry midwifery in Florida from the mid-1970s to 2002, focusing on the "new" Florida midwives and their legislative efforts. The research on which this chapter is based centers around fifty-two interviews with individuals whose personal involvement was significant to the rebirth, growth, and development of what is now a legal and viable profession in Florida. Supplementing the interview data are archival materials collected from participants, state governmental agencies, newspapers, and journals.

I conducted the interviews from the fall of 1999 through spring of 2000. The participants ranged from midwives (including direct-entry midwives, certified nurse-midwives, certified professional midwives, unlicensed midwives, and various combinations of each); midwifery supporters active in the grassroots consumer movement; lawyers who worked pro bono for the midwifery cause; lobbyists, politicians, and state officials who either supported or opposed direct-entry midwifery; and a physician who had a consultation relationship with the midwives in his community. There were many others involved in the evolution of direct-entry midwifery in Florida whose stories are not presented here. It would be impossible to recognize everyone but I acknowledge and appreciate that grassroots movements require enormous amounts of human power.

A HISTORY IN CONTEXT

Florida, like other Southern states in the early 1900s, extensively debated the "midwife problem," especially because its maternal and infant death rates were high compared to the rest of the country. Granny midwives were blamed for these negative statistics. At that time, if someone wanted to be a midwife she simply registered at the office of the circuit court under "Physicians, Midwives, Sextons, Retail Casket Dealers, and Undertakers" (Susie 1988:34). Florida informally regulated its registered midwives under the Bureau of Child Hygiene and Public Health Nursing, created in 1918 as a branch of the State Board of Health (Yagerman 1982). Some public health officials wanted to see Florida's midwives eradicated, while others understood their utility in the rural, low-income communities they served, and for these supporters, midwives' education and control became major goals. The state sought to organize and standardize midwives with a focus on hygiene and birth recording. Through the bureau, midwives received training, obstetrical kits containing silver nitrate to prevent eye infections in newborns, and an instruction manual. Florida's granny midwives had a "close working relationship with the local county health unit" and, according to Susie (1988:63), appreciated the instruction, inspection, and supervision they received from county nurses. As the medical profession developed in Florida, its attitude toward the grannies became increasingly racist and paternalistic: "The grannies were really super people, but they were tolerated by the OB community back then because they were taking care of black people and [the OB community] didn't care what happened to black people," noted Charlie Mahan, an obstetrician who served as State Health Officer for HRS (Department of Health and Rehabilitative Services) during the early 1970s.

The Florida legislature did not address midwifery through statute until 1931, when it passed Florida Statute 485, the Midwifery Act. This law required licensure and state supervision of lay midwives. It established a minimum level of competency and required enough literacy to read the instruction manual and fill out birth certificates. Four thousand midwives (the majority of whom were African-Americans) attended at least one-third of the births in Florida in 1933, primarily for rural, poor, non-white populations (Ely 1933); they were not accorded professional status in the Midwifery Act. "It was never the state's objective to enhance the midwifery profession" (Susie 1988:47); midwifery was encouraged only in areas where it did not compete with existing medical facilities. "Need" was determined by a local private physician and the public health officer. In the 1950s and 1960s, in Florida as in other Southern states, the medical community began to actively discourage most granny midwives from continuing to practice. The midwives lacked internal organization, were not integrated into the health-care system, and relied on the medical community for licensure and permission to practice, all of which made it easy for the health department to forcefully phase them out. In 1964, 191 midwives held Florida licenses; these numbers decreased to fifty-seven in 1974 (Wennlund 1992:37) and to twenty a few years later.

The new middle-class, white, direct-entry midwives shared with the grannies the appellation "lay," various forms of self-training or apprenticeship education, and the experience of opposition from HRS (Susie 1988:64), but the similarities ended there. Geography, race, class, education, and the resultant differential relationships to the health-care system severely limited overlap between the old (poor, black granny) and new (young, white, middle-class) Florida midwife. The granny midwives were primarily located in the Florida Panhandle, while the new midwifery energy originated from areas around Gainesville, St. Augustine, Tampa, and Miami. Their vastly different class and cultural perspectives made it hard for these two groups to relate to each other, despite the deep respect and appreciation the younger generation of midwives felt for the older ones who had kept the tradition of midwifery alive. Using the rhetoric of respect, Joan McTigue acknowledges this disjuncture:

> The women who initiated the movement were pretty fearless and big-hearted, but they really recognized—just as they recognized intuitively how right the things that Ina May Gaskin and Suzanne Arms were saying—they really championed the granny midwives. They really understood this was someone to honor. . . . You can't quite graft it on because it doesn't work but you can pay homage to it.

These issues crested when the new law passed in 1982 and the differences between the African-American and white licensed midwives became exaggerated because of their similar legal standing. Most granny midwives did not benefit from the legal gains achieved by the new Florida midwives.

WOMAN WITH WOMAN
AND THE DAYS OF THE "OLD LAW"

During the 1960s and 1970s, many citizens of the United States felt part of a counterculture. They questioned the authority of various institutionalized systems, including health care. Unsatisfied with the standard treatment they received in hospitals, women wanting natural childbirth, which they could seldom achieve in hospitals, sought new avenues for birthing their babies. An alternative childbirth movement became juxtaposed against medicine's directional shift, as Joan McTigue put it, "away from women-centered birth to being technology-centered birth."

In Florida, small isolated pockets of women started exploring their childbirth options, moving toward out-of-hospital birth in underground communities attended by friends, neighbors, other women who had given birth at home, La Leche League leaders, and childbirth educators. These women were the pioneers of the midwifery renaissance in Florida and, as Joan McTigue stated, became the "backbone of the Midwives Association of Florida." Gradually, individuals started investigating the legal ramifications of midwifery in Florida and found that there was a midwifery law on the books. The Midwifery Act of 1931 was still in existence; it authorized licensure for midwives, with consequences (first-degree misdemeanor) for practicing midwifery without that licensure. It became obvious that "the 1931 Midwifery Act, written to provide only stop-gap supervision until midwives ceased to be part of the health care system, was an inadequate vehicle for establishment of the 'new midwifery' envisioned by natural childbirth advocates" (Yagerman 1982:140). However, fearing prosecution and in the interest of their client's safety, many of the underground midwives sought legalization through licensure under this old law. Its requirements were basically to attend fifteen births under the supervision of a physician within a one-year period, get letters of recommendation from at least two licensed practicing physicians, one of whom had to be the local county medical director, and pass a written and/or oral examination. According to Joan McTigue, one of the first women to get her midwifery license in Florida's new era of midwifery, the regulating agency (HRS) was not cooperative with people inquiring about licensure.

> It was not their intention to give any more licenses out, but it *was* their intention to retire the practice of midwifery and the few granny midwives that were left in the state, and eventually it was their intention to have the law repealed. They were very surprised to find that there were women who were interested in reviving it.

No new midwifery licenses were issued from 1972 to 1976, but between 1977 and mid-1979, HRS received seventy inquiries about licensure. Only nine applications were filed between 1976 and 1980 (House Health Care Committee on Regulatory Reform 1984:7), yet between 1973 and 1980, the percentage of reported midwifery-assisted births in Florida increased from one percent to 2.6 percent (Wennlund 1981).

As noted above, the momentum that brought about the revised midwifery legislation in 1982 began in the late 1960s and early 1970s. Part of the "back to nature" and "self-help" movement included a belief that birth was normal, and a desire on the part of birthing women to have their partners present and to give birth "awake and aware," without restrictive hospital procedures, isolated from support people, being strapped down to delivery tables, and unconscious from general anesthesia. Often their only option was homebirth. Some families used lay midwives; others did it themselves with the aid of books or with friends who were nurses or women who had delivered their own babies. News spread through the grapevine and people interested in midwifery and homebirth began to become aware of each other and meet informally. "There was a groundswell of midwifery activity in the state, just hot-beds of it" (Joan McTigue, interview). Midwife-run prenatal self-help clinics operated in people's backyards and homes, where pregnant women learned and performed prenatal care on each other with the guidance of midwives. "We kind of got a network, like little tendrils of a jellyfish out through the state, and started connecting with other people," said Maryann Malecki, a licensed midwife from the Daytona area.

In need of more organization and desiring to be politically visible, in 1979 Linda Wilson, Margaret Hebson, Gazelle Lange, Justine Clegg, Janice Heller, Sara Pinkman, Joan McTigue, Sam Woods, and others founded the Florida Midwives Association[1] as the state's professional association for midwives. Their purpose was to revamp the outdated 1931 law and promote the training and licensure of non-nurse-midwives in the state. Many of the women practicing midwifery at this time were frustrated and scared about being in the illegal underground, and felt they deserved the opportunity to get a license and training. Sharon Hamilton, a past president of the Midwives Association of Florida (MAF) who originally got involved in the early 1980s when she moved to Florida after practicing midwifery in California, described the organization at this point as being "very vibrant and committed to legalizing midwifery . . . because the only people who were getting licensed were people who sued the state [*State v. McTigue, State v. Baya*]."

With the assistance of attorneys Terry DeMeo and Bruce Winick, and the determination of Linda Wilson and Margaret Hebson, among others, the emerging group analyzed the old midwifery law, looked at related laws from other states (Washington in particular), and worked to write improved legislation regarding midwifery. Bruce and Terry, husband and wife, gave birth to their two children at home in Miami, with the help of local midwives. They were active in the Florida American Civil Liberties Union and concentrated on reproductive rights issues, so the midwifery model of care resonated well with their belief system. They worked pro bono for the midwives' struggle for legalization. In addition to drafting the new statute, Terry gave legal advice where it was needed. Occasionally Terry and her law partner Tom Sherman represented a midwife who was trying to get her license but was running into bureaucratic obstacles, such as Sara Pinkman, who sued HRS in 1981 for the right to take her midwifery exam and obtain a license. Terry expressed that she was inspired by the dedication and effort put forth by the midwives.

Through connections with Terry and Bruce, MAF convinced Senator Jack Gordon and Representative Elaine Gordon to be their sponsors and promote a new midwifery bill that would modernize the 1931 law. Also at this time, MAF asked Beth Swisher, a midwifery consumer and La Leche League leader in the Tallahassee area, to be their lobbyist. Beth's original naïveté is typical of many early participants in legislative activities who had no idea what they were getting into; she said:

> I got a call from the Midwives Association and they asked if I could be their contact person for Senator Gordon and Representative Gordon because they were putting in legislation for the practice of midwifery, and so I did. I had never been to the Capitol before and so when I hung up the phone my husband said, 'What did you just do?' and I said, 'Oh, I don't know honey, I'm just going to be the contact person for Senator Gordon and Representative Gordon.' And from there on I was up at the Capitol

about sixty hours a week. It was absolutely intense. I was so naïve and had no idea about anything to do with lobbying.

Beth worked full time as the midwives' lobbyist from 1982 until the beginning of 1998 and was paid a minimal sum for her tremendous effort; MAF simply did not have the funding to pay her more. Entirely dedicated to midwifery, Beth also opened her home for midwives to stay when they came to the Capitol to lobby.

The members of MAF, through their legislative sponsors, introduced their first bill in the Florida legislature in 1979 and again in 1980, but these attempts failed and they decided to sit out the 1981 session. Members of MAF often went to the Capitol to lobby for their proposed bill. Maryann Malecki explained how lobbying fit in with a midwife's schedule: "We took the pregnant women with us in the caravan. If we had somebody due, we packed all our equipment into a VW camper and took [her] to Tallahassee with us. So we had a myriad of babies and strollers, babies attached to bodies, babies in bellies, all storming Tallahassee numerous times."

One of the most important aspects of the proposed new statute was that it reflected the midwives' firm stand on the idea of independent practice. Through the example of their nurse-midwifery sisters, the midwives understood the vulnerability that practitioners can have when tied to physician supervision. With this awareness, the midwives wanted to practice independently of another health-care professional's authority. "Advocates of the bill stressed its necessity in light of the growing demand for low-cost and more personalized obstetrical care" (Yagerman 1982:141).

The major opponents of midwifery were the Florida Medical Association (FMA) and specialty groups within the FMA, such as the Florida Obstetric and Gynecologic Society and the Florida Pediatric Society. These groups argued that licensure might give midwives permission to practice when they were not qualified or competent health-care providers. Dolores Wennlund, the State Nursing Director of Public Health Nursing during the mid-1970s, noted, "The problem with the lay midwives, though I'm sure that some were not only very committed, but very talented, is that they were outside of the system and if something went wrong they did not have an easy and rapid referral arrangement to get that patient under care." Many doctors were upset with the midwives for "dumping" their emergency patients on them in the hospital emergency rooms and then turning around and suing them or maligning them in the paper.

Nancy Moreau, a lobbyist for the FMA from 1975 till about 1984, and later for the Florida Pediatric Society, echoed Dolores, noting that at least the granny midwives worked through their county health departments and had ties to the medical system, so if their mothers needed further medical care, they had access to it. Nancy stated:

> The contention with the medical establishment was with what we perceived the desires of the lay midwives to be, and that is that they wanted to be out in the community, independent and promoting homebirth . . . and this was distressing because the education of lay midwives is very wanting, they did not have the health-care background that most medical professionals believed was necessary to appropriately evaluate a woman and monitor her throughout her pregnancy and birth.

Nancy expressed the FMA's preference for nurse-midwives: "We felt we had evolved to where we had elevated midwifery to the point where there was at least some nursing background and training and a tie to a higher level professional that could take over and assist should there be any complications in pregnancy or birth." George Palmer, a lobbyist for the FMA during this period, described the strong resistance from physicians to accepting any recommendations from midwives. He sensed that there was a turf battle going on in which the FMA was rallying against another allied health group trying to get a piece of the pie.

It took pressure from the public, lawsuits, and media coverage to force HRS to deal with direct-entry midwifery licensure. Dolores Wennlund said, "The press saw the bureaucrats as the bad guys, regardless of what was going on—so we were the bad guys and the lay midwives were envisioned as the saviors of women." In several cases, midwives had been accused of practicing midwifery without a license, among them a 1979 landmark case involving an unlicensed midwife named Carol Baya from St. Augustine in which a circuit judge ruled on the lack of constitutionality of the old 1931 midwifery law and said it delegated licensing power to doctors, which violated the state constitution. Larry Turner, one of three lawyers on the defendant's side, explained:

> Carol's friends and supporters, who were many, felt that it [the lawsuit] was unfair. She was by all accounts an excellent midwife, had delivered many babies in the St. Augustine area, had tried to become licensed, and was frustrated in that effort because the statute in existence at the time was an old statute . . .

and the medical doctors in her area would not provide supervision for her licensure. It was alleged, and I think probably true, that they didn't want the competition.

Larry believed that the defendant won the case on the grounds that the law was vague and therefore void: "The best defense was to go after the constitutionality and ethicality of the statute itself, which we thought was clearly unconstitutional, in that it unlawfully delegated legislative authority, that is to determine licensing, to the doctors." This implied that there needed to be a new law written, one that would address the current midwifery situation in Florida.

According to Larry, on the day of the trial there was a lot of favorable press covering the event. The courtroom was packed with a couple of hundred children who had been delivered by midwives. Many people were wearing T-shirts promoting midwifery, with phrases like "my daddy caught me" or "I was born at home." Dolores Wennlund, representing HRS, described the midwifery supporters that day as an "unruly group" who were demonstrating all around the courthouse. The clincher was a powerful audiotape of a beautiful homebirth. Larry said, "The judge declared the law unconstitutional and the Secretary of the State's Office had the good judgment not to appeal him, but rather said 'let's back off and redraft the statute.'" "And so it happened that the law, styled to facilitate the occupational phase-out of a portion of the American population, was legally exposed" (Susie 1988:62).

The Baya case served as a catalyst, after which members of MAF and HRS decided to work together to build a new law for licensed midwives. There were other factors besides losses in court that made HRS collaborate with the midwives, such as a steady increase in licensure inquiries, statistics suggesting an increase in homebirths, and negative news coverage of vague allegations that babies were dying during homebirths with untrained or no attendants present. The would-be midwives and consumers used this information to show that there was a demand for out-of-hospital birth and it was incumbent upon the Florida legislature to modernize the midwifery law to answer this demand with safe, well-trained, and regulated midwives. The goal of HRS—to license safe and competent health-care practitioners—required clarification of the old midwifery law. "A safer atmosphere for women was our primary concern," stated Dolores Wennlund. Meetings were held in Tallahassee in 1980 and 1981, and from the midwives' perspective many compromises were made, but independent practice was not one of them.

During this era, citizens had been organizing countrywide into activist groups for various political agendas, giving form and structure to idealism and the belief that people could change the system. Far from idle, in 1981 Florida midwives and consumers with babes in arms visited legislators in their district offices around the state to educate them about midwifery and homebirth. Their message was well received by many legislators from rural areas in central and northern Florida who had themselves been born at home with lay midwives.

In 1982, the Midwifery Practice Act, Florida Statute 467, successfully passed the Florida legislature, thereby endorsing a three-year, direct-entry midwifery education program and state licensing exam. Definitions that were vague in the 1931 law, such as "midwifery" and "normal labor and childbirth," were made clear. This was the first time that formal midwifery education was required in Florida and "the apprenticeship model was virtually discarded" (Susie 1988:63). In addition to the course of study, the applicant was to observe twenty-five births and attend twenty-five more under supervision (Susie 1988:63). A key difference between the old and new laws was the state's legal recognition of the need for parents' freedom of choice in the manner, cost, and setting of their children's births. According to Yagerman, the purpose of the statute was twofold: "to protect the health and welfare of mothers and infants and to make midwifery safe and available to women expecting normal deliveries" (1982:142). Thus, licensed midwifery began to be integrated into the dominant health-care system.

Midwifery supporters felt the law was passed due to several factors—eventual HRS support, consumer power, the political inexperience of the midwives, and the element of surprise. Linda Wilson explained:

> We had nothing to lose so we could step on all the toes we wanted to because we had no school or law behind us. . . . All we had was people power and the ability to say, "we are not going to pay you X amount of dollars to deliver our babies in a way that we don't agree with. We are going to stay at home. We are going to step out of the system." So it was kind of a civil disobedience. . . . We weren't afraid and we were so politically naïve that we didn't really know how the system was supposed to work, so we went in brash and bold and said, "Here we are. You have to listen to us, because we are the people who vote for you."

According to Margaret Hebson, the law passed easily in 1982 because it was not a high-profile topic and the Florida Medical Association was not adequately prepared to counter the grassroots support that had grown for the midwives. The FMA had no lobbyists positioned against the midwives. Terry DeMeo said, "It was a combination of our inexperience and lots of energy. . . . The medical association and anybody else who had a stake in prohibiting it was just kind of unaware of what we were doing." For Linda Wilson, the passing of midwifery legislation was her heartfelt dream come true—a clear indication of the many people involved and invested in midwifery and it was finally gaining momentum. However, she described herself feeling exhausted and discouraged in that moment of glory, after struggling for her own licensure in a system that refused her for political reasons. She decided to step down from her integral role in the midwifery community, confidently knowing that the cause she had fought so hard for was won.

The main opposition to the bill, although ineffective, did come from the Florida Medical Association. Charlie Mahan provided an alternative perspective as to why the Midwifery Practice Act passed.

> The public health folks sat down with [the FMA and the Society for OB/GYNs] and said, "You know, all you're perceived as is somebody who is against something. If you'd leave the midwives alone, and there aren't many of them out there and there is a demand for them, just leave them alone and take on some public health issues, like prenatal care and things along that line." . . . So they sort of left it alone because we convinced them to take on some white hat issues and quit looking like they were beating up on the poor little old midwives.

My interview with Ken Plante, a lobbyist for the FMA during the time the midwifery law passed, gave another angle. Ken recalled a lot of internal disagreement about the 1982 bill. There was a small faction of doctors who wanted the bill to pass in the interest of delivering maternity services to future mothers. There were others who were strictly interested in defining and clarifying the roles of doctor and midwife, so as to avoid more court cases like the Baya trial. A third group within the FMA was "adamantly against anybody being able to practice anything that they [doctors] could practice without that person being a full-blown doctor." When I asked Ken about what motivated the FMA's position against midwifery, he said:

> They start out with the intention of trying to protect the consumers and as the years go by it becomes more of limiting who can come into the market to compete, so it doesn't matter whether you look at doctors, lawyers, real estate people, and so

on. Many of these things are designed to protect the public to a degree, but it is also turf guarding.

Whatever the reason—whether economic or ideological—midwifery was a divisive issue for the FMA. Ken spoke about being on the phone with the president of the FMA thirty minutes before the Health Care Committee meeting was to take place in the Senate and getting the final word to support the midwifery bill as is.

Nevertheless, in a last-minute attempt to gain control, the FMA's legislators managed to attach a two-year Sunset Review provision to the statute. At that time, all statutes that regulated professions, occupations, businesses, industries, or other endeavors in Florida were required to undergo the Sunset Review process,[2] which meant the new law was systematically evaluated by the legislature for termination, modification, or reenactment on a more permanent basis. However, the Sunset Review usually occurred after a five- or ten-year period following the creation of the statute. The midwives never questioned the Sunset Review provision, as they trusted that the new law would be "rubber stamped" in 1984 because their three-year education programs had not even been established yet.

FLUSHED OUT OF THE UNDERGROUND

Following the passage of the Midwifery Practice Act in 1982, the midwifery community took off! Next on the agenda was to create the Advisory Committee of Licensed Midwifery within HRS. The Committee's job was to flesh out the specifics of the practice rules and regulations for the administration and enforcement of the statute and to create educational programs to train midwives as required by the new law. The Advisory Committee also planned to meet regularly to counsel HRS on the problems and needs of current midwifery practice. The Advisory Committee was comprised of two midwives licensed under the old 1931 law, a nurse-midwife, a physician (obstetrician or family physician practicing obstetrics), and a state resident representing a disinterested public citizen. One of the downfalls of the Advisory Committee was that it had consultative responsibility but little authority or power of its own—a situation that continues to be a vulnerable aspect of licensed midwifery in Florida.

The 1982 law retained HRS as the rule-making authority for the midwifery profession, but its power was restricted by the specifics of the law. Whenever a new rule was proposed, testimony would be taken. The rule-making process resulted in bitter fights and seemed another attempt at keeping midwives "as tightly regulated as possible" (McTigue 1989:37) by defining the midwife's scope of practice, her standards, an accountability procedure, and a set of requirements for training programs and licensing. Due to the intense involvement and argument between members, it took the Advisory Committee from July 1982 until January 1984 to finish the Rules and Regulations regarding the education, practice, and regulation of midwifery, which in turn delayed the process of developing midwifery schools.

Under the Midwifery Practice Act, midwives reported directly to the state HRS office in Tallahassee. The county health departments were no longer responsible for licensed midwifery throughout the state, which eliminated the county health nurse role (Susie 1988). This modification was particularly difficult for the older African-American midwives, as they no longer had a liaison to help them stay current on the state's changing expectations of midwives.

> The law's bureaucratic technical jargon alone was enough to impel them [the granny midwives] to voluntarily turn in their licenses. The county nurse, who usually translated the state's edicts as they came down, was no longer in place. And without interpretation, the new law appeared to be only a maze of red tape and thus yet another assault on the weary midwifery profession. (Susie 1988:65)

In addition to the elimination of the "middleman" role of the county health nurse, the new law entitled midwives to more freedom in their scope of practice than the older African-American midwives previously experienced. This was intimidating to them, as was all the detailed paperwork they were required to fill out after each birth they attended. Another consequence of the new law was that the licensed midwife was now vulnerable to malpractice lawsuits, and insurance premiums were too expensive for many rural midwives to afford. Previously the county health departments acted as a legal buffer for midwives, and without this protection, midwives, when encouraged by HRS and "fearful of losing all that they had worked for, turned in their licenses" (Susie 1988:65). MAF attempted to help the African-American midwives with the transition between the old and new law they had created, but the grannies often felt alienated and confused, which resulted in most of them retiring, taking their rich traditions with them to their graves (Susie 1988).

> As had happened so many times before, the needs of the old-style midwife were disregarded in the fluster of compromise that

shaped the new law. Under legal pressure from the medical community, the new midwives were anxious to gain a legal status that would end the random harassment. In the face of strong medical opposition, the midwife proponents settled for a statute for the contemporary model of the institutionally educated nurse-midwife. (Susie 1988:66)

With the 1982 Midwifery Practice Act in place, two new private schools were established, the North Florida School of Midwifery in Gainesville and the South Florida School of Midwifery in Miami. Both the North and South Florida Schools of Midwifery were considered postsecondary vocational schools under the Florida Department of Education Board of Postsecondary Vocational, Technical, Trade and Business Schools. The schools' curricular framework was set up by the state and structured around the three-year direct-entry European model, which trained midwives as specialists in low-risk, noninterventionist birth and emergency procedures (McTigue 1989). Two influential figures involved in the development of the schools' curricula, along with assisting in formulating midwifery's rules, regulations, and scope of practice, were Alan McCloud, head of obstetrics, and Anne Scapone, head of the CNM program, both from the United Kingdom and familiar with direct-entry midwifery, and both at the University of Miami's Jackson Memorial Hospital. The first classes of midwives were largely made up of unlicensed, self-trained, and self-proclaimed midwives who had been in the underground and had worked toward licensure under the old law.

The schools were organized and licensed by the Florida Department of Education without much input from HRS, which was a "bone of contention" according to Dolores Wennlund. Nancy Moreau questioned the quality of the new schools and stated, "Just because you call yourself a school doesn't mean your curriculum is adequate." This was the same concern brought up in my interview with Senator Myers, who said, "If they are going to school, then educate them and include some level of nursing training." He continued, "I was the 'enemy of midwifery' and I really wasn't, I just was trying to bring professionalism there."

The North Florida School of Midwifery was founded by Sharon Wells, Lynn Knox, and Kathy Beall, all three of whom were part of the first class of midwifery students. Sharon received her midwifery license in 1986 and maintains her Florida license today, though she no longer lives in the state. After her trying involvement with legislative efforts in New York, Sharon later became a key member of the Board of the

North American Registry of Midwives and was instrumental in the development of the CPM certification process (see chapter 3).

People active in starting and running the South Florida School of Midwifery included Janice Heller, Margaret Hebson, Linda Wilson, Cindy Ellis, Justine Clegg, Sara Pinkman, Rickie Taylor, and Carol Nelson. In 1982, Carol was the last person to get her midwifery license under the old 1931 law, which she still holds despite not residing there. She was the main preceptor and instructor for the twenty-four students of the South Florida School of Midwifery, seventeen of whom graduated and became licensed. Like Sharon Wells, Carol went on to help develop the CPM and currently serves on NARM's Board of Directors as treasurer and director of the applications department; she also continues her long-standing midwifery practice on the Farm in Tennessee. Carol described the first, intimidating application forms the school received from the Department of Education: "It was this three-inch paper stack that we had to go through and fill out, so we just sat there totally mortified. Then I said, 'Wait a minute, this is just paper, we can do this.' Next we divided up the pile and each took a section home and eventually we compiled it all together." The South Florida School opened in 1984 and the first class graduated in 1987. The original administrator of the school was Linda Wilson, who was succeeded by Justine Clegg, who held the position until the school closed in 1992. Justine later went on to establish a three-year Associate in Science in Midwifery degree program at the Miami-Dade Community College, based on the philosophy and curriculum of the South Florida School of Midwifery. Justine was part of the national midwifery community's Certification Task Force Meetings, which established the criteria for NARM CPM certification, and also served on the first Board of Directors of the Midwifery Education Accreditation Council (MEAC).

On the political front, things had been going smoothly for licensed midwives during this period except for a privacy issue that came up in 1984, when a Miami newspaper, the now defunct *Miami News*, wanted access to midwives' clients' records so it could do a story on midwifery. Apparently all other medical practitioners have an obligation to keep their patient records confidential, so there was a serious fight over whether or not midwives had to make their records available to the popular press. According to attorney Charlene Carres, the midwives argued that "there was a fundamental privacy right that patients had and that shouldn't be violated even in situations of freedom of the press." The case went to the Florida Supreme Court and ultimately the midwives won, with the legal help of attorneys Charlene Carres and

Tom Sherman. The clients of midwives were ruled to have the same privacy rights as do patients of doctors.

Charlene, who worked practically pro bono for the midwives on the privacy issue, became committed to the midwifery cause, continued to offer her legal advice, and in conjunction with Beth Swisher, acted as a MAF lobbyist for several years. She recalled that through her lobbyist role she "got a real taste of how nasty doctors could be about other medical practitioners." Charlene described how the FMA would make allegations about the midwives and homebirth without offering any proof to back up their statements, relying instead on their reputation and authority.

> It was kind of an eye-opener to see that they [FMA lobbyists] really didn't care whether what they were saying had any basis. . . . It's not so much that they were so careless of the truth that they made up statistics or anything in that regard, but they were more untruthful in what they omitted. It was mainly scare tactics.

According to Charlene, the FMA would set up scenarios such as, "What if a woman is in the middle of labor and x, y, z, happens, then the baby will die," but it was never mentioned that this rarely or never happens:

> [Lobbyists] really can't lie at the Capitol and get away with it because once that lie is uncovered you are not trusted anymore. We [lobbyists] really try to be very cautious with other people about the way we present information so that we are not fabricating data or saying blatant lies. It doesn't mean, however, that the way lobbyists present information isn't damaging.

Charlene was a tremendous asset to the midwives, but her subsequent involvement with abortion rights in 1989 became a major concern for MAF. (Abortion is such a controversial and volatile topic that it could tear the midwifery community apart, so while individual midwives may take particular stands, midwifery organizations very consciously stay away from the abortion issue.) Charlene remained connected with midwifery, although to a lesser degree. She legally represented MAF in an action challenging mandatory malpractice attached to a law providing Medicaid reimbursement for homebirth passed in 1997.

Nancy Moreau, former lobbyist for the FMA and current lobbyist for the Florida Pediatric Society, noted how the medical community viewed this period—people were having their children with midwives believing childbirth to be an ethereal, community, and hippie-type of event. All the focus was on the mom and dad, but who spoke for the baby? Nancy said:

> The whole point of childbirth is to bring a healthy human being into this world and you would hope that if you were ever going to be a selfless human being, this is the time that we need to be other-directed and to understand that the most important thing is to ensure that child has every chance of being born without any kind of complication and if there is a complication, it needs to be dealt with in a medical establishment.

Echoing the official position taken by the American Medical Association in 1972 that homebirth is "child abuse," Nancy implied that having a homebirth is a selfish act in which the mother is more concerned about her comfort than the safety of her baby. In this view, the kind of attendant—midwife or physician—matters less than the site of delivery: homebirth is dangerous because of the lack of immediate availability of appropriate backup equipment and staff. When I asked Nancy about the good statistical outcomes midwives report, she distrusted the numbers and claimed that self-reporting does not tell the whole story. She perceived that the expansion of licensed midwives and their clientele meant that they would have a higher chance of encountering complications, which would be dangerous.

Despite the new midwifery statute, HRS maintained its discriminatory attitude against licensed midwives. Tom Sherman, a Miami attorney who helped at least five women get their midwifery licenses, believed that HRS did not like midwives becoming licensed again and sought to "discipline" them for the ways they practiced midwifery. Sara Pinkman noted, "The agency always seemed to have the attitude that licensed midwives were second-class citizens and could be treated with no respect, as if they needed to constantly prove themselves to be okay and in compliance."

The story of Gladys Milton, Florida's most famous black granny midwife, is a prime example of this kind of behavior. Gladys Milton began her path of midwifery in 1958 with the encouragement of her local county health department, which was looking to train midwives to do home deliveries in rural areas. Adding to this prompting, Gladys stated that she was "born to be a midwife…to help God's little ones into the world" (Bovard and Milton 1993:38). Gladys apprenticed with two doctors in her community who ran a clinic and attended births. In 1959 she received her license to practice midwifery and continued to work in the clinic for several years while doing homebirths. In 1976 she built the Eleanor Milton Memorial Birthing Center in Florala, next to her home. At this time, all of Gladys's clients received their prenatal care through the health department, and if they remained low-risk, were given approval to have her attend their births. Being a prominent and experienced midwife, Gladys was asked to serve as the licensed midwife representative on the state advisory board in 1982 after the passage of the new midwifery legislation.

In her book about her career and life, *Why Not Me?*, Gladys stated that in the early 1980s, "just when things were going well for midwifery in Florida, I started to feel like the rug was being pulled out from under me, ever so slowly" (Bovard and Milton 1993:88). Her clientele had changed from poor and needy minority women to more educated white women with insurance. Medical professionals, who before had tolerated Gladys's practice, perceived this situation as an encroachment on their territory with the potential to leave doctors with the complicated deliveries and more malpractice risk. Gladys talked about how "the Health and Rehabilitation Services of Florida, the same agency that invited me to my profession, geared up for what appeared to be a massive battle" (Bovard and Milton 1993:89). Her clients were being treated rudely at the health department. In 1985 the state alleged that her birth center did not abide by state-specified standards, and closed it. It remained closed for almost a year while Gladys and her local community raised money for the needed changes and submitted the appropriate paperwork to pass inspection. "We had a lot of support, but the trouble with HRS never went away" (Bovard and Milton 1993:95). Governor Bob Graham nominated her Woman of the Year in 1988, which was the same year she delivered a stillbirth due to complications of shoulder dystocia. As a result of this loss, her license was suspended before an investigation into the case was completed. Gladys described the letter she received from HRS asking her to retire.

> It was a short and sweet little letter. They told me how much they appreciated my commendable service to the community and thanked me for my humanitarian effort. Then they went on to say that the day of the midwife was over, that Florida didn't need us anymore, and besides, I was too old to continue working [at age 64]. It said things had changed since I started delivering babies, and even though I had been a real asset to the midwifery program, I was now obsolete. (Bovard and Milton 1993:13)

Tom Sherman represented Gladys in her successful hearing against HRS. Members of the midwifery community, including Joan McTigue, Sharon Wells, Justine Clegg, and Beth Rodriquez, helped Tom prepare Gladys's defense. Tom did the case virtually *pro bono* and the midwifery community helped raise money to pay his expenses. However, HRS disregarded the judge's ruling and denied Gladys her license. Tom made an appeal; the midwifery community continued to provide moral and financial support to Gladys, and after two years of waiting while HRS created additional charges to stall the process, Gladys finally regained her license in 1992. In a presentation on the history of Florida midwifery at the 2000 MANA convention in Clearwater Beach, Florida, Jana Borino, Administrative Director of the Florida Traditional School of Midwifery in Gainesville, humorously referred to these events as "the alliance of the grannies and the granolas."

SNIPPED OFF AT THE BUD

During the 1980s, Florida used the Sunset Review process to periodically examine professions and make recommendations if there was a need for regulation, to decide whether the public derived benefits from it, and determine what modifications were needed. Often the state conducted a formal study to investigate the relevant issues. In 1983 the House Health Care Committee on Regulatory Reform conducted a study of midwifery in Florida as part of the Sunset Review process. At the time there were thirty-three licensed midwives and 156 certified nurse-midwives licensed in Florida (House Health Care Committee on Regulatory Reform 1984:5). The committee's conclusions stated that licensed midwives provide safe, effective care that meets a public need, and recommended the statute not be repealed.

> Recognizing the need for parents' freedom of choice in the manner, cost, and setting of their children's births and in the interests of public health, the legislature deemed the regulation of the practice of midwifery in this state to be necessary. The purpose of the legislation is to protect the health and welfare of mothers and infants and to make the practice of midwifery safe and available to those anticipating safe deliveries. (House Health Care Committee on Regulatory Reform 1984:27)

Since the new law passed in 1982, the midwives had busied themselves with creating schools, attracting students, and opening up a lost profession. They had not geared up for the political battle and challenges brought by the 1984 session. The FMA, however, had two years to prepare for a confrontation. They became more organized and boosted their lobbying efforts against midwifery. The opposition to direct-entry midwifery was formidable, much more intense than in 1982. The nurses, hospitals, and insurance companies were all against it. HRS, the agency that regulated midwifery prior and subsequent to 1982, took a very passive role politically. Midwifery became a contentious topic in Tallahassee, the state capital, and the deregulation of the Midwifery Practice Act was a realistic threat. In addition, "Republican Governor Martinez was heavily supported by the doctors and so they [the doctors] had more power than they usually had under Democratic governors" (Charlie Mahan, interview). Throughout the 1984 legislative session, Senator "Doc" Myers worked aggressively to revoke the midwifery statute. Consequently, on the last day of the legislative session, May 31, Senator Myers proposed an amendment that allowed only those midwives currently licensed or enrolled in one of the two midwifery schools to practice legally. In his interview, Senator Myers stated that he was worried that the midwives were starting to handle some of the ten to twenty percent of births that were considered complicated, and that this was dangerous. This concern, along with pressure from the midwifery opposition, may have influenced his decision to propose this amendment.

Bibb Willis, hired by MAF specifically to shepherd the statute safely through the 1984 legislative session, sought to modify the Myers Amendment to include students already enrolled in midwifery programs with the rationale that the schools had been licensed and people had enrolled and paid tuition in good faith. The midwives did not have much political power at that point, so their options were to endorse the amendment with the addition of including current enrollees or pull the whole bill by getting the governor's veto. MAF had to determine how far they could compromise their new law. Some midwives wanted to scrap the 1982 law and come back another year with a more favorable version. Linda Wilson said:

> If the midwifery law was taken off the books for some reason, it's not going to wipe out midwifery because it will just go back underground. There have always been midwives, there will always be midwives, and when you put something underground that's when it really becomes stronger. There is so much more passion for it than there would be if it's aboveground, then it gets refocused.

Others believed something was better than nothing and feared they might not be able to pass legislation in the future. In addition, a significant number of midwives already were licensed, practicing, and dependent on their midwifery earnings for their livelihood, including some of the remaining African-American midwives. In a period of several hours, MAF's regional representatives consulted with midwives in their area and came to the consensus that MAF should oppose any attempts at deregulation. There were just too many licensed midwives practicing who would be out of a job. So the midwives decided to accept the amendment—given the choice of deregulation or compromise, MAF chose the latter with the hope of being able to amend this restriction out of the bill in the following legislative session.

The new version of the Myers amendment was agreed upon. Thus, after 1984, the Midwifery Practice Act only allowed midwives who were licensed as of October 1 and those students enrolled in the two midwifery programs as of the beginning of May 1984 to practice midwifery. All others who were not "grandmothered" in would be considered illegal. This potentially allowed roughly thirty-five midwives to practice legally in Florida (Susie 1988). Looking back at that decision, Beth Swisher recalled that it was an emotional moment. Many midwives wondered what would have happened if they had allowed midwifery to become illegal.

The profession could not grow with the restriction of the Myers Amendment in place. Many midwives, students, and consumers felt burned out after all their effort ended in only a handful of new midwives being allowed to practice legally. They realized it was going to be extremely difficult to have the Myers Amendment repealed. As one midwife described, "It was back to grassroots square one," but only a few individuals had the energy to keep going. This was the first of several times in my research that I noticed a changing of the guard within the ranks of direct-entry midwifery in Florida. Many who had repeatedly sacrificed their time, money, and spirit felt exhausted and needed to rest. Taking their place was a fresh and highly motivated set of leaders, ready to lend their energy for the cause, at least for a while.

THE LONG ROAD TO LEGALITY, AGAIN

After the Myers Amendment was put in place, the schools stayed open to graduate all students who had been enrolled since 1984. For a time, both schools offered midwife assistant programs, as they expected the Myers Amendment to be lifted and to be able to resume training midwives. Eventually the North Florida School closed in 1986, while the

South Florida School kept a license with the Department of Education, but no longer took new students.

It is important to step away from Florida momentarily and look at the relationship of midwives to the medical system on a national level in the mid-1980s to early 1990s. "Many of the original homebirth enthusiasts were no longer in their childbearing years" (McTigue 1989:37). Possibly in response to the alternative birth movement, but definitely for public appeal, hospitals started developing more home-like settings or birthing suites where fathers were permitted to be present for labor and delivery and mothers were able to keep their babies in the room with them. Nurse-midwives were increasingly being employed by these kinds of hospitals to provide a less aggressive approach to birth. There was less use of consciousness-altering medication and general anesthesia, and epidurals were becoming more popular. Breastfeeding started making a comeback after years of heavy propaganda from the infant formula industry. As medical costs increased, insurance companies greatly influenced which caregiver a family could use. Few of these companies reimbursed for licensed midwives; state programs like Medicaid also refused to pay for out-of-hospital midwifery services. Cesarean section rates were climbing and women were fighting through consumer movements to have more vaginal birth(s) after cesarean (VBACs).

MAF and midwifery supporters tried every year for the next eight years to have the Myers Amendment repealed. "It was a political nightmare," stated MAF lobbyist Beth Swisher. The midwives knew they had ten years from 1984 to pass legislation before they had to repeat another Sunset Review process and run the risk of permanently losing the legal status of their profession. "We were really trying to figure out our niche—was it a restraint of trade issue, was it a consumer issue, was it a women's reproductive choice issue?—and we sort of worked it any way we could depending on who the audience was," explained Jana Borino. For Jana, homebirth was a major concern, as she had given birth to three babies at home. But she knew homebirth was a fairly radical concept in the United States, so, Jana continued, MAF "got hip pretty quick to not talking about homebirth, just always casting [midwifery] politically in the birth center movement because that's just easier for our culture to hear."

The opposition lobby from the FMA remained steady and strong, thwarting the midwives' moves by using political tactics such as keeping their bill stalled in committee until it died. One of the ways to kill a bill is to assign it to too many committees, making it unlikely to pass through them all, or to a committee that is totally irrelevant to the proposed bill. Beth Swisher said, "We'd get the sponsors but because the opposition was so strong, the sponsors would figure, 'Well, this isn't going to go anywhere.' When you have limited amounts of legislation that will pass in a year, a sponsor is not going to put time and effort needed to get the bill going if it was going to be killed."

Amy Young, the lobbyist for the Florida Obstetric and Gynecologic Society since 1984, explained the opposition's position: "if anybody wanted to deliver babies, they ought to be trained as a nurse-midwife or as a doctor," repeating the argument against homebirth: "any kind of pregnancy, whether high risk or not . . . can have complications, and it's much better to be in a facility, either an outpatient ambulatory center, a birthing center, or a hospital, where one can have adequate back-up." One of the society's largest concerns centered on the midwives' education and training requirements, especially because they considered the Midwifery Practice Act less stringent than the nurse-midwifery legislation. "I think there are [good and bad] midwives, and [good and bad] doctors, but the best thing you can do to protect our public is to get the highest training, to assure the safety and welfare of the public."

The Florida Nurses Association (FNA) also took an anti–licensed midwifery stance, although it was subtler, according to Sharon Hamilton. Barbara Lumpkin, the Associate Executive Director of the Florida Nurses Association and lobbyist for the nurses, believed direct-entry midwifery was not "their issue." While they supported nurse-midwifery, they had no official association with direct-entry midwives and therefore did not play much of an active role until the early 1990s when the nurses advocated for the licensure of competent practitioners.

HRS demonstrated a passive approach by refusing to give midwifery its support, as did the Florida Chapter of the ACNM, which took no position, a move some saw as reinforcing the stereotype that nurse-midwifery was no different than obstetric nursing (McTigue 1989). All of this opposition resulted in legislators who were potentially supportive of midwifery would not touch the issue.

The situation seemed dismal for licensed midwives. Their political strategies were not working and they did not have the numbers, money, and influence their opponents possessed. Some midwives went on to get nursing training and became CNMs, who had more job security. Sharon Hamilton, who became president of MAF in 1986, recounted the frustration felt by the midwifery community:

> We would try and try. We would write letters, make phone calls, everything that we could think of to make progress but we were

really blockaded by the powers that be because we had no help from the governor and we had strong opposition in the health-care committee, which is where we would be "agendaed" and be heard.

The 1990s brought a breath of fresh air. Lawton Chiles, a midwifery-friendly Democrat, was elected Governor and the legislators at the Capitol were reshuffled. Midwifery is not a partisan issue, explained Sharon Hamilton:

> It truly is a bipartisan issue because with the Republicans you have respect for the family, respect for individual rights, and government out of your personal business type of philosophy. And midwifery appeals to Democrats for the reason that they tend to be more liberal. On both sides there is support based on the principles of the party, besides that it is a health issue.

Momentum for midwifery was growing again and "it seemed like we were really slowly but surely making inroads" (Justine Clegg). A multitude of factors led to the reopening of the Midwifery Practice Act in 1992. On an economic level, the victory was a true David and Goliath story: the FMA spent somewhere around $4 million fighting midwifery, while MAF spent about $40,000 dollars promoting it, as Sharon Hamilton explained. When I asked Joan McTigue how it happened she said, "It was just sort of a miracle, a set of defeats culminating in a victory." Joan later told me in a more serious tone that it was because "a small dedicated group remained faithful to the vision."

Becky Martin, who had three "wonderful" homebirths with midwives, initially became involved in the midwifery scene because of her desire to be a midwife and because she wanted other people to be able to have the positive experience she had with midwives. Passionate about bringing midwifery into the public eye, Becky compiled a packet of research articles and other scientific information pertaining to midwifery and sent copies to national talk shows, as well as to publications and organizations related to midwifery and homebirth. Surprisingly, Geraldo Rivera responded by doing a show on homebirth. Continuing in this direction, Becky began attending Friends of Midwives meetings in Tampa. Friends of Midwives groups were primarily consumer-based organizations that arose around licensed midwives, forming local chapters in various parts of the state. Other people involved with Friends of Midwives were midwives' assistants who wanted the law changed so they could realize their career dreams as midwives, but these individual groups were not networked together. Becky and other pro-midwife consumers in her area started their own Friends of Midwives, called the Gulf Coast Friends of Midwives. As Becky became more active in the politics of midwifery, she traveled to MAF meetings around Florida and learned more about other Friends of Midwives groups. "We started sharing information and looking at what was going on and what I saw was that we were all doing the same thing over again, you know, reinventing the wheel."

Demonstrating her networking and organizational ability, Becky hosted the first Florida Friends of Midwives meeting at her house in the summer of 1989.

> We came in with all our different ideas and our different connections and energy and said, "The midwives have been working to get this law changed for years now and it's not going anywhere. We need to, as consumers and as people who want to be midwives, get involved on a very big level and demand from our legislators that they fix this law so there can be more midwives, so people can go to school and that there will be midwives for our children. That it is an option that we want and that it's not illegal, it's not unsafe, it's done in many parts of the world, and it's OK."

The new statewide group functioned as a clearinghouse for publishing materials, such as flyers and newsletters, which were to be mutually used among the groups. This made it easier for local Friends of Midwives to get their message out and get people active and organized. Its representatives wrote letters, made calls, visited their legislators, put on workshops, and held a variety of fundraising events to support their local midwives. Membership was free and it was extremely grassroots oriented.

> None of us ever had any kind of training or education in doing any of this kind of stuff, we were just flying by the seat of our pants and doing what seemed right and what seemed needed to be doing and it was like She [spirit] was guiding us where we needed to be. . . . If something is supposed to happen with a lot of hard work and we were there to do the work. Finally it happened and it was wonderful! (Becky Martin, interview)

Becky clearly communicated that the Florida Friends of Midwives understood that midwifery and out-of-hospital birth was not for everyone, but it was something they wanted available, and they wanted it to be safe, legal, and regulated by the state.

Becky found herself "stunned by the vehemence of the opposition." For example, the Florida Friends of Midwives inadvertently discovered that the opposition—which generally meant the FMA, the Florida Obstetric and Gynecologic Society, the Florida Nurses Association (FNA), and others—sent a letter to all the legislators in the state that portrayed midwives negatively. Objecting to the misrepresentation, the Florida Friends of Midwives drafted a follow-up letter that addressed each point and proved it invalid, sending it to all the people who had received the first letter.

Through the influence of Representative Elaine Gordon, the Senate Committee on Health and Rehabilitative Services agreed to do a study called the Sunrise Report. The study looked at reopening licensure of lay (the term direct-entry was not yet widely used) midwives in the context of the need for additional maternity care providers and the level of skill and training deemed minimally necessary for providers of these services (Senate Committee on Health and Rehabilitative Services 1991). The study was done during the 1990 interim period and focused on the practice of licensed midwives in Florida between 1984 and 1990. It examined the various aspects of midwifery based on questionnaires sent to all the parties involved. Staff also contacted individuals in other states and performed an extensive review of vital statistics data relevant to the issue. The results were summarized in a report to the legislature, which came out in 1990. "This study was objective and credible and removed a lot of the arguments which were purely partisan in nature by the opposition: turf guarding really" (McTigue 1992:20).

The Sunrise Report found licensed midwives' safety record comparable to CNMs and physicians; it also determined that the public could benefit from increasing the number of licensed midwives. In addition, it stated that the 1982 law should be reopened with additions strengthening education requirements, and suggested Medicaid pay for prenatal and postpartum care provided by licensed midwives (Rooks 1997). The study recommended that midwifery be moved out of HRS and into the Department of Business and Professional Regulation (DBPR), the agency that regulated all the other health care professions in Florida. Another conclusion of the study was that "the state can regulate licensed midwives in such a way as to not adversely affect the competitive market while still protecting the public's health" (Senate Committee on Health and Rehabilitative Services 1991:63). After its completion, the staff director wrote a model bill that incorporated all the results of the study, which was voted to become a proposed committee bill sponsored by the Senate Committee on Health and Rehabilitative Services. Despite the study's favorable stance toward midwifery, passage of the bill was not a given. "What was so frustrating was that both the Sunset Review in '84 and the Sunrise Report in '90 were so positive, it was almost as if you'd say, 'Who could argue with this? Of course they are going to open up licensing again.' It's the politics that get in the way of rational thought" (Beth Swisher, interview).

The political struggle between MAF and the FMA has not always been clear. Justine Clegg described that in 1991, Senator Ben Graber, an obstetrician from South Florida, introduced a piece of legislation called the Graber Amendment, which would have required midwives to have five years of education, work under the supervision of a physician, and be regulated under the Board of Medicine. The Graber Amendment was first introduced at a Senate Health Care Committee meeting and presented as if the midwives and the FMA had created it jointly. In fact, the midwives had never seen it before and would never support an amendment restricting their freedom. When the midwives investigated, they discovered that members of the opposition had called legislators pretending to be midwifery supporters and communicated their approval of the amendment. If not for the watchdog effort by several politically active midwives, and help from Ann Gannon and Charlene Carres of the National Organization of Women (NOW), the Graber Amendment might have passed. Instead it died before it got to the Senate. The Graber Amendment was a compromise amendment and was difficult for midwifery supporters in the legislature to turn down. Even the midwives' Senate sponsor seemed eager to accept the amendment. However, it contradicted everything the midwives had been fighting for all along, and had no support from the midwives around the state. As a result of this incident, the Senate Health Care Committee charged the FMA to meet with the midwives to produce legislation both sides could agree on.

In the summer of 1991, three interorganizational meetings were arranged between MAF and the FMA. Their agendas dealt with educating and communicating with the end result of writing a mutually agreed-upon bill. The meetings "collectively resulted in first-time, direct dialogue between these groups [MAF and the FMA] and produced substantive exchanges about mutual perceptions, concerns, and expectations" (Senate Committee on Health and Rehabilitative Services 1991:11). Concrete training requirements were created and MAF committed to developing educational programs based on these models (Senate Committee on Health and Rehabilitative Services 1991). Several of my research participants relayed an interesting story to me about the first meeting. Ina May Gaskin, a national pillar in the midwifery community and an experienced midwife, came to speak about midwifery and showed her videos on shoulder dystocia and breech births. Justine Clegg said:

> Of course the doctors were glued to the screen. They were fascinated, which frustrated the nurses all to hell and gone because the doctors were dialoging with Ina May. "How do you do this? How do you do that?" like equals, because ultimately when you put politics aside and you're delivering babies, the doctors and the midwives will share tricks with each other.

At the meetings, the midwives wrote a far broader bill than the one that passed in 1982. This bill placed midwifery under the Department of Business and Professional Regulation (DBPR) with other health-care practitioners, where it was believed they might have more power. According to Beth Swisher, the meetings were productive with both sides understanding each other better; however some members of the opposition still absolutely did not support midwifery. The level of rapport between the two groups was improved but not ideal for professionals who must interact (Senate Committee on Health and Rehabilitative Services 1991).

People's passionate belief in midwifery seemed to lead to their political activity on the issue. Depth of consumer presence, which neither MAF nor its lobbyists could replicate, was a critical piece in passing midwifery legislation and was appreciated by many midwives I interviewed. The grassroots organizations really "galvanized consumers because you know the real power with the legislature is [the] consumer" (Justine Clegg, interview). Another midwife said, "An active grassroots movement means a great deal in state politics" (McTigue 1992:23). Becky Martin explained the consumer impact with respect to midwifery legislation:

> It was just getting the consumer involved and motivated, in my view, is what turned things around because midwives are special interest. When you have constituents calling their legislators saying they'd better fix the law so there can be midwives in their communities and have the phone ringing ten times a day saying that kind of stuff, they eventually start to listen. It's because people spoke out!

The 1990s represented a decade of national health care reform. Governor Lawton Chiles was a powerful advocate of this cause; one of the first things he did in office was to set up the Healthy Start program. He saw midwives as part of the solution to access and cost containment problems with maternity care in Florida. At one of the first Healthy Start organizational meetings in Tallahassee, Anne Richter, Alice Poe (the director of the nurse-midwifery program at the University of Florida), and Justine Clegg were invited to present their ideas to the committee as to how midwives could be used in Florida to meet consumer needs. From Governor Chiles's perspective, there was a need for more health care providers in Florida. A significant number of women were without prenatal care. His daughter Rhea Chiles explained to me that in his opinion, expanding the practice of midwifery was one of the answers: "It was a way to save babies and get women the health care they needed while providing them with a practitioner they could relate to that would be part of their culture and/or community." Becky Martin added, "he had family experience to know—he had grandchildren he could bounce on his knee that were caught by licensed midwives, so he knew they provided a valuable service and was always very supportive."

Char Lynn Daughtry and other activist midwives encouraged midwifery supporters to visit their legislators. One of their projects was sending postcards designed by MAF to local legislators that said, "Congratulations on a New Constituent!" announcing that another healthy baby had been born with a licensed midwife in their district. Because of her relationship with Rhea Chiles, Char Lynn had a significant impact and influence. Rhea delivered her first baby at the Tallahassee Birth Center with licensed midwives, and her second baby with Char Lynn at her birth center, and as a result Char Lynn was close to the governor's family. Char Lynn described visiting the governor's mansion and spending time talking about women's issues with the governor's wife. Apparently Mrs. Chiles was anxious to do something for midwifery and ended up putting together a certificate of appreciation, signed by the governor, to all the physicians and nurse-midwives who worked with licensed midwives.

Becky Martin described to me the exciting events surrounding Governor Chiles's son and daughter-in-law who were having a baby and planning on a hospital delivery with a local obstetrician. The couple lived on Anna Maria Island, off the coast of Tampa. One night her water broke and out came feet, signaling a footling breech presentation. They called an ambulance. When it arrived the paramedics followed their protocols for an obstetrical emergency and immediately called for backup. Doreen Virginiac, a retired licensed midwife, was on the backup ambulance. Along with her years of midwifery experience, she had received additional EMT training in Texas. It took ten minutes for

Doreen's squad to arrive at the home. Becky said, "Doreen walked into the room and immediately saw what was going on and knew that the first ambulance crew had done the opposite thing from what they should have done." The baby had been born except for the head. They had cut a huge episiotomy and were trying to pull the baby up and out by the feet. Doreen stepped in, repositioned the woman, did the appropriate maneuvers for a breech delivery (which involve putting the baby's head in a flexed position so the neck will not be damaged) and was able to easily complete the delivery. "Doreen saved [the baby's] life and Senator Chiles came down and gave her a Guardian Angel award" (Becky Martin, interview).

At the time this dramatic birth took place, Lawton Chiles was serving his third term in the U.S. Senate. When he decided to run for governor in 1990, the midwifery community was excited at the prospect of a midwifery-friendly governor. The first day Senator Chiles declared his candidacy, MAF sent a check for $100 to his campaign, the largest donation allowable. Around the state, midwives and consumers worked on his campaign, knowing if he won the gubernatorial election it would be a great benefit to licensed midwives and would go a long way in helping to get the legislation passed. The governor's support continued throughout the eight years of his administration, as he signed proclamations recognizing an International Midwives Day and a Licensed Midwives Awareness Week in Florida. Governor Chiles was a powerful state figure and the midwives' alliance with him significantly contributed to the successful passage of midwifery legislation in 1992. "We would have never gotten anywhere without the governor," stated Sharon Hamilton.

MAF recognized that 1992 would be a crucial year for getting the midwifery bill passed. In addition to Beth Swisher, they decided they needed a male lobbyist with influence and experience with the legislature. In 1992 they hired Bob Levy from a powerful professional lobbying firm with strong ties to many of the maternal and child health advocacy groups. Bob had been involved with the midwifery issue for about ten years, and he had been active with women's choice issues and often represented the Florida Nurses Association (FNA). Bob was able to convince the FNA not to lobby against licensed midwifery, which proved to be a great advantage. Previously, MAF relied on the full-time lobbying efforts of Beth Swisher, who although not the sole lobbyist for MAF in 1992, was still instrumental. "We would never have passed the law without Beth because she stuck at it for years and years and was a tremendous supporter," said Sharon Hamilton. Beth was able to help Bob understand and prepare for the lobbying tactics of the FMA and FOGS lobbyists, which Bob, a seasoned lobbyist of many years, said he had never previously encountered. Although he was more expensive, Bob "got the midwives' bill on the agendas of organizations that had generally dismissed us as 'old hippies' or too concerned with a small number of middle-class consumers" (McTigue 1992:20). Another factor that helped the midwives was that it was a peak time for women serving in the legislature. This impacted which issues were put on the agenda, with emphasis given to social concerns over financial ones.

When I asked Bob how the bill passed in 1992, he claimed it had to do with powerful support from Bo Johnson, the Rules Chair of the Florida House of Representatives; Kip Jackson, Bo's legislative assistant; and Elaine Bloom, the Chair of the House Health Care Committee and Speaker Pro Tem. Bo and Elaine were actually born with a midwife; Kip also had an extensive background with midwifery. The three of them convened regular meetings with the different parties and expressed their desire to pass midwifery legislation.

> We enlisted very broad support, from North Florida conservative white male Democrats to conservative Republican members, and traditional Southern Democrats to the Midwestern Republicans to Cuban members, black members, Jewish members, and women. Finally we were just able over the years to build up enough steam and strength to kind of dispel the mythology surrounding midwifery and get the legislation passed. (Kip Jackson, interview)

Kip described strong resistance from the FMA, whose members still claimed midwifery was not safe and would lead to the deaths of women and children, but Kip saw it as a pro-choice issue, "a woman's right to give birth to her child in her home with proper medical care and support backup with well-trained midwives." Kip observed that the majority of the world gives birth with midwives and questioned why Florida should be any different: "the best thing we could do medically was to try to support an idea that allowed the very natural rhythm of a woman's body to function . . . and not have all this medical intervention every step of the way." Bob Levy added, "I think having leadership supporting your position is hard to oppose."

Also aiding in the bill's passage was the fact that the FMA was concerned with more pressing issues at that time, such as self-referrals. This decreased the focus on midwifery and implied that if the FMA really did not want the bill to pass, it would have fought harder. Reflecting on the political scene in the Capitol, Bob stated, "Almost every battle of substance in Tallahassee is about money," and Kip agreed:

> There were those in the medical community that felt like this threatened their bread and butter . . . it was the idea that midwives are going to come in here and do something not only for poor women who couldn't afford the high costs but middle- or upper-class women with a great deal of money would make these choices and they would lose revenue. Economically it was good for the government if women choose to have homebirths with a midwife because the costs are far less and then consequently you also maintain the available dollars and resources to help those women and children that really do need radical medical intervention to save their lives.

In an attempt to make contact with and educate politicians on the issues concerning midwifery, Becky Martin and the Florida Friends of Midwives sent a questionnaire to every senator and representative. The last questions asked if they would sponsor or cosponsor legislation that would reopen midwifery. Becky remembers being at her home one evening when Representative Daryl Jones from Miami called her regarding the questionnaire. She described it as a "fabulous" talk, as he was very curious about midwifery and related issues. Daryl was already somewhat familiar with midwifery; he had friends who were active with the issue in the Miami area, and his oldest child was delivered by a nurse-midwife. Becky, Daryl, and members of MAF arranged several meetings, and eventually Daryl ended up sponsoring the midwifery bill in the House in 1992. At first the midwives were hesitant to work with Daryl because he was a freshman politician, but the commitment and attention he brought to their cause were unlikely to be replicated by a more senior member. "It's not common to get somebody who really has a fire in their heart," said MAF president Sharon Hamilton about Daryl. Julie Snyder, a homebirth mother who organized a consumer advocacy group in Miami (the Midwifery Access Project) and served as treasurer of MAF, commented that he was "quick to understand the issues and notice where the danger points lay; he really did a good job representing us." Daryl devoted many hours to finding common ground between the midwives and the FMA.

When I asked Daryl Jones why he sponsored the bill, he told me that he thought midwifery would be beneficial for the state of Florida because the care midwives provided was high quality with good results. His initial plan was to bring the different groups (MAF, FMA, and FNA) together to talk about the issues, but the meeting proved chaotic and emotional. So he decided to meet with the groups separately, as a middleman, going back and forth between them working on finding a compromise that all could support. The FMA brought forward the same argument they had often used, that midwives had inadequate training, making even low-risk births dangerous. Daryl perceived the true problem to be economic turf. The FMA's view, according to Daryl, was that "if lay midwives were allowed to be licensed and were allowed to circulate through their training programs, then the obstetricians would be left with only the high-risk cases. So every potential client would be a potential lawsuit and their jobs would be more stressful." The FMA never openly brought up this competition issue, Daryl thought, because it is in the best interests of physicians and not constituents.

One of Daryl's strategies was to keep the negotiations solely between the FMA and MAF. With this motive, he convinced the nurse-midwives not to get involved, and to remain neutral. Another of Daryl's objectives was to keep the FMA's emotions low-key so they would not lobby the entire legislature; as it was, they were only working on about five out of 120 members. Daryl said he was lobbying all of the members, putting together educational bullet sheets for members who were unfamiliar with midwifery, and changing certain parts of the bill with which legislators had problems.

> I was lobbying members and educating them so that by the time the bill got to the floor, every member had heard the story two or three times prior to their voting for it. When the doctors came in at the last minute and tried to interject themselves and say, "this will not work because of this and that," I had already answered their questions a couple of times and [the legislators remembered], so they didn't trust the answers that came from the doctors anymore. . . . We knew who was for us, we knew who was in the middle, and we knew who was against us, and so we were counting votes the entire time. I knew when we got to the floor that I was going to win!

Another part of Daryl's confidence came from his knowledge that Governor Chiles supported the bill and had even persuaded some of the members to back it. The fact that the governor was personally invested in the issue meant there was no veto threat, which gave the bill a huge advantage. Daryl expressed to me that opening up the Midwifery Practice Act in 1992 was the hardest thing he has done in the legislature, but that he really wanted to see it through.

Helen Gordon-Davis, a longtime advocate for midwifery legislation, sponsored the bill in the Senate. Helen was strong on women's issues and promoted the midwifery bill in that light. She described one of the more powerful Senators getting up and speaking about how he had been born at home, how that was responsible for him being so healthy, how wonderful midwifery is, and why the Senate should open up the Midwifery Practice Act. Helen said, "He was a man that took everything personally and if they had voted against him, he would have been a very dangerous enemy." Anticlimactically, compared to the House, the midwifery legislation passed the Senate with all but one member voting for it. Jeanne Madrid, a licensed midwife present in the Senate that day stated, "Helen Gordon-Davis threw kisses up to us [midwifery supporters] up in the balcony and we were like ohhhh." Justine Clegg described the emotions she felt as she witnessed the legislation being passed: "I remember walking out and collapsing in Beth Swisher's arms and I just started crying and I couldn't stop. I was just crying and crying and people were coming up asking if I was all right. Beth told them, 'Her bill just passed and we worked thirteen years on it!' And they were like, 'Oh, we understand, good for you, good work!'"

Throughout this marathon struggle, the leaders of MAF never gave up on their commitment to resuscitate direct-entry midwifery in Florida. MAF members drafted position papers, lobbied, held fundraisers, and did anything they could to gather support and educate politicians. Sharon Hamilton talked about how passing legislation is a process of educating legislators, establishing a base of support within the legislature, and building an activist consumer movement through letters and phone calls. Sharon offered some of her insights from her years of political participation:

> The thing I discovered about being a lobbyist and about being the president of the midwives association and about being in Tallahassee was how I finally came to see the legislature as a three-dimensional chess game. Most of us, the common citizens, only see it on a one-dimensional level. Our perception of it is very flat. Then as you get into it a little bit more, you get a little more varied understanding of it and you see that there is a lot of "you scratch my back and I'll scratch yours" stuff going on. So you see how it actually begins to work. The third level is the level that nobody sees, only the legislators, and that's the stuff that goes on "behind closed doors." Of course, all this was before the Sunshine Amendment passed.

Sharon described herself as a risk taker, not in terms of her midwifery practice, but with respect to the politics of midwifery. "As a leader, you hope you can inspire people to follow you and take the road that is going to be the most beneficial for the entire group. You really have to have a sense of what is best for the group and what is best for midwifery."

As a statute, the Midwifery Practice Act of 1992 was relatively broad, with the assumption that the more specific rules of practicing midwifery would be further defined in the Florida Administrative Code by the associated state department with the advice of the Council of Licensed Midwifery. The law was based on World Health Organization (WHO) standards and successful European direct-entry midwifery programs, and stated that licensed midwives are autonomous maternity care providers for healthy, low-risk pregnant women during the childbearing year. Midwifery rules provide risk screening criteria for entry into midwifery care and describe what care is to be provided during pregnancy, labor, delivery, and the postpartum period, including ongoing risk assessment and specific conditions requiring physician consultation, referral, and transfer of care. Criteria for assessing the safety and suitability of the client's home for childbirth are also given. Risk factors such as smoking, anemia, previous cesarean section, multiple gestation, non-vertex presentation past thirty-seven weeks, and so forth, have assigned numbers. If a client has a risk score of three, the midwife shall consult with a physician who has obstetrical hospital privileges, and if there is a joint determination that the woman can be expected to have a normal pregnancy, labor, and birth, the midwife may provide services to that client. This potentially opens up midwifery practice to controversial groups such as women desiring VBACs or with breech presentations if midwives can find supportive physicians; multiple gestation is an automatic transfer of care. However, few if any obstetricians are referring clients back to licensed midwives for the above cases. Women without significant risk factors never need to see a physician, although many midwives prefer that their clients meet the backup doctor at least once during pregnancy. A midwife may provide collaborative prenatal and postpartal care to pregnant women not at low risk in their pregnancy, labor, and delivery within a written protocol of a physician currently licensed. Licensed midwives in Florida are able to work in a variety of settings including home, birth center, and hospital. They must renew their license every two years; the process includes submitting a statistical report for their practice, completing continuing education credits, and holding professional liability insurance.[3] Midwifery clients must sign an informed consent document and an emergency care plan is prepared for both mother and baby in case problems arise during pregnancy, delivery, or in the postpartum period. As a result of legislation passed in 1988, licensed midwives are eligible for HMO and third-party reimbursement for all out-of-hospital birth.[4]

In order to become a licensed midwife in Florida, an applicant must graduate from an approved midwifery program, have a written plan for the management of emergencies, pass NARM's national certification examination,[5] and show proof of having liability insurance. Midwives can also follow the "Licensure by Endorsement" route. Approved midwifery programs in Florida must be conducted in an accredited public institution or licensed by the Florida Department of Education's Board of Non-public Career Education, and be approved by (and meet accreditation requirements as determined by) the Florida Department of Health's Council of Licensed Midwifery. These are intensive three-year programs of academic and clinical education whose educational requirements are founded upon the core competencies of the American College of Nurse-Midwives (ACNM) and the Midwives Alliance of North America (MANA). Clinical requirements for graduation are to observe twenty-five women in the intrapartal period; undertake, with the supervision of a preceptor, the care of fifty women in each of the antepartal, intrapartal, and postpartal periods (the same woman need not be seen through all three periods); and perform newborn exams and assessments of fifty babies. Well-woman gynecology is also part of the scope of education. (For more information about Florida licensed midwives including laws, rules, and licensure requirements, visit www. doh.state.fl.us/mqa/midwifery/mw_home.html.) A Licensed Midwife in Florida does not automatically gain the status of Certified Professional Midwife (CPM); however with state licensure, many of the requirements for the CPM are met (go to www.narm.org to view "How to Become a CPM").

DEVELOPING A PROFESSION: THE PRIVILEGES AND PRICES OF SWIMMING IN THE MAINSTREAM

After the 1992 legislation passed, the Department of Business and Professional Regulation (DBPR) took the place of HRS and was in charge of midwifery. Switching to DBPR meant midwifery was required to be self-sufficient; in other words, licensure fees needed to cover the profession's regulation expenses. However, due to the small number of licensed midwives in the state, debt started accumulating. In response, licensing fees increased, but still did not meet the costs incurred. The debt issue has proved to be an important threat to the profession: by the end of the 1990s, the debt was over $500,000 and remains a problem today. At present, midwifery, along with the other health care professions in Florida, is regulated by the Department of Health.

Under the new law, practice rules had to be revised by the Council of Licensed Midwifery, and in that process a significant mistake was uncovered. Rules are meant to clarify law, and they have to be directly related to each other; this is termed *statutory authority*. There must be statutory authority for every rule; if there is not, the rule is considered as having been written with *unbridled discretion*. There was a rule drawn up after the 1982 law that required midwifery clients to have two visits with a physician, in their first and third trimesters, so that the client could be approved for midwifery care outside the hospital; some thought this necessary for client safety. When this rule was being evaluated to determine if it needed to be updated, a lawyer at the council meeting spoke up and asked, "Where is the statutory authority for this rule?" Apparently there was none—it was unfounded and did not relate back to the law—and thus it was written with unbridled discretion. When this rule was originally written, the midwives had a limited understanding of law and simply accepted it as legitimate. At that point, the midwives were working hard to survive, and questioning the validity of those details never occurred to them. Becky Martin told me how much trouble midwives had in complying with this rule. Sometimes the midwives would travel across the state to find physicians who would agree to do these prenatal checkups. The eventual nullification of this rule removed a significant obstacle in licensed midwives' practice.

The Florida Midwifery Resource Center was established in 1992 after the passage of the law, with the support of an implementation grant from the Robert Wood Johnson Foundation to the University of Florida College of Medicine. The purpose of the Resource Center was to help birth centers and midwifery grow in Florida. Toward this end, it set the "Call to Action" goals of having "fifty percent of healthy pregnant women cared for by midwives by the year 2000" and "to promote the development of family centered free standing birth centers" (Florida Midwifery Resource Center brochure). At the time the Center started, the original funding body believed there were "very few licensed midwives who were going to set up within an academic system...and were not going to make a major impact on what's happening" (interview Anne Richter), so the funding was more aimed at supporting nurse-midwifery. Anne Richter, who at the time was Deputy Director of the Midwifery Resource Center, admitted that they put more emphasis on nurse-midwives, in part because CNMs attend more births than licensed midwives (LMs). Anne stressed that one of the goals of the center is to "reduce infant mortality and to improve health care for women, so we're going to go where most of the action on births is." She said that they have been able to "go a little bit broader but right now [1999] we don't have much money." Before closing its doors due to a lack of funding, the center published a guide to all the birth centers in Florida, as well as a directory of CNMs and LMs in Florida.

In 1992 with the passage of the Midwifery Practice Act, the midwifery community seemed to breathe a great sigh of relief and enjoy their long-awaited success. It was a time for rest and rebuilding, and to think about the future. Jana Borino said:

> So the law passed and there was much renewed excitement and energy about "what do we do next" and really, I don't think anybody had ever really entertained the thought of what we would do next. We were so hyperfocused on getting the law changed and opening licensure that it was only in our wildest dreams to think about what to do next.

This period marked the second wave of leadership transition within direct-entry midwifery in Florida. The Friends of Midwives groups disintegrated. Many of the people who had been activists were now preparing to attend midwifery school, and many of the midwives who had become licensed in the 1980s continued to take an active role in implementing the new law, especially with regard to education and regulation. The grassroots movement ebbed and flowed, rematerializing only when something threatening appeared on the horizon.

Reestablishing educational programs became a top priority. In 1993, Justine Clegg was asked to attend the Florida Department of Education Leveling Committee meeting to decide what degree the state would require for the midwifery educational program. The midwifery regulations mandated a three-year, ninety-credit program and made it clear that postsecondary vocational schools, as well as degree-granting institutions, could provide midwifery programs. The typical associate degree program is two years, sixty credits long, while the typical baccalaureate degree program is four years, 120 credits long—and making this choice was a hotly debated topic among the midwives. A baccalaureate degree would gain greater credibility and respect and be more credit efficient, yet an associate degree would make midwifery education more affordable. Most in the midwifery community felt they would have greater control and access at the associate degree level, so they gave this as their preference to the leveling committee. From a national perspective, this decision may have closed the door to a pivotal opportunity to create a liaison with the American College of Nurse-Midwives through education.

The National School of Technology (NST), a technical school in the Miami area, had expressed an interest in providing a midwifery program and subsequently sponsored the first midwifery program after the 1992 legislation passed (Marguerite Epstein, interview). Led by Patti Starkman, Debbie Marin, and later Shari Daniels, the program began in November 1993 and graduated its first class in May 1995. These NST graduates were the first midwifery students in Florida to take the NARM exam for their state licensure, in August 1995 (Marguerite Epstein, interview). However, the NST midwifery program was short-lived; due to economic reasons it was cancelled after it graduated a second class in 1996. Shari Daniels went on to independently open the Miami Beach Maternity Center (now the Miami Maternity Center) and International School of Midwifery (ISOM), where she and her students currently attend around twenty births per month and are frequently featured in a national television series, *House of Babies.*

Justine Clegg met with consumers, midwives, and aspiring midwives in South Florida to consider whether to reopen the South Florida School of Midwifery or to place the program in an existing institution. Back in 1990, Justine, representing the South Florida School of Midwifery and Sharon Hamilton, president of MAF at the time, met with the Deans of Nursing and Allied Health at Miami-Dade Community College (MDCC) to interest the college in starting a midwifery program. MDCC responded that they could not consider starting a midwifery program until licensure was once again available. So it was not until the 1992 law passed, and after much negotiation between Justine and MDCC, that they agreed to begin the process of developing a midwifery program. Justine's decision to pursue the initiative with MDCC was born out of her conviction that women need access to affordable education with college credits that "articulate"—meaning that they are readily accepted by other institutions toward additional degrees.

Justine put together an advisory committee of midwives and associates and began working with MDCC to adapt the curriculum and course objectives from the South Florida School of Midwifery into an Associate of Science in Midwifery Degree program. Despite internal opposition within the college, most notably from the nursing department, in the fall of 1993 MDCC accepted the proposal to establish the only direct-entry midwifery undergraduate degree program in a state institution in the country. (www.mdc.edu/medical/Nursing/Programs/ Midwifery_Prog/main.htm.) Justine was hired as Chair in early 1994 to write the syllabi for the courses, hire faculty, purchase equipment and supplies, and select the first class, which was enrolled in August of 1994. To earn the degree, students must take thirty-four credits (one year) of general education and basic science courses similar to nursing prerequisites, and an additional fifty-six credits (two years) of core midwifery courses. MDCC midwifery students are eligible for federal financial aid.

Miami-Dade Community College is the largest postsecondary institution in the United States, with a student body comprised of a high percentage of women, minorities, inner city, and English-as-second-language individuals. Sharon Hamilton, a clinical preceptor for the Miami-Dade program, stated that "you need to have a short program that is inexpensive and you need to have it in a setting that is going to be supportive to single moms and people who are going back into education late in life and that means Miami-Dade Community College." The college has produced graduates from the African-American, Latin American, and Caribbean communities, who serve women with cultural competency in their own languages, which broadens the licensed midwifery population beyond the white middle-class midwives of the 1980s, bringing it full circle to all the people.

The Florida School of Traditional Midwifery in Gainesville was incorporated in the fall of 1993, licensed by the Department of Education, and approved by the Department of Health on the recommendation of the Council of Licensed Midwifery in May of 1994 (www.midwiferyschool.org). The process of planning the school took two years. Jana Borino, one of the school's founding members, described her role: "I had been the central organizer in this part of the state, and I was organizing the meetings to talk about having a school but nobody was coming forward with the energy or the interest in putting together a school, so I became that person." On the advice of Joan McTigue, in 1993 Jana attended a National Coalition of Midwifery Educators meeting to connect with others involved in midwifery education and learn how to create a midwifery school. Jana recruited Becky Martin to be her partner and together with the help of Karen Kearns, Joanna Varadi, and Susan Shapiro, they became the founding board members of the Florida School of Traditional Midwifery. Jana commented:

> We put it out there that we were opening a school and I talked to no fewer than 800 people directly in the middle of dinner, in the

> middle of changing diapers, when I was trying to get out of the door to take my kids to an activity . . . but we got the word out. People believed in us, people supported us, and it happened!

Women "came out of the woodwork" at meetings for prospective students, all wanting to attend the new midwifery school.

Another major milestone in the development of direct-entry midwifery in Florida particularly relevant in today's health-care world dealt with third-party reimbursement and malpractice insurance. In 1988, with the help of MAF lobbyist Beth Swisher, a law quietly passed requiring insurance reimbursement for licensed midwives, and in 1992 birth centers became reimbursable by Medicaid. When the Midwifery Practice Act passed in 1992, Medicaid reimbursement for homebirths was specifically excluded, which MAF agreed to in order to gain the support of Charlie Mahan, the State Health Officer. Yet getting Medicaid reimbursement for homebirths was critical to the survival of midwifery, because midwives often serve low-income women. Sharon Hamilton informed me that the Medicaid issue was not "glamorous" compared to legalizing midwifery, and the consumer support was significantly less than had existed for the legalization fight. "It was still very complicated in that how do you get this passed when you don't have the kind of public support you once had?"

Working on the Medicaid/homebirth issue was Beth Swisher, longtime midwifery lobbyist, with the help of professional lobbyist Bob Cerra, who got involved with midwifery in 1994 through an internship at Mixon and Associates. The argument against Medicaid reimbursement for homebirths was basically that the opposition did not want the state to have a financial incentive to force poor mothers to have births at home and get what they thought of as "substandard care." However, since 1992 Governor Chiles had increased welfare programs related to prenatal care and increased the income level that made a family eligible to receive Medicaid benefits. Supporters of Medicaid reimbursement for homebirths took the stance that just because a woman is poor does not mean she is high risk and not reimbursing for homebirths limited that population's choices of where to give birth.

After trying unsuccessfully to get the Medicaid for homebirth bill included in larger comprehensive health care packages, in 1996 MAF and Bob Cerra decided to have the bill stand on its own. Finding a sponsor in the House was a challenge, but eventually, through a connection licensed midwife Jeanne Madrid had established with freshman Representative Paula Dockery the year before, MAF secured a bill sponsor. Daryl Jones, a Senator at that point, supported the bill in the Senate.

Negotiations around the bill were charged. It became clear that in order for it to pass, the opposition lobby required a revision that included language about malpractice insurance. Up until then, licensed midwives were not required to carry malpractice insurance. However, Amy Young, the lobbyist for the Florida Obstetric and Gynecologic Society, believed that the state should not be paying Medicaid money to midwives when they did not have malpractice insurance (Bob Cerra, interview). In our interview, Amy expressed her opinion that the midwives "greedily" wanted more income through Medicaid dollars, but that they should not even be doing Medicaid births anyway because these women are typically a high-risk group.

Back in 1992 when the midwifery bill was being voted on in the Florida House of Representatives, an amendment by Representative Ben Graber designed to force midwives to carry malpractice insurance was defeated by Daryl Jones. MAF believed it was just a matter of time before midwives would be required to carry malpractice insurance, and agreed to accept the revised bill as a trade-off for several reasons: malpractice insurance was then affordable, the addition of Medicaid birth reimbursement would pay the premium, and the midwifery law included a requirement that the state Joint Underwriting Association (JUA) would have to secure malpractice insurance for midwives if it was otherwise unavailable, so that in the long term, mandatory malpractice insurance could not close down the practice of licensed midwifery.

The midwives accepted the revised bill, which was heard by the House Health Care Committee and successfully passed through the rest of the legislative process. Bob Cerra remembered that when the bill came up, "we had conference calls, sent out letters, and had multiple pollings about whether we were going to pass this bill the way it was [in revised form] or not." Sharon Hamilton recalled that making the decision to accept the revised bill and agree to place licensed midwives under the financial burden of malpractice insurance was one of the more difficult moments of being president of MAF and resulted in a lot of controversy within the midwives' association. Sharon said, "We decided that malpractice insurance was inevitable. Pretty much every other health-care practitioner is required to have malpractice insurance, so we decided that getting the Medicaid reimbursement was worth having the malpractice insurance."

After agreeing to the proposed legislation, in the eleventh hour, the opposition attempted to make licensed midwives carry malpractice insurance for an inflated amount of coverage equivalent to that of obstetricians. The opposition also refused to accept the standard insurance exemptions. In response to these unrealistic demands, the midwives ended up filing a legal challenge, essentially suing the state with the legal assistance of Charlene Carres. After several years of litigation, the midwives won the case: the malpractice insurance requirement was set at an acceptable level, the same amount required for CNMs, and was to take place upon initial activation or licensure renewal past 1997. This gave licensed midwives two years to collect Medicaid-funded deliveries before they had to pay for malpractice insurance. In 2004, Alan Huber (then chief financial officer of the Miami Beach Maternity Center and President of the Florida Association of Birth Centers), after years of lobbying, was successful in his efforts to make Blue Cross/Blue Shield insurance coverage available to any Florida birth center that applies for it.

Bob Cerra continues to represent MAF in Tallahassee as their primary lobbyist. In the last few years, his responsibilities have included monitoring the current situation and making sure there are no major issues or bills in the works that would negatively affect the practice of licensed midwives. He described his job as "protecting," while he encourages the midwives to build up the grassroots network with legislative members and promote their cause as much as possible.

Ironically, there are both privileges and prices that have come about through the licensure of direct-entry midwives in Florida. With the 1992 Midwifery Practice Act in place, midwives have gained the right to practice a legitimate profession that is recognized by the state and the nation, one that is autonomous for low-risk women, and is reimbursable by Medicaid and private insurance. When clients develop complications, midwives can openly reveal their identities and present their records, making for a safer and more efficient transfer of care into the medical model. Midwives collaborate freely with other health care and related professions, making it possible to best meet their clients' needs.

However, Florida licensed midwives also face challenges. Along with legitimacy comes the fear of institutionalization and control by outside forces, especially those typically hostile to midwifery. Some may argue the practice rules are too strict, giving away midwives' power in certain circumstances. Despite third-party reimbursement, the burdens of affording licensure fees and carrying mandatory malpractice insurance are heavy, and both run the risk of increasing, forcing smaller midwifery practices out of business. Florida midwives also have a historical memory from the legislation passed in 1984 that their hard-earned victories can be taken away. Political figures come and go, yet powerful opposition groups continue to exert their pressure. Under Governor Chiles's administration, licensed midwifery was awarded some protection, but sadly he passed away in 1998 just a few weeks before his second term in office. The politics of midwifery are a constant battle and one that is essential for survival.

As of July 2004, 174 licenses had been issued to direct-entry midwives in Florida (for current information about individual Florida licensed midwives: www.doh.state.fl.us/irm00praes/praslist.asp). In early 2003 there were approximately 750 CNMs in Florida; seventy percent to seventy-five percent belong to the American College of Nurse-Midwifery (personal correspondence with George Hamilton, ACNM, February 10, 2003). The most recent state birth statistics come from 2002 Florida Vital Statistics data (see www.doh.state.fl.us/planning_eval/intro.html for *Vital Statistical Annual Reports* for 1996 through 2002). These numbers are ambiguous with respect to out-of-hospital and midwife-attended births since there are no distinctions between the types of midwives and homebirth as a category is not specified. Yet it can be assumed that nurse-midwives primarily work in hospital settings and licensed midwives make up the majority of out-of-hospital attendees. In general for 2002, midwives attended 11.26 percent (22,849) of births in hospitals and 97.15 percent (785) of births in birth centers. There were 1,094 births that happened in other places such as homes, and 791 births that were documented as being at an unknown place (Florida Department of Health 2003:22). Of the 205,580 total births in Florida in 2002, 0.93 percent (1,902) happened in birth centers and in other named places (Florida Department of Health 2003:22). By 2003, the majority of Florida birth centers were run by Florida licensed midwives. Recently, birth certificate data for Florida has been updated to be more specific concerning birth attendant and location, which will hopefully in turn improve the accuracy of these reports.

CONCLUSION: THE VALUE OF HISTORY

Never doubt that a small group of dedicated concerned citizens can change the world. Indeed, it is the only thing that ever has.

—Margaret Mead

Midwives in the United States have a history of being displaced by the medical profession. The cause of their disappearance was partly related to their traditional practices, which did not keep pace with society's demand for increased medical technology, and also due to their lack of organization and financial resources, all attributes needed to survive in the face of powerful opponents. Other practitioners who are located outside the mainstream health-care system face these same challenges. Predominantly female, midwives have also encountered resistance related to their status as women.

Emerging out of the late 1960s and 1970s came a group of women consciously deciding to birth their babies far from the norm of the standard hospital and obstetrician experience. Because they were members of the middle class, educated, mostly white, and knowledgeable of their rights as consumers in this country, their choices made an impact. They understood that it was not enough to go against a system; rather, it was necessary to change that system to better meet their needs. They wanted to be competent midwives, but not nurse-midwives, as they saw that path going in the direction of further subordination. They wanted to be trained, independent, and legal. To achieve these goals they had to do what their midwife predecessors did not: organize, become politically active, and generate a national infrastructure that could be adapted to the needs of a given state. This infrastructure had to include a solid written knowledge base, an accrediting agency for direct-entry midwifery educational programs (MEAC), and a process for national certification that included pathways for both institutionally and apprentice-trained midwives to demonstrate their knowledge, skills, and experience (NARM). Having established these national processes, they had to take the next steps to earn credibility and obtain national recognition: MEAC is recognized by the U.S. Department of Education, and NARM is recognized by the National Organization for Competency Assurance.

None of the women involved at this early stage in the development of licensed midwifery had much experience with grassroots groups, law, politics, or the health care system. They learned about networking, fund raising, legal terminology, lobbying, the official and unofficial workings of the political process, and health professionalism mostly through innocent common sense, self-study, trial and error, and the occasional help of someone in the field. These women had to add this information to their midwifery bags along with their compassion and traditional motherwit. When I interviewed Florida midwives currently practicing, I recognized that most of them seem to have a basic grasp of law and politics relative to their profession, and almost all of them have participated in the state professional organization and made contact with their local legislators.

The value of history lies in what individuals do with the historical information. Realizing where you came from can help you fully see where you are. In this way the journey, with all its transformations, can be appreciated and honored while past mistakes can be avoided. In my interviews, I noted that almost all midwifery supporters were thankful someone was recording their experiences during this difficult journey toward legalization and legitimization. They talked about how important it was to them that the emerging midwives of the future know how direct-entry midwifery in Florida began, and that the path to licensure was not always as smooth as it is now. Direct-entry midwifery in Florida at the dawn of the millennium is one of the best examples of how this style of midwifery has moved from being an unorganized, illegal underground operation into a legitimate profession that has gained endorsement from the state, a population of health practitioners, and insurance companies. Sharon Wells stated:

> I tell you Florida was a great experience for me, it's one of the ones I consider a win. I'm glad I was a part of the whole initial movement there. . . . Florida is the law I hold up as the model law, it works really well and it has a lot of latitude built into it and I like the Florida school model, I just think it's good.

Yet despite the distance direct-entry midwifery has traveled, it remains an alternative choice for a minority of women, and the medical opposition remains alert to opportunities to rid the playing field of its competitors. The heart of direct-entry midwifery and the pressures these midwives face constitute conflicting influences they must vigilantly work to hold together.

TIMELINE: A BRIEF HISTORY OF LICENSED MIDWIFERY IN FLORIDA

1931 Midwifery Act (Florida Statute 485) is passed and 1,400 lay midwives become licensed

1933 Approximately 4,000 midwives serve Florida families

1964 191 midwives hold Florida licenses

1974 57 midwives hold Florida licenses

1979 Florida Midwives' Association (FMA) is formed, then later changed its name to the Midwives Association of Florida (MAF) when it realized FMA was the acronym for the Florida Medical Association

1982 Midwifery Practice Act (Florida Statute 467) is passed; two-year Sunset Review Study is mandated

1983 North Florida School of Midwifery in Gainesville opens and takes their first (and only) class of midwifery students; the

Sunset Review Study is conducted and recommends the continuation of licensed midwifery

1984 South Florida School of Midwifery in Miami opens and takes their first (and only) class of midwifery students; the Myers Amendment is passed

1988 Licensed midwives are included in state legislation mandating insurance companies reimburse for midwifery services

1989 Florida Friends of Midwives is formed

1990 Senate Committee on Health and Rehabilitative Services Study (Sunrise Report) is completed and recommends reopening midwifery licensure

1992 New midwifery legislation (Florida Statute 467) is passed; Medicaid reimburses birth centers

1993 Council of Licensed Midwifery develops Rules and Regulations; National School of Technology accepts first class of midwifery students

1994 Miami-Dade Community College becomes the only public institution in the United States to offer a degree for licensed midwives

1995 Florida School of Traditional Midwifery accepts first class of midwifery students

1997 Medicaid reimbursement for homebirth; malpractice insurance required for licensed midwives

2004 Blue Cross agrees to include Florida birth centers in their network in all categories

ACKNOWLEDGMENTS

I would like to thank the editors, Robbie Davis-Floyd and Christine Barbara Johnson, for their guidance through the publication process. I am also grateful for the sage advice and comments of some of those who lived the history I attempt to portray here: Joan McTigue, Linda Wilson, Margaret Hebson, Justine Clegg, Sharon Hamilton, Jana Borino, Beth Swisher, Becky Martin, and Carol Nelson. I would be remiss not to mention the loving appreciation I feel toward my husband, who always has supported me and looked after our children as I wove this story together.

I dedicate this chapter to the many wonderful people I interviewed for my master's research, especially the midwives. It is my intention that the new generations of midwives understand and be thankful for the effort, courage, and wisdom of the women who preceded them.

ENDNOTES

1. Several years later the Florida Midwives Association (FMA) changed its name to the Midwives Association of Florida (MAF) to avoid confusion with the Florida Medical Association (FMA).
2. The Sunset Review was abolished in 1992.
3. Since 1997 licensed midwives have been required to carry liability insurance.
4. However, licensed midwives were not able to collect Medicaid reimbursement for homebirth until 1997.
5. The NARM national certification exam was used as the Florida state exam beginning in 1995.

REFERENCES

Bovard, Wendy, and Gladys Milton. 1993. *Why Not Me?: The Story of Gladys Milton, Midwife.* Summertown, TN: The Book Publishing Company.

Denmark, Melissa 2002. "The Evolution of Direct-Entry Midwifery in Florida, 1975–1999." Master's thesis. University of Florida.

Ely, Joyce. 1933. Statement made in minutes of meeting of state health officials, series 904, box I, *Essays on Midwifery 1931–1946*, Florida State Archives, Tallahassee, FL: Bureau of Archives and Records Management.

Florida Department of Health. 2003. Table B-4: Resident Live Births by Type of Place of Delivery and Attendant, by County, Florida, 2002. In *Florida Vital Statistics Annual Report 2002*, 22. Tallahassee: Florida Department of Health.

———. 2004. Licensed Midwifery homepage. http://www.doh.state.fl.us/mqa/midwifery/mw_home.html, accessed July 19, 2004.

———. 2004. "Public Health Statistics." http://www.doh.state.fl.us/planning_eval/intro.html, accessed July 19, 2004.

———. 2004. "Search for Health Care Provider Information." http://ww2.doh.state.fl.us/irm00praes/praslist.asp, accessed July 19, 2004.

Florida School of Traditional Midwifery (FSTM). 2004. FSTM homepage. Electronic document, http://www.midwiferyschool.org, accessed July 19, 2004.

Hamilton, George. Membership manager ACNM, personal correspondence by e-mail on February 10, 2003.

House Health Care Committee on Regulatory Reform. 1984. Sunset Review of Chapter 467, Florida Statutes, Midwifery Practice Act. Tallahassee, FL.

McTigue, Joan. 1989. "The Aborting of Direct-Entry Midwifery in Florida." *Midwifery Today* 9:36–37.

———. 1992. "A Change in the Status of Licensed Midwifery in Florida." *Birth Gazette* 8(3):20, 23.

Miami-Dade Community College. 2004. "Midwifery Program." www.mdc.edu/medical/Nursing/Programs/Midwifery_Prog/main.htm, accessed July 19, 2004.

North American Registry of Midwives (NARM). 2004. NARM homepage. http://www.narm.org, accessed July 19, 2004.

Rooks, Judith. 1997. *Midwifery and Childbirth in America.* Philadelphia, PA: Temple University Press.

Senate Committee on Health and Rehabilitative Services. 1991. *A Study of the Practice of Lay Midwifery Chapter 467, Florida Statutes.* Tallahassee, FL.

Susie, Debra. 1988. *In the Way of Our Grandmothers: A Cultural View of Twentieth-Century Midwifery in Florida.* Athens: University of Georgia Press.

Wennlund, Dolores. 1981. "The Issue: Midwifery." Unpublished manuscript, Florida Department of Health and Rehabilitative Services, Health Program Office.

———. 1992. *Annals of Public Health Nursing in Florida.* Tallahassee: Health and Rehabilitative Services.

Yagerman, Katherine. 1982. "Legitimacy for the Florida Midwife: The Midwifery Practice Act." *University of Miami Law Review* 37(1):123–150.

5

MINNESOTA DIRECT-ENTRY MIDWIVES: ACHIEVING LEGISLATIVE SUCCESS THROUGH FOCUSING ON FAMILIES, SAFETY, AND WOMEN'S RIGHTS

Mary M. Lay and Kerry Dixon

- Initial Success: The Midwifery Study Advisory Group • Failed Efforts: The License Rule Writing Group • The Minnesota Midwifery Licensing Law: A Grassroots Effort Succeeds • Victory of Minnesota Midwives: The Minnesota Direct-Entry Midwifery Statute • The Challenges Ahead: Lessons from the Minnesota Story • Timeline of Licensed Midwifery in Minnesota

Dorothy gave birth to her first two children in a hospital setting with the help of nurse-midwives. The care was "wonderful" and caused Dorothy to come to a conclusion: she "just knew that she wanted to do midwifery."[1] But the more she read, the more she realized that "her heart belonged to traditional midwifery" rather than nurse-midwifery. She wanted to give the continuity of care and the individual attention that clinically-based practitioners could not provide. Although her second birth in the hospital was a "deeply sacred experience," the setting prevented her from enjoying its full potential. She says, "Partly that limitation came from sharing this family moment in a strange place with people I couldn't personally choose to attend me."

Traditional or direct-entry midwives [2] such as Dorothy believe that birth should empower the woman—to help her come into her own sense of self, a journey made difficult by medical caregivers who might assume control of the birth. "But midwifery isn't an easy door to knock on," Dorothy found. Eventually she was asked to births by friends and then volunteered as labor support for single women and teen mothers who were birthing in the hospital. Direct-entry midwifery was very much underground when Dorothy first began to explore the practice in late 1980s. "But the whole time I was reading," Dorothy said. She then began an apprenticeship with a local midwife. After a certain point, the local community of midwives gave its blessing for Dorothy to move into the role of primary midwife. By 1995 Dorothy had attended over fifty-three births, by 2000 over 200 births: "Any experience I can get," she seeks, "because I feel that it's so essential. I feel real lucky. I have been to births with six or seven midwives. I have seen a lot of different styles of practice. Some people think that it takes less time to become a traditional midwife than to become a nurse-midwife. But to be a truly good midwife, you have to continue to study and learn." Dorothy eventually became copresident of the Minnesota Midwives' Guild and established her own direct-entry midwifery practice for homebirth parents in the Twin Cities.

Presently, the direct-entry midwives of Minnesota like Dorothy enjoy one of the most liberal midwifery licensing laws within the United States. The journey to this status, however, was hard-fought and dependent on the endurance and strategic skills of the midwives themselves, their home-birth clients, and a couple of friendly but persuasive state legislators. The opposition the Minnesota midwives encountered along the way reveals the extent to which the hegemonic medical community seeks to maintain its professional jurisdiction through claimed ownership of scientific knowledge and birth technologies. However, through a grassroots and collaborative effort with their homebirth clients, the Minnesota direct-entry midwives overcame this opposition to their own authoritative knowledge about birth and gained the legal status they enjoy today. Dorothy became one of the first licensed DEMs within the state.

The grassroots effort that helped bring legal status to Minnesota midwives was led, to a great extent, by their local homebirth clients. Patsy exemplifies the journey to homebirth of some of these clients. A friend of Patsy's had two of her children at home, and Patsy was interested in having a "natural" first birth herself in a nonhospital setting.

She contacted the International Cesarean Awareness Network to learn more about natural birth and meet the midwives involved in this group. When Patsy became pregnant, she took a childbirth class and began to make the very personal decision about which midwife would meet her needs. In the end, she had instead a "wonderful" hospital birth with "most of the good stuff of a homebirth" with the help of a labor support person who was trained as a midwife, but so newly off her apprenticeship that she was not taking first-time moms at that point. Patsy went on to have her second child at home. Patsy's attitudes about homebirth and midwifery come from her appreciation of such things as how much time in the prenatal stage midwives are willing to spend with their clients during each visit—an hour and a half with a midwife versus ten minutes in the doctor's office. Midwives "also tend to work with understanding a women's psychology and not just her physical reality of pregnancy," says Patsy. And, during birth, midwives offer continuous care, no shift changes, as one might experience in the hospital. When preparing for the homebirth of her second child, people would say to Patsy, "You're so brave to do a homebirth," but Patsy says she trusts the process of birth, and her body to do it. So, to Patsy, others seem brave to want a hospital birth. "A soul is coming into our family," says Patsy. "It is a sacred moment to be reverenced and celebrated—not just another event in someone's workday, one more down, 'how many to go and by the way, how was your weekend,' and 'excuse me, but I think the woman next door needs a C-section, doc, can you come?'"

To Dorothy and Patsy, direct-entry midwifery and homebirth offer the opportunity for each woman to "design" her own birthing experience—to choose the location, the support people, the atmosphere—and to rely on her own knowledge and confidence in her body to see her through the process. Midwives such as Dorothy decided that licensing would bring advantages to their practices: the ability to advertise, to follow protocols that were sanctioned by the state, to have legal access to antihemorrhagic drugs and other means to make birth safe, and to be recognized by medical professionals who might serve as consultants or backup to midwifery care and homebirth. However, they also wanted to preserve the philosophies and knowledge systems of homebirth midwifery. And their clients, like Patsy, were willing to fight to help them do so.

Dorothy, Patsy, and the other Minnesota midwives and homebirth clients who fought the battle for licensing did so within a unique setting. Minnesota is known for its liberalism and social welfare programs, yet also for its strong medical communities. Politically, the state is often characterized as "bipolar"—with equally strong liberal and conservative leanings. For example, in the late 1990s Minnesota was represented in the U.S. Senate by Paul Wellstone, an outspoken liberal, and Rod Grams, a staunch conservative.

In trying to explain the liberal leanings of the state, during the 1998 governor's race that elected former professional wrestler and National Reform Party candidate Jesse Ventura, the St. Paul *Pioneer Press* characterized past state leadership as having created a "moralistic and activist vision of government," a belief that "enlightened government can and must uphold society's standards of fairness and decency in an increasingly changeable, competitive and impersonal world."[3] Quoting from historian John Haynes, the article characterized Minnesota in the 1920s as "being politically divided between "progressivism with a left wing" and "progressivism with a right wing." In the 1930s, the Farmer-Labor Party united farmers and industrial workers around their dislike of big business and elected governor Floyd B. Olson, who declared, "I am not a liberal . . . I am a radical." Olson convinced legislators to support state relief for the destitute and a moratorium on farm foreclosures, and supported labor during a particularly violent truckers' strike. The Minnesota Democrats and the Farmer-Labor parties merged in the 1940s to form the DFL (Democratic-Farmer-Labor Party), a new party led by Hubert Humphrey that reacted to then-governor Harold Stassen's Republicanism. However, Stassen himself was a reformer of sorts, initiating a "new day" Republicanism that "looked like an undated rebirth of progressivism—earnest, moralistic, practical." The Minnesota precinct caucus system still reinforces that local and progressive involvement in state government when neighbors gather to reach consensus on resolutions and representatives to send to the district conventions. Within this liberal and progressive political atmosphere, Minnesota midwives could be optimistic about there being a state-sanctioned place for their practices.

However, Minnesota also has a well-established and renowned medical community. For example, the state is home to the Mayo Clinic, the internationally known medical site that promotes clinical care and groundbreaking research. The two physicians who founded the Mayo Clinic "envisioned a system in which patient care was continually improved through research and new knowledge passed on to the next generation through education."[4] The Mayo system treats almost a half a million patients annually and employs more than 2,000 physicians. Moreover, the primary agency that the Minnesota midwives would have to deal with, should they become licensed, was the Minnesota Board of Medical Practice. The board is made up of eleven physicians and five members of the public (all appointed by the governor), and licenses 14,000 physicians. The board's primary mission is to "protect the public by: (1) extending the privilege to practice to qualified applicants, and (2) investigating complaints relating to the competency or behavior of individual licensees or registrants."[5] Physicians associated with the Mayo Clinic, the University of Minnesota Medical School, and the many hospital systems within the state serve on the board.[6] The Minnesota Medical Association monitors the board and lobbies to maintain what the association envisions as safe, quality health care within the state. To become licensed, the Minnesota midwives would have to convince the board and the Minnesota Medical Association lobbyists that their practices were safe and would not harm Minnesota citizens. The midwives would also have to function in an environment that normally granted a great deal of status to medical knowledge systems.

There were, however, some indications that alternative systems could function within this medical stronghold, perhaps because of liberal leanings within the state. For example, at the University of Minnesota Hospital and Clinic, a new Center for Spirituality and Healing was established in 1995. The mission of the center is to "facilitate the integration of biomedical, complementary, cross-cultural and spiritual aspects of care."[7] The center promotes a holistic, integrated model of care delivery and early on became involved in advocating changes in the education of health professionals. In 1997 the center was positioned as a freestanding unit within the Academic Health Center at the university. The University of Minnesota Medical School had achieved fame in such research areas as cancer, AIDS, and transplant drugs, and promoted itself as now entering the "revolution in molecular medicine and genetics."[8] This medical/academic stronghold also found a place for alternative approaches to healing.

Dorothy, Patsy, and other DEMs and their homebirth clients sought the status that licensing would bring to midwifery practice by first entering into public conversations with the Board of Medical Practice and with state legislators, conversations that were closely monitored by the state medical communities. When this effort was unsuccessful, they employed a strategy appropriate in Minnesota—a grassroots effort that became almost a social movement, employing local forces but also calling upon national support from midwifery professional organizations.

Complicating the midwives' and their homebirth clients' efforts were issues of gender and power. Power among professional systems is established when specific jurisdictional boundaries distinguish one practice from another and when these boundaries are recognized by professional and governmental organizations, such as the Board of Medical Practice. The jurisdictional boundaries reflect exclusive knowledge systems of particular professions. In some professions, such as medicine, jurisdictional boundaries are also based on claimed ownership of science and technology. Therefore, newly emerging and competing professions must fight for status by establishing their own exclusive knowledge systems or by successfully encroaching upon the systems of the dominant professions.[9] The boundaries of medical caregivers within Minnesota were well-established within institutions such as the Mayo Clinic, the University of Minnesota Medical Schools, and the Minnesota Medical Association. The Board of Medical Practice recognized these boundaries and disciplined those caregivers who did not follow proper protocols for practice within those boundaries. The Minnesota midwives asked to cross boundaries in order to become licensed—to maintain their own knowledge systems and yet have access and contribute to those claimed by the medical community.

Moreover, Minnesota midwives' knowledge about birth is gendered. Their knowledge systems come from their own embodied knowledge when they become mothers, from their experiential knowledge as they attend other mothers, and from the authoritative knowledge passed on to them during their apprenticeships and training. Their communities are populated with women, and the midwives consider themselves to a great extent the "guardians of certain choices and options" in women's rights (Lay 2000:178). Their sense of power often comes not from professional power or status granted by state agencies, but from the birth experience itself. As one midwife said, "I was completely blown away by how powerful birth was and how empowering it was to become a mother . . . it was a time I knew that I could take on the world" (Lay 2000:176). It is this sense of personal power that the midwives want to pass on to their homebirth clients: a power or belief in their bodies and in their spirits. However, to succeed in becoming licensed by the state, they had to gain other sources of power and status while still safeguarding their midwifery knowledge systems.

In this chapter, we describe how, during the journey to achieving this liberal licensing law, the Minnesota midwives and their supporters first lost everything they fought for—and then how they reversed this defeat. The journey to licensing for the DEMs of Minnesota over the last ten years falls into three stages:

- public hearings in 1991 and 1992 during which the rhetorical strategies of Minnesota Midwives' Guild members successfully marked them as safe and careful caregivers;

- rule-writing meetings from 1993 through 1995 during which a bid for access to the tools of science and technology, an encroachment into the professional boundaries of medicine, led to failure for the midwives; and finally
- grassroots efforts led by Minnesota Families for Midwifery and state legislators that successfully led to the writing and passage of the Minnesota midwifery licensing law.

This last stage demonstrates how a marginal, experiential, gender-based knowledge system was able to gain legitimacy and destabilize the hegemonic, technologically-based medical system by moving into the larger social system to gain recognition and support. We end this chapter with a summary of the current Minnesota midwifery law and how it provides room for both autonomy and state sanction.

INITIAL SUCCESS:
THE MIDWIFERY STUDY ADVISORY GROUP

In October 1991, the Minnesota Board of Medical Practice and the Department of Health called together midwives, physicians, homebirth parents, and other interested parties to determine whether the state should regulate what its midwives were then calling "traditional" midwifery. (The term direct-entry came into wider use by professionalizing homebirth midwives in the mid-1990s; see chapter 1.) Charged with licensing traditional midwives by Minnesota statute, the Board of Medical Practice had not granted such a license since 1938, stating that no appropriate school of midwifery or licensing examination existed. Without clear regulations, Minnesota midwives were continually subject to possible investigation for practicing medicine without a license, a felony that carries fines and possible jail time. The group formed by the Board of Medical Practice engaged both in formal testimony and then in open debate to determine whether regulating traditional midwifery was needed to safeguard Minnesota citizens. The hearings resulted in a temporary victory for the members of the Minnesota Midwives' Guild because they were able to portray themselves as professionals who carefully screened out high-risk clients and yet were able to speak the language of medical caregivers. Their goals were to gain state recognition through licensing or certification, and to be able to practice openly. Their success depended on identifying a group of "others" who were less medically astute, who accepted homebirth clients based on their religious faith or more open rebellion against the medical community, seemingly regardless of risk. Identifying an "other" diverted any negative attention of medical caregivers and state agencies from the Guild midwife to the non-Guild midwife, thus moving the Guild midwife and her practice into the category of "normal" or acceptable caregiver.

The professionalizing midwives and their representatives distinguished themselves from the suspect imagery of midwifery—the "herbs-and-candles" myths of the "past." Key spokespeople created comparisons between these midwives and medical caregivers; for example, where medical knowledge depends on case studies, midwifery knowledge is passed on through birth stories and peer review. Each means of educating is appropriate for the particular practice and has comparable legitimacy, the midwives argued. For example, one speaker noted that birth stories and peer review constituted "a very useful way of teaching. It's similar to the way that doctors used to teach in many ways, an anecdotal, case by case tradition" (Lay 2000:82).[10] Moreover, throughout this first stage of public meetings, the image of the safe and knowledgeable midwife was the Guild midwife, the midwife who not only spent about 100 hours per birth with each client, but who also followed the Guild's *Standards of Care and Certification Guide*, a document that would eventually be referenced in the Minnesota midwifery licensing law.

The Guild midwives had to overcome not only the myths about unsafe and mystical midwifery, but also had to react against the image of birth proposed by a pathologist and OB/GYN from the University of Minnesota. Rachel Waters reported on the Minnesota Obstetrics Management Initiative or MOMI project, which identified some 25,000 risk factors out of a random sampling of 5,000 hospital births between May 1988 and May 1989. Moreover, Waters portrayed the typical homebirth client in Minnesota as poor, possibly anemic, with a "great number of infections" (Lay 2000:90).

Fortunately, the Minnesota Midwives' Guild selected one of their more medically educated members to follow Waters. Rita Ortiz, who also holds a nursing degree, quoted often from the Guild's *Standards of Care and Certification Guide* and described how she limited the number of births she would attend, based not only on the careful screening process of Guild midwives, who would not attend high-risk clients, but also on her own level of stress. After reading the long list of contraindications for homebirth that the Guild followed, Ortiz asserted, "Unlike most other caregivers, we try to send people away as opposed to get them to come to us" (Lay 2000:93). She identified the typical homebirth clients in Minnesota as middle-class, well educated, healthy, and thoughtful. Moreover, Ortiz could speak the language of the dominant medical profession, as well as articulate the philosophy of midwifery—for example, she spoke not only of nutritional concerns but also of the various medical means of controlling postpartum hemorrhage. Ortiz's testimony was followed by that of two midwives who served the Christian fellowship community. Instead of stressing the screening process used to identify high-risk clients, these midwives asserted that every woman has a right to birth at home if she reached that decision spiritually: "Every woman should have the choice to stay home or not. . . . We talk about protecting the public but to tell a woman she cannot stay home, I do not know how that is protecting her [as she will stay home anyway]" (Lay 2000:97). As Ortiz and others had so successfully created the image of the careful Guild midwife, who used her knowledge to screen for risk, the midwives who would sit with any woman who felt she was called to birth at home provided a clear image of the "other."

The members of the Midwifery Study Advisory Group and the representative from the Department of Health who would write the group's final report were convinced that while some midwives might be suspect, the Guild midwives practiced safely. For example, the final report said, "Not all homebirth attendants meet MMG [Minnesota Midwives' Guild] standards, and members of the Midwifery Study Advisory Group expressed serious concerns about the practices of these 'other' midwives" (Minnesota Department of Health 1992:ix). The report defined a scope of practice for out-of-hospital midwifery that matched that of the Guild's *Standards of Care* and recommended an advisory council, upon which midwives would serve, to oversee any complaints about homebirth practices. The report also recommended that midwives sign birth certificates and recommended limited liability for health care providers who accepted transports from homebirth clients who encountered difficulty, thus acknowledging midwives as appropriate birth attendants within a cooperative system.

With this final report, it would seem that the Minnesota direct-entry midwives had achieved most of the professional recognition they sought, even though they were not yet to be licensed. However, the rhetorical success of identifying the "other," non-Guild midwife, and the consequent status gained by the Guild midwives was lost once the report was taken outside of the closed forum of the Midwifery Study Advisory Group and presented to the Minnesota Senate and House of Representatives. The companion bills based on the report were considered too controversial within the wider legislative community and never reached the floor for a vote. Consequently, the Minnesota midwives were left in that gray area of the law—unable to become licensed but not prevented from practicing.

FAILED EFFORTS: THE LICENSE RULE WRITING GROUP

In the next stage of the midwives' efforts to become licensed, a larger public forum heard their concerns—a forum carefully monitored by the Minnesota Medical Association and the Minnesota OB/GYN Society. At this point the midwives seemed to encroach upon the jurisdiction of the medical communities when they asked for legally sanctioned access to some of the tools of science and technology, and lost the ground they had gained in the Midwifery Study Advisory Group.

In the fall of 1993, one county attorney wrote to the Minnesota Speaker of the House to insist that the Board of Medical Practice fulfill its obligation to oversee midwives to ensure quality care, and so the issue of licensing began to be publicly debated again. The Minnesota Midwives' Guild informed the Board that a branch of the Midwives Alliance of North America (MANA), the midwives' national organization, had developed an examination that might be appropriate for states to use as a licensing exam. The North American Registry of Midwives (NARM) exam was being pilot-tested with experienced midwives nationally. MANA had a long-term vision to establish a national credential, with entry-level requirements, around which homebirth midwives throughout the country could unify. In December 1993, the Board of Medical Practice responded by gathering direct-entry midwives, nurses, physicians, nurse-midwives, homebirth parents, and attorneys to write collaboratively the rules and regulations to license DEMs—the License Rule Writing Group.

Although the rule writing group met for almost two years, the first indication of trouble in the process came in April 1994, when the group began to write the scope of practice and contraindications section. Members representing such distinct groups as the Minnesota OB/GYN Society, the Minnesota Nurses Association, the Minnesota Midwives' Guild, and the Twin Cities chapter of the American College of Nurse-Midwives brought to the group carefully worded drafts of specific rules under discussion. When the rule group members discussed contraindications for midwifery care and homebirth, they were confronted with three proposed drafts—one from the Minnesota OB/GYN Society, one from a physician writing independently, and one from the Guild.

The Guild's list of contraindications included both twins and breech births, despite the fact that these were conditions some Minnesota midwives felt they were skilled in handling at home. Twins tend to be smaller or underweight, and often one twin might be in the breech position. Breech babies approach the birth canal feet or rump first, rather than head first, and might suffer oxygen deprivation and other problems, as the head is delivered last. Some midwives are quite skilled in turning breech babies manually to the vertex or the head-down position before birth. However, in preparing their list of contraindications, the Guild members had decided that they were willing to give up breeches and twins, considered high risk by many medical caregivers, to demonstrate their willingness to narrow their practices in order to gain licensure. But some of the midwives were unwilling to make this compromise. "Almost the only people in this country who know how to deliver breeches [vaginally] are traditional midwives. They do a lot of them. And they do know how to deliver them. A lot of twins are born at home, very safely," one midwife claimed (Lay 2000:141).[11] Breeches and twins did not appear on the contraindications list proposed by the Minnesota OB/GYN Society representative or the independent physician—perhaps because they were initially unaware that midwives were attending mothers with these conditions.

The possible exclusion of breeches and twins from any prohibited conditions for homebirth alarmed medical caregivers. And the next meeting of the rule writing group brought even greater controversy when the group discussed the scope of practice section of the licensing rules. Guild midwives wanted to carry oxygen, essential for neonatal resuscitation, as well as pitocin (a drug effective in stopping postpartum hemorrhage), and they wanted these tools listed in the midwifery scope of practice section of their licensing rules and regulations. They felt that they were more likely to need these tools than they were to attend a breech baby or a set of twins. They also wanted to perform emergency episiotomies (a cut in the perineal tissue to allow a distressed baby's head to be more easily delivered), and the midwives wanted to suture first- and second-degree perineal tearing. Although midwives like Dorothy had never had to do an episiotomy, even though she had attended many healthy-sized babies, Dorothy thought that some day she might have to. Moreover, midwives do everything they can to prevent a tear to the perineum, but sometimes tears happen despite the midwives' precautions, and they wanted to avoid having to send the mother to the hospital for suturing. But these were procedures that some medical caregivers defined as diagnostic, surgical, and pharmaceutical, requiring formal education, testing, and supervision to perform adequately, they believed. The procedures and the education needed to perform them fell solidly within the jurisdictional boundaries of medical care, claimed the Minnesota Medical Association and other groups monitoring the rule writing group's decisions.

Because of these two controversial meetings, the Board of Medical Practice became convinced that the midwifery licensing rules and regulations would not pass the scrutiny of the wider medical community. Moreover, the board began to raise objections to the NARM exam. NARM was in the process of testing and revising the exam, but up to this point only the most experienced midwives had taken the exam—and none of them had failed. NARM was also in the process of adding a hands-on skills test to the written test (see chapter 3). Nevertheless, the board judged the current version of the exam inadequate and shut down the rule writing process.

Then, in 1995, the revised NARM exam became more widely available, and MANA was actively recruiting entry-level midwives to take the exam. Also, the exam had been proven to have valid standards and contained a clinical component. The Minnesota Board of Medical Practice itself had invested several thousand dollars in having the exam psychometrically validated. The Minnesota Midwives' Guild approached Senator Sandy Pappas, a homebirth parent, who made a series of phone calls. Consequently, the Guild and a national representative from the NARM board were invited to attend a full meeting of the Board of Medical Practice to present birth statistics compiled by MANA's statistics committee, and to defend the latest version of the NARM exam. The Board of Medical Practice then formed the Midwifery Regulation Task force, a small group that met in 1997 and 1998 to write a scope of practice for direct-entry midwifery. But now there were strong calls for physician oversight of midwifery practice, and the midwives objected that few of them could convince liability-conscious physicians to provide them with backup care. And so the licensing effort again failed.

The board warned that if the midwives were not licensed but continued to practice, even though NARM might certify them as Certified Professional Midwives (CPMs), they would be practicing medicine without a license. Then in the spring and later in the fall of 1998, two Minnesota direct-entry midwives were criminally investigated by the Attorney General's Office at the request of the Board of Medical Practice and advised by their attorneys to suspend their practices. Although these investigations of possible "criminal activity" ended up costing one midwife $7,000 and the other $2,000 in legal fees, they also would eventually unite the midwives against what they perceived as a "common enemy."

The rhetorical strategies of identifying an "other" and speaking the language of medical science failed in the new larger and more public forum of the rule writing group. The voices of the other midwives, particularly those who did not want to compromise by excluding twins and breeches from their practices, made the midwifery community seem divided and chaotic. And the midwives who wanted access to the tools of science and technology appeared to be encroaching on medical jurisdiction boundaries. Midwifery knowledge systems, decided medical caregivers, could not include pharmaceuticals, episiotomies, and suturing. Finally, when confronted with potential physician oversight of their practices, the midwives saw the impossibility of finding the needed number of cooperative physicians and the potential threat to their autonomy. After two of their own came under investigation, the midwives, exhausted and discouraged, were uncertain about the next step.

THE MINNESOTA MIDWIFERY LICENSING LAW: A GRASSROOTS EFFORT SUCCEEDS

Even though the midwives had failed to gain licensing status through the Midwifery Study Advisory Group and the rule writing effort, they had become very adept at gaining access to the public forum. Moreover, they had a powerful legislative ally in Senator Sandy Pappas, a well-known liberal Democrat. Pappas had tried to get the Midwifery Study Advisory Group recommendations through the legislature, but couldn't garner the support to push the bills through. However, now she had moved from the conservative-dominated House to the liberal-dominated Senate and had more visibility and political clout. Moreover, she still had the connections in the House to mount a bipartisan effort on behalf of the midwives. Finally, NARM could now credential CPMs and thus MANA could support local bids for power and status. In October and November 1998, advisors within MANA urged the Minnesota midwives to pursue licensure through legislation. "We didn't have a choice," said Dorothy. There was no going back now that midwives were being criminally investigated. But even more important, the investigations of the two midwives had also pushed consumers into action. A town meeting drawing over 100 people was held to discuss, among other issues, how burned out midwives such as Dorothy were feeling: "It was the consumer's turn to do something." Without the involvement of the homebirth parents—the Minnesota citizens, whom the Board of Medical Practice was charged to protect—the midwives would find it difficult to continue fighting. Finally, the midwives and their supporters chose a new strategy—articulating their position from the point of view of the consumer, rather than distinguishing between the "good" and the "other" midwife.

Minnesota Families for Midwifery (MfM) had formed in 1996 from parenting groups. Now homebirth parents like Patsy offered to write a licensing bill and to help coordinate lobbying efforts. The MfM, Senator Pappas, and the local direct-entry midwives drafted a bill, pulling text from the various pieces of writing the midwives had done within the groups formed by the Board of Medical Practice and from other states' statutes. Portions were also created anew to address the political concerns the midwives, consumers, and legislators might express. Senator Pappas asked House representative Jim Abeler, a conservative chiropractor and homebirth father, to sponsor a companion midwifery bill. The effort to license the midwives would be bipartisan.

The most important strategy would be to make licensing a public concern and a safety concern—and so a legislative concern. To do so, MfM and the midwives would have to reach the greater Minnesota population. These groups had to learn to lobby at the state capital, to create appeals that legislators would be interested in, and to get large numbers of citizens to contact their representatives on behalf of the midwives. Moreover, they had to decide how to handle the hot issues of breech and twin births, antihemorrhagic drugs, episiotomies, and suturing—the issues that had contributed to the failure of earlier efforts. The midwives would have to appear to be united around these issues and, to make the legislators care, they would have to dramatize their passion about midwifery and homebirth.

Senator Pappas conducted a lobbying workshop for MfM and the midwives. Within packets to be distributed at the Capitol, the group identified key talking points to appeal to the legislators and provided answers to frequently asked questions, articles and statistics on the safety of homebirth, and an outline of the bills. One key point would be the issue of access. They wanted their legislators to ask, "How come Minnesota citizens presently cannot have access to midwifery care? How can they have access to any necessary medical tests and backup if they wish a homebirth?" Moreover, it was particularly important that MfM members portray themselves as the common, rather than the uncommon or "other" citizen: "I am just a regular person—not too unusual—and I want these options as to where I want to birth. I am not too far left or far right—not hippie or religious. I am in the mainstream." To garner support for the bills, MfM and the midwives stressed that licensing would better guarantee safety and training. Midwifery clients would be able not only to work with a direct-entry midwife but also have the medical tests and procedures that might ensure a safe birth in each case. Informed consent would ensure that the parents would take on the responsibility for their choices. Finally, the public would be protected by uniform standards for midwifery practice. MfM sent postcards to consumers, providing the names and phone numbers of legislators and urging the consumers to ask their representatives to support the bill. MfM members also traveled to Duluth, Fargo, Mankato, and other towns to meet with consumers and legislators.

MfM and the midwives agreed that no one would speak of the hot issues that had dissolved the Board of Medical Practice rule writing meetings. About breeches and twins, "We did our best to never bring it up," noted Patsy. Other techniques such as episiotomies, suturing, and the use of pitocin could be defended as safety measures, but the conditions that so alarmed the medical community must not be raised. Midwifery Now!, an umbrella group of CPMs and non-CPMs, was created specifically for this legislative effort. Dedicated to keeping licensing voluntary rather than mandatory, Midwifery Now! presented a united face for homebirth midwifery. Midwives who wished to follow the dictates of their specific communities, such as the Christian fellowship community, could decide not to become licensed. The proposed legislation would not even mention breeches, twins, or vaginal birth after cesarean (VBAC), but instead refers to the Guild's *Standards of Care and Certification Guide* for how to respond to these conditions. The 1995 edition of the *Standards of Care* listed breech babies in first-time mothers and multiple gestations with one or more baby presenting other than vertex as contraindications for homebirth. "Suspected" multiple gestation required medical consultation; and "known" multiple gestation when the mother still wanted a homebirth, breech presentation at term, and prior cesarean birth required consultation with other certified midwives. "Unforeseen" multiple and breech presentations required transport to the hospital unless the expected birth time was shorter than the projected transport time (Minnesota Midwives' Guild 1995: Appendices A-E). To a great extent, reference to the *Standards of Care* allowed the midwifery community to create and rely upon its own authoritative knowledge about birth—and gave the individual midwife flexibility and autonomy in designing her own protocols.

To emphasize their passion about midwifery care and homebirth, the midwives arranged to pack the committee hearings with homebirth parents and children. But one of those typical Minnesota blizzards began to rage the first day of the committee hearings. Nonetheless, almost eighty parents made long commutes in the snow and wind. Parents constantly took fussy children out in the hallway and then came back in again—there was no mistaking their physical presence. For Dorothy, it was a moving moment: "It was really beautiful to see these families that I had helped. I thought, 'OK, I can give up more of my life to do this—to further this.'" Homebirth parents began to share their stories with the legislators: one spoke about receiving a termination letter from her physician because she was planning a homebirth; another told of being denied blood work and ultrasounds because she was working with direct-entry midwives rather than physicians. How could birth be safe if consumers could not have access to these screening techniques? "Consumer protection is what legislators are interested in. So that was our focus," Patsy noted. Supportive physicians also testified, but not with the passion of the homebirth families. And those homebirth babies, safe and healthy, testified by their physical presence. The bills passed through the committee votes, and when the bills were merged for final vote, the language of the Abeler bill, the version that made licensing voluntary rather than mandatory, dominated.

MfM and the midwives faced two final obstacles—reaction from the Board of Medical Practice and potential veto by Governor Ventura. At that point, MfM and the midwives had a stroke of luck. At the same time that the companion bills were being debated in the committee hearings, the Board of Medical Practice, the Minnesota Medical Association, and the Minnesota Nurses Association were involved in a fight over advanced practice nursing. Focused on this larger group of practitioners, the board had no time to lobby against the bill as it had against earlier versions in the 1980s. Ventura signed the bill, which became law in July 1999. Ventura's signing of the bill is somewhat of a mystery. The explanation probably lies in two areas: Ventura really believed in a hands-off government for the state, leaving more individual choice; the second reason probably comes from Ventura's tendency to pay most attention to concerns that interested him and that matched his campaign promises. Midwifery undoubtedly did not get much of his attention, either in the positive or the negative.

VICTORY OF MINNESOTA MIDWIVES: THE MINNESOTA DIRECT-ENTRY MIDWIFERY STATUTE

The Minnesota statute determining the licensing process and requirements for DEMs acknowledges both local and national midwifery organizations.[12] Thus, the law grants a certain degree of authority and self-governance to the midwives themselves. For example, a midwife seeking to be licensed by the state must submit a diploma from an educational program approved or accredited by the Midwifery Education and Accreditation Council (MEAC), the accrediting body of the Midwives Alliance of North America (MANA), or evidence of having completed an apprenticeship. She must also submit a credential from NARM attesting that she has passed the NARM exam (Minnesota Statutes Section 147D.17, Subd. 1). She must have in place a medical consultation plan, and "[t]he conditions requiring the implementation of the medical consultation plan must meet at the minimum the conditions established by the Minnesota Midwives' Guild in the *Standards of Care and Certification Guide*, the most recent edition" (Minnesota Statutes Section 147D.11, Subd. b). However, given this language and the current vagueness of the *Standards of Care*, some procedures could also be interpreted as falling within the "community standards," which are written and practiced in the medical model. Finally, an advisory council makes recommendations to the Board of Medical Practice on standards, distribution of information, enforcement, educational programs, complaints and disciplinary actions, and reviews applications and recommends granting or denying licensure or license renewal. Four of the five members of this advisory council are appointed from lists of names submitted by Midwifery Now! or MfM.[13] Thus, many of these statutory features seem to recognize the authoritative knowledge about birth generated within direct-entry midwifery communities.

The scope of practice section of the Minnesota statute also grants authority to DEMs by placing few restrictions on their practices. The scope of practice section states that direct-entry midwifery involves "attending and supporting the natural process of labor and birth," conducting "initial and ongoing assessment for suitability of traditional midwifery care," "coordinating with a licensed health care provider" for routine testing, and supporting postpartum care (Minnesota Statutes Section 147D.03, Subd. 2). Most licensed midwives do routine prenatal blood work for clients and decide on other tests on a case-by-case basis. Most important, the statute introduces these features of practice with the words: "includes, but is not limited to." Individual midwives may then create their own protocols, as long as they avoid "unauthorized care." Unauthorized care consists of only three actions: removing placenta accreta, "assisting of childbirth by artificial or mechanical means," or using any surgical instruments except to "sever the umbilical cord or repair a first- or second-degree perineal laceration" (Minnesota Statutes Section 147D.03, Subd. 3). Therefore, the midwives need not send a homebirth mother to the hospital for suturing of first- and second-degree perineal tears during birth, and they are allowed to diagnose the degree of tearing.

The statute recognizes a less formal relationship between the direct-entry midwife and medical caregivers than between the nurse-midwife and physicians, whose practices reflect the hierarchy of authority within hospitals. The licensed DEM must prepare a written plan with each client "to ensure continuity of care throughout the pregnancy, labor, and delivery," and that plan must "incorporate the conditions under which the medical consultation plan, including the transfer of care or transport of the client, may be implemented" (Minnesota Statutes Section 147D.05, Subd. 2). The statute leaves it up to the midwife to screen for any contraindications for homebirth and then transfer care to a licensed health-care provider. Thus, the Minnesota-licensed DEM maintains a great deal of autonomy over her own practice, and having the state formally recognize midwifery makes it harder for other professionals to dismiss licensed midwives.

Licensed midwives do have to provide their clients with an informed consent form, which includes the following:

> We realize that there are risks associated with birth, including the risk of death or disability of either mother or child. We understand that a situation may arise, which requires emergency medical care and that it may not be possible to transport the mother and/or baby to the hospital in time to benefit from such care. We fully accept the outcome and consequences of our decision to have a licensed traditional midwife attend us during pregnancy and at our birth. We realize that our licensed traditional midwife is not licensed to practice medicine. We are not seeking a licensed physician or certified nurse-midwife as the primary caregiver for this pregnancy, and we understand that our licensed traditional midwife shall inform us of any observed signs or symptoms of disease, which may require evaluation, care, or treatment by a medical practitioner. We agree that we are totally responsible for obtaining qualified medical assistance for the care of any disease or pathological condition. (Minnesota Statutes Section 147D.07 Subd. 2.9)

This form places the responsibility for any unforeseen risk firmly on the shoulders of the homebirth parent. Although midwives are charged with alerting their clients to conditions that require medical attention, clients must assume the responsibility of seeking that attention or the risk of rejecting it.

The licensed DEM in Minnesota does have access to the tools and procedures of medical science and technology. She may not only suture perineal tearing, but also has the responsibility for administering vitamin K (either orally or through intramuscular injection), oxygen, and a prophylactic eye agent. Moreover, in emergencies she may administer antihemorrhagic drugs such as pitocin (Minnesota Statutes Section

147D.09 Subd. b). Administration of antihemorrhagic drugs is quite important to midwives practicing in rural areas where transport to the hospital for postpartum hemorrhages might take much too long.

However, as liberal as this licensing law might seem, the Minnesota midwives regret that the current version of the law does not specifically allow an option for birth centers or reference third-party reimbursement.

Currently, licensed DEMs in Minnesota like Dorothy have a great deal of freedom to develop their own protocols, which may include suturing minor perineal tears and administering antihemorrhagic drugs. They have legally sanctioned access to these surgical and pharmaceutical tools and the ability to purchase them. They screen out clients they deem too high-risk for homebirth, but the specifics of their medical consultation plans are determined by their own community's standards of care. They remain autonomous, initiating transfer or transport to an alternative care venue after conducting their own screening processes. Their clients take responsibility for unforeseen risks, and the midwives' own national organization provides the licensing exam. These licensed midwives find that their work is validated to a certain degree because the very fact that they are licensed says that they have agreed upon a standard of accountability. And licensing is *voluntary* in Minnesota. If a midwife chooses to practice without a license, currently there is no penalty.

THE CHALLENGES AHEAD:
LESSONS FROM THE MINNESOTA STORY

Within the midwifery licensing bill, MfM, Midwifery Now!, and the Minnesota direct-entry midwives seem to have the best of all worlds. Those midwives who wish to become licensed can; and those midwives who were rhetorically identified as "other" in the public hearings in the 1990s can practice without licensure if they wish. In fact, although the majority of homebirths in the state are attended by licensed midwives, the majority of DEMs remain unlicensed in Minnesota. The midwives who want access to pharmaceuticals have that access through licensing and those who wish to perform episiotomies or suture can do so. The midwives' own professional community seems to have the authority to make decisions about VBACs, breeches, and twins.

However, in January 2000 a piece of legislation was written by the Board of Medical Practice, supported by a key staff member in the governor's office, and was introduced by Senator John Hottinger, chair of the Health and Family Security Committee. "This was too easy," Dorothy said. "Everyone was on the lookout for it, because they hadn't licensed anyone [yet]." The Hottinger bill would make licensing mandatory. It would limit direct-entry midwifery care to the home, closing down the opportunity for birth centers. The 1999 law stated that the practice of direct-entry midwifery included but was not limited to five essential aspects of practice; the proposed bill would limit the practice of midwifery to these five points. Added to the "medical consultation plan" would be the word "agreement": "An applicant must have a written consultation agreement with a physician who is licensed under chapter 147 or a nurse who is licensed under chapter 148 and certified as a nurse-midwife" ("A Bill" 2000). Therefore, the midwives would face required physician oversight of their practices. Finally, the Midwifery Advisory Council would be restructured to have nine members rather than five, the additional members representing physicians appointed by the Minnesota Medical Association, nurse-midwives appointed by the Minnesota Nurses Association, and the public.

MfM and the midwives again went into action. They took advantage of Governor Ventura's popular bus tours of the state and greeted the governor with signs saying "Support Midwifery." As Dorothy said, "Everywhere he went in these small towns we would have someone show up with signs." He would say, "But I have nothing against midwifery!" Ventura's office received so many calls in support of the midwifery bill that it made his "top ten topics" list for the week—quite a change from his initial apparent lack of attention when signing the law.

One of the midwives called for a meeting with Senator Hottinger in early February, where she argued that the proposed bill should not be heard. As head of the health committee and author of the bill, Hottinger had the power to choose whether the bill would come up for discussion. "Give us a chance," the midwives asked, "to see if it's going to work." Hottinger, a friend and office mate of Senator Pappas, decided that the House committee would not hear the bill. The 1999 law would therefore not be open to change—for the moment. In February 2000, the Midwifery Advisory Council recommended the first group of applicants for licensing. The Board of Medical Practice met in early July 2000 and licensed the applicants.

At present, the factions within the direct-entry midwifery community are not in complete agreement and might again haunt the midwives in the future. The Minnesota Midwives' Guild no longer exists; it has been replaced, in part, by the Minnesota Council of Certified Professional Midwives (MCCPM), members of which must either be CPMs or student midwives apprenticing with a CPM. The Minnesota Midwives' Guild's *Standards of Care and Certification Guide* is now under revision. Midwifery Now! continues to exist and to recommend candidates to the advisory council. It has been quite problematic that as of fall 2000, no members of MCCPM belonged to Midwifery Now!, but the CPM and non-CPM midwives within the state were sharing ideas for updating the *Standards of Care.* On the other hand, there is still very little coordinated collaboration between the CNMs and the DEMs within the state, although respectful exchanges continue between individual midwives. The CNMs experienced conflict in their own community over approach and timing when they attempted to put forth enabling legislation for birth centers in 2000. CNMs may perceive the DEMs as presently having more autonomy, but the DEMs perceive nurse-midwives as enjoying more protection from their own licensing process and organization rather than through the Board of Medical Practice. Moreover, some Minnesota midwives are content not to be licensed—the "other" continues, therefore, to exist.

Such divisions might invite the scrutiny of the Board of Medical Practice again. In fact, in July 2001 the Board of Medical Practice informed Dorothy that it was intending to try to make licensing mandatory through 2002 legislation. Some of the midwives might support mandatory licensing if, given the troubled history of interaction, the board is not the licensing body. On the other hand, some licensed midwives have indicated that they might choose not to renew their licenses because they feel that this status makes them too vulnerable to scrutiny by the board—and they feel that they have no protection from this scrutiny. Some of those midwives who remain opposed to mandatory licensing plan to "slip back underground" should it ever come about, but others state they would support mandatory licensing if there were an inclusion about birth centers and third-party reimbursement in such a revision. Finally, it's too early to tell, they say, to what extent the licensed midwives' knowledge of birth is truly acknowledged in the health-care community.

Direct-entry midwives in the United States must constantly battle to gain broad legal acknowledgment of their authoritative knowledge about birth. When they also ask for access to the current tools and procedures of medical science and technology, they often confront the medical community head on. By claiming exclusive access to these tools and procedures, the medical community maintains its distinct professional jurisdictional boundaries. In asking to suture, to administer pitocin, and to distinguish between degrees of perineal tearing, the midwifery community seems to be encroaching on these boundaries. And when the midwifery community publicly displays its divisions, that community becomes less able to articulate its needs and more vulnerable to scrutiny and criticism.

But homebirth consumers have a powerful voice. State legislatures are charged with supporting and protecting their citizens and their families. When Minnesota homebirth clients united to support their midwives and to demand access to medical technologies even when choosing a homebirth, their voices were heard. The midwives also benefited greatly from the help of Senator Sandy Pappas, not only a powerful legislator but also someone who could speak personally of the benefits of midwifery and homebirth. Pappas's decision to make the midwifery legislative effort bipartisan was strategically wise and paid off in an unexpected way, in that the more liberal version of the companion bills passed. Perhaps one of the most remarkable aspects of the current Minnesota midwifery law is that it assigns decisions about how to handle breeches, twins, and VBACs to the midwives themselves, through a formal recognition of their own *Standards of Care and Certification Guide.* Yet it is important to remember that potentially major opponents were distracted when the bill came forward, and the law is still vulnerable to revision, as evidenced by the Hottinger bill proposed less than a year after the midwifery law was passed.

The Minnesota midwifery law came about through the grassroots organizing and lobbying efforts of homebirth clients and midwives. They focused on families, safety, and the rights of all citizens—and in doing so maintained their autonomy and gained access to tools and procedures frequently claimed by the hegemonic forces of the medical community. Of all the midwives' strategies, the strategy of unification proved to be the best.

TIMELINE OF LICENSED MIDWIFERY IN MINNESOTA

1906 Minnesota Statute 4983 allows for the licensure of midwives upon production of a diploma from a school of midwifery recognized by the Board of Medical Examiners (BME) or after examination of the applicant. The fee for license is $1 for diploma holders and $2 for those who sit for the exam.

1924 118 licensed midwives (although BME and Board of Health felt this did not represent the true number of practicing midwives).

1938 Midwife license issued to Ebba Kirschbaum, who eventually became Minnesota's last licensed midwife, until her death in 1984. In this decade, the BME stops licensing midwives due to "lack of exam."

Late 1960s and early 1970s La Leche League leaders, childbirth educators, and determined do-it-yourselfers restart the homebirth movement.

1975 Genesis, a group of direct-entry midwives within Minnesota, is founded.

1980 Birth Community, Inc. (BCI), an organization of consumers and midwives started, an affiliate of the International Association of Parents & Professionals for Safe Alternatives in Childbirth.

1985 Minnesota Association of Midwives is established with members mostly outside of the metropolitan area of Minneapolis.

1988 Minnesota Midwives Guild (MMG) replaces Genesis as a self-governing, peer-reviewed group of direct-entry midwives, and Minnesota Association of Midwives merges to form one statewide group.

1991–1992 Public hearings and meetings of the Midwifery Study Advisory Group are sponsored by the Department of Heath and the Board of Medical Practice (BMP) to determine whether Minnesota direct-entry midwives should be regulated.

1991–1992 Consumers unite under the name Parents Coalition for Homebirth, for the purpose of having their voices heard as part of the advisory group.

1992 Final report of the Midwifery Study Advisory Group recommends that direct-entry midwives be regulated in some way, and that MMG standards serve as a model for all midwives in Minnesota.

1992 BCI, whose membership has dropped off in recent years, formally disbands.

1993 License Rule Writing Group is constituted by the BMP to write the rules for licensing direct-entry midwives in the state. This group includes any interested midwives, student midwives, and consumers, as well as representatives of nursing, nurse-midwifery, medicine, and the attorney general's office.

1994 BMP suspends the License Rule Writing Group based on a number of complaints, particularly from the established medical communities.

1994 BMP reconvenes the License Rule Writing Group and presents a draft of the rules that limits practices of direct-entry midwives.

1994 BMP invests several thousand dollars in having NARM exam psychometrically validated but then suspends the License Rule Writing Group once more when it discovers that licensing fees would exceed the direct-entry midwives' abilities to pay.

1995 An organized consumer voice is called for and the Minnesota Friends of Midwives is founded.

1997 MMG's Epidemiological Study of Midwife-Attended Home-births in Minnesota 1990-1996, prepared by the MANA Statistics and Research Committee (under Ken C. Johnson and Betty-Anne Daviss-Putt) is presented to the BMP.

1997 Participating members of MMG vote to disband their organization and become Minnesota Council of Certified Professional Midwives (MCCPM) to align with the NARM credential and have formal membership agreements.

1997 Largely based on the study presentation and the work of NARM on a national level, the BMP forms the Midwifery Regulation Task Force, which meets over the next year to write the scope of practice section for licensing direct-entry midwives. MCCPM, the only professional direct-entry midwife organization in the state, is invited to participate.

1997 Midwifery Regulation Task Force fails when there are strong calls for physician oversight of midwifery practice, which would negatively affect physician liability and limit backup for midwives.

1997 Minnesota Friends of Midwives morphs into Minnesota Families for Midwifery to support direct-entry midwifery as a member group of the national Citizen's for Midwifery organization.

1998 Two direct-entry midwives, one a certified professional midwife (CPM) and the other a traditional midwife, are criminally investigated by the state attorney general's office and advised to suspend their practices.

1998 Midwifery Now! is created as an umbrella for other midwives to support new legislative and grassroots efforts, and the state's direct-entry midwives are now represented by two groups: MCCPM and Midwifery Now!

1998 Minnesota Statute, Chapter 147D, sponsored by Senator Sandy Pappas and Representative Jim Abeler, is signed into law by Governor Jesse Ventura, reactivating the 1906 licensing law and making licensing an option for direct-entry midwives who are CPMs.

1999 The Midwifery Advisory Council, constituted under the statute, recommends the first group of applicants for licensing.

1999 The BMP meets in July to begin the licensing process for the first applicants.

2000   Licenses given to nine midwives for the first time in over 60 years in Minnesota! Fee is $100.

2002   The Stork's Nest, a freestanding birth center, is opened in Moorhead, MN, by Jill Kent, the first licensed direct-entry midwife in the state under the updated law.

2004   The Stork's Nest closes due to third-party reimbursement issues.

2005   Minnesota has twelve licensed midwives (who must be CPMs) plus seven CPMs. True number of direct-entry midwives is unknown, but estimates would suggest another twelve who are not credentialed.

ENDNOTES

1. Except for Minnesota legislators and other officials, whose names are a matter of public record, we have assigned pseudonyms to all people featured in this chapter. Personal information and quotations are based on interviews and correspondence completed between June and August 2000.

2. Within this chapter, most frequently we simply use the term midwife to refer to direct-entry or traditional midwives and use nurse-midwife for those who enter the practice of midwifery through the profession of nursing. Most direct-entry midwives enter midwifery "directly" through apprenticeship and/or vocational midwifery schools. These midwives might also be NARM-certified CPMs. Minnesota midwives are some-what unusual in that some continue to refer to themselves as "traditional." In other locations, in the past, midwives used the term "lay" rather than "traditional" midwife to distinguish themselves from nurse-midwives. Now, however, the term direct-entry is almost universally used in the United States. In part, the word traditional was imposed upon the midwives by the Minnesota medical community, which in their deliberations, seemed to resist the term direct-entry. However, some of the midwives who have practiced in the state before and after licensing, which included recognition of NARM certification, continue to use traditional on occasion. We have retained this use, even though it seems inconsistent, in the quotations we present in this chapter.

3. D. J. Tice. "Great Governors." Published on the Pioneer Plant, the website of the St. Paul *Pioneer Press*, 11/01/98. http://www.stpaulpioneerpress.com/archive/stassen/110198century.htm. (There are two major newspapers in the Twin Cities—the St. Paul *Pioneer Press* and the Minneapolis *Star Tribune*.)

4. The mission and the history of the Mayo Clinic can be found at its web-site, http://www.mayo.edu/.

5. This and other information about the Minnesota Board of Medical Practice can be found at http://www.bmp.state.mn.us/.

6. For example, in June 2001, serving on the board was Steven I. Altchuler, a psychiatrist in practice at the Mayo Clinic, and Carl S. Smith, the chief of urology at the Hennepin County Medical Center and a member of the graduate faculty in the biomedical engineering program at the University of Minnesota.

7. Information on the Center for Spirituality and Healing can be found at http://www.csh.umn.edu/.

8. From the Dean's "Welcome" to the University of Minnesota Medical School, http://www.med.umn.edu/main/deanwelcome.html, June 13, 2001.

9. For more information on professional boundaries, see Andrew Abbott, 1988, *The System of Professions: An Essay on the Division of Expert Labor.* Chicago: University of Chicago Press.

10. For a more detailed review of the Midwifery Study Advisory Group, see chapter 4 of Lay 2000.

11. Statistically there are just not that many breeches and twin births, but the parameters of normality are quite complicated in such conditions. The breech position might be detected prior to birth or it might come as a surprise, and breech births are best addressed if the baby is of average or smallish size. Again, because the majority of twin births don't reach term, many midwives would screen out these pregnancies from homebirth for that reason alone.

12. See http:///www.revisor.leg.state.mn.us/stats/147D for the complete text of this law.

13. The advisory board consists of one licensed physician who "has been or is currently consulting with licensed traditional midwives, appointed from a list of names submitted to the board by the Minnesota Medical Association," three direct-entry midwives "appointed from a list of names submitted by to the board by Midwifery Now!" and one homebirth parent "appointed from a list of names submitted to the board by Minnesota Families for Midwifery" (Minnesota Statutes Section 147D.25, Subd. 1).

REFERENCES

A Bill for an Act Relating to Health; Modifying Midwifery Requirements; Amending *Minnesota Statutes 1999 Supplement,* Sections 147D.03, Subd 1 and 2; 147D.11; 147D.17, Subd 1, and by Adding a Subd; and 147D.25, Subd 1. (January 28, 2000).

Lay, Mary M. 2000. *The Rhetoric of Midwifery: Gender, Knowledge, and Power.* New Brunswick, NJ: Rutgers University Press.

Minnesota Department of Health. June 7, 1992. *Regulation of Traditional Midwifery in Minnesota: Considerations & Recommendations. A Report to the Minnesota Board of Medical Practice.*

Minnesota Midwives' Guild. September 1995. *Standards of Care and Certification Guide.*

Minnesota Statutes, Chapter 147D: Section 147D.01 Definitions; Section 147D.03 Midwifery; Section 147D.05 Professional conduct; Section 147D.07 Informed consent; Section 147D.09 Limitations of practice; Section 147D.11 Medical consultation plan; Section 147D.13 Reporting; Section 147D.15 Protected titles; Section 147D.17 Licensure requirements; Section 147D.19 Board action on applications for licensure; Section 147D.21 Continuing education requirements; Section 147D.23 Discipline; reporting; Section 147D.25 Advisory council on licensed traditional midwifery; Section 147D.27 Fees (July 1999).

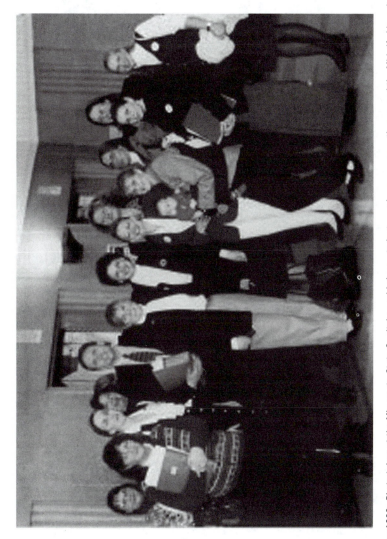

Fig. 5.1 January 1999–Photo taken at the Minnesota State Capitol as midwives, students, and consumers gather around the Midwife Licensing bill authors, Representative Jim Abeler and Senator Sandra Pappas. Both authors are homebirth parents. Photographer: Kerry Dixon.

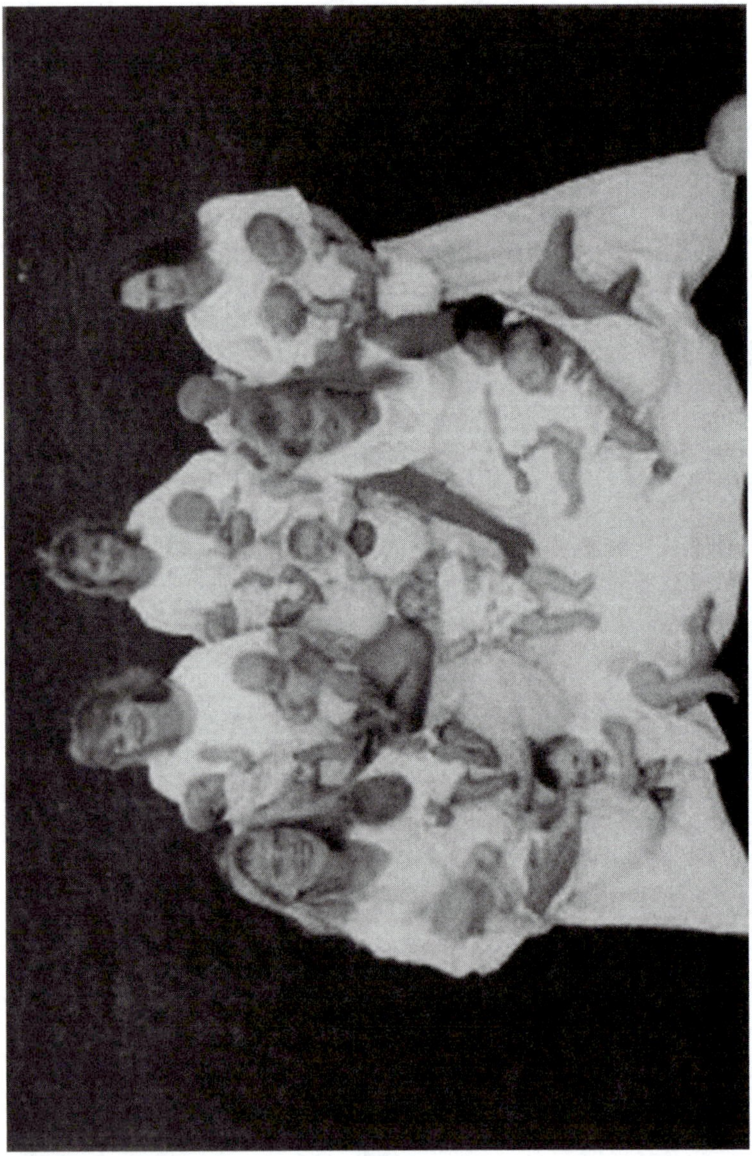

Fig. 5.2 Spring 1997~Midwives and Friends of Midwives homebirth babies. Photographer: Dan Dennehy.

6

RISKS, COSTS, AND EFFECTS OF HOMEBIRTH MIDWIFERY LEGISLATION IN COLORADO

Susan Erikson with Amy Colo

• Introduction • Methodology • Situated Praxis • Colorado Midwifery Organizations • Politicizing Danger, Constructing Risk • Current Regulation • The Costs of Midwifery Legislation in Colorado • Epilogue • Timeline of Events in Colorado Midwifery

INTRODUCTION

Homebirth midwifery has been legal in Colorado now for more than a decade, becoming law in May 1993.[1] The law was renewed by the state legislature in 2000, passing through the state House and Senate without a fight. Colorado Governor Bill Owens signed the law renewing the legalization of direct-entry (homebirth) midwives on June 5, 2001, and homebirth midwifery care remains a legal option for Colorado women. In 2001, there were forty practicing registered homebirth midwives in the state who attended 566 births (DORA 2001).[2]

At first glance, then, homebirth midwifery in Colorado appears secure from legal, professional, and consumer vantage points, but a closer examination reveals a much more complicated situation. This chapter is about the law's renewal process and the costs and effects of legalization on the Colorado homebirth midwifery community and the midwifery arts. Since 1991, when the homebirth midwives began the legislative campaign that resulted in the current law, homebirth midwives in Colorado have been kept on a short legal tether, forced to return to the legislature *three times in nine years,* twice for formal sunset reviews[3] of their law. Compared to other states where homebirth midwifery is regulated, Colorado homebirth midwives have the greatest restriction on the scope of care they can legally provide (e.g., medications, suturing, IV fluids; see appendix). Most significantly, legalization has had its costs: the legal wrangling and the legislative fight required (beginning with ineffectual initial attempts at legalization in the mid-1980s) has resulted in a fractious homebirth midwifery community and a decidedly more obstetrically oriented practice of midwifery.

Midwifery culture itself is the subject of our chapter as we attempt to account for the costs—to the art of midwifery and the midwifery community itself—of waging a legalization campaign. Our chapter uses both the public face of midwifery[4] in Colorado and the behind-the-scenes controversies among the midwives themselves (over scope of care and educational requirements) to illustrate what can happen when midwifery "goes public." With our analysis we do not mean to imply that Colorado midwives would be better off without the legal status and professionalization that resulted from the legislative fight, but rather that the process of legalization served as a catalyst for *particular* types of changes—some of which were welcome, some unwelcome—within Colorado midwifery culture. The smooth passage of the 2001 bill, in fact, belies the professional (and unduly personal) chasms within the Colorado homebirth midwifery community, as well as aspects of the midwifery arts that have been, if not quite lost, then strategically removed from public view.

METHODOLOGY

Our primary research data come from participant observation conducted formally and informally since 1992; a survey questionnaire; and informal and semistructured interviews conducted with registered midwives, legislators, lobbyists, nurse-midwives, representatives of the Colorado Department of Regulatory Agencies, and the Colorado governor's office. Survey and interview data for this chapter were collected in 1996 and 1997 and between 2000 and 2002. Secondary sources include historical texts, public legislative records, and Colorado Midwifery Association (CMA) newsletters and communications.

A seven-question survey was sent out to all thirty-two registered midwives in Colorado in March 2001. The survey had a return rate of forty-one percent. Several returned surveys were supplemented with multipage responses to questions asked, and a few respondents preferred to respond via telephone. Two midwives requested formal telephone interviews. Face-to-face, semi-structured interviews were formally conducted with eight informants. Interviews generally lasted between one and two hours. Interviews were transcribed, and the comments included in this chapter are excerpts from those transcripts. Although our survey data represents midwives' opinions from throughout the state, geographical distance and budgetary constraints limited our ability to interview midwives much beyond the Denver-Boulder metropolitan area.

Like many other researchers of midwifery, we conducted "interested" research (see MacDonald and Bourgeault 2001). Both of us maintain long-term personal and professional commitments to midwifery, and we both had our children with midwives when midwifery was not legally sanctioned by the state. Amy has been professionally involved with the Colorado midwifery community since 1991 when she began her midwifery training, and she became a registered midwife in 1998. She is a member of the CMA as well as one of its past presidents, serving from 1995 to 1997. Susan was first introduced to the midwifery community in Boulder County in 1992 when she sought out a homebirth midwife to assist her in the birth of her first child. Although homebirth midwifery was illegal and underground in 1992, the midwifery network was easy enough to access if one knew alternative health-care practitioners in Boulder County. In 1996 and 1997, Susan conducted a research project on the effects of midwifery legalization on actual practice, and some of that research is drawn on in this chapter. In sum, Amy's professional experience as a midwife, Susan's academic engagement with the topic, and their personal experiences of homebirth constitute the departure points for this chapter.

SITUATED PRAXIS

The legal history of homebirth midwifery in Colorado has followed a pattern found in many other U.S. states—once legal and unregulated, then illegal, now legal and regulated with a limited scope of practice. As detailed in Patricia Godeke Tjaden's (1984:154) excellent thesis on Colorado midwifery, at the turn of the twentieth century, midwifery in Colorado "was regarded as a service to the community." Until 1915 when the state began to require licensure, midwifery in Colorado was legal, unlicensed, and unregulated; midwives, like physicians, simply had to register with the state to practice. Following the 1915 passage of laws regulating midwifery, however, a licensed midwife could practice independently, though she was not legally allowed to use drugs or instruments. Over the following decades, midwifery came under attack from the allopathic medical community. In 1941 midwifery licensure was discontinued completely, in effect setting in place a phasing out of the legal practice of midwifery in Colorado. In 1976, all references to midwifery were stricken from the legal record, and it became illegal for any midwife to assist women in childbirth. Although certified nurse-midwives lobbied successfully to amend the Medical Practice Act in 1977 so that they could provide birthing services under the supervision of a physician, homebirth midwifery remained illegal until 1993.

In Colorado today, homebirth with midwives in attendance accounts for only about one percent of all births. Colorado physicians maintain the largest share of birth-assisting privilege, attending about 55,000 births annually (CDPHE [Colorado Department of Public Health and Environment] 2002). The 226 certified nurse-midwives (ACNM [American College of Nurse-Midwives] 2002) in Colorado, who provide prenatal care and assist women giving birth in hospitals and birth centers, attended approximately 7,000 births in 2000 (CDPHE 2002). By comparison, in 2001 Colorado's forty homebirth midwives assisted in a total of 566 births at home (DORA 2002). While numerically the 2001 data are a significant increase from the twenty-three homebirth midwives who assisted 345 women who gave birth at home in 1995 (DORA 2002), when Colorado's population growth between 1995 and 2001 is factored in, the percentage of homebirths has remained fairly constant, about one percent of all births. What has changed, however, is that nearly all homebirths (ninety percent) are now attended by registered midwives, indicating that homebirth has been effectively brought under regulatory control (DORA 2002; Karberg, personal communication).

Homebirth midwives in Colorado are a diverse group. Many of the differences among them correlate to the demographic, economic, and political distinctions of Colorado itself. Demographically, most homebirth midwives work in the eastern foothills of the Rocky Mountains—the Boulder-Denver-Colorado Springs corridor—where most Coloradoans live. But there are also a number of homebirth midwives practicing on the western side of the Continental Divide, along what is called the western slope. The fewest number of homebirth midwives work in the southern regions of the state, the dry, desert-like Four Corners and San Juan Valley regions. Economically, the Boulder-Denver-Colorado Springs corridor is most affluent, but politically this stretch along the eastern foothills of the Rockies could not be more different.

Northernmost Boulder is politically liberal; Denver is a more moderate aggregate by virtue of being home to both politically conservative and liberal factions; and Colorado Springs is politically and religiously conservative. Most of Colorado's Christian homebirth midwives practice in the Colorado Springs area.

Historically, there has also been a great deal of variation in midwives' interaction with the law. One midwife put it this way:

> Most of the practicing midwives here have no idea what happened twenty to thirty years ago or what the "witch hunts" were like. They have no idea what it was like to worry about the cops coming to your door or the DA [District Attorney] wanting to arrest us all. They think it has always been a "good time" to practice here. We (those of us from other parts of the state) have always said that "Boulder is another planet" and is NOT at all indicative of practice in other locations in Colorado. Unfortunately most people think Boulder *is* Colorado. NOT! (Emily, 2001, homebirth midwife for twenty-eight years)

So while we expected some internal variation among the midwives as a group, an unexpected result of our study was the identification of an *ideological hierarchy of orientation* among the midwives.[5] This hierarchy is not acknowledged in midwifery discourses as a hierarchy per se—either within or outside of the midwifery community—but midwives use it to categorize one another in discussions, and actively reference its existence as if it were something quite literal. This hierarchy corresponds to a continuum of legitimization, a point we elaborate upon below. Of course, ideological orientations are hardly unique to the profession of midwifery. In any profession, one's ideological orientation helps one to identify like-minded colleagues for both professional and personal support, and is an inevitable result of personal proclivity, education, and experience.

For Colorado homebirth midwives, however, the tent, if you will, under which midwives organized was ideologically inclusive in the early years of their professionalization. It grew progressively less tolerant of difference as the professional organization, the Colorado Midwives Association (CMA), matured. The legalization process raised the stakes, and as a result, Colorado homebirth midwives came to self-sanction much more aggressively than the regulatory agencies charged with their oversight. Further, legalization has meant that some ideological orientations were more politically advantageous than others. Whether a midwife's practice is shaped by an ideological orientation in keeping with, for example, the mainstream medical model, the Wise-Woman model of care (Weed 1989), Christian midwifery tenets, or even if she locates herself astride several categories, her primary ideological orientation locates her along a *continuum of legitimization.*

There is no question that the hierarchy of orientation for midwives themselves reflects the Colorado legislature's hierarchical valuation of the healing arts: mainstream allopathic obstetrical medicine supersedes the midwifery arts, and within the midwifery arts, there is a further hierarchical breakdown that few legislators or the public realize exists. As far as the legislators were concerned, the public face of homebirth midwifery in Colorado was that of a more mainstream, obstetrically sympathetic midwifery. Showing that particular face of midwifery was a politically strategic move, orchestrated by the CMA and their lobbyist to rebut the stereotype of, to quote a CMA lobbyist, "Big Bertha, the Midwife."

> I think that sometimes when you go to make an argument to a legislator, you better have somebody who is not going to rely solely on the Mother Earth folk wisdom of yesteryear, because that plays into the stereotype of many people who are not keen on midwifery. You don't want to reinforce their worst fears. (CMA lobbyist, 2001)

Deliberately cultivating a particular public face of midwifery is nothing new. Tjaden comments on a 1982 CMA newsletter article, written at the same time as the CMA's first legalization effort, recruiting midwives for the CMA's Speaker's Bureau, whose job it was to educate the public about homebirth midwifery:

> [She should be an] "'articulate, experienced speaker, have a good professional vocabulary, dress professionally, be supportive of midwives and a good debater.' . . . It is apparent from this statement that members of the CMA are extremely concerned about their public image; they do not want to be perceived as counterculture types." (Tjaden 1984:214–215)

While there is nothing duplicitous in this concern, it should also be recognized that its effects were not neutral. Such a concern marginalized midwives who did not fit the Colorado Legislative Assembly's conventions—at minimum, stockings, heels, and "big hair," as one midwife reported—for meaningful participation in the legislative process. A CMA lobbyist reported that a legislator teased him about keeping "all the gals wearing Birkenstocks delivering babies in the woods" hidden from view. In the next section we explore what the legislative process has meant for Colorado midwives who, well, *do* wear comfortable shoes and who want midwifery law to reflect what they feel is special about the art of midwifery.

COLORADO MIDWIFERY ORGANIZATIONS

Currently, there are several organized factions of homebirth midwives in Colorado, which we will describe in more detail, but the 1993 legalization of homebirth midwifery in Colorado is almost exclusively due to the work done by the Colorado Midwives Association (CMA). Originally formed by midwives in 1979 to provide continuing education opportunities (study groups, conferences, workshops), the CMA took up the issue of legalization in 1982. In 1983, in a first effort to legalize homebirth midwifery in Colorado, the CMA submitted a bill to the Colorado Legislative Assembly, titled Concerning Midwifery, which argued that midwifery was not the practice of medicine and therefore should not be regulated as such. The bill died in committee. By many accounts, political naïveté killed CMA's first legalizing effort. As one midwife summarized it, "Bad choice of sponsor, poorly written bill, totally wrong line-up of witnesses, totally wrong posture" (Margaret,[6] homebirth midwife for twenty-nine years, 1997[7]).

During the next two decades, political organizing continued and took its toll on the CMA, an organization that was already marked by the political and economic distinctions of Colorado. Until the second wave of legalization in the early 1990s, the CMA had been quite inclusive. The trajectories of homebirth midwifery professionalization in Colorado had allowed for multiple orientations of practice and there was a general sense of acceptance among the members. The process of legalization, however, raised the stakes and increased the fractionalization of the organization. This was perhaps an inevitable result of the maturation of both the CMA as an organization and the homebirth legalization movement—younger, smaller organizations and movements *need* to be inclusive—but fractionalization also occurred because the process of legalization forced a *valuation* of the various orientations of homebirth midwifery.

Within the CMA, there is a small group of politically seasoned midwives who know how to work the legislative system (and are very good at it) and other midwives who remain less politicized. The less politicized midwives were usually less political by choice. Several reported being "sickened" by politics. Others, though, reported being forced into a less politicized role by exclusion, and it was the exclusionary practices that intensified a fractionalization of the CMA. The politically seasoned midwives, who for the most part were and continue to be the CMA leadership, maintained a stranglehold on the political process. They had been charting the political waters for years, knew which way each state senator and representative was likely to vote, and had, with the help of their lobbyist, strategized each and every move of the legislative effort. They had sacrificed both personally and professionally to make midwifery legal, cutting back on their individual practices and working twelve-hour days (in stockings and high-heels, as one pointed out) lobbying Colorado legislators. By virtue of their experience and political acumen, and in no small part, their personal sacrifice, they felt justified to manage the legislative process and expected the membership to rubber-stamp their decisions. Midwives who questioned the strategy or wanted the law more accurately to reflect what midwives actually do were considered obstructionist. In one instance, at a meeting about the legislative strategy, a midwife member who was taking notes and posing challenging questions was deemed "troublesome" and asked to leave by the CMA leadership.

It is no surprise then that additional midwifery organizations formed in Colorado. The most vocal and well-organized alternative is the Colorado Alliance of Independent Midwives (CAIM) with about fifty members. (CMA membership is about 100.) There is also a Colorado Christian Midwives Alliance (CCMA) that has been serving as an organizational center for Christian midwives practicing primarily along the Denver-Colorado Springs corridor. Other groups have come and gone, like the Boulder Alliance of Midwives (BAM), which began in 2001 with the intention of serving the political and professional needs of both homebirth- and certified nurse-midwives (CNMs). Although the intentions of this alliance were good, members discovered there was not enough common ground with regard to needs to sustain the organization.

During the 2000 legislative effort, the CAIM drafted a formal Position Statement on Direct-Entry Midwifery Legislation (CAIM 2000). In the early committee meetings, before the bill left committee, CAIM testified in favor of, among other things, licensing midwifery (rather than, as is currently the case, "registering" midwives with all the requirements of licensure); expanding the scope of midwifery care; and using the Certified Professional Midwife (CPM) certification as an education standard. CAIM leadership had hoped to work collaboratively with the CMA, especially on the issue of scope of practice, but the political aims of CAIM and the CMA were considered to be oppositional by the CMA. The politically experienced CMA leadership pitted themselves against the more ambitious CAIM members, and a CAIM member described the CMA's reception of CAIM's presence at those early committee meetings as "hostile and contentious." The stage was set for further fractionalization of the Colorado homebirth midwifery community.

POLITICIZING DANGER, CONSTRUCTING RISK

In this section we explore how notions of danger and risk informed the legalization strategies of the CMA in their campaign to keep homebirth midwifery legal in Colorado. Usually public discourses about midwives and risk focus on the "riskiness" of midwifery care itself—the "what if" medical contentions waged about the risks to the woman and baby of giving birth at home. That perception of risk was certainly at work for the House and Senate committee legislators who had to decide whether the proposed bill would be voted on by the whole legislative body, but other perceptions of risk were also operative, and as it turns out, much more detrimental to the cohesiveness of the homebirth midwifery community. In the recent legislation regarding homebirth, the CMA leadership assumed that if their legislative efforts failed, midwifery would become illegal. The CMA, on the advice of their primary lobbyist, operated as if the renewal bill risked defeat, and a fight to expand the scope of practice would mean losing the legal right to practice. The CMA charted a low-risk political course because they perceived high-consequence cost to campaigning for an expansion of scope of practice. The bill, we were told repeatedly by CMA leadership, risked defeat if the CMA pushed for too much.

In her scholarship on risk, Mary Douglas (1992:58) theorizes that:

> [Individuals] have set up their institutions as decision processors which shut out some options and put others in a favorable light. Individuals make basic choices between joining and not joining institutions of different kinds. They then engage in continuous monitoring of the institutional machinery. The big choices reach them in the form of questions whether to reinforce authority or to subvert it.

Douglas's work is relevant here in two ways. First, for the Colorado midwives, some options were shut out while others were put in a favorable light. The CMA is subject to the rules, regulations, and politics of an institution, the Colorado Legislative Assembly. Institutionally speaking, the Colorado legislature requires certain operative norms for the successful passage of a bill. The institution requires compliance with procedural (read political) norms that may be outside the usual professional realm of midwives. Such compliance places some childbirth options (e.g., hospital birth) in a favorable light and shuts down others (e.g., homebirth). Thus it forces what we term a *Stepfordization* of homebirth midwifery—a Stepford wife–like change from a emphasis on full-bodied, full-scale midwifery knowledge to a more restrictive and falsely narrow representation of midwives' ways of knowing. Homebirth midwifery is forced to appear to be something much less than it is in order to be palatable to the legislators. The institution regulates homebirth midwifery in such a way as to shape its public face, and also to alter the art of midwifery itself, a point we address in greater detail in the last section of this chapter.

Second, the CMA also acted as an institution. Throughout the legislative process, CMA's leadership acted as an institutional surrogate, itself shutting out some options and putting others in a favorable light. CMA's identification of what was at risk shaped collective action. One midwife identified the effect of CMA's assumption of risk this way:

> Never once did people—midwives and consumers—get asked [by the CMA], "How would you like to see midwifery improved?" They were only asked, "Do you want to stay legal?" So when you start a discussion from that point of view, it shapes the whole story. (Samantha, homebirth midwife for six years, 2001)

Midwives who challenged the political strategies of the CMA were perceived as dangerous and responsible for putting the legality of homebirth midwifery at risk. "Asking for too much" and "bringing too much attention to midwifery practice" were perceived by the CMA leadership as threatening the legality of midwifery in Colorado. This left midwives who had a different vision of what legal midwifery in Colorado could look like, all of whom were CMA members but not among the leadership, with no other option but to subvert the institution by "not joining" and forming another group.

How real was the risk? Measuring risk is a complex process, but several indicators suggest the risk of homebirth midwifery becoming illegal during the 2000 sunset review was next to nonexistent. In the House, the final bill passed by a vast majority (sixty to five). In the Senate, where the bill was first introduced (the Senate being the more advantageous place in which to introduce a bill), it passed unanimously (thirty-five to zero). One of the CMA's most brilliant exhibitions of political craft was their selection of the bill's sponsor, the chairman of the Senate Health, Environment, Children and Families Committee (HECF). Alienating the chairman by opposing his bill was not something medical lobbyists and medical societies were likely to do. (As a CMA lobbyist put it, "How angry do you want to make the chairman of the committee that all your bills are going to?") The Department of Regulatory Agencies (DORA), the state agency responsible for oversight of registered homebirth midwives, testified in support of an expansion of practice as well as an increase in educational requirements. Although a CMA lobbyist claimed that "the threat of a governor's veto was the biggest factor" deterring the CMA from fighting for an expansion of practice, a House Representative who voted in favor of the bill assessed the actual risk of a governor's veto as "slight to nonexistent." Telephone interviews with officials in the Governor's Legislative Liaison Office also indicated that

> [T]here was never any talk of a veto. . . . The DORA [Department of Regulatory Agencies, Midwifery Registration Office] program is recognized as a good program that provides the necessary oversight. . . . This governor has enough respect for the process across the street [in the Legislature] that he wouldn't have vetoed it. He doesn't veto many bills to begin with.[8] (Official in Governor's Legislative Liaison Office)

And while our contacts in the Governor's Office thought that the right to carry pitocin would have been the most problematic aspect of an expansion of practice, the legality of midwifery was not at stake, only pitocin's inclusion in the bill. One contact specifically said, "Pitocin wouldn't have even made it out of committee, but Vitamin K and Rhogham, they probably would have gotten through."

We interviewed midwives who felt their legality was unquestionably at risk, as well as those who questioned the assumption that homebirth midwifery could become illegal. One midwife categorized the threat to legally practicing homebirth midwifery this way:

> Single most important issue: staying legal. The bill as it stands seems okay, but knowing legislation can be real different in practice, I am waiting to see what really pans out from it. The [homebirth midwives] in New York got screwed royally after supporting a bill they thought would help them practice. Instead, it got them arrested. (Emily, 2001, homebirth midwife

for twenty-eight years) [See chapter 2 for a description of events in New York.]

Another midwife pointed out why the CMA advocated a bill that did not ask for an expansion of practice which, she felt, would have required a short-term (two to three years) rather than long-term (ten years) Sunset Review deadline:

> We want to be renewed and we want to be renewed for ten years. None of this three-year [Sunset Review] stuff. That is another way the medical community wears us down. We don't have the money to be renewed every three years. We can't do it.... So we wanted ten years and we can't do that with meds. We think the meds are the right thing to do, but what we really want is to be legal for ten years. (Linda, homebirth midwife for twenty years, 2001)

On the other hand, two midwives from CAIM thought:

> [Although] just maintaining our legal status has been put forth as the only issue we can hope to address in this legislative session, I find no evidence to support the fears that this program is in any danger of being discontinued. There has been no testimony or written recommendation that the state make the practice of homebirth midwifery illegal. Maintaining our status as legally authorized practitioners is a minimalist bottom line to which we all agree. Yet there is much more to which we can aspire. (Nancy, homebirth midwife for six years, 2001)
>
> At the beginning, what the midwives did was amazing, but what didn't happen after was that people didn't make a paradigm shift from "Oh, we're illegal, we're hunted" to "Oh, we're legal now and how do we want to have a presence in the world?" ... [Making midwifery illegal] was never the choice. . . . I was at the first hearing. No one recommended making it illegal again . . . .The doctors didn't, the nurse-midwives didn't, the nursing association didn't. They all testified for staying legal. (Samantha, homebirth midwife for seven years, 2001)

Clearly there is a generational difference between the midwives who lived through the days when midwifery was illegal and those who felt they could afford to dream. Samantha characterized the generation gap like this:

> People who'd been practicing midwifery when it was illegal—once it became legal, they became complacent. . . . Not to have the stress of being put in jail, I understand that. But that's not who I am and not who many of the midwives are today. I started my practice when we were legal and so I don't live from that place of "this is enough." I want something bigger. (Samantha, homebirth midwife for seven years, 2001)

It could very well be that some of the contentiousness evidenced within the homebirth midwifery community is due to a reluctance to pass the legislative mantle on to this next, more ambitious generation. Of course, such reluctance is not exclusive to the leadership of the CMA. Anthropologists have long taken note of the relationship between senior and junior members of communities. Rosaldo (1989) describes the relationship as a "reciprocity" arrangement with seniors holding knowledge, juniors possessing passion, and each secretly admiring that of the other. Although the senior and junior members of the Colorado homebirth midwifery community do not fall neatly into categories of those with knowledge and those with passion, Rosaldo's description is apt here: legislative savvy, political expertise, and institutional memory in this last round of legislation held more sway than a passion for change. But inevitably junior members become more senior, and senior members at some point relinquish their power to the next generation.

CURRENT REGULATION

The law Colorado Governor Bill Owens signed in June of 2001 maintained the legal status of homebirth midwives.[9] The final bill did not include an expansion of practice. Specifically, neither the carrying and use of intramuscular (IM) medications to stop a hemorrhage, nor the right to suture first-and second-degree perineal lacerations had been included in the bill. Educational requirements, however, were increased (See tables 6.1 and 6.2).

Table 6.1 Midwifery Practice and Educational Standards before and after 2001 Legislation

	Suturing	Rhogam	Antihemorrhagic Medications	Intramuscular Medications[a]	Educational requirements
Before Bill Passage	Illegal	Illegal	Illegal	Illegal	See table 6.2
After Bill Passage	Illegal	Illegal	Illegal	Illegal	Increased

[a]Intramuscular medications include pitocin, methergine, Rhogam, and vitamin K, all prescriptive medications.

Table 6.2 Midwifery Educational Standards before and after 2001 Legislation

	Births	Clinical Site	Formal Education	Apprenticeship Required
Before Bill Passage	60	Home	Variable	Yes
After Bill Passage	60	Unspecified	MEAC, CPM, PEP	No

There is a bitter irony in the requirements of the current law: Midwives have more educational requirements than before the latest Sunset Review, but they did not receive a concomitant expansion of practice. Originally, DORA recommended increasing educational requirements in order to justify its recommendation that midwives be able to administer medications. DORA also recommended a five-year Sunset Review date to revisit the new medication privilege (See table 6.3 for a comparison of medication authorizations by state). The CMA, for whom continued legality and a ten-year Sunset Review date were of highest priority, recommended no expansion of practice and supported the increased educational requirements once they were in the bill. CAIM recommended an expansion of practice and that the North American Registry of Midwives' (NARM) Certified Professional Midwife (CPM) standards serve as educational requirements. Of the three most contentious aspects of the bill (administration of medication and suturing, and additional educational requirements) only the increase of educational requirements made it into the final draft of the bill.

Putting the issues of medications and suturing aside, the new educational requirements have raised concerns for advocates of the traditional midwifery arts. There are now two routes to meeting the new educational standards: graduation from an accredited midwifery education program approved by the Midwifery Education Accreditation Council (MEAC), or "a substantially equivalent" education approved by the Colorado Director of Registrations. Substantially equivalency is achieved by (1) certification as a CPM through NARM; (2) certification from NARM's Portfolio Evaluation Process (PEP), an avenue that allows for apprenticeship to serve as a primary educational means; or (3) utilizing either (1) or (2) and having a credential review performed by the International Credentialing Associates (ICA) or International Consultants of Delaware (ICD). Some midwives fear the new requirements signal a departure from the apprenticeship training model and mark a move toward the more standardized and obstetrically-based training offered by formalized educational settings. Homebirth midwives may still have apprenticeship training as long as they use NARM's PEP process (see chapter 3) to acquire educational certification. The intent

Table 6.3 Comparison of Medication Authorizations by State (DORA 2000)

State	Eye Prophylaxis	Pitocin	Methergine	Vitamin K	Rhogam	O$_2$	IV	Local Anesthesia	Suturing
AK	Yes	Yes	Yes	Yes	Yes	Yes	Yes	Yes	Yes
AR	No	No	No	No	No	No	No	No	Yes
AZ	Yes	Yes	Yes	Yes	Yes	Yes	No	Yes	Yes
CA	Yes	Yes	Yes	Yes	Yes	Yes	Yes	No	No
CO	Yes	No	No	No	No	Yes	No	No	No
FL[a]	Yes	Yes	Yes	Yes	Yes	Yes	Yes	Yes	Yes
LA	Yes	Yes	Yes	Yes	No	Yes	No	Yes	Yes
MN[a]	Yes	Yes	Yes	Yes	No	Yes	No	Yes	Yes
MT[a]	Yes	Yes	No	Yes	Yes	No	Yes	Yes	Yes
NH	Yes	Yes	Yes	Yes	Yes	Yes	Yes	Yes	Yes
NM	Yes	Yes	Yes	Yes	Yes	Yes	Yes	Yes	Yes
OR	Yes	Yes	Yes	Yes	No	Yes	No	No	No
SC	Yes	Yes	No	No	No	Yes	No	No	No
TX[a]	Yes	No	No	No	No	Yes	No	No	No
WA[b]	Yes	Yes	Yes	Yes	Yes	Yes	Yes	Yes	Yes

[a] Other medications must be authorized by a physician.

[b] The director may authorize additional medications. Epinephrine, magnesium sulfate, rubella vaccine have been authorized.

of this requirement was to preserve some flexibility in homebirth midwifery education. But the term "substantially equivalent education approved by the Director of Regulations" (DORA Rules and Regulations: Rule 2), empowers the director to determine exactly what "substantially equivalent" means.

In the latest amending of the bill, requirements that practical experience be gained through apprenticeship and specifically in a home setting were deleted. Now, all sixty births required for registration could conceivably be attended at a clinic, an environment that includes more technology and personnel than is available at home. Several midwives expressed concern that the apprentice model of training was not preserved as the primary training model, and that midwifery arts would be gradually replaced by more obstetric-centric midwifery practice. Additionally, the expense of obtaining midwifery training will clearly be greater than in the past. While MEAC programs provide the academic component of training, student midwives in Colorado must still obtain clinical experience through an apprenticeship in either a homebirth or birth center practice, as there is no MEAC-accredited program or school in Colorado. The clinical aspect of training continues to be the most difficult to arrange due to the limited pool of both clinical opportunities and

preceptor midwives in Colorado. It is yet to be seen how these requirements will affect the ability of midwives to obtain their education in
Colorado.

THE COSTS OF MIDWIFERY LEGISLATION
IN COLORADO

The tangible costs of midwifery legislation (raising the $77,000 the
CMA has paid in lobbying debts since 1992, paying for mailings and
phone calls, commuting to and from the Capitol) translate very literally
into a substantial investment in keeping homebirth midwifery as a legal
birthing option for Coloradoans. This section, however, focuses on the
intangible costs of legislation. As already discussed, legislation has left
its mark on the homebirth midwifery community, but perhaps more
insidiously it has altered the public practice of the homebirth midwifery arts. Again, as we stated in the introduction, we do not mean to
imply with our analysis that Colorado midwives would be better off
without the legal status and professionalization that resulted from the
legislative fight, but rather that the process of legalization served as a
catalyst for *particular* types of changes, some of them costly, within
Colorado homebirth midwifery culture.

In 1997, when the first phase of this research project was conducted,
the central research question was how had legalization affected practice? At that phase, Susan focused on how the seemingly innocuous
process of regulating women's birth-giving options infuses the art of
midwifery with a number of new concerns. As one midwife told Susan:

> When I was illegal, whatever I did was illegal. I could do twins or
> breeches or whatever I did. It didn't matter because I was already
> illegal. Now I have something I want to protect: being legal.
> (Barbara, homebirth midwife for sixteen years, 1997)

The dilemma for many of the midwives was whether to continue doing
what they knew how to do, including stopping hemorrhages with
intramuscular pitocin, external version, and delivering breeches and
twins—aspects of the midwifery arts that not only serve as a standard
of care but which are also skills and knowledge lost to the mainstream
obstetrical community.

Breech birth is a good example of a prohibited practice that poses an
interesting dilemma for midwives, particularly those who practiced
before legalization. Experienced midwives know how to deliver most
breech babies vaginally. Most obstetricians do not. The fact that senior

midwives like Ina May Gaskin are occasionally invited to medical schools to teach about breech delivery attests to the fact that midwives preserve a particular kind of knowledge about birth—knowledge not necessarily held by obstetricians. One of the most senior midwives expressed it this way:

> We still know how to do things that maybe doctors don't even know how to do, that we can take care of at home because our whole training was to use our hands, intuition, and our common sense. (Mary, homebirth midwife for nineteen years, 1997)

This being the case, midwives have to choose between following the letter of the law and practicing what they and the parents believe is best for all concerned. The ideological spaces and birth arts that homebirth midwives preserve are significant, yet legalization has forced many midwives to abandon some midwifery arts practices, or at the very least strategically remove certain practices from public view. Legalization has forced homebirth midwifery to appear to be something much less than it is in order to be palatable to legislators.

The push for an expansion of practice was, at heart, an attempt to bring the law and practice into sync.

> The biggest thing for me was I thought that the scope of practice should be expanded to really reflect the way we practice. It is a standard of care that we carry emergency anti-hemorrhagic drugs. (Samantha, homebirth midwife for seven years, 2001)

In interviews, several midwives expressed frustration with the fact that they are regulated by people who do not understand midwifery arts. Many midwives are currently practicing a much broader scope of midwifery care than is legally sanctioned, and felt it unnecessary to fight for regulations that more accurately reflected what they do.

> We'd have to make such a commitment for the law to reflect what we actually do. And could we actually provide better care with an improved law? No! (Kathy, homebirth midwife for ten years, 2001)

An interesting parallel can be made between the homebirth midwifery regulating process and cross-cultural encounters more generally. Between the 1940s and 1980s, homebirth midwives in Colorado were illegal and practiced in isolation—a modernist isolation replete with access to modern medicine when they needed it, but an isolation nonetheless, which enabled their culture to flourish with little outside influence. Then, in the mid-1980s, the cross-cultural contact necessitated by the legalization effort entailed not only the cultivation of a public face of homebirth midwifery that would be deemed acceptable, but also an evaluation of midwifery practices by the dominant paradigm—allopathic obstetrics. A power differential required changes not only in midwifery practice and behavior, but also in how midwives are educated. A colonization metaphor would go too far here, but to say that the encounter was neutral is equally inadequate.

Midwives with the social capital—formal education, upbringing, socioeconomic standing and financial resources—to subvert the dominant paradigm have less at stake and less to fear from operating outside the law. But not all homebirth midwives are equally empowered in this scenario, and as with most laws, it is the people without social capital that the law must protect. A law that reflects what midwives actually *do* would benefit these midwives the most.

EPILOGUE

After the law passed, DORA, as the agency charged with program oversight, was required to hold a Rules and Regulations Hearing to review their plan for implementation of the law. DORA sent out information letters and invitations to this public hearing to all the registered homebirth midwives. The information letter mentioned DORA's intention to include restrictions on vaginal births after cesarean (VBACs), an item that, according to the program administrator, DORA expected would generate much interest and activism within the homebirth midwifery community. In fact, both the CMA and CAIM testified in support of striking VBAC restrictions from the Rules and Regulations. This time the fractionalization that has been so emotionally distressing and time consuming *served* the larger goals of the homebirth midwifery community in Colorado. CMA and CAIM testimonies, different though they were, complemented each other well, and the VBAC restriction was lifted.

The bitterness that had sparked the fractionalization of the Colorado homebirth midwifery community may not be a distant enough memory for the midwives themselves to appreciate the value of now having more than a single public face of homebirth midwifery in Colorado. But homebirth midwifery as a legal practice in Colorado is stronger because it no longer relies solely on the strength of one small group of women shouldering the legislative burden. Legislation has had its costs.

What remains to be seen is the extent to which homebirth midwives in Colorado will allow the process of legislation to chip away at what is special about the homebirth midwifery arts, and whether they will work to instantiate the actual scope of midwifery practice as a matter of public record.

TIMELINE OF EVENTS IN COLORADO MIDWIFERY

1915 Introduction in Colorado of midwifery licensure, required for the practice of midwifery arts.

1941 Midwifery licensure was discontinued completely, in effect phasing out the legal practice of midwifery in Colorado.

1976 All references to midwifery were stricken from the legal record. While it remained legal for women to give birth at home, it became illegal in Colorado for midwives to assist women in childbirth.

1979 Colorado Midwifery Association (CMA) formed.

1982 CMA takes up the issue of legalizing homebirth midwifery through the legislature. The proposed bill, which argued that midwifery is not the practice of medicine, dies in committee.

1991 CMA takes up the issue of legalizing homebirth midwifery through the legislature.

1993 Homebirth midwifery legalized in Colorado.

1995 First Sunset Review of midwifery legalization. Midwifery legality sustained.

2000 Colorado Alliance of Independent Midwives (CAIM) formed, catalyzed, in part, by fractious internal CMA politics.

2000 Second Sunset Review of midwifery legalization. Midwifery legality sustained, but the expansion of practice advocated by CAIM not realized.

2003 Training for midwifery solely through apprenticeships no longer satisfies legal requirements. MEAC-approved education is preferred training. Credentials review through NARM's Portfolio Evaluation Process is possible, but not encouraged.

ACKNOWLEDGMENTS

We are indebted to the many Colorado homebirth midwives who completed survey questions, granted interviews, and corresponded by e-mail with us during the 1997 and 2001 research phases. Additionally, we gratefully acknowledge the assistance of the Colorado Midwives Association (CMA) and Colorado Alliance of Independent Midwives

(CAIM) leadership, various civil servants within Colorado state agencies who provided data, statistics, and interpretation of the legalization process, as well as other key but unnamed people who were instrumental to the legislative process.

ENDNOTES

1. Homebirth midwifery was legal in Colorado until 1976, when all references to midwifery were stricken from the legal records. Beginning in 1915, the law became increasingly restrictive, and by the 1940s, homebirth midwifery was virtually unpracticable under the law.
2. Homebirth and homebirth midwifery statistics are collected by both the Midwifery Registration Office of the Department of Regulatory Agencies (DORA) and the Colorado Department of Public Health and Environment (CDPHE). The numbers cited here are from DORA. CDPHE typically reports fewer births attended by midwives, by about 100, but there are sociopolitical reasons for this. CDPHE data is dependent on data filed for birth certificates, which requires identifying an attendant. Some midwives list "husband," "self," or "other" as the attendant as a matter of childbirth politics.
3. By definition, a Sunset Review of a law is a review by legislative committees and regulatory agencies. Not all laws are subject to such a review, but those that are, will be automatically terminated by a specified date unless extended by legislative action. The 1992 law (which went into effect May 1993) was sunsetted until 1995. That renewal was sunsetted until 2000.
4. The "public face of midwifery" is a term originated by Robbie Davis-Floyd who organized an American Anthropology Association conference panel in 2000 with that title.
5. These categorical orientations are not meant to be discrete or totalizing. For most midwives, there is overlap from category to category.
6. All names are pseudonyms.
7. Relevant and informative citations from the 1997 interviews Susan conducted are included in this article.
8. In fact, of the 476 measures that passed through both houses of the legislature in 2001, Governor Owens vetoed fourteen or three percent.
9. The law (statute) and official rules and regulations can be found at the Department of Regulatory Agencies (DORA) Office of Midwifery Registration webpage: http://www.dora.state.co.us/midwives/.

REFERENCES

Colorado Association of Independent Midwives (CAIM). 2000. Position Statement on Direct-Entry Midwifery Legislation. Available from CAIM.

Colorado Department of Public Health and Environment (CDPHE). 2002. *Colorado Vital Statistics, 2000.* Colorado Health Statistics Section. Denver, Colorado.

Douglas, Mary. 1992. *Risk and Blame: Essays in Cultural Theory.* London: Routledge.

Erikson, Susan. 1997. "Culture Change: Implications of Midwifery Legislation–A Case Study." Paper presented at the joint meeting of the Society for Applied Anthropology and the Society for Medical Anthropology, Seattle, Washington, March.

Karberg, Beth. 2002. Personal communication on September 9, 2002.

MacDonald, Margaret, and Ivy Lynn Bourgeault. 2001. "The Politics of Representation: Doing and Writing Interested Research on Midwifery." *Resources for Feminist Research* 28(1/2):151–168.

Rosaldo, Michelle. 1989. *Knowledge and Passion: Ilongot Notions of the Self & Social Life.* Cambridge: Cambridge University Press.

State of Colorado, Department of Regulatory Agencies (DORA). 2000. "Colorado Midwives Registration Program: 2000 Sunset Review." Denver, Colorado.

————. 2002. Midwives Registration Office. Special information request. Denver, Colorado.

Tjaden, Patricia Godeke. 1984. *Delivering Babies Underground: A Study of Illegal Midwifery and Elective Home Births.* PhD dissertation. University of Colorado-Boulder.

Weed, Susun S. 1989. *Wise Woman Herbal: Healing Wise.* Woodstock, NY: Ash Tree Publishing.

Appendix 1 Direct-Entry Midwifery Regulated Scope of Care: By State

State	Medicaid	Prescription Meds[a]	Suturing	IV Fluids
Alaska	*	*	*	*with transport
Arkansas			*	
Arizona	*	*	*	*
California	*	*	*	*
Colorado				
Florida	*	*b	*	*b
Louisiana		*	*	*
Minnesota		*	*	
Montana		*	*	
New Hampshire	*	*	*	*
New Mexico	*	*c	*	*
Oregon	*	*	*	
South Carolina	*	*		
Tennessee				
Texas		*c	*	*d
Vermont				
Washington	*	*e	*	*

Source: Table compiled by Beth Karberg, MS, RM, CPM, Fort Collins, Colorado, and Elizabeth Moore, RM, CPM, Boulder, Colorado, 2002. Colorado Alliance of Independent Midwives (CAIM), Denver. Original information collected from published statutes, regulations, and phone interviews. Originally published 2000, updated in March 2002.

[a] Prescription Medications: Intramuscular pitocin, Rhogam, vitamin K, eye prophylaxis unless otherwise noted.

[b] Florida licensed midwives also administer intrapartum IV antibiotics for Group B Streptococcus.

[c] Midwives authorized to administer medications as prescribed by a physician in New Mexico and Texas.

[d] Texas midwives administer IV fluids with a physician's orders.

[e] Washington licensed midwives also authorized to administer epinephrine, magnesium sulfate, and rubella vaccine as well as other prescription medications the director deems necessary for the safe practice of midwifery.

7

"EVERY BREATH IS POLITICAL, EVERY WOMAN'S LIFE A STATEMENT": CROSS-CLASS ORGANIZING FOR MIDWIFERY IN VIRGINIA

Christa Craven

• Preface: Breaking News • Introduction • Methods and Demographics • Birthing Histories in Virginia • Public Discourses Concerning the Legalization of Direct-Entry Midwifery • Negotiating Diverse Desires for Homebirth in Grassroots Organizing • The Future of Grassroots Organizing for Midwifery: Scholarship and Advocacy Strategies • Timeline of Legislative History of Midwifery in Virginia

PREFACE: BREAKING NEWS

I am excited to report that as this chapter goes to press, Virginia Governor Mark Warner has signed legislation to license Certified Professional Midwives! The CPM licensure law goes into effect on July 1, 2005 and establishes an Advisory Board to develop regulations for CPMs under the Board of Medicine. The Advisory Board will consist of "three Certified Professional Midwives, one doctor of medicine or osteopathy or certified nurse-midwife who is licensed to practice in the Commonwealth and who has experience in out-of-hospital birth settings, and one citizen who has used out-of-hospital midwifery services" (Commonwealth of Virginia 2005). Importantly, the bill ensures independent practice for CPMs and does not require mothers to be assessed by another health-care professional in order to seek midwifery care. Thus, the physician supervision requirement, which has prevented out-of-hospital practice for many nurse-midwives in Virginia, will not affect CPMs under this law.

Another victory for Virginia midwives is that, despite the efforts of some legislators to require malpractice insurance for CPMs—a financial constraint for independent practitioners that is not required for independently practicing physicians or other medical personnel in Virginia—the law passed without this stipulation. Rather, licensed midwives will be required to *disclose* malpractice or liability insurance coverage to clients—along with other background information, including their training and experience, their written protocol for medical emergencies, and the procedures to file complaints with the Board of Medicine. One drawback of the bill is that it prohibits the possession and administration of controlled substances, including oxygen. Most midwives and citizens agreed, however, that this was acceptable in order to pass the CPM licensure bill and could be dealt with through future legislation. More information on the law may be obtained at the Virginia General Assembly's Legislative Information System at http://leg1.state.va.us/ (see also Commonwealth of Virginia 2005).

The passage of the CPM licensure law in Virginia followed over eight years of grassroots organizing and lobbying for similar bills. One particularly valuable strategy during the year before the legislation passed was an effort by Virginia Friends of Midwives to compile a database of members, organized by legislative district. This allowed organizers to target key legislators by mobilizing constituents to contact their local representatives. This chapter focuses on other efforts that occurred prior to the passage of this legislation, as midwives and homebirth families mobilized throughout the state to demand legal access to midwives.

INTRODUCTION

Midwives were obviously attractive to many people, for they usually charged much less than a doctor and often provided such other services as housecleaning, laundry, and postnatal care of the mother and child for several days, while the more expensive doctor usually attended only the birth.... Many [women] disliked clinics, which marked them as charity cases, and most could afford a midwife.

> —**Richard W. Wertz and Dorothy C. Wertz, Lying-In: A History of Childbirth in America (1979: 212)**

Beginning with the movement to improve maternal and infant health in the United States during the early 1900s, efforts to eliminate homebirth in the name of biomedical progress were complicated by women's cultural, emotional, and economic attachments to midwives in their communities, as well as federal and state policies that denied access to medical care for women of color and poor women (Cobb 1981; Dougherty 1982; Susie 1988; Mathews 1992; Fraser 1995, 1998). While the opening quote was written to describe the fact that midwives were an attractive option for recent immigrants to the United States in the early 1900s, it also evokes the continued concern with affordability and personalized care that many women who seek the services of midwives at the dawn of the twenty-first century share. The majority of U.S. women gained access to medical care by the late twentieth century, but many low-income women continue to struggle for access to affordable quality health care in an increasingly stratified and privatized health-care market (Nelson 1983; Morgen 1988, 2002; Mullings 1989; Whiteford 1996; Lazarus 1997; Rapp 1999; Maskovsky 2000; Klassen 2001). As state, biomedical, and commercial interest in alternative health care continues to grow (DeVries 1996; Baer 2001), there is also increased potential for access to contemporary midwifery services to become similarly stratified—particularly as high-end clinics market midwives as a luxury birth care option to privately insured consumers (Susie 1988:71–72). In Virginia and many other states, however, women and families from a broad range of economic backgrounds are becoming politically mobilized to maintain and enhance access to affordable midwives in their communities.

This chapter explores the development of a cross-class movement for midwifery in Virginia and suggests ways that improving birth care for low-income women may be an important strategy for midwifery advocacy efforts. First, I outline the history of midwifery in Virginia, paying particular attention to the race and class rhetoric used in attempts to eradicate midwives in the early 1900s, the eventual criminalization of non-nurse-midwives in 1977, increased state investigations of midwives in the late 1990s, and the current grassroots organizing that developed in response. I follow in section two with a review of the public discourse around midwifery, highlighting the often harsh and demeaning narratives of homebirth experience told to state officials and the public by biomedical personnel. In section three I examine how different desires concerning medical care and uneven access to basic health-care services for women in Virginia have influenced their hopes for the future of midwifery care. While all home-birthers have been forced to respond to charges by state and medical officials that they are irresponsible mothers, the diverse motivations driving women and families to seek midwifery care can complicate the development of effective advocacy strategies. For example, Virginia midwifery advocates disagree over lobbying efforts that emphasize the professionalization of midwives and focus on homebirthers as middle-class consumers. In the final section of this chapter, I suggest that scholars studying midwifery, as well as grassroots organizers, remain attentive to the diverse reasons that women seek midwives and work toward developing advocacy strategies that reflect their shared desire for midwifery care. The cross-class appeal of midwifery services has the potential to be an important factor in strategies to improve care for low-income women, as well as expand the legal options to make mid-wives available to all families.

METHODS AND DEMOGRAPHICS

The research I present in this chapter is drawn from an ongoing field study of political mobilization around midwifery in Virginia. Since 1999, I have participated in grassroots advocacy groups for the support of midwifery, such as Virginia Friends of Midwives and the Commonwealth Midwives Alliance. From January to May 1999, I worked at Birthcare and Women's Health, a nurse-midwifery practice specializing in homebirth. I have also attended legal proceedings during the prosecution of an underground midwife, participated on national and local listservs regarding midwifery politics, and taped and transcribed numerous debates over direct-entry midwifery (DEM) in the Virginia General Assembly.[1] Throughout my fieldwork, I have practiced what Lynn Wilson (1988) calls "activist anthropology," in that I support the goals of the movement I study: particularly as it relates to increasing access to homebirth and midwives in Virginia.

Similar to national statistics on homebirthers (Declerq et al. 1995:480), many of the participants in my study were white and from middle-class backgrounds, particularly those who became involved in public activism for midwifery services. Participants also included a significant number of low-income homebirthers, some of whom had become politically active and others who maintained access to midwives via local community networks. Though I did not consciously seek out participants from particular class backgrounds, a cross-class movement for midwifery in Virginia became evident in the broad range of reported annual incomes among participants, ranging from as low as $6,000 to $250,000 plus. Two-thirds of the forty midwifery advocates I interviewed lived in households that fell below the median income levels for their county (U.S. Census Bureau 2000a) and nearly one-quarter lived in households that fell below the federal poverty line (U.S. Census Bureau 2000b).

My research included documenting a cultural history of efforts to maintain and enhance access to midwives in Virginia from the early 1900s to the present (Craven 2003a). For this, I relied heavily on historical sources to trace the participation of African-American women in the support of Virginia midwives. Notably, in light of the rich history of African-American midwives in Virginia, which I will outline in the following section, African-American women's voices are largely absent in contemporary legislative debates over midwifery in the Commonwealth. *Mama's Little Baby: The Black Woman's Guide to Pregnancy, Birth and the Babies First Year* suggests that contemporary African-American women who have homebirths swear by them, but that many, "influenced by parents and grandparents who worked hard to give us a better life, still consider giving birth at home 'going backward'" (Brown and Toussaint 1998:94). As anthropologist Gertrude Fraser explains, African-American women's rejection of homebirth at the turn of the twenty-first century speaks to the successful dissemination of hegemonic narratives of racial stereotypes and poverty during the early 1900s:

> I am convinced that the almost total success of the dominant ideology among African American women, especially among the middle class, came in large part because these women wanted to distance themselves from the pejorative racial stereotypes used to characterize the traditional midwife and those who depended on her skills. Going to the hospital or using a doctor at home became a marker of status among African American women. Ironically, the relatively inexpensive service of the midwife became less desirable because it was seen as an indication of poverty and "backwardness," and perhaps even as a measure of a woman's "insensibility" to the welfare of her unborn child. (1998:103)

African-American homebirthers in my study echoed this explanation when describing the reactions of family and friends regarding their choice to give birth with midwives at home; few supported midwives in the public arena.

BIRTHING HISTORIES IN VIRGINIA[2]
The Midwifery "Problem"

As was common for midwives in the early twentieth century throughout the United States, Virginia midwives found themselves at the center of a movement to eliminate nonmedical health care providers. While Virginia state and medical officials agreed that midwives were detrimental to medical progress and general public well-being, the limited availability of physicians and hospitals to most African-American and rural, poor white women made it impossible to completely eliminate midwives outright (Plecker 1925). Instead, W. A. Plecker, a physician and county registrar of vital statistics, established a pilot program to license, regulate, and monitor midwives between 1900 and 1912. By 1918, the Commonwealth legislature enacted a law to ensure the supervision of all Virginia midwives under the jurisdiction of the Bureau of Vital Statistics, requiring both licensure and registration (Bennett 1925). Although the intent of this legislation was ostensibly to monitor reproductive health and create a more accurate record of vital statistics in the Commonwealth, it also discouraged midwives from practicing because of increased surveillance, literacy requirements, and bureaucratic structure of reporting births (Fraser 1998:63). Furthermore, laws regulating and "supervising" midwifery during the early part of the twentieth century "inevitably mixed arguments about the need to reduce maternal and infant mortality and to improve health care with those confirming the importance of maintaining the racial and social order" (Fraser 1998:72). For example, laws for the "preservation of racial integrity," passed in 1924, required the midwife to report the race of each child born under her supervision during a time when interracial marriage was illegal and mixed-race children born of white women incriminated and risked violent repercussions on African-American men and the larger African-American community (Fraser 1998:72). At the same time, the falsification of such information was a felony, punishable by a year in the state penitentiary for the midwife.

Despite the divisive political hierarchy of race emerging in the Virginia legislature through "racial integrity laws" and the like, on a grassroots level, racial integration occurred through the widespread use of African-American midwives in both black and white communities. Gertrude Fraser's ethnographic and historical research on African-American midwives in Virginia offers several examples of the interracial and cross-class professional relationships that developed in the 1930s:

> Poor whites [came] "into the yard" to solicit medical advice . . .
> as well as middle-class women who hired this well-respected
> [African-American] midwife to attend them. . . . Another
> woman speaking of her aunt remembered that "she had just as
> many white people that she delivered for as she had black and
> she took care of them. And she had some of the richest people
> here in Green River County." (1998:188)

In spite of the social networks maintained by midwives in communities throughout Virginia, federally sponsored public health programs and the increasingly stringent policing of midwives conducted by public health nurses precipitated the steady decline of midwifery throughout the century. While Virginia kept no official records of the women who used midwives at the turn of the twentieth century, medical officials suggested that thousands of midwives were serving a variety of communities prior to the widespread use of physicians and hospitals for childbirth. One physician praised the local health departments that had "done a splendid piece of work by reducing the number of midwives in the state from nine thousand very ignorant and dirty creatures, to four thousand eight hundred and forty [by the 1920s], only one thousand two hundred and thirty-three of whom are really active" (Baughman 1928:749). These numbers continued to fall to around 1,000 in 1950 and approximately 600 by the 1960s (Commonwealth of Virginia, Department of Health, Center for Health Statistics, as cited in Commonwealth of Virginia, Joint Commission on Health Care 2000a:4 [hereafter referred to as JCHC]). Although this decrease corresponds with national trends, the transition reflected different developments among different constituencies of women.

Not surprisingly, early campaigns against homebirth and midwives were directed at the white women who could afford physicians' services; indeed, urban white women of all classes, and rural, affluent, and middle-class white women were the first to choose physicians over midwives in Virginia (Fraser 1998:95). For these women, physicians and hospitals were purported to alleviate pain in childbirth (through medication) and maintain an appropriately sanitary environment. As hospital birth became more mainstream for white women, middle-class urban African-American women began to deliver in hospitals as physicians allowed,[3] and it was mainly rural, poor women of all races who continued to use midwives into the mid-1900s (Fraser 1998:88). Even into the 1950s and 1960s, Claudine Curry Smith, the last African-American lay midwife to practice in the Lower Northern Neck of Virginia (near the Chesapeake Bay), explained how the racial divide in health care continued:

> Most of the White people had their doctors come to the house—they had the money to pay the doctor. Black people just didn't have the doctor's money. Midwives were cheaper. Insurance didn't cover having a midwife come. So, they'd pay out of their pocket. I delivered some White too, but the ones that did it said they'd rather have a midwife than go to the hospital. (Smith and Roberson 1994:23)

Criminalizing Lay Midwifery and the Subsequent Resurgence of Homebirth

Virginia's confidence in biomedical progress prompted the Virginia General Assembly's 1962 decision to move regulation of midwives to the Virginia Department of Health (VDH)—in what a VDH representative later characterized as an attempt to further limit midwifery practice to "rural, underserved areas, minority women, and poor, uninsured women" (Stern 1999:4). In 1976, the General Assembly enacted legislation that limited the practice of non-nurse midwifery to those who were permitted to practice by the VDH prior to January 1, 1977. No DEMs have been licensed in the Commonwealth of Virginia since that date. Thus, in 1977, the remunerated practice of midwifery by a non-medically trained practitioner became a criminal offense in the state. In addition, this law enabled certified nurse-midwives (CNMs) to practice, with certain restrictions (such as the provision for practice under the supervision of a physician), through joint regulation by the boards of medicine and nursing.

Interestingly, my interviews with women utilizing and/or offering midwifery services during the 1970s indicate that most were unaware of this legislation. Because this law was not widely enforced for nearly twenty years, some midwives continued to provide homebirth services well into the 1990s before realizing that receiving compensation for their services was a criminal offense. In fact, during this time, even unlicensed midwives who were aware of the laws criminalizing their practice felt safe continuing—and often publicizing—their homebirth services. For example, Sherry Willis, who offered homebirth services in the Blue Ridge Mountains of northern Virginia, told a reporter that she preferred "the autonomy of her form of midwifery" to that of physician-supervised nurse-midwifery (Strobel 1990:27–28). The reporter continued, "She has never been sued, and, she says, has no fear of legal repercussions. No baby has ever died in her care" (Strobel 1990:27–28). Similarly, Carol Cahours, an unlicensed midwife who practiced in central Virginia during the 1990s, told a reporter, "Everyone knows I'm here"; ironically, the article was entitled "Unlicensed Midwives Can't Practice Legally under Virginia Statute" (Pegram 1996:B-5).

While many DEMs disregarded the laws that were designed to eliminate their practice, others questioned their legal application. One DEM who had practiced legally in Texas and California, but had switched to offering birthing talks and facilitating childbirth support groups when she moved to the Northern Neck of Virginia, explained to a reporter:

> Present Virginia laws define midwifery as being present at the time of birth and receiving payment for this. Payment could be anything: a goat, a painting, money, even just a thank-you. A licensed nurse-midwife may only facilitate labor and birth under the direct supervision of a physician. Obviously, the definitions of midwifery are a bit unclarified here. What if you suggested that a laboring woman drink a cup of tea or take a walk? What if you took her blood pressure for her at her request? Is this practicing midwifery or medicine? (Stacey Newby as cited in Norris 1995:74)

During the mid- to late 1990s, the state began to answer these questions by intensifying investigations (and in several cases the criminal prosecution) of underground midwives and those who assisted them.

Midwives Forced from Practice

As a result of highly publicized judicial proceedings against illegally practicing midwives in the late 1990s, many women I interviewed found it difficult to access homebirth services in their geographical areas. Others expressed concern regarding the tenuous legal situation of hiring midwives in the wake of state investigations. In one case, Martha Hughes, a CPM who formerly practiced in Virginia, had attended over 200 homebirths but stopped practicing after her arrest in a manslaughter case regarding a baby who died after a homebirth she assisted in 1995. While the charges were eventually dropped because the baby's parents would not cooperate with the prosecution, maintaining that their midwife had done all she could to save their baby, Hughes's practice remains closed; she now works as a part-time waitress in Rappahannock County. Following Hughes's early retirement, several former and potential clients were not able to have homebirths because they were unable to find available practitioners to attend them (Neuberger 1999b:A-1).

Similarly, after charges were brought against DEM Cynthia Caillagh, a prominent homebirth midwife who had attended 2,500 births throughout the southeastern and central areas of the Commonwealth, many women in her region found themselves without an attendant for their homebirths. In 1999, Caillagh and her assistant, Elizabeth Haw, were charged with involuntary manslaughter, practicing midwifery without a license, and practicing medicine without a license in Stafford County following the death of their client Julia Peters in 1997. The medical examiner's report cited postpartum hemorrhage as the cause of death, but Caillagh and Haw's attorneys, as well as their supporters, maintained that the cause of Peters's death was open to question. Before the trial, supporters suggested that the lab report documenting Peters's hemoglobin and hematocrit levels—9.8 and 22, respectively—did not support the diagnosis of postpartum hemorrhage (Voices for Healthcare Rights Fund 2000a) and that the delayed issuance of the medical examiner's report (eight months after the date of death) was significant to the defense's case (Neuberger 1999a).[4]

Nearly three years after Peters's death, the case ended in a plea bargain on May 5, 2000. The irony that the decision came on International Midwives Day (and on the eve of what Governor Jim Gilmore had proclaimed as Virginia Midwives Day) was not lost on Caillagh and Haw's supporters (Voices for Healthcare Rights Fund 2000b). The prosecution dropped the manslaughter charge—which would have required a full trial—in part because of the publicity around defense attorney Peter Greenspun's case, involving expert witnesses to testify against the medical examiner's report (Krishnamurthy 2000b:A-1) and in part because Daren Peters, Julie Peters's husband, maintained that the midwives "did their job" and refused to cooperate with prosecutors (Hall 1998; Glod and White 1999:B01). Caillagh pleaded guilty to practicing midwifery without a license, practicing medicine without a license (based on testimony regarding her use of pitocin and her performance of an internal vaginal exam), and the neglect of an incapacitated adult.[5] Haw pled guilty to practicing midwifery without a license. Both received suspended jail sentences, were fined $2,500 and $500, respectively, and promised to stop delivering babies unless the state law was changed. In a press release following the trial, Caillagh (2000) indicated that the prosecutions' agreement to drop charges against Julie Peters's mother-in-law,

Claire Peters, and reduce charges against Elizabeth Haw weighed heavily in her decision to plead guilty to the three misdemeanors.

Several participants in my study also told me lengthy stories about being reported to the state by hostile physicians or health-care officials, but asked that I not include their full stories for fear that they may still be under investigation by the state. Recalling her investigation, one DEM was told:

> "You will either receive a summons to go to court . . . and go through a prosecution trial or you'll receive a letter dismissing your case. When either one of those two things happen, it's closed and until either of those two things happen it's not." Neither of those have happened and it's been [many years], so it's an open case and they do that. They love to keep them open because then what [they're] waiting for, Christa, is . . . if something happens at a birth and that gets brought to the public eye, that's when I will be prosecuted. (Unnamed participant, personal communication, 2001)

This midwife joked that for identification purposes, "my first name is 'The' and my last name is 'Midwife.' That keeps me from getting prosecuted."

In the wake of these indictments, many other DEMs found themselves increasingly more cautious for fear of similar criminal investigation. One advocate explained, "The midwives are quitting and they're scared. And people are choosing unattended homebirths instead of choosing to have somebody with them with experience because they don't want to go to the hospital. This is an access problem, this is a problem of being able to choose somebody to help you" (Terri Jacobs, personal communication, August 7, 2001).[6] One former midwife, who now works as an artist in Virginia, cites the tenuous legal position of midwives as a prime reason for her decision to stop practicing: "There were a couple of instances that made me realize things could go a different direction and [people] could cause me a lot of trouble. And my partner wasn't very supportive. He was always giving me grief about 'why are you doing this?' ... My freedoms could be taken away from me" (Rebecca Ullman, personal communication, August 7, 2001). Some midwives, such as Rosy Farlam, who recently received her national CPM credential, have chosen to move out of the state (in her case, to Vermont) in order to practice in a legal environment. As other aspiring midwives have considered their options for training, many have rejected paths to becoming a DEM for fear of legal trouble.

The only reason that I became a nurse-midwife is that I found out that [it was] the only way to be a legal midwife in Virginia. And I did not want to go to nursing school. I never wanted to be a nurse. I wanted to be a midwife. But I also knew that it was unlikely that I would ever live any place besides Virginia and that I was not willing to operate outside the law. (Kate Kaplan, personal communication, June 4, 2001)

Even as legally practicing CNMs, however, Virginia midwives have not been immune to harassment by medical and state officials in recent years. For example, the CNM-run birth center in Charlottesville closed in the late 1990s because its midwives could no longer secure physician supervision for their practice: "After the Board of Medicine ruled that the supervising physician was too far away, the only birth center in Charlottesville was forced to close and a homebirth midwife had to close her practice as well, abruptly leaving an entire community without the access they had come to rely on" (author's transcription, Ellen Hamblet, presentation to the Board of Medicine, August 3, 2001). Other CNMs have not been able to find jobs practicing midwifery: the Taskforce on the Study of Obstetric Access and Certified Nurse-Midwives indicated that at least one-third of Virginia CNMs were practicing outside of their chosen profession in 1991 (Commonwealth of Virginia, Department of Health Professions and Virginia Health Planning Board, Task Force on the Study of Obstetric Access and Certified Nurse-Midwives 1992:10; hereafter referred to as the Task Force).

Although a handful of obstetricians, osteopaths, and CNMs provide homebirth services in some areas of the commonwealth, they are often unable to keep up with the volume of women seeking their care. For example, Veronica Nelson, a doula in northern Virginia at Birthcare and Women's Health, a practice of five CNMs that offers homebirths and birth center births to eighteen to twenty-five clients a month, reported to an organizing listserv:

just getting back this morning from a hugely medically intervened OB/hospital birth—client had wanted to use a homebirth midwife after we talked in January (and even still when I got to her home yesterday morning), but you know how that goes . . . the [homebirth] CNMs were booked. (Listserv message, March 26, 2001)

The growing desire for homebirth among women in the Commonwealth is also evident in health statistics on Other Midwives, a category designated by the VDH to distinguish both legally and illegally practicing non-nurse-midwives from legally practicing CNMs. Although the numbers of births attended by "other midwives" initially declined after the 1977 law criminalizing non-nurse midwifery, decreasing to a low of thirty-five in 1985, they steadily increased from that point, growing to 155 in 1995, 303 in 1997, and to 500 births in 2000 (Commonwealth of Virginia, Department of Health, Vital Records & Health Statistics 1995, 1997, 2000; JCHC 2000a:5).

Recent Political Mobilization

The increasing demand for midwife-attended homebirth, coupled with state investigations into the practices of unlicensed midwives, has been the catalyst for the recent surge of grassroots organizing among homebirth mothers and families in Virginia. Practicing DEMs in the Commonwealth initially remained relatively quiet on the political front because of their tenuous legal status. As a result, the Virginia movement has gained a national reputation as an example of the "Consumer Movement for Midwifery."[7] In states where DEM is illegal or not legally defined, grassroots political efforts among homebirthers have become increasingly important because unlicensed midwives who become visible and/or politically active risk incrimination and arrest by the state.

In fact, several grassroots organizations were created to raise funds and support midwives who were being investigated or prosecuted. One such group was Voices for Healthcare Rights Fund (Voices), founded in 1998 in response to the arrest of Cynthia Caillagh. Voices members focused primarily on offering financial and organizational support to Caillagh and her assistant, Elizabeth Haw. In addition, Voices took an active role in encouraging attendance at legislative hearings and promoting awareness regarding activism to challenge the illegal status of DEMs in the Commonwealth. A fundraising letter from Voices read:

> We, as an organization founded by families and consumers, believe that we have the right to make informed decisions about our healthcare. . . . Without the ability to retain the practitioner of our choice, informed healthcare decisions become meaningless. If our practitioners have been prosecuted and legislatively controlled to the point of extinction, then we as consumers can only stand to lose. (Voices for Healthcare Rights Fund 1999)

Other local groups, such as Harrisonburg Advocates for the Midwifery Model of Care, Richmond Families for Birthing Alternatives, Families for Natural Living near Williamsburg, Midwifery Options for Mothers in Northern Virginia, and statewide organizations such as Virginia Friends of Midwives (formerly Virginia Birthing Freedom), the Commonwealth Midwives Alliance, the Virginia Midwifery Coalition, Mothers United for Midwifery, the international web-based Childbirthsolutions.com, and an umbrella group, the Virginia Coalition of Midwives, have also addressed local issues of access in specific communities, supported particular practitioners, promoted education about midwifery and homebirth, and encouraged cooperation and consensus among the various groups in the state. In the interests of brevity, I will focus my discussion on the statewide group that became the largest grassroots advocacy organization for midwifery in Virginia.

Shortly after the formation of Voices in Virginia Beach, Virginia Birthing Freedom (VBF) was organized in southwestern Virginia, near Roanoke. VBF began as a relatively small group of midwifery supporters and grew to include a listserv of over 400 supporters around Virginia. A VBF fundraising letter described their purpose as follows:

> VBF began . . . as a grassroots organization of citizens who sensed a compelling need to expand the available options for giving birth in Virginia. . . . VBF's primary, but not exclusive, goal is to convince the Virginia General Assembly to mandate licensure for the Certified Professional Midwife (CPM). We face stiff opposition from the medical lobby, which insists in its writings and at public hearings that homebirth is unsafe for any woman at any time. They have power, money and access, but we have something far more valuable: facts, and families. (Listserv message, Danielle Adams, December 16, 2000)[8]

In 1998, VBF brought the issue of increased public interest in DEM to the attention of the General Assembly by proposing a study resolution regarding the practice of midwifery in Virginia. This prompted the JCHC Midwifery Subcommittee, with assistance from the Department of Health Professions and the VDH, to conduct a study to examine "the advisability of legalizing the practice of midwifery in the Commonwealth" (Commonwealth of Virginia 1999). To gauge public support for legislation regarding DEMs, the subcommittee held three public hearings, all of which generated a sizeable response from midwifery proponents. Of the sixty-three individuals speaking at the meetings in Dublin (at New River Valley Community College), Fairfax (at George

Mason University), and Newport News (at Christopher Newport University), sixty-one spoke in favor of legalizing DEM. These included mothers and fathers whose births had been attended by midwives, Virginia's only legally practicing DEM,[9] several CNMs, and representatives of grassroots organizations supporting midwifery. Similarly, the committee received twenty-three written public comments from individuals and organizations, twenty-two of which supported the legalization of midwifery. Despite a plea for physician participation in this process ("to get reasonable legislation . . . on direct-entry midwives"), in a publication by the Virginia Obstetrical and Gynecological Society and the Virginia Chapter of the American College of Obstetricians and Gynecologists (Gerheart 1999:2), only two representatives from these groups spoke at public hearings and only one representative from the Medical Society of Virginia sent a letter opposing legislation (Murray 1999a:10, 1999b:5). In total, the JCHC received comments from 192 citizens, 183 of whom explicitly supported the licensure of CPMs (JCHC 2000b:1–2): "Following the public comments period, the Joint Commission also received a petition signed by 124 citizens requesting 'the General Assembly to decriminalize the practice of home-based midwifery. This includes legalizing the Certified Professional Midwife'" (JCHC 2000b:3) [see chapters 1 and 3 for a description of the creation of the CPM]. Ultimately, the JCHC Midwifery Subcommittee voted to recommend that a bill be introduced to allow CPMs to become legal practitioners in Virginia.

Although VBF initiated legislation to legalize CPMs in the 1999 General Assembly session, it gained little support from the medical community, and midwifery advocates found themselves frustrated by the continued inclusion of a provision mandating physician supervision of all midwives. While the JCHC had recommended that a bill be introduced, it became a disadvantage that no seal of approval was given to a particular piece of legislation. Again in 2000, 2001, and 2002, VBF presented revised bills to legalize CPMs to the General Assembly, and again, facing opposition from the Virginia Chapter of the American College of Obstetricians and Gynecologists (VA-ACOG), the Medical Society of Virginia (MSV), the VDH, the Department of Health Professions, and the Commonwealth's chief medical examiner, the bills failed.

In 2002, VBF reorganized and became Virginia Friends of Midwives (VFOM) reflecting a change in leadership in response to "the need for a more inclusive identity as the movement to improve access to midwives has grown [and] to reflect a new commitment to working with likeminded groups of other consumers and midwives" (Virginia Friends of Midwives

2003). In 2003, VFOM joined with DEMs in the Commonwealth Midwives Alliance to lobby for a bill to strike down the 1977 law, which had effectively criminalized non-nurse midwifery in Virginia for the past twenty-six years (Commonwealth of Virginia 2003: HB 1961). Without significant opposition, House Bill 1961 passed, removing the 1977 definition of the lay midwife. Further, the bill exempted "individuals who are not registered as nurses" from registration and permit requirements. While these changes mean that DEMs can no longer be charged with "practicing midwifery without a license" in Virginia, the legislation did not allow DEMs to become licensed or permitted by the state, and thus does not protect them from being charged with practicing medicine or nurse-midwifery without a license. In both 2003 and 2004, legislators defeated additional bills to legalize CPMs through the Board of Medicine, and organizers continue to work on new legislation to regulate and protect the practice of DEMs and CNMs. (For updates on recent developments, see http://www.vfom.com.)

PUBLIC DISCOURSES CONCERNING THE LEGALIZATION OF DIRECT-ENTRY MIDWIFERY

Because homebirthers made their interest in access to midwives public in 1998, legislative debates about the viability of legalizing direct-entry midwifery in Virginia have caused much controversy both inside and outside the Commonwealth, joining national and international debates over the legitimation of particular childbirth practices and the state's role in safeguarding and/or regulating motherhood. These debates have involved a variety of actors, including lobbyists from health-care advocacy groups, policy experts from national and international health organizations, and representatives from medical associations.

In addition to the work of grassroots organizers, the efforts to legalize direct-entry midwifery in Virginia have drawn support from individual CNMs and nurses, as well as official support from several organizations of health professionals. The Virginia Chapter of the American College of Nurse-Midwives (VACNM) initially supported efforts to legalize direct-entry midwifery through either one of the two existing national certification processes (see chapter 1). At a public hearing in 1999, a representative of VACNM issued this statement:

> In order to protect the public and increase access to health care, the American College of Nurse-Midwives, Virginia Chapter, supports regulation of direct-entry midwifery through licensure. Licensure should require certification by examination

through the North American Registry of Midwives or the American College of Nurse-Midwives. (As reported in JCHC 2000a:8–9)

Notably, this support broke from the national ACNM policy, which has consistently opposed the licensure of any midwives who are not certified by their organization. Individual Virginia CNMs also spoke at hearings and wrote to members of the JCHC in support of legislation to legalize CPMs. Rosemary J. Taibbi wrote:

I am a Virginia certified nurse-midwife (CNM) who provides homebirth services. I also was a consumer of homebirth services provided by a direct-entry midwife (DEM). . . . It is now time for Virginia to step forward in legalizing direct-entry midwives and allowing families safe access to the midwifery model of care that is provided by CNMs and DEMs in the home and birth center settings. (As reported in JCHC 2000a:8–9)

Many CNMs recognize the importance of autonomous midwifery practice, particularly for practitioners who offer out-of-hospital birth care. Several CNMs also practiced as DEMs in Virginia before becoming nurse-midwives (to comply with state regulations); these practitioners remain prominent members of statewide midwifery organizations. Since 1999, many of these individual CNMs have maintained their support of legislation to license CPMs, but VACNM has not conferred their official support. When I asked CNMs in my study about this shift, most highlighted Virginia CNMs' tenuous relationship with individual physicians and medical organizations in the state, expressing concerns about reprisal by the physicians who supervise them (and therefore determine whether or not they are able to practice).

While a few physicians have supported direct-entry midwifery legislation in Virginia, physicians' organizations have been undivided in their opposition. Notably, much of the individual physician support cited by grassroots advocates has been from outside the Commonwealth. For instance, Marsden Wagner, former director of the Women's and Children's Health Program in the European office of the World Health Organization, presented the following arguments in favor of legalizing DEM to the Virginia General Assembly:

Since homebirth and direct-entry midwifery are perfectly safe options, [a majority of] state legislatures have concluded that it is the right of each woman and her family to choose such options. State laws must guarantee families the freedom to choose homebirth by recognizing the type of midwifery which focuses principally on out-of-hospital birth, direct-entry midwifery.... State legislatures are also concerned with guaranteeing an open marketplace and fair competition, including in health care services. To exclude direct-entry midwives from practice is to allow a scientifically unjustified monopoly of doctors and nurse-midwives. (As recorded at http://www.vbfree.org, February 15, 1998)

Unanimously, however, the Virginia Obstetricians and Gynecologists Society, the MSV, and the VA-ACOG have opposed legislation. The VA-ACOG reiterated the ACOG statement of policy on homebirth, which dates to 1979:

Labor and delivery, while a physiologic process, clearly present potential hazards to mother and fetus before and after birth. These hazards require standards of safety which are provided in the hospital setting and cannot be matched in the home situation.

We support those actions that improve the experience of the family while continuing to provide the mother and her infant with accepted standards of safety available only in hospitals which conform to the standards as outlined by the American Academy of Pediatricians and the American College of Obstetricians and Gynecologists. (as cited in JCHC 2000a:9)

Additionally, health and professional organizations such as the VDH, the Department of Health Professions, public health directors, the state medical examiner, and the Trial Lawyers Association have voiced their opposition to legislation to legalize the CPM in Virginia. Representing the VDH, Commissioner Dr. Anne Peterson explained to the Health, Welfare and Institutions (HWI) Committee:

Philosophically I am in support of the services that nurse- and lay-midwives provide, but this bill does not protect the safety [of mothers and babies], and [does not have] built into it the enforceability that we need to have for any health care provider. (Author's transcription, January 30, 2001)

Despite efforts on the part of grassroots advocates to differentiate between DEMs and the term "lay-midwife," which they feel is a pejorative term that smacks of the prejudicial treatment of midwives during the early twentieth century, medical and state personnel have continued to routinely employ the term lay-midwives to describe nationally certified CPMs, as well as midwives who are not certified, licensed, or registered in the Commonwealth. In another example, a representative of the Virginia OB/GYN Society described CPMs as "lay-midwives" in an article directed toward lawmakers; he used the term synonymously with "medically uneducated and medically untrained laypersons" (LeHew 2000:12).

Indeed, physicians' organizations and health directors in Virginia have voiced some of the most important ideological blocks to contemporary legislation. While midwifery advocates have offered copious national as well as international studies speaking to the safety of home-birth with midwives, questions regarding the training and outcomes of United States–based DEMs have been at the forefront of public debate. Furthermore, bureaucratic details, such as whether CPMs would be licensed under the Board of Health Professions, the Board of Health, the Board of Nursing, or the Board of Medicine have been an ongoing concern. In conjunction with the issues specific to the licensure of midwifery, advocates also battle the long-standing conservatism regarding reproductive rights in the Commonwealth. Health-care advocates, newspaper reporters, and researchers have been quick to highlight Virginia's regrettable record concerning eugenic sterilizations and the denial and then restriction of contraceptive and abortion services to Virginia women (Lombardo 1982; Fraser 1998; Condit 2000; Hardin 2000). The argument for midwifery as "a woman's right to choose" has not proved effective in Virginia, as it has in many other states.

Above all, however, issues of risk and safety have permeated both medical and legislative opposition to the legalization of DEMs. During the 2001 HWI committee meeting to vote on legislation to legalize the CPM, Dr. John Partridge, representing the MSV, the Virginia OB/GYN Society, and the VA-ACOG, invoked the authority of medical science to suggest a "natural" medical jurisdiction over the birth process:

> Modern medicine has brought maternity care to an ever safer level and loosening the standard would place mothers and babies at risk. . . . Birth is, by nature, a medical event. [Home-birth is] a slippery slope—like driving a car without brakes. You may do okay on level ground with no turns, but when the road starts going downhill, and you start making some turns, it gets very dicey. . . . Isn't it logical to think hospitals and

doctors have made birth safer? [I hope that you will] preserve the public health of mothers and babies by preserving the current statutes. [You will hear mothers talk about preserving *their* right to choose, but I ask you,] what about the *baby's* choice? (Author's transcription, February 8, 2000)

What is most notable about Dr. Partridge's final question is the adoption of markedly different philosophical tenets and values than those of the midwifery model (Davis-Floyd and Davis 1997). While midwives position the locus of responsibility for childbirth with the woman and her family, Dr. Partridge situates the responsibility of a baby's safety firmly outside the mother, suggesting state and/or medical safeguarding of the "baby's choice." As legal expert Suzanne Suarez explains, this strategy has proved doubly effective in blocking legislation to legalize midwives in many areas because the statement places the power and authority of "good" outcomes with physicians and the state, while "bad" outcomes remain the responsibility of the mother:

> The fallacy-ridden dominant belief that "homebirth is dangerous" makes it relatively easy for the medical lobby to convince lawmakers that pregnant women who reject doctor control endanger themselves and their babies and that midwives are safe practitioners only if they are nurses. Physicians cite the safety of the infant (and, secondarily, the mother) as a primary concern. Doctors have successfully prioritized the rights of the unborn and maintained control over birth against the wishes of the parents who pay their fees. Ironically, consumers are afforded little control even though they, not the physicians, bear the ultimate responsibility of pregnancy and birth. (Suarez 1993:320–321)

Homebirth mother Fern Jackson echoed this frustration on a Virginia listserv supporting midwives: "If legislators feel (or can say they feel) that they're protecting babies from the bad decisions made by their selfish mothers (grrrr), all the logic in the world won't prevail against that" (listserv message, February 14, 2000). As homebirthers are forced to respond to the medical claims that they are irresponsible mothers, organizers also face internal concerns over how lawmakers will respond to the diversity of reasons women and families in Virginia desire homebirth.

NEGOTIATING DIVERSE DESIRES FOR HOMEBIRTH IN GRASSROOTS ORGANIZING

In many ways, the Virginia movement for midwifery, as well as national advocacy for midwifery, is a profoundly diverse effort, particularly in terms of religion and political affiliation. Fundamentalist Christians often stand alongside pagans and Buddhists at rallies, and Democrats, Republicans, Greens, and Libertarians put aside political differences to hold signs that read "Affordable Healthcare Begins with Midwifery." As a result of this diversity, however, homebirthers are not always in agreement with the lobbying strategies put forth for midwifery. Some advocates have voiced displeasure with efforts to legalize CPMs—sometimes even on the floor of the General Assembly. Some have suggested a political platform defining the right to choose *any* midwife as a religious freedom, drawing on the Virginia Statute for Religious Freedom (Commonwealth of Virginia 2002: §57–1). These advocates argue that many religious groups, such as the Quakers, the Amish, Muslims, and Christian Scientists, believe that birth should occur in the home and/or with only women in attendance. Many advocates cite Mennonite midwife Faith Gibson, the founder of the American College of Domiciliary Midwives, as she defines the role of the midwife as a witness to an act of God.

> The true role of the midwife is to deliver the mother to deliverability at which point a truly spontaneous birth becomes an act of God, no matter who[se] hands are on the baby—the mother herself, the father, a physician, midwife or simply a soft surface. . . . spontaneous birth of this kind is an Act of God, it is a sacred and a social event—not a medical one. (Gibson 1994)

A Virginia advocate echoed this sentiment: "it is my belief that the parents are given true autonomy by God Himself to determine what is a proper [birthing] environment" (listserv message, Dana Smith, March 18, 2000). Advocates report compelling individual lobbying efforts in this regard, but the issue of religious freedom has remained largely untouched on the floor of the General Assembly. (See chapter 5 by Mary Lay and Kerry Dixon for an example of how such religious voices were silenced during midwifery legislative efforts in Minnesota.) As a national midwifery organizer cautioned, religious exemption "generally appl[ies] to midwives who practice in a religious or ethnic community and perform their servi[c]es for no fee" (listserv message, Rita Olsen, August 9, 1999). Importantly, connections among contemporary legislation and the historical practices of religious practitioners, African-American granny midwives, and the hippie roots of the natural childbirth movement are often rejected by political organizers in public conversations with legislators and health officials. By and large, grassroots organizers have found it politically advantageous to distinguish these fringe groups from the new wave of professionalized midwives (see Reid 1995; Davis-Floyd 1997, 1998, chapter 1, this volume; Lay 2000; and Klassen 2001 for further discussion of this phenomenon).

Other grassroots organizers have brought up concerns that legislators might see their movement as primarily rural and poor, as was historically the case for homebirthers in Virginia in the early twentieth century. One well-educated, middle-class homebirth mother explained, "A couple people would come from more rural counties and be kind of, not really what you wanted there fighting for midwifery because they kind of perpetuated the stereotype" (personal communication, Carla Grayson, April 14, 2002). During interviews with low-income homebirthers, many highlighted the challenges of cross-class organizing when they felt that "choosing" a midwife for financial reasons put them at odds with other advocates.

> Every time that I [mentioned that] I homebirthed because I was poor . . . this one woman who always stands up [at meetings] and says, "But that's not the only reason," because they don't want to hear that within the movement. I am told not to say it's because I was poor [that I had a homebirth] because that makes you look dumb. . . . Most of the people I've seen in this movement had a lot and have had the opportunity to say they were taken care of by their parents. And I didn't come from that class. I wasn't even brought up to go to college. It wasn't an issue in my house. When I look at people in this movement, they're older, have one child, want to get the most they can out of this experience, and I think that's great, I do. Where I grew up, children were part of life, you didn't dwell about it. You were lucky to have health insurance so you could go to that doctor and do everything that looks good, you know, get [your children] all immunized on time and [make sure] they all looked nice and clean so they could get a good shot of having the teachers at school look at them. . . . The other people [in the midwifery movement] were able to travel, didn't stay in one area, have seen other ways of life, grew up in California and are in Virginia now. . . . It's definitely a social thing of having money, having

time to read the books, and be able to take care of yourself. I know it's by the grace of God that I know what I do, because I did not have those opportunities. (Personal communication, Paula Queen, April 17, 2002)

Anthropologists have highlighted ways in which women of diverse racial and class backgrounds have played major roles in political movements, though their strategies for political action have often been noticeably different.

> Although in recent years middle-class women have made inroads into the arena of electoral politics, most of the substantive reforms benefiting working-class women have emerged from battles waged in extra-electoral terrains—the office, the factory, the hospital, the church, or the streets. And legislative reforms have emerged, for the most part, in response to pressure from grassroots activity. (Bookman and Morgan 1988:4)

Some homebirthers, especially those in rural areas, have emphasized how political action may also be constituted in the act of seeking maternity care outside the norm of the hospital. In response to assumptions that many women, including rural women in Amish and Mennonite communities, do not wish to be involved in political action toward gaining access to midwives, Terri Jacobs wrote to a grassroots organizing listserv, "having a homebirth makes you a political creature by default, like-it-or-not" (listserv message, October 10, 2000). Echoing this sentiment, Evie Diaz suggests that women's lack of access to midwives in many communities, and the intensified prosecution of community-based midwives in others, makes "every breath political and every woman's life a statement" (personal communication, February 3, 2000). Like Bookman and Morgan (1988), what these advocates call for is a broader definition of what is considered "political," including the collective and individual action that goes on outside the state legislature and Internet-based political discussion lists. While complicated negotiations over advocacy strategies demonstrate how religious and class-based differences have the potential to cause schisms within the midwifery movement, I suggest in conclusion that the cross-class appeal of midwifery services may also be an important point for advocates and lobbyists to highlight for legislators as one way to improve access to prenatal care for low-income women.

THE FUTURE OF GRASSROOTS ORGANIZING
FOR MIDWIFERY:
SCHOLARSHIP AND ADVOCACY STRATEGIES

In this chapter, I have highlighted the cross-class political mobilization for midwifery in Virginia and examined how contemporary grassroots organizing efforts reflect different ways that women have responded to restricted birth care options, as well as biomedical and state attacks on their desire for homebirth and midwifery care. As Virginians continue to seek out homebirth services for a variety of reasons—including dissatisfaction with biomedical care, the desire for personalized treatment, and financial concerns—the maintenance of this cross-class movement will require both grassroots organizers and scholars to further interrogate the advocacy and organizing strategies adopted in support of midwifery.

For example, terminology, such as homebirth as a "consumer's right" and the "right to choose" midwives can divide advocates around religious issues as well as economic disparities. As one homebirth father explained, he did not participate in local grassroots organizing because unlike what he calls "normal midwife consumers," it was restricted economic resources that encouraged his family to make the "choice" to hire a local midwife: "We're not like the normal midwife consumers or clients. . . . it's also a financial issue with midwifery, in choosing midwifery too. We didn't have health insurance and didn't have income to be able to afford a hospital birth, couldn't figure out a way to do it. It was really dragging us down and midwives were very reasonable (personal communication, Kevin Rogers, August 8, 2001). In addition, the advent of the Internet as a crucial source of community support for midwifery in Virginia has introduced significant opportunities for grassroots-organizing efforts, but also presented challenges to cross-class organizing. On the positive side, the Internet affords anonymity for advocates who feel at risk of incrimination regarding reproductive choices. It also offers an inexpensive method for the distribution of political materials and provides a forum for discussion across geographical boundaries regarding the details of advocacy strategies. At the same time, the use of the Internet as a primary organizing tool reinforces the digital divide of class-based politics in Virginia. Particularly among low-income, rural women in my study, supporters of midwifery expressed concern that their ability to advocate was limited by their lack of access to the Internet, in addition to the financial restrictions that kept them from attending legislative hearings and advocacy meetings in other areas of the state. The formation and preservation of locally based groups will remain essential to furthering statewide political mobilization involving economically and geographically diverse participants.

For grassroots organizers, it may also be useful to consider the strengths of advocating for midwifery as one way to improve the health care of low-income women in Virginia. As one study of access to obstetrical care in Virginia summarized:

> The majority of [local health directors] cited significant problems in obtaining prenatal and delivery services for medically indigent patients and Medicaid recipients. Most reported a dearth of providers willing to accept Medicaid reimbursement and some noted a total lack of support for prenatal care by community physicians who were unwilling to serve uninsured patients. (Task Force 1992:8)

Moreover, in fifty-one of Virginia's ninety-nine counties, the local health department was the only source of perinatal health care, including both prenatal and intrapartal (labor and delivery) care. As a result, the Task Force recommended that the Virginia legislature support the expansion of the practice of nurse-midwives throughout the state. These recommendations resulted in the creation of the Master's Degree Program in Nurse-Midwifery at Shenandoah University in 1997, and the implementation of a scholarship program through the Department of Health for nurse practitioner and nurse-midwifery programs.[10] It may useful for DEMs in Virginia and other states to consider similar strategies. In Florida, for example, sounding "a general alarm over the state's infant mortality rate" and concurrently suggesting that the positive outcomes of midwife-attended childbirth would be a low-cost solution to the problem became integral to passing a bill that secured licensure for DEMs in 1992 (Miller 1999:370).

While legislative, institutional, and social roadblocks continue to punctuate the experiences of midwives and homebirthers throughout the United States, it is my hope that midwifery advocates will continue to find new ways to benefit from the strengths of their cross-class movement. I am continually inspired by the words of one determined advocate:

> Every time I feel this is getting to be too much, I think about having to tell my daughters, "I gave up...it was too hard." No way! I know I will remember for the rest of my life being part of a true grassroots effort to change something that urgently

needed changing. (Fern Jackson, listserv message, March 9, 2001)

TIMELINE OF THE LEGISLATIVE HISTORY OF MIDWIFERY IN VIRGINIA

1918 The Virginia General Assembly (GA) passed legislation requiring regulation of all midwives under the Bureau of Vital Statistics. (This legislation was in response to pressures to eliminate midwives—the GA decided to monitor midwives, especially in regards to their usefulness in rural areas and their registration of birth certificates.) Virginia kept no official records of midwives at the turn of the twentieth century, but one physician estimated that 9,000 midwives were practicing throughout the state in the early 1900s (Baughman 1928:749).

1950s Health departments began to require pregnant women to get a card from a physician to approve a midwife-assisted delivery. By this time, approximately 1,000 midwives remained in practice, according to the Virginia Department of Health (VDH).

1962 The GA passed legislation to move regulation of midwives to the VDH. The VDH registered around 600 midwives.

1974 The VDH restricted applications for a midwife permit to registered nurses.

1976 The GA enacted legislation that limited the practice of non-nurse midwifery to those who were permitted by the VDH prior to January 1, 1977. The number of registered midwives quickly fell to around 100 in the 1980s and slowly decreased to just five in 1999. During the same year, the GA also introduced legislation to license nurse-midwives as CNMs through joint regulation by the Boards of Medicine and Nursing. Unlike non-nurse-midwives, CNMs were required to work under a physician's supervision.

1992 The Department of Health Professions and Virginia Health Planning Board appointed the Task Force on the Study of Obstetric Access and Certified Nurse-Midwives. Task Force recommendations resulted in the creation of the Master's Degree Program in Nurse-Midwifery at Shenandoah University in 1997 and the implementation of a scholarship program through the Department of Health for nurse practitioner and nurse-midwifery programs. By the early 1990s, approximately eighty CNMs were practicing in Virginia and more than 180 CNMs were licensed by 2002.

1995   The Virginia Department of Health appointed the Non-Nurse-Midwife Regulation Advisory Group to review the rules and regulations governing the practice of permitted non-nurse-midwives in Virginia (those midwives who had been permitted prior to 1977 and had maintained their permits). The advisory group recommended that the existing regulations be retained and the previously permitted non-nurse-midwives remained regulated by the VDH.

1997   The GA enacted legislation that mandated direct insurance reimbursement (including Medicaid) for CNMs.

1998   A Study Resolution was introduced to the GA to study maternity care in out-of-hospital settings, but was rejected because it called for the creation of a special subcommittee (all study resolutions were rejected that year).

1999   Two identical bills and one study resolution were introduced to the GA. The bills would have registered and permitted lay midwives under the regulations set forth prior to 1977. No action was taken on the bills, but the Study Resolution to examine "the advisability of legalizing direct-entry midwifery" passed.

2000   As a result of the Study Resolution, the Joint Commission on Health Care (JCHC) conducted a Midwifery Study and recommended that the GA introduce legislation to legalize the practice of direct-entry midwifery by licensing individuals who are Certified Professional Midwives (CPMs). Two identical bills were also introduced in 2000, which would have licensed DEMs through the Board of Health Professions (however, the CPM certification, which was supported by the JCHC, was not mentioned in the bills). One bill was defeated and the other carried over to the 2001 session.

2001   A revised version encompassing the two bills from 2000 was defeated, and the last midwife who had retained her pre-1977 permit moved out of state.

2002   Three bills to license midwives as CPMs, DEMs, or LMs (respectively), and one study resolution that would have would have put the onus of recommending "the appropriate degree of regulation" for DEMs on the Board of Health Professions were introduced and defeated.

2003   A bill to remove the 1977 definition of the lay midwife and exempt "individuals who are not registered as nurses" from registration and permit requirements passed. It did not provide for licensure or regulation, and an additional bill to do so and a study resolution were defeated.

2004   One bill to license CPMs was defeated and another bill and a study resolution were tabled during the January legislative session. During the summer, the governor commissioned the Work Group on Rural Obstetric Care. Midwives mobilized quickly to nominate both a CPM and a CNM to the Work Group (both were appointed by the Governor). Midwives and midwifery advocates also spoke at public hearings for the work group and sent letters about the need for both licensing CPMs and removing restrictions on CNMs to facilitate more access to midwives throughout the state. The final report recommended the institution of a pilot program to allow CNMs to practice in collaboration and consultation with physicians (as opposed to a supervisory relationship) in medically underserved areas (Governor's Work Group 2004:66–69). The report also recommended the eventual elimination of supervision requirements from all CNM practice. The report discussed the educational requirements for both CNMs and CPMs and cited studies indicating positive outcomes for midwife-attended home and hospital births (Governor's Work Group 2004:69–71). The report reads: "The work group acknowledges that based on testimony it received, many consumers would like to have the option of a home birth attended by a certified professional midwife. The Work Group considered the option of recommending licensure for certified professional midwives but did not recommend that such action be taken at this time. Instead the Work Group chose to focus its recommendations on certified nurse-midwives who are already licensed in Virginia" (Governor's Work Group 2004:71).

2005   Legislation allowing non-nurse-midwives to be licensed by the Virginia Board of Medicine as Certified Professional Midwives passed. This law was effective July 1, 2005.

ACKNOWLEDGMENTS

It was a pleasure and a privilege to contribute to this collection and I am especially grateful for the critical, yet kind, comments on earlier drafts of this chapter from Robbie Davis-Floyd and Christine Barbara Johnson. I would also like to thank the countless midwifery advocates and midwives in Virginia who have taken time to share their wisdom with me and allow me to look critically at their important work for the rights of women and families to choose midwifery as an option for birth care; I would particularly like to thank Alice Bailes, Steve Cochran, Juliana Fehr, Ellen Hamblet, Marsha Jackson, Jessica Jordan, Leslie Payne, Brynne Potter, Katie Prown, Patty Ogden, D'Anne Remocaldo, Lois Smith, and Trinlie Wood. The list of other friends and colleagues who joined me in conversation about this research is also far too long to print here; in particular, I am indebted to Bill Leap, Susan Virginia Mead, Brenda Murphy, Krissi Jimroglou, Jeff Maskovsky, Teo Owen, Sabiyha Prince, Heidi Schultz, Maria Vesperi, and Brett Williams for their comments on this chapter. I am also grateful for an American University College of Arts and Sciences Doctoral Dissertation Fellowship, which supported portions of the research for this project.

ENDNOTES

1. Among Virginia midwives and advocates, as in many states (Davis-Floyd 1998), "direct-entry midwifery" has become a common phrase to describe an often-diverse group of birth care providers. These often include nationally credentialed certified professional midwives and certified midwives, as well as those who label themselves traditional midwives, domiciliary midwives, and community-based midwives.

2. Virginia's history of midwifery is rich with narratives from many different women's published and unpublished accounts. Several published historical accounts are useful for further reading: see Claudine Curry Smith and Mildred Roberson's (1994) *Memories of a Black Lay Midwife* and their later, significantly revised version (2003) *My Bag Was Always Packed: The Life and Times of a Virginia Midwife*, Karen Cecil Smith's (2003) *Orlean Puckett 1844-1939: The Life of a Mountain Midwife*, Gertrude Fraser's (1998) *African American Midwifery in the South: Dialogues of Birth, Race, and Memory*, based on her ethnographic fieldwork in Virginia; Virginia certified nurse-midwife Juliana van Olphen-Fehr's (1998) *Diary of a Midwife: The Power of Positive Childbearing*, and a more extensive version of the history I provide here, which is available on the Virginia Friends of Midwives website at http://www.vfom.org/history.doc.

3. In Virginia, African Americans were denied care in hospitals during the early to mid-1900s and continued to face segregation in childbirth clinics until after the passage of the Civil Rights Act in 1964. Virginia's largest public hospital, the Medical College of Virginia Hospital in Richmond, had a separate building for African-Americans, the St. Phillips Hospital, until 1965 (Smith and Roberson 2003:6).

4. Critics of the prosecution also questioned the impartiality of Chief State Medical Examiner Marcella Fierro, who was married to a prominent Richmond obstetrician (Krishnamurthy 2000a: B-4); both had vocally opposed the licensure of DEMs. Fierro reported to lawmakers at a Health, Welfare, and Institutions Subcommittee meeting regarding the licensure of DEMs in 2001, "We do see, each year, a few deaths where there was no physician involved, where the woman, generally it is due to postpartum hemorrhage, where this has not been recognized and the woman has been allowed to bleed for hours and hours and hours and then dies of shock" (author's transcription, January 30, 2001). Following a legislator's request for specific statistics regarding

maternal deaths as a result of homebirths with midwives, Fierro was unable to substantiate her claims, repeating several times, "We don't have figures for that" (author's transcription, January 30, 2001).

5. The final change, the violation of a statute governing care provided to incapacitated persons, is most commonly brought to bear in cases intended to protect patients in mental institutions and nursing homes. This sets a disturbing precedent; by Virginia case law, the definition of an *incapacitated person* now includes a pregnant woman in labor.

6. Quotations from personal interviews are identified by pseudonyms to protect the privacy of participants in my study. However, statements that were made at public events (such as hearings at the Virginia General Assembly) or quoted in the media are attributed to the speaker.

7. Many midwives and midwifery advocates in Virginia, as well as nationally and internationally, have adopted the term *consumer* to distinguish women who seek access to midwifery care from midwives themselves. I have argued elsewhere (Craven 2003b; 2005) that consumer rights strategies toward legalizing midwives may ultimately alienate low-income homebirthers who feel unable to participate in political efforts that focus on choices they may not be able to afford. Still, many middle-class advocates see benefits to this term as politically palatable as they vie for the right to legally choose DEM services. Additionally, many advocates reject the term *activist* to describe their involvement in attempts to legalize DEM; *consumer* has become the most widely agreed-upon term to differentiate these groups and individuals from practicing midwives.

8. I have received permission from the authors of all listserv quotations to include them in this chapter. In all quotations from written sources (i.e., letters, reports, websites, listserv messages, and newspaper articles), I have left grammar, punctuation, spelling, and the like as it appeared in the original text, except in cases where omissions or additions (in brackets) make the text more clear.

9. Adella Scott Wilson was the last legally permitted lay midwife in Virginia, who assisted in approximately 2,000 births in the Virginia Beach area during her thirty-four years of practice (Forster 2000: A4). Since she was licensed prior to the 1977 law that restricted the practice of midwifery to nurse-midwives, Wilson maintained her lay midwifery license until 2001 when she retired and moved out of the state.

10. Recipients of the nurse practitioner/nurse-midwife scholarship must attend a program in Virginia and commit to full-time practice in a state-designated "medically underserved area" for a period of years following their education that is equal to the number of annual scholarships the student received. If the recipient fails to complete the program, withdraws, moves out of state, or elects to work in an area that is not considered medically underserved, the full amount of the scholarship, plus an annual interest charge, must be repaid immediately (Commonwealth of Virginia, Department of Health 2003).

REFERENCES

Baer, Hans. 2001. *Biomedicine and Alternative Healing Systems in America: Issues of Class, Race, Ethnicity, and Gender.* Madison, WI: University of Wisconsin Press.

Baughman, Greer. 1928. "A Preliminary Report Upon the Midwife Situation in Virginia." *Virginia Medical Monthly* 54:748–751.

Bennett, Emily. 1925. "Midwife Work in Virginia." *Public Health Nurse* 17:523–526.

Bookman, Ann, and Sandra Morgen. 1988. *Women and the Politics of Empowerment.* Philadelphia, PA: Temple University Press.

Brown, Dennis, and Pamela A. Toussaint. 1998. *Mama's Little Baby: The Black Woman's Guide to Pregnancy, Childbirth, and the Baby's First Year.* New York: Plume.

Caillagh, Cynthia L. 2000. Press release, May 5.

Cobb, Ann Kuckelman. 1981. "Incorporation and Change: The Case of the Midwife in the United States." *Medical Anthropology* 5:73–88.

Commonwealth of Virginia. 1999. Study; direct-entry midwifery. Chief Patron Phillip A. Hamilton. Passed, March 22: House Joint Resolution 646, http://leg1.state.va.us/cgi-bin/legp504.exe?ses=991&typ=bil&val= hj646, accessed July 26, 2003.

———. 2002. Code of Virginia, http://leg1.state.va.us/000/ src.htm, accessed March 10 (last updated August 13, 2002).

———. 2003. Health; practice of midwifery. Chief Patron Phillip A. Hamilton. Passed, January 8, effective July 1: House Bill 1961, http://leg1.state.va.us/cgi-bin/legp504. exe?031+sum+HB1961, accessed July 26, 2003.

———. 2005. Midwifery; licensure. Chief Patron Frederick M. Quayle. Passed March 29, effective July 1. Senate Bill 1259. Electronic Document, http://leg1.state.va.us/cgi-bin/legp504.exe?ses=051&typ=bil &val=sb1259, accessed April 21, 2005.

Commonwealth of Virginia, Department of Health. 1995. Recorded Live Births by Attendant and Facility of Birth by Race of Mother, Virginia, Table 18. Vital Records & Health Statistics. Unpublished, photocopied, faxed by Robert Magiotti, September 4, 2002:IV-14.

———. 1997. Recorded Live Births by Attendant and Facility of Birth by Race of Mother, Virginia, Table 88. Unpublished, photocopied, faxed by Robert Magiotti, September 4, 2002:IV-53.

———. 2000. Recorded Live Births by Attendant and Facility of Birth by Race of Mother, Virginia, Table 88. Unpublished, photocopied, faxed by Robert Magiotti, September 4, 2002:IV-59.

———. 2003. Virginia's Nurse Practitioner/Nurse-Midwife Scholarship Program Application, http://www.vdh.state.va.us/primcare/center/pdfs/VDH29.pdf, accessed August 18, 2003.

Commonwealth of Virginia, Department of Health Professions and Virginia Health Planning Board, Task Force on the Study of Obstetric Access and Certified Nurse-Midwives. 1992. The Potential for Expansion of the Practice of Nurse-Midwives, House Document No. 12. Richmond: Commonwealth of Virginia.

Commonwealth of Virginia, Joint Commission on Health Care. 2000a. Midwifery Study Pursuant to HJR 646, House Document No. 76. Richmond: Commonwealth of Virginia.

———. 2000b. Summary of Public Comments: Midwifery Study (HJR 646). Richmond: Commonwealth of Virginia.

Condit, Deirdre. 2000 (February 1). Presentation at Women, Birth, Politics, and Power. Virginia Commonwealth University, Richmond, Virginia.

Craven, Christa. 2003a. "Educated, Eliminated, Criminalized and Rediscovered: A History of Midwives and Grassroots Organizing for Midwifery in Virginia." Virginia Friends of Midwives, http://www.vfom.org/history.doc.

———. 2003b. "Expectations of Motherhood: Citizenship and Political Mobilization for Midwifery in Virginia." Ph.D. diss., Department of Anthropology, American University.

———. 2005. "Is Reproductive Healthcare Access a 'Consumer Rights' Issue?: Questioning Activist Strategies under Neoliberal Governance." *Anthropology News* 46(1):16, 19.

Davis-Floyd, Robbie. 1992. *Birth as an American Rite of Passage.* Berkeley: University of California Press.

———. 1997. "Birth of a Dream, Death of a Dream: The Development of Direct-Entry Midwifery in New York." Paper presented at the Joint Meetings of the Society for Applied Anthropology and the Society for Medical Anthropology, Seattle, Washington.

———. 1998. "The Ups, Downs, and Interlinkages of Nurse- and Direct-Entry Midwifery: Status, Practice, and Education." In *Pathways to Becoming a Midwife: Getting an Education.* Eugene, OR: Midwifery Today.

Davis-Floyd, Robbie, and Elizabeth Davis. 1997. "Intuition as Authoritative Knowledge in Midwifery and Home-Birth." In *Childbirth and Authoritative Knowledge,* ed. Robbie Davis-Floyd and Carolyn Sargent, 315–350. Berkeley: University of California Press.

Declerq, Eugene R., Lisa L. Paine, and Michael R. Winter. 1995. "Home Birth in the United States, 1989–1992: A Longitudinal Descriptive Report of National Birth Certificate Data." *Journal of Nurse-Midwifery* 40 (6): 474–482.

DeVries, Raymond G. 1996. *Making Midwives Legal: Childbirth, Medicine, and the Law,* 2d ed. (orig. *Regulating Birth: Midwives, Medicine, and the Law Philadelphia: Temple University Press, 1986*). Columbus: Ohio State University Press.

Dougherty, Molly. 1982. "Southern Midwifery and Organized Health Care: Systems in Conflict." *Medical Anthropology* 6:114–126.

Forster, Laura. 2000. "Welcome Home: Home Birth Creates Intimacy for Some, Controversy for Others." *Potomac News: Manassas Journal Messenger* (serving the Prince Georges Region), November 26, A1, A4.

Fraser, Gertrude. 1995. "Modern Bodies, Modern Minds: Midwifery and Reproductive Change in an African American Community." In *Conceiving the New World Order: The Global Politics of Reproduction,* ed. Faye Ginsburg and Rayna Rapp, 42–58. Berkeley: University of California Press.

———. 1998. *African American Midwifery in the South: Dialogues of Birth, Race and Memory.* Cambridge: Harvard University Press.

Gerheart, Melanie. 1999. *Joint Commission on Health Care to Study Lay Midwives and Obstetrical Education in Med Schools.* Virginia Section Review, a joint publication of the Virginia Obstetrical and Gynecological Society and the Virginia Section of The American College of Obstetricians and Gynecologists (spring):2.

Gibson, Faith. 1994 (December 25). "The Goodly Art of Orifice Maintenance." http://www.goodnewsnet.org/practice/calling.htm. Originally published in the *Newsletter of Midwives' Association of North America.*

Ginsburg, Faye, and Rayna Rapp, eds. 1995. *Conceiving the New World Order: The Global Politics of Reproduction.* Berkeley: University of California Press.

Governor's Work Group on Rural Obstetrical Care. 2004. Executive Directive 2, *Report of the Governor's Work Group on Rural Obstetrical Care,* October 29. http://www.vdh.virginia.gov/COMMISH/OBFinal_Report.pdf, accessed May 9, 2005.

Glod, Maria, and Josh White. 1999. "Midwives Charged in Death of Va. Woman." *Washington Post,* January 21, B01.

Hall, Jim. 1998. "Death and its Consequences, Cradle & Grave (Part 5)." *The Free Lance-Star,* Fredericksburg, Virginia, January 30, A1, A14.

Hardin, Peter. 2000. "Eugenics Affected Va. Law: Theory Advocated Social Engineering." *Richmond Times-Dispatch,* March 5, A-13.

Hyatt, Susan Brin. 1999. "Poverty and the Medicalisation of Motherhood." In *Sex, Gender and Health,* ed. Teresa M. Pollard and Susan Brin Hyatt, 94–117. New York: Cambridge University Press.

Klassen, Pamela E. 2001. *Blessed Events: Religion and Homebirth in America.* Princeton, NJ: Princeton University Press.

Krishnamurthy, Kiran. 2000a. "Midwife Expected to Enter Guilty Plea." *Richmond Times-Dispatch,* May 5, B-4.

———. 2000b. "Unlicensed Midwives Get Jail Sentences." *Richmond Times-Dispatch,* May 6, A-1.

Lay, Mary M. 2000. *The Rhetoric of Midwifery: Gender, Knowledge, and Power.* New Brunswick, NJ: Rutgers University Press.

Lazarus, Ellen. 1997. "What Do Women Want? Issues of Choice, Control, and Class in American Pregnancy and Childbirth." In *Childbirth and Authoritative Knowledge,* ed. Robbie Davis-Floyd and Carolyn Sargent, 132–158. Berkeley: University of California Press.

LeHew, Willette L. 2000 (summer). "An Obstetrician's View on Lay Midwives and Home Delivery." *Virginia Capitol Connections Quarterly Magazine* 6(3):12–13.

Lombardo, Paul. 1982. "Eugenic Sterilization in Virginia: Aubrey Strode and the Case of *Buck v. Bell.*" Ph.D. thesis, School of Education, University of Virginia.

Martin, Emily. 1987. *The Woman in the Body: A Cultural Analysis of Reproduction.* Boston, MA: Beacon Press.

Maskovsky, Jeff. 2000. "'Managing' The Poor: Neoliberalism, Medicaid HMOs and the Triumph of Consumerism among the Poor." *Medical Anthropology* 19(2):127–172.

Mathews, Holly F. 1992. "Killing the Medical Self-Help Tradition Among African Americans: The Case of Lay Midwifery in North Carolina, 1912–1983." In *African Americans in the South: Issues of Race, Class, and Gender,* ed. Hans Baer and Yvonne Jones, 60–78. Athens: University of Georgia Press.

Miller, M. Linda. 1999. "Public Argument and Legislative Debate in the Rhetorical Construction of Public Policy: The Case of Florida Midwifery Legislation." *The Quarterly Journal of Speech* 85 (4): 361–379.

Morgen, Sandra. 1988. "'It's the Whole Power of the City Against Us!': The Development of Political Consciousness in a Women's Health Care Coalition." In *Women and the Politics of Empowerment,* ed. Ann Bookman and Sandra Morgen, 97–115. Philadelphia, PA: Temple University Press.

———. 2002. *Into Our Own Hands: The Women's Health Movement in the United States, 1969–1990.* New Brunswick, NJ: Rutgers University Press.

Mullings, Leith. 1989. "Inequality and African American Health Status: Policies and Prospects." In *Race: 20th Century Dilemmas, 21st Century Prognoses,* ed. Winston A. Van Horne, 154–182. Madison: University of Wisconsin Press.

Murray, William L. 1999a (July 27). Direct Entry Midwifery Study: Presentation to the Joint Commission on Health Care Midwifery Subcommittee. General Assembly, Richmond, Virginia.

———. 1999b (August 6). Staff Follow-up from Last Meeting: Presentation to the Joint Commission on Health Care Midwifery Subcommittee. General Assembly, Richmond, Virginia.

Nelson, Margaret. 1986. "Birth and Social Class." In *The American Way of Birth,* ed. Pamela S. Eakins, 142–174. Philadelphia, PA: Temple University Press.

Neuberger, Christine. 1999a. "Officials Explain Charges against Two Midwives." *Richmond Times Dispatch* (web version), January 29.

———. 1999b. "Traditional Midwife Extols Value, Rewards She Discovered." *Richmond Times-Dispatch,* March 1, A-1.

Norris, Lynn. 1995. "Birthrites: Midwife Brings Art to Life." *Riverviews: Northcumberland Echo and Westmoreland and Northern Neck News,* July, 72, 74.

Pegram, Cynthia T. 1996. "Unlicensed Midwives Can't Practice Legally Under Virginia Statute." *The News & Advance,* Lynchburg, Virginia, August 18, B-1, B-5.

Plecker, W. A. 1925. "Virginia Makes Efforts to Solve Midwife Problem." *Nation's Health* 8(12):809–811.

Rapp, Rayna. 1997. "Constructing Amniocentesis: Maternal and Medical Discourses." In *Situated Lives: Gender and Culture in Everyday Life,* ed. Louise Lamphere, Helena Ragoné, and Patricia Zavella, 128–141. New York: Routledge.

———. 1999. *Testing Women, Testing the Fetus: The Social Impact of Amniocentesis in America.* New York: Routledge.

Reid, Margaret. 1995. "Sisterhood and Professionalization: A Case Study of the American Lay Midwife." In *Women as Healers: Cross-Cultural Perspectives*, ed. Carol Shepherd McClain, 219–238. New Brunswick, NJ: Rutgers University Press.

Smith, Claudine Curry, and Mildred Baker Roberson. 1994. *Memories of a Black Lay Midwife from Northern Neck Virginia*. Lisle, Illinois: Tucker Publications.

———. 2003. *My Bag Was Always Packed: The Life and Times of a Virginia Midwife*. Bloomington, IN: First Books.

Smith, Karen Cecil. 2003. *Orlean Puckett 1844–1939: The Life of a Mountain Midwife*. Boone, NC: Parkway Publishers.

Stern, Howard. 1999. A Public Health Perspective on Midwifery by the Director of the Office of Family Health Services, Virginia Department of Health. A presentation to the Commonwealth of Virginia, General Assembly, Joint Commission on Health Care. Richmond, Virginia, August 10.

Strobel, Jennifer. 1990. "Going Back to the Roots, Midwives: A Tradition Reborn (Part 2)." *The Free Lance-Star*, Fredericksburg, Virginia, March 15, 27–28.

Suarez, Suzanne Hope. 1993. "Midwifery is Not the Practice of Medicine." *Yale Journal of Law and Feminism* 5:315–364.

Susie, Debra Anne. 1988. *In the Way of Our Grandmothers: A Cultural View of Twentieth-Century Midwifery in Florida*. Athens: University of Georgia Press.

U.S. Bureau of the Census. 2000a. *Income and Poverty in 1999, Virginia, by County*, http://factfinder.census.gov, accessed January 24, 2003.

———. 2000b. *Poverty Thresholds in 1999 by Size of Family and Number of Related Children under 18 Years Old*, http://factfinder.census.gov, accessed January 24, 2003.

Van Olphen-Fehr, Juliana. 1998. *Diary of a Midwife: The Power of Positive Childbearing*. Westport, CT: Bergin and Garvey.

Virginia Friends of Midwives. 2003. Virginia Friends of Midwives homepage, http://www.vfom.org, accessed July 6, 2003 (last updated June 23, 2003).

Voices for Healthcare Rights Fund. 1999. *Alternative Healthcare Practitioners: Endangered Species*. Fundraising Brochure. Toano, Virginia: Voices for Healthcare Rights Fund.

———. 2000a. Stafford Case against Midwives Unravels amidst New Questions. Press release, May 2.

———. 2000b. Midwives Vindicated on Midwives Day. Press release, May 5.

Wertz, Richard W. and Dorothy Wertz. 1979. *Lying-In: A History of Childbirth in America*. New York: Free Press.

Whiteford, Linda M. 1996. "Political Economy, Gender, and the Social Production of Health and Illness." In *Gender and Health: An International Perspective*, ed. Carolyn F. Sargent and Caroline B. Brettell, 242–259. Upper Saddle River, NJ: Prentice Hall.

Wilson, Lynn. 1988. "Epistemology and Power: Rethinking Ethnography at Greenham." In *Anthropology for the 90s*, ed. Jonetta Cole, 42–57. New York: Free Press.

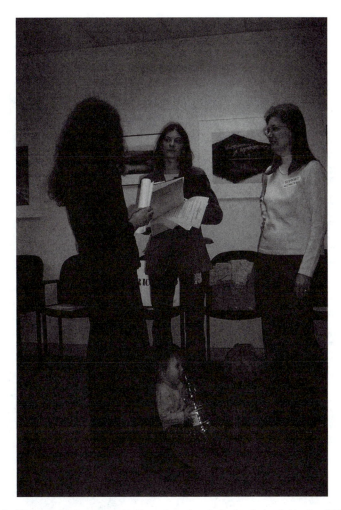

Fig. 7.1   Virginia midwives and midwifery advocates strategize during Lobby Day 2005 in the Virginia General Assembly. Photographer: Christa Craven.

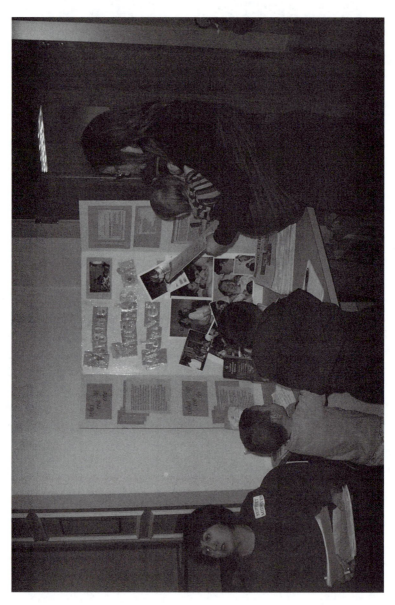

Fig. 7.2 Homebirth moms and kids check out the Virginia Friends of Midwives display for legislators on Lobby Day 2005. Photographer: Christa Craven.

8

"I'M LIVING MY POLITICS": LEGALIZING AND LICENSING DIRECT-ENTRY MIDWIVES IN IOWA

Carolyn A. Hough

• **Introduction** • **Professionalizing Biomedical Alternatives** • **Emerging from the Underground: Making Direct-Entry Midwifery Public** • **The Professional Politics of Direct-Entry Midwifery** • **Critical Differences: Perspectives on Legalization and Licensing** • **Spiritual/Professional: Forging New Self-Definitions** • **Questioning Authority: Client Responsibility and Midwife Accountability** • **Conclusion: Looking Toward the Future** • **Postscript** • **Timeline of Direct-Entry Midwifery in Iowa**

INTRODUCTION

During the summer of 1999, Iowa's statewide direct-entry midwifery association drafted and submitted a scope-of-practice review application to the state's Department of Public Health. This review process marked a major step toward enacting legislation that would legalize and license direct-entry midwifery in the state, and generated a wide range of responses from midwives themselves[1]—from impassioned approval to staunch rejection of legalization and regulation efforts.

Within the context of the licensing debate, the meaning of midwifery and being a midwife has become an increasingly salient issue for these direct-entry midwives (DEMs) as they face an uncertain future that may bring a restructuring of their practices. This chapter will examine sites of multiple meaning within narrative accounts elicited from Iowa midwives, which demonstrate the complexities of their efforts at self-definition and how these complexities affect their desire for, or opposition to, legislation and regulation.

PROFESSIONALIZING BIOMEDICAL ALTERNATIVES

The presence of certified nurse-midwives (CNMs) in hospital settings and the professionalization efforts of DEMs have increased the sites of contact between midwifery and the biomedical system, which dominates health care in the United States. Biomedical hegemony, along with most other forms of professional monopoly, can be understood in part as the constant construction and maintenance of prohibitive boundaries. As sociologist Eliot Freidson has observed, "Knowledge itself does not give special power: only *exclusive* knowledge gives power to its possessors" (1973:28). The professional hegemony and relative autonomy of biomedicine in the United States are maintained through the consent of the state, which views medical professionals as the experts best suited to evaluate and govern the provision of health care, and allows these practitioners to erect and enforce professional boundaries (Freidson 1970; 1973).

Yet the power of biomedical professionalism should not be understood as completely totalizing. As Margaret Lock and Patricia Kaufert assert, "hegemony is not a given, nor simply a product of oppressive forces or class difference, but is realized only through negotiation among competing forces" (1998:4). The key notion here is that biomedical domination does not go unchallenged, and the professional supremacy of allopathic physicians is continually tested by both internal and external forces. Irving K. Zola and Stephen Miller (1973) articulate the contemporary challenges to biomedical hegemony, which emerge from within the ranks of biomedicine itself. The specialization that has taken place among physicians threatens to splinter their professional unity, as does an increased technical division of labor, which serves to separate physicians from their patients. Zola and Miller view this delegation of responsibility as a dissolution of physicians' professional clout, and a distribution of exclusive wisdom that strengthens the knowledge claims of auxiliary health-care providers.

The distribution of knowledge and decision-making authority is a result of external as well as internal pressures due to the rise of managed care in the United States. David Mechanic addresses the increasing bureaucratization of biomedicine, which often reconfigures who has ultimate control over a patient's care, stating:

Physicians who work in bureaucratic settings usually continue to regard themselves as autonomous professionals, and they resist many of the demands that would alter their role as agent of the patient. But despite such resistance, the requirements of many of the physicians' roles in organizations create strong incentives and pressures that may be inconsistent with the individual patient's interests. . . . Indeed, the definition of the physician's employment, under some circumstances, transforms the definition of who the client is. (1976:53)

Raymond DeVries has specifically addressed how managed care has the potential to draw midwifery's low-tech and relatively inexpensive approaches further into the mainstream (1996:167–168). Despite this potential, however, DeVries emphasizes the fact that this threat to the authority of the physician has thus far had little impact on the state of midwifery in both hospital and out-of-hospital settings:

Watching from the sidelines, the remnants of the alternative birth movement were convinced that the clinically irrational resistance of physicians to midwives (i.e., an opposition to midwives stemming not from questions of safety but from fear of competition) could not survive the cool rationality of business managers. . . . In 1996, ten years into the managed care revolution, physicians continue to lose control to administrators. The medical citadel is crumbling, and yet, almost inexplicably, childbirth remains in the hands of obstetricians. (1996:xiii–xiv)

Yet the bureaucratization of biomedicine and the iatrogenic results that accompany its practice have opened the door to a revival of alternative/holistic medicine[2] in the United States and Western Europe, where one may seek health care from nonbiomedical practitioners to complement or replace more customary allopathic care (Baer, Singer, and Susser 1997:215). This increasing demand for alternatives to standard biomedical approaches has engendered a co-option of holistic methods, which are transformed for the hospital setting. One such adaptation is the *hospital alternative birth center*, which attempts to simulate a homebirth setting. Though these birth centers may provide comfortable furnishings and soft lighting, they have been criticized for their high delivery-room transfer rate and lack of commitment to noninterventionist care.[3]

As alternative health-care modalities have achieved popularity and success, their practitioners have increasingly begun to professionalize in order to achieve credibility and establish authority—a trend that has not escaped the attention of medical anthropologists and sociologists (Baer 1984, 1989; Baer et al. 1998; Cant and Sharma 1996). While this push for professionalization points to breaches in biomedical dominance, it can also indicate a willingness on the part of these practitioners to sacrifice a holistic perspective on health and healing for a more reductionist model that resembles allopathy (Baer 1989:1103–1104). For this very reason, these professional projects are usually not undertaken with unanimous internal endorsement. In the case of British homeopaths, Sarah Cant and Ursula Sharma (1996:583) address the uneasy junction between establishing exclusive professional knowledge and maintaining non-hierarchical relationships with patients through which knowledge of homeopathic treatments and philosophies of care have been dispersed—a process that has saved homeopathy from obscurity.

EMERGING FROM THE UNDERGROUND: MAKING DIRECT-ENTRY MIDWIFERY PUBLIC

The legalization and professionalization process undertaken by direct-entry midwives in Iowa raises some important questions, which guided this research. Do all of Iowa's direct-entry midwives share the same positive outlook on legislative change? In what ways do midwives feel that legalization will affect their practices or their perceptions of themselves as practitioners? What problems will licensure solve for DEMs? What problems might it create? I sought answers to these questions by conducting semistructured interviews with direct-entry midwives working in Iowa,[4] and by attending monthly meetings of the statewide direct-entry midwifery organization, the Iowa Midwives Association (IMA).

At the first IMA meeting I attended, I met most of the midwives interviewed for this project. The informal gathering took place in one midwife's living room, where a dozen practicing midwives, apprentices, and dedicated homebirth supporters had convened to discuss, debate, commiserate, and share a meal together. One midwife addressed the possibility of the organization purchasing educational videos on homebirth produced by DEMs, as well as creating their own short promotional film to show on local public access television. Another expressed the anxiety she had been feeling over an upcoming interview with local news media on the topic of midwifery. She, as well as the other midwives present, were concerned that the editing process prior to broadcast could distort her statements and reinforce negative stereotypes of midwives as unsafe practitioners in such a powerful public forum.

Both of these conversational threads addressed how direct-entry midwives should engage a wider audience to promote the idea that giving birth in one's home without extraneous biomedical intervention is as safe or safer than giving birth in a hospital with an obstetrician. This concern was further emphasized when the meeting's agenda turned to the drafting of a scope of practice review application for the Iowa state legislature, a major step toward the production of legislation that could potentially legalize direct-entry midwifery throughout the state and establish the certified professional midwife (CPM) credential, as outlined by the North American Registry of Midwives (NARM), as a licensing standard.

Currently, under a state's attorney's opinion published in 1978, "an unlicensed 'midwife' who administers to or treats pregnancies and delivers babies, whether within or without a licensed physician's supervision, can be considered to be practicing medicine and surgery without a license" (Iowa Attorney General 1978:371). It is this legal interpretation that has prohibited the practice of direct-entry midwifery in Iowa. The scope of practice application discussed by the midwives would be sent to Des Moines, the state capital, to be formally reviewed by a board consisting of one physician, one direct-entry midwife, one "impartial" health-care professional, and two consumers, who would decide whether or not the applicants had satisfied the criteria laid out by the Department of Public Health.[5] The committee could approve the application, grant approval with revisions, or deny the application. Their recommendations in the form of a final report would then be passed down to the director of the Department of Public Health, affected health regulatory boards, and the Iowa General Assembly in time for the start of the next legislative session. At this early summer meeting, the midwives attempted to hammer out both major and minor sticking points as the application deadline loomed large.

The room's atmosphere seemed excited and eager, but also a bit battle weary—this was not the first time the midwives' organization had attempted legislative action to achieve legal status. According to Marianne,[6] a senior midwife and chief lobbyist for the group, the first attempt to legalize direct-entry midwifery began in 1994 when midwives contacted the Attorney General's office through a state representative to petition a review of the 1978 opinion. That request was denied and the midwives were told that their efforts should be redirected into legislative measures that would overturn the Attorney General's opinion.

As a first step toward drafting legislation, the midwives' association inquired about decriminalizing direct-entry midwifery and allowing midwives to register with, but not be regulated by, the state, but this option was rejected by the Department of Public Health. At the same time, the midwives founded a consumer activist group called Iowans for Birth Options and began grassroots initiatives to familiarize the public as well as health-care professionals with homebirth and traditional midwifery practices. Meanwhile, faced with internal disagreement over issues of licensure and regulation, the process of drafting legislation was slowed and the first bill to propose legalization and licensure in Iowa was submitted late in the 1998 legislative session. Because of its late submission date, the bill made little progress, but was resubmitted early for the 1999 legislative session, during which IMA representatives spoke before the House Health and Human Resources Committee. To attempt to move the bill out of committee, the midwives made biweekly lobbying trips to Des Moines. Their appeals at the statehouse, however, were outmatched by written responses from physicians encouraging their representatives to vote against this legislation. The bill's sponsor then allowed the legislation to sit in committee through the end of the session and authorized the scope of practice review process, which was then voted into reality after additional lobbying. While this review had been approved and a small group of DEMs were preparing the application, the consequences of this process were still being debated within the Iowa Midwives Association.

THE PROFESSIONAL POLITICS
OF DIRECT-ENTRY MIDWIFERY

In their study of direct-entry midwifery groups that institute self-certification as a means to internally regulate midwives at the state level, Irene Butter and Bonnie Kay query, "Are lay midwives' groups the beginnings of new professional organizations which eventually will become part of the dominant system or do they model themselves more closely after alternative women's health groups?" (1990:1329). On one hand, DEMs may survive as alternative practitioners by forming groups that resemble the collectives that grew out of the Women's Health Movement (see Ruzek 1977) of the 1960s and 1970s outside of the sphere of biomedicine, or they may survive by fashioning their organizations after the medical model, becoming subordinate within the biomedical hierarchy of physicians and nurses (Butter and Kay 1990:1330).

Butter and Kay draw a sharp distinction between the empowerment-based, consensus-driven women's health model and the bureaucratic, professionally-oriented biomedical model, but this dualism fails to adequately reflect the complexity of the situation I observed among Iowa's DEMs as they pursued legalization and licensure. While the DEMs I interviewed spoke of being "spiritually called" to midwifery, they also stressed the importance of their professionalism and credibility as practitioners. Though they hoped to level the power imbalances inherent within the biomedical doctor/patient relationship in their interactions with clients, at times they also asserted their authority as ultimate decision makers.[7] Recognizing the importance of demonstrating the safety and competence of midwifery care to their biomedical colleagues, they are also driven by their own passion for homebirth and by the desires of their clients for individualized and noninterventionist care at home.

This type of negotiation has been referred to as *postmodern midwifery* by anthropologist Robbie Davis-Floyd, who comments:

> The postmodern midwife knows the limitations and strengths of the biomedical system and of her own, and moves fluidly between them to serve the women she attends. She plays with the paradigms, working to ensure that her culture of midwifery is not subsumed by biomedicine. She is a shape-shifter—she knows how to subvert the medical system while appearing to comply with it, a bridge-builder, making alliances with biomedicine where possible, and a networker. (Davis-Floyd, Cosminsky, and Pigg 2001:112)

I hope to build upon this view of contemporary midwifery to develop a perspective on the power dynamics that both necessitate and constrain resistant practices. Additional constructions of resistance and negotiation can be used to investigate the midwives' location between these two poles.

For example, feminist anthropological accounts of resistant practices have benefited from the careful inspection of "the romance of resistance" by Lila Abu-Lughod (1990) and others (Lock and Kaufert 1998; Ortner 1995; Ong 1997). While embracing the value of resistance as an analytical tool, Abu-Lughod calls for a reapplication of resistance as a "diagnostic of power" rather than a catch-all category that "collapse[s] distinctions between forms of resistance and foreclose[s] certain questions about the workings of power" (Abu-Lughod 1990:42). Though the Foucauldian analysis, from which Abu-Lughod draws her criticism, argues that resistance is a necessary consequence of power, it also claims that resistance is never exterior to the power relations being opposed. This position demands that anthropological accounts bring into critical focus the connections and interactions between those who are resistant and the structures they resist.

Sherry Ortner (1995) critically comments upon and adds to Abu-Lughod's ideas by suggesting that ethnographic accounts of resistance must draw attention to the messy internal politics and complex subjectivities of those who appear to be collectively resistant to dominant structures. Stratified by class, gender, race, age and opinion, oppositional groups must not be hastily homogenized by the anthropologist. She argues:

> Overall, the lack of an adequate sense of prior ongoing politics among subalterns must inevitably contribute to an inadequate analysis of resistance itself. Many people do not get caught up in resistance movements, and this is not simply an effect of fear, naïve enthrallment to the priests, or narrow self-interest. Nor does it make collaborators of all the non-participants. Moreover, individual acts of resistance, as well as large-scale resistance movements, are often themselves conflicted, internally contradictory, and affectively ambivalent, in large part due to these internal political complexities. (Ortner 1995:179)

This paper will build upon Davis-Floyd's conception of postmodern midwifery by incorporating these critical perspectives on the tensions engendered by resistant practices in order to understand how activism and professionalization have shaped and transformed the meanings of midwifery in Iowa.

Midwifery Activism: Common Goals and Shared Understandings

As I began the fieldwork for this project, I was immediately drawn to the political process that had been set in motion within the midwives association. I wanted to discover how these women had developed such a bold commitment to homebirth and how they felt that legalization would affect their practices and direct-entry midwifery in Iowa more broadly. The interviews elicited women's accounts of how they became midwives, how they practice midwifery, and how these practices may be similar to or different from the biomedical model. Each midwife spoke frankly about important life events and transitions, framing her life through the breakthroughs and triumphs as well as the setbacks and heartbreaks she had experienced as a midwife.

In *Contested Lives: The Abortion Debate in an American Community,* Faye Ginsburg states:

> the [American] cultural system requires that the individual constitute himself or herself in order to achieve a social identity, and that the means available for achieving identity are through

voluntary affiliations with others in a group that offers a comprehensive reframing of the place of the self in the social world. In this model, "individual" and "community" are not oppositional givens in American culture, but indeterminate constructs that take on definition through each other. (1998:221)

Ginsburg applied this model of identity formation via group membership and activism to women in Fargo, North Dakota, who were active in pro-choice or pro-life groups. Recognizing that for these activists, their sense of personal identity and their role in the abortion debate were intimately intertwined, she asked, "How . . . did they see their own lives in relation to their current activism on the abortion issue? The result was a set of life stories—narratively shaped fragments of more comprehensive life histories" (133).

Midwives' stories can also be read as the accounts of activists. While midwives must engage the political system when seeking legalization and licensure, their political prerogatives extend far beyond lobbying state representatives to further advance the cause of professionalization. As discussed previously, Freidson contends that the process of attaining and maintaining professional dominance is political. He bases this claim on the knowledge that professional authority is derived from the power of the government and is attained through legislative measures. Not only must a group seeking professionalization initially appeal to the sensibilities of elected officials, its members must also further establish themselves as a special interest group once professional status has been achieved (Freidson 1973:29). While this evaluation of the process may certainly apply in part to the professionalization of alternative health-care practitioners, including direct-entry midwives, Freidson's conception of the political fails to include the more radical and less normalizing aspects of the professional project for these groups. The legalization and professionalization process that has been undertaken by direct-entry midwives across the country is not political merely because it petitions state governments, but also because it is a form of midwifery activism.

Many of the direct-entry midwives I interviewed saw their work as transformative for individual clients and their families and for the world at large. One midwife asserted, "I became a midwife because I wanted to help women own that experience [childbirth], take back that gift, and be able to just experience the wonder of it themselves, without giving that over to society in the form of doctors, hospitals, modern medicine, and so on." Another midwife explained, "I really believe that babies who are born in a gentle environment without interventions, with their mothers totally present and family members, is just really a way to change the future generations of the planet."

But midwifery politics extend beyond a simple belief in women's abilities to give birth unassisted by biomedical technology, a stance that affects and can be affected by other facets of direct-entry midwives' worldviews. Many of the midwives I spoke with expressly decried what they see as the excesses of consumerism and conspicuous consumption within American culture. Other anthropologists have investigated the positive correlation between American consumer capitalism and a proliferation of technologies to be consumed within the context of pregnancy and childbirth, from ultrasonography to cesarean sections scheduled around the calendars of mothers-to-be (Davis-Floyd 1996; Taylor 1992). In this vein, Paula, a direct-entry midwife and homeopath, made the connection between families who are looking to detach themselves from this way of living and the stripped-down practices of DEMs:

> I suppose I don't share the same value system of upper-middle class people perhaps. They strive toward . . . a higher standard of living. If anything it's the opposite. We strive for a simpler way of life and . . . getting rid of rather than adding on things, and so that's probably, you know, the kind of client I attract.

Though one might argue that homebirth clients are still consumers of midwifery care, this care is relatively low-tech and inexpensive, and can even be compensated through bartering. [8]

The role of biomedical technologies used in direct-entry midwifery care is complex and may be best understood as a form of political pragmatism. Lock and Kaufert conceptualize this as a mechanism used by women toward realization of their goals, contending that, "If the apparent benefits outweigh the costs to themselves, and if the technology serves their own ends, then most women will avail themselves of what is offered" (1998:2). Direct-entry midwives resist the routine implementation of high-tech obstetrical interventions such as sonography, continuous electronic fetal monitoring, and epidurals, yet all of the midwives I interviewed incorporate some biomedical technologies into their practices. One such device is the handheld Doppler, an electronic instrument that allows the midwife to monitor fetal heart tones during labor. This permits the client to labor in whatever position she chooses, including submerged in water, options not as readily available to a client being monitored via fetoscope.[9] Because the Doppler is non-restrictive and even provides a wider range of choices to women in terms of where and how they labor and give birth, its use is advantageous to DEMs who want their clients to labor as effectively[10] and as comfortably as possible. This technology is, therefore, not implemented for its own sake, but because it advances the aims of direct-entry midwives within a politicized context.

The midwives also expressed a reluctance to cede authority to powerful and widely accepted or unquestioned beliefs about child care. Over half of the midwives I interviewed in Iowa were home-schooling or at one time home-schooled their children. At the first midwifery meeting I attended, one DEM brought an anti-circumcision poster to give to a friend, and when I later interviewed this same midwife, she wore a T-shirt that bore an anti-circumcision message. Other midwives invoked the dangers of immunizing children through means other than breastfeeding. Supporting a woman's decision to give birth outside the hospital setting, using herbal, homeopathic, or naturopathic remedies rather than pharmaceuticals, speaking out against conspicuous consumption—in all of these scenarios midwifery activism stands in opposition to aspects of the biomedical/capitalist system. As direct-entry midwifery in the United States moves toward professionalism via legalization and licensure, however, midwives are increasingly faced with the challenge of negotiating their relationship to mainstream biomedicine.

While it is easy to see everyday midwifery practice as a critique of biomedical approaches to pregnancy and childbirth that evokes a degree of unity among direct-entry midwives, the legalization cause can be both solidifying and divisive. Letter writing and lobbying can ally the personal concerns of individual midwives with the collective aims of the midwifery organization, creating a strong and united front. All of the midwives I interviewed spoke out against the financial, legal, and emotional obstacles they faced as underground practitioners. However, solidarity is only possible if these individual midwives feel that the proposed solution—legalization and licensure—would best solve their problems and those of the collective without creating a new set of equally challenging obstacles.

CRITICAL DIFFERENCES: PERSPECTIVES ON LEGALIZATION AND LICENSING

As a newcomer to the midwifery organization, I initially thought that the women I met were united in solidarity because of their shared dedication to women and childbirth, and because of their frustration that homebirth had been pushed underground and shunned by, and in favor of, the medical mainstream. Their desire, it appeared, was to rectify this situation through outright political activism. As the summer wore on, however, and I began to talk with these midwives individually, I came to understand that my initial impression of the meeting's dynamics masked multifaceted debates and personal struggles over the future of direct-entry midwifery, which issued from each interview.

Through an introduction by an Iowa direct-entry apprentice, I had the opportunity to meet a midwife currently practicing in Wisconsin, a state where direct-entry midwifery is "gray" (alegal), that is, not regulated by the state but not considered illegal. Although Wisconsin's midwives are not currently pursuing regulation efforts, Lydia's deliberative statement on her internal conflict over legalization and licensure can serve as a preface to the perspectives of Iowa midwives who are currently in the belly of the proverbial beast:

> I always wonder, "Why is midwifery different than any other profession?" I mean, you need a license just to collect money for cutting someone's hair and why is midwifery different? Why? Is it because it's a sisterhood that's always been involved in healing and helping the community? You know, in some people's minds, more of a spiritual calling. And do we have the right to be completely free to practice however we want and come from wherever we want? . . . I know a midwife that believes that, "If you think you're a midwife, you are and you have a right to practice." Or are we supposed to buckle up and be like the rest of the United States? Every single other profession out there, from chef to cutting hair to cutting fingernails requires licensing, and why? I have no idea, truly, what I believe. Why should we be different? And it's like, on one hand I do believe we should be different, but I don't know why. I can't define why.

Several of the DEMs practicing in Iowa were a bit more explicit in their oppositional stance toward regulation by the state. Rachel describes herself as a "traditional midwife"[11] and she had been in practice for close to twenty years when I interviewed her. Her path to midwifery began with the out-of-hospital birth of her first child. Soon after, she began to be invited to births, first as a photographer and then as an apprentice midwife. Rachel frames this chain of events as the result of her search for spiritual direction and guidance after her daughter's birth, and she has pursued midwifery ever since. Her involvement in the midwifery organization has waned over the years, especially since the group began pursuing legalization. As our interview began to wind down, she emphasized her increasing disenchantment with the political powers with which she would have greater contact if midwifery were legal and regulated, stating:

> There's various times in my life when I've been more political, and at this point the politics of it, just seeing what's coming down in the government, the system, the President and all of that—how can I hold that to any kind of stock with the work that I'm doing? I'm doing the work [midwifery] that God has given me so that goes beyond all of that other stuff for me. . . . I'm not looking to that to give me something because I already have it. I don't want them to give me more than I already have. I'm doing the work that has been given to me. . . . I feel that I'm living it, I'm living my politics.

Rachel's objections reflect the idea that midwifery should not be confused with the practice of biomedicine (Suarez 1993). Though it is all but impossible for direct-entry midwives to practice without a fair amount of interaction with biomedical practitioners, settings, and tools (Weitz and Sullivan 1985, 1986; Lay, this volume), the philosophies of care and values that separate the two are of utmost importance to Rachel. Legislative change would blur the sharp boundaries between DEMs as practitioners who reject obstetrical knowledge and the biomedical status quo, and the physicians and legislators who have thus far upheld these standards (Reid 1989:235).

Rachel's brand of midwifery activism is played out in the everyday, in the rhythm and pace her daily life has taken on because she is a midwife. This level of engagement with a social movement, in this case the U.S. midwifery or homebirth movement, has been referred to as participation in a "submerged network" wherein members self-consciously and presently engage in changes they would like to see made in the future (Schneirov and Geczik 1996). These actions may be described as "largely invisible since they are embedded in everyday life and not openly engaged in political acts like demonstrations, sit-ins, petitioning, and the like" (Schneirov and Geczik 1996:630). While she acknowledges once being more involved in public, political acts, Rachel defines her politics in contrast to an engagement with mainstream medicine and the state. Rather than seeking new rights and privileges from these powerful sources, she strives for autonomy and distance from them.

Eliza, a young midwife who had been in practice for five years at the time of our interview, describes herself as a "fence-rider" in terms of legislative efforts. After her first child was delivered by cesarean section, Eliza began searching out alternatives to obstetrical care and delivered her second baby at home with direct-entry midwives in attendance. She then worked toward certification as a childbirth educator and began attending homebirths in that capacity before beginning an apprenticeship with the midwives who had helped her give birth at home.[12] Eliza feels that legal recognition would lead to a greater number of women having homebirths, which fits into her hopeful vision of a more perfect world. This positive change, however, is weighed against the restrictions she envisions with the introduction of regulations for direct-entry practices:

> I would like it to be decriminalized, but at the same time it just seems like playing into that whole medical mindset, you know? Midwifery's just this normal, mammal thing to do. . . . I feel like midwives are going to be arrested if it's legal. I feel like we're going to be very restricted in what we can do. Especially for me it's doing VBACs, which is vaginal birth after cesarean. Because my first baby was a cesarean and I think it's very important that we do VBACs at home and I think that they would say we cannot.

Furthermore, she fears that obtaining licenses will lead midwives to lose sight of the beliefs that led them to a homebirth practice. Eliza herself is concerned that she would sell out and refuse VBAC clients in order to preserve her legal and regulated status. These fears resonate with Baer's (1989) contention that mainstream legitimization of alternative medical practices leads to accommodation to biomedical beliefs and practices.

The strength of the commitment that binds direct-entry midwives to their clients has been partially explained by their shared secret of illegal activity. DeVries argues that "the relationship between the unlicensed midwife and her client reflects its illegal nature. . . . The midwife is providing a necessary service that she and the expectant parents believe in and yet that is defined as illegal, allowing for a sense of unification behind a 'cause'" (1996:110, see also Reid 1989). The homebirth cause has made clients extremely protective of their midwives even when bad outcomes occur, and has propelled midwives to take legal, financial, and personal risks for their clients.

The more pragmatic side of Eliza's concerns relating to restriction of practice and arrest are certainly not unfounded: midwifery legislation has not always unequivocally benefited direct-entry midwives. During the summer of 1999, the Minnesota state legislature signed into law a bill that made the CPM the direct-entry midwifery licensing standard (see Lay, this volume). No less than eight months later, another bill was drafted by a state senator, which would severely limit CPMs' scope of practice. According to the consumer organization Minnesota Families for Midwifery, this proposed legislation would:

> require a physician's oversight of a midwife's practice. For insurance and political reasons, it would be practically an impossibility for a midwife to find a physician who would agree to such a relationship. This part of the bill alone would end traditional midwifery in this state. There are three other main changes that this bill proposes to the current legislation: doing away with the possibility of birthing centers, making licensure mandatory, and expanding the advisory council (which currently includes three midwives, one consumer and one physician) to include three midwives, two physicians, one nurse-midwife, one consumer and two "members of the public." In other words, the traditional midwives would be outnumbered on a council that is in place to regulate the midwives' profession. (2000)

Passing legislation to legalize and license direct-entry midwifery is only a first step toward validation and autonomy for DEMs, and clearly this process does not guarantee that licensed midwives will not be caught between their own personal standards of safe practice and the state's restrictions on the scope of midwifery practice.

Lydia, a midwife from Wisconsin, discussed the difficulties some of her fellow midwives who work in a licensed state endure during hospital transports:

> I have friends in Colorado who practice and, now that it's legal there, the doctors are all over their charts, looking for problems, looking for stuff that they've done illegally. So they lie on their charts. You know, they have to. Now that they're "legal," now they're being scrutinized in ways that they never were and they have to lie about good care that they gave because they're not allowed to give pitocin.[13] [*sarcastically*] What kind of law is that? Let's set up a law and then set up protocols so that you have to practice unsafely.

Even though licensure may build bridges among direct-entry midwives, new homebirth clients, and mainstream biomedicine, it does not ensure a midwife's right to practice according to her own standards and the protocols she had while unlicensed and underground.

Despite these objections to seeking licensure through the state legislature, most of the midwives I interviewed believe that legalization and regulation will help create a more secure future for direct-entry midwifery and allow midwives to gain respect and recognition. Their justifications of these changes complement the criticisms of legalization offered by other midwives. Rather than focusing on the potentially restrictive effects of regulation, several midwives pinpointed potential sites of expansion and legitimization for legal midwifery practice, from insurance reimbursement to open collaboration with physicians to establishing a direct-entry midwifery school in Iowa.

While some midwives fear that DEMs who are competent and practice safely will be arrested if they choose not to be certified, pro-legalization midwives point out that there is currently no formal peer review process in Iowa to identify underskilled or incompetent midwives. This aspect of the licensing issue was highlighted by Sandra, who had been practicing as a direct-entry midwife for twenty years. As a college student, she researched the history of obstetrics and midwifery for a women's studies course and became interested in pursuing an education in midwifery. The CNM route was closed to her because she did not want to attend nursing school, so she looked internationally for her training and chose a program in the United Kingdom. After her formal education was complete, Sandra worked both for the National Health Service in the hospital setting and in private practice as a homebirth midwife in the United Kingdom, where certified midwives have practiced legally under regulation in all settings since 1902 (Donnison 1977).[14] Before returning to the United States she explained her dedication to legislation that would regulate DEMs in Iowa:

> This is a profession where you could kill somebody or let them die or do them harm. And I don't want to be regulated by doctors, but it needs regulation. I would like to be able to, if I am really concerned about somebody's practice, to have somebody to talk to who could do something about it. Right now there's nothing. Either you turn them in and they get slapped with a class-D felony or you do nothing. Who's going to turn them in under those circumstances? You know, it doesn't have to be so extreme. With peer review, which is meant to be the process, you can hopefully communicate that they may need to modify some of their practice, that it's not good enough.

SPIRITUAL/PROFESSIONAL:
FORGING NEW SELF-DEFINITIONS

This range of perspectives on the legalization and licensure of direct-entry midwifery in Iowa is also connected to midwives' attitudes toward professionalization because the two processes go hand in hand. When many of these women spoke of their personal journeys to midwifery and reflected on their experiences with homebirth and their clients, they incorporated concepts of spirituality, intuition, and vocation. All but one midwife I interviewed referred to midwifery as her calling or vocation. Many added that midwifery cannot be as easily separated from the rest of one's life as a more conventional nine-to-five occupation. It is easy to cede this point when one considers that most DEMs work within their homes with their families in tow, and base a good deal of their advice to clients on their own experiences as pregnant women, wives, and mothers. However, when the interviews shifted to a discussion of legalization and licensure, the midwives stressed the importance of professionalism, competence, and credibility.

Eileen had been practicing as a midwife for just over a year when we met at her interview, though she has served as a doula[15] for eighteen years. Before pursuing midwifery, she had worked as a secretary, a banker, and a hospital administrator, but she had always felt that a large portion of her life would be dedicated to birth. She emphasized:

> You know, it's not something that's just attractive or curious to me, it's my life. It is my life. I will do it—if I could not do it, I could not live. I would not want to. . . . I know it's strange sounding but it is very empowering for me to be, to help another woman be empowered by a positive birth experience, so it's a spiritual kind of thing. It goes beyond words.

But these spiritual, organic aspects of her relationship to her calling are not in the foreground when she addresses the importance of midwifery regulation: "I do think that there needs to be some regulation because there are midwives out there who lack the expertise to handle situations that could arise that could prove to be fatal. . . . I think we owe it to ourselves and our profession at large to be accountable and knowledgeable," as well as developing a backup relationship with an obstetrician, "I think it adds to my entire credibility and my professionalism so I would strive for that."

Eileen's statements about professionalization are made more complex when one considers the ways her life has been, and continues to be, connected to biomedicine. On the one hand, her own professional experiences as a hospital administrator allowed her to see the negative effects of the alienating uses of knowledge within the biomedical context:

> The exposure that I had in hospital administration let me see that patients have the right to decline options, have the right to complain about their care providers, have a right to complain that they're overcharged. Every patient should request to see their bill, things like that. And prior to that experience, I was blindly going along like the rest of the world thinking, "this is the way it is, this is the way it has to be."

On the other hand, her husband is a physician, and as Eileen explained, he would be "the happiest man in the world" if she decided to pursue a nurse-midwifery degree rather than continue working as a DEM. Also, her calling has generated friction within her social circle, which is comprised of individuals who have a more mainstream outlook on biomedicine:

> Considering that most of my friends are doctors or doctors' wives, you know, I just don't talk about it in front of them. You know, [with] some of them I do because they know if I can't make it to a function because I had a birth, they know. Everyone knows that I do this. Nobody talks about it because they know it's illegal, and I have friends who think I'm absolutely nuts. They think that my husband is absolutely nuts for allowing me to do this, but you know, that's how they look at it.

Though her own experiences as a doula, a midwife, and a hospital administrator have made her critical of the alienating dimensions of biomedical professionalism, her family and friends are invested in the dominant medical model. These aspects of Eileen's life suggest a complicated view of biomedical authority that is mediated by her understanding of midwifery as both an organic and spiritual calling and a legitimate profession.

Paula, a strong supporter of licensure, has been practicing as a midwife for just over a decade; she is also an alternative-healing practitioner. Currently in the process of earning her CPM, she also teaches midwifery classes. In her interview, Paula reemphasized Eileen's notion of "calling," when she told me, "a midwife is a midwife inside of herself, in the deepest part of herself. And you can't make that. You can't make a midwife if she's not already a midwife. And in the process of a midwife going through her education, it's more of a remembering. It's more of a recollection than it is a training."

Later, Paula discussed with me her prominent role in the drafting of the scope of practice review and her hope that legalization and licensure in Iowa will allow her to open a school for DEMs that would provide low-cost care for women and a clinical site for apprentice midwives. Paula also added that she believes professionalism is a key concept that currently divides CNMs and DEMs:

> Because everything we do as midwives is a reflection of who we are as people, just as the way a woman gives birth is a reflection of who she is as a person…and until that's acknowledged by CNMs, nothing's going to change in terms of our merging together to form this great, you know, unity and diversity. Because most CNMs can't seem to acknowledge that. You know, for them, it seems to me, it's much more of a profession. You know, they are usually very proud of the fact that they're professionals, and we can't separate ourselves from the work that we do.

She believes that DEMs will maintain their "pioneering kind of independent spirit" in the midst of professionalization, should midwifery become licensed in Iowa. Though she firmly believes that DEMs will reject an alignment with allopathic medicine that some see as an imminent result of instituting midwifery as a profession (DeVries 1985, 1996), Paula nonetheless contends that seeking the validation of midwifery through legislative measures is necessary to insure acceptable standards of competency among DEMs. She resolves the seeming contradiction in her views by arguing that the professionalization of *midwifery* will not professionalize direct-entry *midwives* themselves.

Both Eileen's and Paula's accounts demonstrate that unilateral understandings of one's identity as a direct-entry midwife and the meanings of direct-entry midwifery's present and future are increasingly unworkable as legal recognition and wider acceptance are sought. Their investment in raising the standard for midwives is paralleled by their certainty that legalization and licensure will not fundamentally alter their commitment to midwifery as a calling and as an alternative to both obstetrics and nurse-midwifery.

QUESTIONING AUTHORITY: CLIENT RESPONSIBILITY AND MIDWIFE ACCOUNTABILITY

The multiple meanings of direct-entry midwifery also surfaced in the context of practitioner–client relationships, specifically in the negotiation of issues of responsibility for, and authority over, the health of homebirth clients. The notion that individuals who seek out direct-entry midwifery care should be well informed and willing to be fully accountable for the health care decisions they make during their pregnancy, as well as the eventual outcome of their pregnancy, was a constant in all of the interviews I conducted. Placing responsibility in the clients' hands is a marked shift from biomedical care in which expectant women and/or couples are denied decision-making power (Butter and Kay 1990:1331).

Accompanying client responsibility, however, is the midwife's ultimate liability for a bad outcome. DEMs who attend homebirths in Iowa are protected neither by the law nor by malpractice insurance. Though clients can pursue legal action against their midwife, the majority of charges brought against DEMs originate with physicians, indicating that a midwife puts herself in jeopardy any time she transfers a client to hospital care where attending physicians may feel that her care had been incompetent and irresponsible (DeVries 1985:120).[16]

Denise is a DEM who is pursuing a CNM degree, "kicking and screaming the whole way," so she might practice legally in Iowa. She is also concurrently working toward her CPM because she feels that this credential will better represent her philosophy of care and homebirth training. When I asked her, "What inspired you to become a midwife?" she responded:

> I think that I have always been a midwife in my heart, even as far back as I can remember, being in kindergarten. I knew I needed to work with mothers and babies, but it wasn't until my first pregnancy that I discovered the profession of midwifery through a really bad first birth [in the hospital].

As we discussed the issue of responsibility during homebirth, she had this to say about empowering clients with decision making:

> They have the right to decide how they want it done, they have the right to say no. They must also accept the responsibility for the outcome, and I think that is an important point that other health-care providers can learn from traditional midwives to reduce their own risk of liability. If you help the client accept responsibility and empower them to make their own choices, they are going to be much less likely to file lawsuits and look for someone else to blame.

Denise views this distribution of responsibility not only as a means to balance power in the client–practitioner relationship, but also as a *professional* and personal strategy to avoid the potential legal and financial consequences of a bad outcome.

She invokes two important features of direct-entry midwifery care as it is currently practiced in Iowa: midwives believe that women and their families have the right to decide where and how they will deliver their children, and midwives are not privy to any legal or financial safety nets as practitioners. Denise's words are echoed in other midwives' accounts. Rachel stated, "For us, we need the cream of the crop, the healthiest women because we want women taking responsibility for their own births. And because they are taking responsibility for that, we are there to monitor safety and backup, so we don't take that responsibility." Paula explained, "I have [the client] sign [an informed consent form], and that says that she takes full responsibility for this pregnancy and birth and that she understands that there are risks involved no matter what the birth setting and that she will not hold me liable in any way." Eileen commented, "In homebirth you have to take a more personal accountability for everything that goes on in your birth and it surprises some people to know that, to realize that they have to be more involved in this birth than they would if they went to a hospital."

However, when DEMs believe that clients have not been taking adequate responsibility for their health they have the option of "risking out" their client: discontinuing midwifery care if they feel that the client's behaviors may lead to complications during labor and delivery that would fall outside their range of capabilities as low-tech, minimal intervention practitioners.[17] Many midwives had stories to tell about ties with clients that needed to be severed for this reason. "We've had clients that we've had to risk out very late in the pregnancy because they lied or were not following recommendations and the physical exam showed other than that," Denise noted.

> Yes, I had one client . . . that I took care of throughout the pregnancy, and I actually did some labor-sitting during false labor for her. When she thought she was going into labor I actually spent the night at her house, and it became obvious when I was there that she hadn't been eating. . . . The baby wasn't growing at all, and so I did explain to the mother that I didn't think it was safe.

If the midwife feels that her client is not adequately maintaining her health, her own authority and knowledge as the health-care provider allow her to discontinue care. While DEMs emphasize the importance of client responsibility, this does not indicate a hands-off approach. Clients are meant to be decision makers and authorities in their own right, yet they are not free to choose behaviors that the midwife could label irresponsible. Within this context, midwives can and do exercise a fair amount of authority.

As Iowa's direct-entry midwives seek legalization and professionalization, it seems that the complex value placed on client responsibility, in light of the family's rights and the midwife's ultimate accountability, may be substantially transformed. If legalized, will midwives increasingly take on decision-making authority for fear of losing their licensure and damaging direct-entry midwifery's new professionalism, or will the budding credibility of DEMs in the eyes of the state established through legalization make room for a model of the client–practitioner relationship that does not mirror biomedicine? Will legal and financial (if insurance is made available) safety nets reduce the need for client responsibility or will these measures dispel personal anxieties and encourage a shared sense of authority between midwives and clients? At this point, the answers to such questions remain to be seen in Iowa. Regardless of these answers, however, one can be certain that direct-entry midwifery's new relationships with biomedicine and the state will further transform the meanings that these women attach to their identities as midwives and the practices attached to these identities.

CONCLUSION: LOOKING TOWARD THE FUTURE

For direct-entry midwives in the United States today, the pursuit of legalization and licensure in states where their practices are presently prohibited or not clearly defined by law is not merely a professionalizing process but a deeply political process as well. In Iowa, these efforts are motivated by the belief that women and their families should have the right to pursue an alternative to biomedical obstetric or nurse-midwifery care, and an understanding that direct-entry midwives must be competent and accountable health care practitioners.

Yet these political views reflect an opposition to biomedical norms that becomes blurred through this very process of becoming "legitimate" practitioners. Working through the system to gain credibility can be seen as a process of negotiation and resistance, and one must be careful to implement these terms in a way that truly reflects the realities and repercussions that accompany the professionalization of alternative health practices. In this chapter I have explored the internal debate within the Iowa Midwives Association and the multifaceted feelings of its members about the legalization process, which complicate any notion of a unified resistance to biomedicine.

The initiative to legitimize direct-entry midwifery through legislative action has produced a shift in the meanings midwives attach to themselves *as* midwives, which is reflected in the complex accounts of personal and professional identity, and responsibility as practitioners that Iowa DEMs recounted to me. These transformations, it seems, will be furthered by the (potential) actualization of direct-entry midwifery professionalization in the state. Whether legislative change will allow midwives to retain their independence, bringing about further resistance to biomedicine, or whether it will bring midwives' alternative practices and philosophies of care under restrictive scrutiny by biomedicine and the state remains to be seen.

POSTSCRIPT[18]

After the conclusion of my research with Iowa's direct-entry midwives in 1999, the efforts of the IMA to gain a new level of recognition and respect for direct-entry midwives in Iowa persisted. The scope of practice review took place between August 1999 and February 2000 and the committee concluded that direct-entry midwifery should be legalized within the state, and that all practicing DEMs should hold the Certified Professional Midwife (CPM) or Certified Midwife (CM) credential,[19] and that they should register with the Iowa Department of Public Health. Though the committee did not approve of all aspects of the IMA's application, including the ability to assist in VBACs and carry oxygen and pitocin to births, their decision on the legalization of direct-entry midwifery prompted the IMA to submit legislation to this effect to the Iowa House of Representatives. Strong opposition by physicians and the Iowa Medical Society (IMS) continued, the legalization bill died in committee, and it has yet to be reintroduced. The Attorney General's opinion of 1978, which holds direct-entry midwifery to be the practice of medicine without a license in the state of Iowa and therefore a class-D felony, still stands.

As this chapter has shown, the pursuit of legislative means by the IMA to legalize DEMs in Iowa has been contentious. Some midwives have been unwaveringly wary of or opposed to this political process from the beginning, while others became disillusioned during the preparation of the scope of practice review, and still others continue to have faith in the legislative project despite its shortcomings. The IMA remains an active organization and though its members have, currently (and perhaps temporarily) discontinued attempts to legalize through legislation, Iowa's DEMs continue to discuss and debate future pathways to legalization as well as decriminalization of direct-entry midwifery in the state through an overturning of the Attorney General's opinion.

TIMELINE OF DIRECT-ENTRY MIDWIFERY IN IOWA

1978   An Iowa state's attorney's opinion declares that unlicensed midwives can be considered to be practicing medicine and surgery without a license.

1994   DEMs petition through a state representative for the 1978 opinion to be reviewed. Their request is denied.

1996   The Iowa Midwives Association (IMA) is formed from Midwives Alliance of Midwest America (MAMA), and the consumer advocacy group Iowans for Birth Options (IBO) is established. Scope-of-practice reviews for health professionals are instituted in Iowa.

1998   Legislation drafted by the IMA to legalize direct-entry midwifery is submitted to the Iowa House of Representatives and is sent to the Human Resources Committee. The bill is submitted late in the legislative session and the IMA is encouraged to resubmit it the following year.

1999   The legalization bill is resubmitted and a scope of practice review application is presented to the Iowa Department of Public Health by the IMA.

2000   The scope of practice committee declares that direct-entry midwifery should be legalized and that midwives with the Certified Professional Midwife (CPM) or Certified Midwife (CM) credential should be registered with the state's Department of Public Health. New legalization legislation based on the committee's recommendations is drafted and submitted by the IMA, but the bill dies in committee. This legislation has not yet been reintroduced.

ACKNOWLEDGMENT

I wish to thank the University of Iowa Student Government's Research Grants Committee for funding the master's fieldwork on which this chapter is based.

ENDNOTES

1. Within this chapter, the terms "midwife," "midwives," and "midwifery" refer to direct-entry midwives and the practice of direct-entry midwifery.

2. Alternative/holistic medicine is a broad category used to describe health-care systems that reject the reductionism of allopathy in favor of individualized, low-tech care "in which biochemical processes, emotional states, beliefs, lifestyle practices (especially nutrition) and spiritual phenomena are thought to be interconnected" (Schneirov and Geczik 1996:629).

3. The results of DeVries's (1983) study of West Coast hospital alternative birth centers discovered that the average rate of transfer from birth center to traditional delivery room was 22.58 percent, a surprisingly high figure considering that women who chose the alternative birth center were screened for normalcy throughout their pregnancies. He also cited a study of Washington state birth centers, which showed that protocols allowing high-tech interventions such as electronic fetal monitoring and analgesic/anesthetic pain management in these alternative settings are extremely common (DeVries 1983:7).

4. In all, I interviewed twelve direct-entry midwives for this project. These midwives are a snowball sample derived from a list of practicing DEMs in Iowa provided by the Midwives Alliance of North America. One of these initial contacts informed me of the Iowa Midwives Association meeting where I met many of my informants. Ten of the twelve midwives live and work in Iowa. Of these, one was an apprentice and one was currently not practicing though still active in the midwifery community. The two other DEMs I interviewed live and work in Wisconsin and were introduced to me by a former apprentice currently living in Iowa. Each interview lasted from one to three hours, and I audio tape-recorded and transcribed all interviews.

5. The criteria that must be met by a scope-of-practice review application in Iowa are fourfold. For the committee to recommend legislative change that would legalize and license DEMs, the IMA needed to prove that "the present condition creates a situation of actual or potential harm or danger to the public, the proposed change does not impose any significant new harm or danger to the public, the public health, safety and welfare are reasonably expected to benefit from the requested change, the public health cannot be effectively protected by other more cost-effective means" (Iowa Department of Public Health 2000:1).

6. All names of midwives used in this paper are pseudonyms.

7. The term *client* rather than *patient* was used consistently throughout all of the interviews, highlighting the fact that DEMs resist the terminology of biomedicine and do not consider pregnancy a pathological state that would allow them to characterize the women in their care as sick patients.

8. Direct-entry midwives in Iowa are not financially compensated by clients' health insurance. To offset or, on occasion, replace cash payments, many midwives will barter their services for other services or goods. Some midwives bartered for home repair (carpentry, drywalling) or auto repair work, butchered livestock, and quilts, among other things.

9. A fetoscope is a device, much like a stethoscope, that allows the midwife to hear fetal heart tones. Some of the midwives involved in this research bring both a Doppler and a fetoscope to births. Some preferred using a fetoscope regularly because it allows a more hands-on approach to fetal monitoring, and Denise commented, "A Doppler amplifies the rate of sound, but it doesn't let you hear the heartbeats directly and with a fetoscope, you can train your ear to pick up the little subtle nuances of how strong the heartbeat is, whether there is a murmur present which there almost always is in a fetus . . . and you really need to be able to hear that when the baby is inside the mother so that you have the comparison afterwards. A Doppler is easier because the sound is louder. It's easier of you don't have a trained ear. It can also pick up the heartbeat when the baby's in a real difficult position. So, there is a need for both."

10. Ambulating and changing positions is encouraged by midwives to promote the progression of labor (see Gaskin 1996).

11. When I asked Rachel why she preferred the term "traditional midwife" she said, "I think it more describes the way that we practice, the way that I practice in that we come to it through traditional means which would be apprenticing with other midwives and self-study. And what we bring to midwifery, of course, is a lot of traditional

skills and thoughts and theory mixed with the best of what modern convenience, modern society has to offer us. So we kind of make a blend of what's out there today and the wisdom that's always been there."

12. Direct-entry apprenticeships vary in length. Eliza, for example, had been working as an apprentice for five years at the time of our interview and she had recently begun attending births as a primary attendant, though she mostly continued to go to births with the senior midwives with whom she apprenticed.

13. Pitocin (oxytocin) is a synthetic hormone used by midwives as the ultimate measure to prevent excessive bleeding during the third stage of labor at home. Herbs and manual compression of the uterus are other, less interventive techniques used by DEMs. Pitocin is used in hospital settings to augment labor and to prevent hemorrhage.

14. In addition to interviewing midwives who practice in Iowa and Wisconsin, I also interviewed a friend of Sandra's who currently has a homebirth practice in the United Kingdom. She explained, "The law in England is that a woman can give birth completely unattended. She can catch her own baby. She's perfectly entitled to do that. But, if she's going to choose an attendant, it must be a doctor or a midwife. . . . And that's really to protect against lay midwifery [practicing midwifery with no formal training] because that's completely illegal in Britain."

15. A doula is defined by Rooks as "a woman who attends births in order to support the mother and assist the primary birth attendant (whether a physician or a midwife)" (1997:10). Eileen's experiences as a doula have been primarily in the hospital setting, but she had also more recently begun to provide doula services at homebirths.

16. Midwives are not the only ones at risk if complications arise during an out-of-hospital birth. Anna Lowenhaupt Tsing (1990) addresses the phenomena of women charged with perinatal endangerment in the context of unassisted birth.

17. Direct-entry midwives provide care for women they consider to have low-risk pregnancies. Though risk-screening protocols are variable and flexible, all of the midwives I interviewed take detailed medical histories of each prospective client to spot potential risks, and they will not provide primary care for pregnancies involving twins, a breech presentation at birth, or women with serious, chronic medical problems such as heart disease, insulin-dependent diabetes, or kidney disease. DEMs will also consider psychological factors and their personal compatibility with clients as justification for risking out.

18. Special thanks to Rixa Freeze who was able to provide additional information on legalization and legislative efforts that have taken place within the IMA since the year 2000.

19. The CM credential was created by the American College of Nurse-Midwives (ACNM) and has a set of educational and clinical requirements that differ in certain respects from those of the CPM (see chapters 1–3, this volume).

REFERENCES

Abu-Lughod, Lila. 1990. "The Romance of Resistance: Tracing Transformations of Power through Bedouin Women." *American Ethnologist* 17(1):41–55.

Baer, Hans. 1984. "The Drive for Professionalization in British Osteopathy." *Social Science & Medicine* 19(7):717–725.

———. 1989. "The American Dominative Medical System as a Reflection of Social Relations in the Larger Society." *Social Science and Medicine* 28(11):1103–1112.

Baer, Hans, Cindy Jen, Lucia M. Tanassi, Christopher Tsia, and Helen Wahbeh. 1989. "The Drive for Professionalization in Acupuncture: A Preliminary View from the San Francisco Bay Area." *Social Science and Medicine* 46(4–5):533–537.

Baer, Hans, Merrill Singer, and Ida Susser. 1997. *Medical Anthropology and the World System: A Critical Perspective.* Westport, CT: Bergin & Garvey.

Butter, Irene H., and Bonnie J. Kay. 1990. "Self-Certification in Lay Midwives' Organizations: A Vehicle for Professional Autonomy." *Social Science and Medicine* 30(12):1329–1339.

Cant, Sarah, and Ursula Sharma. 1996. "Demarcation and Transformation within Homoeopathic Knowledge: A Strategy of Professionalization." *Social Science and Medicine* 42(4):579–588.

Davis-Floyd, Robbie E. 1996. "The Technocratic Body and the Organic Body: Hegemony and Heresy in Women's Birth Choices." In *Gender and Health,* ed. Carolyn Sargent and Caroline Brettell, 123–66. Upper Saddle River, NJ: Prentice Hall.

———. 1998. "The Ups, Downs and Interlinkages of Nurse- and Direct-Entry Midwifery: Status, Practice, and Education." In *Pathways to Becoming a Midwife: Getting an Education,* ed. Midwifery Today, 1–40. Eugene, OR: Midwifery Today.

Davis-Floyd, Robbie, Sheila Cosminsky, and Stacy Leigh Pigg. 2001. "Daughters of Time: The Shifting Identities of Contemporary Midwives." *Medical Anthropology* 20(2–3):112.

Davis-Floyd, Robbie E., and Elizabeth Davis. 1996. "Intuition as Authoritative Knowledge in Midwifery and Home Birth." In *Childbirth and Authoritative Knowledge,* ed. Robbie E. Davis-Floyd and Carolyn F. Sargent, 315–349. Berkeley: University of California Press.

DeVries, Raymond. 1983. "Image and Reality: An Evaluation of Hospital Alternative Birth Centers." *Journal of Nurse Midwifery* 28(3):3–9.

———. 1984. *Regulating Birth: Medicine, Midwives and the Law.* Philadelphia, PA: Temple University Press.

———. 1996. *Making Midwives Legal: Childbirth, Medicine and the Law.* Columbus: Ohio State University Press.

Donnison, Jean. 1977. *Midwives and Medical Men.* London: Heinemann.

Freidson, Eliot. 1970. *Profession of Medicine.* New York: Dodd, Mead & Co.

———. 1973. "Professions and the Occupational Principle." In *The Professions and Their Prospects,* ed. Eliot Freidson, 19–38. Beverly Hills, CA: Sage.

Gaskin, Ina May. 1996. "Intuition and the Emergence of Midwifery as Authoritative Knowledge." *Medical Anthropology Quarterly* 10(2):295–298.

Ginsburg, Faye. 1998. *Contested Lives: The Abortion Debate in an American Community.* Berkeley: University of California Press.

Hough, Carolyn. 1999. "Dangerous Intersections: Examining Nurse-Midwives' Perceptions of Risk in Home and Hospital Birth." Paper presented at the 121st Meeting of the American Ethnological Society, Portland, Oregon.

Iowa Attorney General. 1978. "Midwifery." In *Report of the Attorney General of Iowa,* 371–373, 399. Des Moines, Iowa.

Iowa Department of Public Health. 2000. *Report of the Midwifery Scope of Practice Committee,* Des Moines, Iowa.

Lock, Margaret, and Patricia Kaufert. 1998. Introduction to *Pragmatic Women and Body Politics,* ed. Margaret Lock and Patricia Kaufert. New York: Cambridge University Press.

Mechanic, David. 1976. *The Growth of Bureaucratic Medicine.* New York: John Wiley & Sons.

Minnesota Families for Midwifery. 2000. Minnesota Families for Midwifery homepage, http://www.mfmidwifery.org/legal.html.

Ong, Aihwa. 1997. "Spirits of Resistance." In *Situated Lives: Gender and Culture in Everyday Life.* ed. Louise Lamphere, Helena Ragone, and Patricia Zavella, 355–370. New York: Routledge.

Ortner, Sherry B. 1995. "Resistance and the Problem of Ethnographic Refusal." *Comparative Studies in Society and History* 37(1):173–193.

Reid, Margaret. 1989. "Sisterhood and Professionalization: A Case Study of the American Lay Midwife." In *Women as Healers*, ed. Carol Shepherd McClain, 219–238. New Brunswick, NJ: Rutgers University Press.

Rooks, Judith Pence. 1997. *Midwifery and Childbirth in America*. Philadelphia, PA: Temple University Press.

Rothman, Barbara Katz. 1981. "Awake and Aware or False Consciousness: The Co-optation of Childbirth Reform in America." In *Childbirth: Alternatives to Medical Control*. Shelly Romalis, 150–180. Austin: University of Texas Press.

Ruzek, Sheryl Burt. 1977. *The Women's Health Movement*. New York: Praeger.

Schneirov, Matthew, and Jonathan David Geczik. 1995. "A Diagnosis for Our Times: Alternative Health's Submerged Networks and the Transformation of Identities." *Sociological Quarterly* 37(4):627–644.

Suarez, Suzanne Hope. 1993. "Midwifery Is Not the Practice of Medicine." *Yale Journal of Law and Feminism* 5(3):315–365.

Taylor, Janelle S. 1992. "The Public Fetus and the Family Car: From Abortion Politics to a Volvo Advertisement." *Public Culture* 4(2):67–80.

Tsing, Anna Lowenhaupt. 1989. "Monster Stories: Women Charged with Perinatal Endangerment." In *Uncertain Terms: Negotiating Gender in American Culture*, ed. Faye Ginsburg and Anna Tsing, 282–299. Boston, MA: Beacon.

Weitz, Rose, and Deborah Sullivan. 1985. "Licensed Lay Midwifery and the Medical Model of Childbirth." *Sociology of Health and Illness* 7(1):36–54.

———. 1985. *Labor Pains: Modern Midwives and Home Birth*. New Haven, CT.: Yale University Press.

Zola, Irving Kenneth, and Stephen J. Miller. 1973. "The Erosion of Medicine from Within." In *The Professions and Their Prospects*, ed. Eliot Freidson, 153–172. Beverly Hills, CA: Sage.

9

CREATING A WAY OUT OF NO WAY: MIDWIFERY IN MASSACHUSETTS

Christine Barbara Johnson

- Introduction: The Legal Status of Nurse- and Direct-Entry Midwives in Massachusetts • Overturning Historical Precedent • A Unified Midwifery Model • Creating a Way out of No Way, Again?
- Timeline of Midwifery History in Massachusetts

INTRODUCTION: THE LEGAL STATUS OF NURSE- AND DIRECT-ENTRY MIDWIVES IN MASSACHUSETTS

This chapter examines the historical and present struggles of midwives in Massachusetts as they interact with medical and political-legal structures in their attempts to establish professional credibility. Since 1907, when Massachusetts became the first state to declare midwifery the practice of medicine, physicians had been the only licensed prenatal care/birth practitioners. In the early 1970s both direct-entry and nurse-midwives began their own respective battles to become prenatal care/ birth providers. The Massachusetts Medical Society used its social, political, and economic hegemony to prevent both groups of midwives from administering prenatal care and attending births.

The medical lobby battled fiercely to block licensure of nurse-midwives and in the eleventh hour mobilized enough political power to pressure the governor into vetoing the new nurse-midwifery legislation. However, ultimately the Medical Society failed and the nurse-midwives triumphed. In 1977, Massachusetts became one of the last states to pass a bill legalizing CNMs. Direct-entry midwives (DEMs) occupied a more structurally ambiguous position than their nurse-midwifery counterparts. DEMs operated within the private sector, outside the jurisdiction of medicine, by educating themselves in home study groups as well as attending births at home. The 1907 law declaring midwifery the practice of medicine left these midwives vulnerable to legal sanction that could criminalize their activities. As homebirth became increasingly popular and the press responded with favorable coverage, the Medical Society marshaled all its resources, this time backed by legal precedent, in an attempt to outlaw this emergent group of practitioners. Once again they failed. In 1985, midwifery was declared separate and distinct from the practice of medicine.

Massachusetts history illustrates how articulate counterclaims to medical definitions of reality can successfully challenge the professional physician monopoly, both from within and from outside mainstream medical institutions. This stage in Massachusetts history highlights the fluid nature of institutions and institutional definitions of the situation. That is, from this case study it can be deduced that while it is critical not to underestimate structural constraints, it is equally vital not to reify these structures. New health-care ideas and practices can emerge precisely because institutions are both created and re-created through everyday negotiation, interpretation, and social interaction.

Autonomy vs. Legitimacy: Joining Forces

Analysis of present midwifery struggles demonstrates how even successful challenges to a medical monopoly do not automatically alter professional physician dominance. When newly licensed health-care practitioners are brought within the professional jurisdiction of medicine, and those who operate outside this jurisdiction are blocked from gaining licensure, the threat these alternative care providers pose can be neutralized. In Massachusetts, nurse-midwives are licensed maternity care practitioners, and their practice is closely tied to physicians, thus severely limiting their professional autonomy. Direct-entry midwives have gained their autonomy at the expense of professional legitimacy. That is, they operate outside the jurisdiction of medicine by attending births at home but remain unlicensed, marginal practitioners.

Under the present circumstances, neither type of midwife can achieve legitimacy and autonomous professional status simultaneously. To alter this state of affairs, DEMs and CNMs have put aside their professional rivalries and joined forces to initiate a bill that would license all midwives as independent professionals. If they succeed, Massachusetts will make national history by becoming the first state in the country to have a joint board of midwifery pertaining to all types of certified midwives—CNMs, CMs, and CPMs. Ironically, professional medical opposition, which has successfully constrained the practice of all midwifery in Massachusetts, has been the catalyst for spearheading the first united midwifery legislative effort in the country. In this case, circumstances favoring initial medical dominance may ultimately produce the very conditions that undermine medical control over birth.

OVERTURNING HISTORICAL PRECEDENT[1]
The Legalization of Nurse-Midwifery

By 1975, women choosing to give birth at home in Massachusetts had become a recognizable and growing minority. The press took note, and in 1977 the *Boston Globe* featured an article in its Sunday magazine entitled "Home Births." The heading beneath the title stated, "Advocates argue that hospitals overdo delivery; that modern technology creates its own needs, and that hospitals gear themselves and all patients—unnecessarily—for the high-risk mothers and babies." The article noted that "enough rage and frustration has rubbed off on enough women so that [homebirth couples] are part of a new movement." The piece concluded with a section on "Birth-related procedures that are called overused" (*Boston Sunday Globe,* October 16, 1977). Widespread dissatisfaction with standard medical birth protocols culminated in three types of alternative prenatal care/birth practitioners. The first consisted of women who initiated self-study groups and simultaneously began attending births at home. The second was a group of birth attendants who worked with family practitioners to attend births at home. The final group was composed of women who sought to practice nurse-midwifery legally.

In 1973 nurse-midwives initiated a bill to gain licensure. In order to block this attempt at legalization, the medical society argued that CNMs were unqualified birth attendants. One legislator stated that when the nurse-midwifery licensing legislation was introduced "physicians were very opposed [not only to homebirth and lay midwives[2]] but also to birth centers and nurse-midwives. The docs used the 'public safety' argument to say that birth centers should not exist and certified nurse-midwives should not be licensed" (Massachusetts legislator, interview, 1984). The legislators responded to the intense lobbying efforts of the Massachusetts Medical Society and blocked passage of the nurse-midwifery licensing bill for four years.

Frequently, alliances among different segments of the power elite, which enable them to act as a consolidated block, are temporary. Outside pressures intervene to create a conflict of interest among these groups, thereby altering the balance of power. In this case, the larger sociopolitical context created a framework for the legislature to act in opposition to the medical lobby. The fact that by 1977 almost every state but Massachusetts had legalized nurse-midwifery created a legal precedent for the legislature to act, and delegitimated the medical community's "public safety" objection.

In addition to national precedent, local constituent pressure mounted to demand that nurse-midwives be legalized. Under these circumstances, legislators found it in their own political best interest to legalize CNMs. In order to keep their conflicts from entering the public domain, these institutional gatekeepers decided to settle the matter privately. In this case, a group of senators and representatives who supported the bill called for a private meeting with key representatives of the Massachusetts Medical Society who opposed the bill. This meeting resulted in a verbal agreement. The bill would go forward unimpeded if it was made clear that these midwives would remain under professional medical jurisdiction. According to the terms of the private agreement, the medical society would not oppose the bill if the legislation clearly stated that CNMs were legally prohibited from attending homebirths. Such private backroom meetings show how, in the final analysis, deals can be made behind closed doors in which a bill can be rewritten without any participation from the parties who initiated the bill. Further, there is no guarantee that private deals will be honored once they enter the political realm.

The legislature passed the licensing bill in 1977, with the stipulation that CNMs would be licensed to practice only in medical facilities. While the members of the medical society did not oppose the bill during the legislative process, they did intervene at the administrative level in an attempt to kill the bill. This action created animosity between this group of legislators and the medical society. As one senator emphasized, "The docs double-crossed us and pressured the governor to veto the bill" (Massachusetts Senator, private interview, 1984). A turf battle between the legislators and the medical society ensued. The legislators were ultimately triumphant because it rapidly became evident that there was a groundswell of public support for the bill. Operating within this larger social context, the legislators were able to override the governor's veto. CNMs were now licensed, but they could only legally practice within medical institutions under physician supervision.

Physicians and Homebirth Practice: "A Hostile Environment"

With the nurse-midwife "threat" contained, the medical society cast a watchful eye toward the lay midwives and the few physician/birth attendant teams attending homebirths. The biggest threat to medical definitions of homebirth as medically unsound came from the "errant" members of the medical community itself. In April 1982, a birth attended by a family practitioner/birth attendant team ended in a neonatal death. This incident provided the conditions for the medical gate-keepers to mobilize against the homebirth physicians in an attempt to eliminate any semblance of medical support for homebirth. The chief of obstetrics at a major Boston hospital registered a formal complaint with the Board of Registration in Medicine, charging that the death would have been preventable in the hospital. In addition, the state medical examiner filed complaints with the Board of Registration in Medicine and the Massachusetts Medical Society asking them to determine if the death was site-dependent. Both the Board of Registration and the medical society immediately undertook their own investigations. During this period, another homebirth physician was contacted by the chief of obstetrics at the hospital where he retained privileges and informed that he was in jeopardy of losing these privileges unless he refrained from participation in homebirth. Fearing what the loss of these privileges would do to his medical practice, he stopped participating in homebirths.

No investigations demonstrate that the death attended by the other homebirth physician was site-dependent. If the birth had taken place in the hospital it was equally likely that the outcome would have been the same. All complaints were eventually dropped, but this physician also withdrew from the homebirth arena because he was unwilling to practice in such a "hostile environment." Interestingly, while fierce political pressure was unsuccessful in preventing the legalization of nurse-midwifery, the same intensity of political pressure was successful when applied to "wayward" physicians. The medical society succeeded in eliminating the physician-attended homebirth alternative.

Lay Midwifery: The Practice of Medicine?

With both the nurse-midwifery and physician threats contained, the medical society turned its full gaze toward lay midwifery. Lay midwifery in Massachusetts had no clear legal status and the controversy over physician-attended homebirth had initiated a public discussion over what constituted the practice of medicine. A prominent magazine quoted key medical professionals who authoritatively stated that attending birth is the practice of medicine: "Hospital authorities declare with certainty that delivering a baby is indeed practicing medicine" (*Boston Magazine*, 1982:216). Lay midwives publicly stressed that birth could not appropriately be considered the practice of medicine, but privately they worried about the implications of the 1907 law, which had outlawed midwifery as the practice of medicine. The lines had been drawn for the upcoming debate over who had the legitimate right to define the reality of the situation: Is midwifery the unauthorized practice of medicine or is midwifery a type of health care that is distinct from medicine?

The Case of Janet Leigh and the Formation of the Massachusetts Midwives Association In September 1982 another homebirth death occurred, this one attended by a nurse and a homebirth midwife, Janet Leigh. The homebirth Leigh had been attending was complicated by a prolapsed cord (a potentially hazardous condition in which the cord precedes the baby into the birth canal and may be stretched or crushed, threatening the baby's oxygen supply). The midwife put the birthing woman in the knee-chest position, held her hand in the birth canal to keep the baby's weight off the cord, and called an ambulance to transport the woman to the hospital for a cesarean section. Everything the midwife did was according to medical protocol. When three emergency medical technicians (EMTs) arrived on the scene they forcibly prevented Leigh from proceeding with the lifesaving practice. Further, they refused to listen to her recommendations for continuing the same procedure. They spent critical moments arguing with the midwife about her credentials and insisting that she would not be allowed to enter the ambulance without showing proper credentials. The only way Leigh was able to gain entrance into the ambulance was by showing her RN (registered nurse) license.

This turn of events provided the means for the medical community to mobilize their resources in an attempt to declare lay midwifery the practice of medicine and thereby annihilate this emergent group of health-care providers. The effort commenced with the hospital to which the case had been transferred bringing a complaint against the midwife to the Board of Registration in Nursing. In 1983 formal charges were brought against Janet Leigh. The form the case took is peculiar to this state.

During this period in Massachusetts history, it was estimated by both those inside and outside the movement that about half of the lay midwives practicing also held a nursing license. While neither the medical society nor the Nursing Board had any direct authority over the lay midwives, the Board of Registration in Nursing (BORN) did have direct censure and jurisdiction over its licensees. Janet Leigh was also a nurse with a current license. A direct case could be brought against her by the BORN, and this action would send a political message to the other lay midwives retaining their RN licenses. Janet Leigh was of special concern to the board because she had practiced as an obstetrical nurse for a number of years at a major Boston hospital before turning to independent midwifery.

In May 1983, the BORN charged Janet Leigh with deceit, malpractice, and gross misconduct, ordering her to appear at an upcoming hearing stating why her nursing license should not be revoked (Board of Registration in Nursing, Order to Show Just Cause, May 1983). The charges involved three broad issues. The first issue involved the competence of the lay midwife in question, and by implication the competence of lay midwifery in general. In other words, did the lay midwife use improper procedure when dealing with a prolapsed cord, thus opening herself to charges of malpractice? The second issue was the use of a medical degree (in the form of an RN license) to confer on lay midwifery a legitimacy that it did not possess. That is, did the lay midwife in question use her nursing license to misrepresent herself as a certified nurse-midwife? The third issue concerned the ability of a medical professional to engage in a practice the Board of Registration in Nursing and the Board of Registration of Medicine considered to be the practice of medicine without a license. Specifically, can a nurse legally practice lay midwifery without having been first certified by the Board of Nursing as a nurse-midwife? (Board of Registration in Nursing, Order to Show Cause, May 1983).

Instead of shattering the movement, these perilous circumstances resulted in a new vitality and redirection. The loosely organized Massachusetts homebirth movement became a more cohesive and outwardly directed network. Previous to Leigh's troubles, midwives had no regular organized contact, and consumer groups were primarily engaged in childbirth education. Midwives were the first to respond, and shortly after the hospital charges were brought to the Board of Registration in Nursing, they began to meet on a regular basis: "We [midwives] had met in study groups for a while, but it never lasted. Janet Leigh's case, when she came under investigation, was a real legal threat. It mobilized us into action and that took the form of holding further meetings and developing standards" (*Midwife Advocate*, winter 1987). This group soon became the Massachusetts Midwives Alliance (MMA).

Judging from the amount of medical opposition the nurse-midwives faced in their bid for licensing, the Massachusetts lay midwives knew they would be up against formidable medical power. Following the formation of the MMA, the midwives discussed the need to generate a noteworthy political counterpressure to keep the nursing board from spearheading an effort to eliminate lay midwifery by having it declared the practice of medicine. Their clients were their best available resource, and so the midwives turned to them, asking for an organized consumer support group. A homebirth consumer discusses the formation of this new statewide consumer group:

> When the Nursing Board [brought formal charges] things really got going here in Massachusetts. The [midwives who were organizing] asked their clients to form a consumer group. . . . The midwives decided that existing organizations could not handle the state lobbying effort that they felt would now be needed.

In November 1983, this statewide consumer group formed and called itself the Massachusetts Friends of Midwives (MFOM). The group organized around survival issues—to keep midwives in business.[3]

In October 1983, just prior to the official formation of MFOM in November 1983, the Nursing Board held their formal adjudicatory hearing. During the hearing, evidence was presented that the midwife had indeed used proper procedure, but that the emergency medical technicians (EMT) arriving on the scene disregarded her advice and instituted improper procedures. A physician testifying for Janet Leigh noted that if the technicians had followed her instructions, the baby might have lived. Regarding the issue of misrepresentation, the technicians had written on their report that the midwife had told them that she was a nurse-midwife. The board considered this misrepresentation because to be a nurse and a lay midwife is not the same as being a certified nurse-midwife, which is separate and distinct, requiring specific qualifications not possessed by either nurses or lay midwives.

The technicians testified that the midwife may have said that she was a nurse on one occasion and a midwife on another, but it was determined that she was only permitted entrance into the ambulance after showing her registered nursing license. As for the third charge, the board suggested that because nursing was under its jurisdiction, only nurses certified by the board were eligible to practice midwifery and all nurses practicing midwifery without the board's express approval were doing so illegitimately (board of Registration in Nursing, Adjudicatory Hearing, October 1983).

The board publicly executed its decision in January 1984:

> After consideration of all the evidence presented at the hearing...the Board on the basis of all the evidence, makes the

following conclusions of the law: 1. Guilty of deceit for falsely representing self as a nurse-midwife. 2. Two counts of gross misconduct: a. Commonwealth vs. Porn: b. Failing to apply for authorization and awareness of [the Nurse Practice Act]. Therefore, on the basis of these findings of fact and conclusion of the law, the Board rules that the license be suspended. The period of suspension should be at least one year. (Commonwealth of Massachusetts, Division of Registration, board of Registration in Nursing, January 1984)

In the decision the board dropped the charge of improper procedure and the malpractice charges associated with it, noting, "Janet Leigh was prepared for a home delivery" (the Commonwealth of Massachusetts, Division of Registration, Board of Registration in Nursing, January, 1984). Pursuing this type of incompetence charge very probably would have led not to prosecution against the lay midwife, but prosecution against the paramedical professionals arriving at the scene. Such prosecution entailed the potential political danger of exonerating medically illegitimate practitioners while indicting legitimate medical personnel. However, the board clearly sought to remove the medical legitimacy that a nursing degree granted to homebirth by charging the independent midwife with deceit and gross misconduct. Consequently the board used the emergency medical technician's report to charge Leigh with deceit. The members of the board cited the emergency medical technician's report at the time of the incident, "Emergency Medical Technician's record states: Nurse-Midwife Janet Leigh on scene" (Commonwealth of Massachusetts, Division of Registration, Board of Registration of Nursing, January 1984). They did so despite verbal testimony by the EMT that the midwife might not have misrepresented herself as a nurse-midwife.

What had particularly disturbed the board was the idea that the lay midwife had used her nursing credentials to gain entry into the ambulance:

> An ambulance was dispatched [to the scene and the ambulance department] policy requires positive identification of anyone, who at the scene, claims to be a nurse or physician and wants to continue to participate in the actual care of the patient. . . . Janet Leigh showed her registered nurse license to gain access into the ambulance. (Commonwealth of Massachusetts, Division of Registration, Board of Registration in Nursing, January 1984)

The board also made reference to Leigh's previous work in the area of obstetrical nursing, declaring that this type of expertise could not be transferable to the practice of lay midwifery:

> Janet Leigh worked from 1970–1977 as a registered nurse for various agencies in different capacities, however, most of the positions were in Obstetrical Nursing. . . . Nursing Staff Privileges DOES NOT include the function of delivering babies. . . . Janet Leigh lacks the 'appropriate education' as defined in the statutes . . . (Commonwealth of Massachusetts, Division of Registration, Board of Registration in Nursing, January 1984, emphasis in original)

In order to put a halt to the preceding practice and further underscore the point that the legitimacy of a nursing degree (especially one with special expertise in obstetrical nursing) could not imbue lay midwifery with a legitimacy that it did not deserve, the board cited the midwife with two gross misconduct charges. The charges were based upon the board's interpretation of existing nursing statutes and a 1907 Massachusetts Supreme Court decision (*Commonwealth v. Porn*), based on which they implied (but never stated) that only certified nurse-midwives could practice midwifery. These grounds for misconduct were simply cited with no explanation offered. The nature of these charges was ambiguous—did they mean that only nurses could not practice lay midwifery, but that those without a nursing degree could do so, or did they mean that all midwifery was illegitimate and probably illegal, meaning that the Board of Nursing had jurisdiction over all midwifery? Reference to *Commonwealth v. Porn* case as the first basis for the charges of gross misconduct insinuated that the practice of lay midwifery was the practice of medicine.

The Case of Hannah Porn *Commonwealth v. Porn* involved a case against a Finnish immigrant midwife, Hannah Porn, brought before the Supreme Judicial Court in Massachusetts in October 1907. Like Janet Leigh, Porn was a nurse who practiced lay midwifery. She had been formally trained as a midwife in her native country of Finland, but could obtain no legal recognition of this training when she immigrated to the United States. Nevertheless, she continued to serve her Finnish immigrant community as a midwife, in spite of a great deal of harassment from the medical community, until she died (see DeClerq 1994 for a full explication of the Hannah Porn case). The judgment of the court found Porn guilty of practicing medicine without a license:

> Where trained nurse practiced obstetrics and used printed prescriptions for alleviating suffering and other conditions incident thereto, together with the usual obstetrical instruments when they were necessary, she not being licensed to practice medicine, was guilty of violating Rev. Las, c. 76 & 8, providing that whoever, not being lawfully authorized to practice medicine, shall attempt to practice medicine in any of its branches. (*Commonwealth v. Porn*, Supreme Judicial Court, 1907)

Homebirth advocates had long been leery of the implications of this law, fearing that it could be interpreted in a way that would designate the practice of lay midwifery as the practice of medicine. In fact, lay midwives had contacted a legal expert after the case against a family practitioner forced all physicians out of the home and back into the hospital. The midwives hoped to begin a judicial action making lay midwifery legal in Massachusetts. The legal advice sought at the time suggested that *Commonwealth v. Porn* would probably be used successfully to interpret lay midwifery as the practice of medicine (Homebirth consumer advocate, interview, 1984). After discussion, the midwives concluded that it was politically dangerous to proactively initiate a reinterpretation of the 1907 law, which could be used to criminalize their activities. The lay midwives believed that they had no choice but to continue practicing under these legally precarious conditions.

Researchers, in concurrence with the legal expert consulted by the lay midwives, had interpreted *Commonwealth v. Porn* to mean that the practice of lay midwifery in this state was the practice of medicine, and therefore assumed that lay midwifery in Massachusetts was illegal (Sallomi 1982:16; DeVries 1985:152). The BORN, by citing *Commonwealth v. Porn* as the first justification for gross misconduct charges against lay midwife Janet Leigh, had set the stage for possible legal obliteration of lay midwifery in Massachusetts. The ominous and very real nature of this possibility became obvious soon after, when the Massachusetts Attorney General's Office began investigating another lay midwife. Investigations by this office usually resulted in criminal charges.

The Midwives' Legislative and Judicial Response: Midwifery Is Not the Practice of Medicine In response to these frontal assaults on lay midwifery, the new statewide consumer group MFOM and the recently formed MMA initiated their own political strategy at two levels: legislative and judicial. Lay midwife Janet Leigh hired a lawyer and began the fight to retain her nursing license. Her lawyer, who was also one of her homebirth clients, was articulate, politically savvy, and dedicated to the survival of lay midwifery. In light of recent events, her lawyer felt that they had been backed into a corner where it was no longer possible to refrain from attempting to legally redefine the implications of the 1907 law. Accordingly, he decided to take a proactive position and submit Janet's case to a Massachusetts Supreme Court justice. In private communications with me, her lawyer conveyed his trepidation that the Hannah Porn law could be used to declare midwifery the practice of medicine. However, he was quick to add that under the present set of circumstances, the best chance for successful redefinition and reinterpretation of the law was to take the initiative rather than wait to be declared illegal by default.

Janet Leigh's initiation of the judicial action was far from unique; it formed part of a national trend. Researchers analyzing childbirth activists during these years pointed out that "litigation emerged in the eighties as the primary weapon for advocates of childbirth reform" (Edwards and Waldorf, 1984:179). However, such judicial initiation was not without risk. Current statutes reflected a bias toward mainstream medical definitions of the situation. This put lay midwifery at a disadvantage because current medical standards did not support homebirth as a viable option (Annas 1984). On the other hand, the risks involved in midwifery litigation could be offset by remaining aware that the law is more than an automatic product of professional medical constructions of reality. That is, "while medicine shapes the laws that govern it, those laws have an independent impact on medicine. Recognition of the interdependence of law and medicine places them in a larger social and cultural context and acknowledges that both institutions are shaped by that context" (DeVries 1985:11). Accordingly, DeVries's research at the time indicated that within the larger national context, the courts had begun to demonstrate a reluctance to prosecute alternative health-care providers because they did not want to deprive individuals of health care by eliminating their options. MMA and MFOM also entered the legislative arena. Again, this course of action was not unique during these years. Across the nation, lay midwives had been introducing regulatory and licensing bills before their legislatures in an attempt to gain legal recognition (Sullivan and Weitz, 1988; Sallomi et al., DeVries, 1985).

The stimulus for legislative action in Massachusetts was primarily to support the judicial action. Homebirth advocates were becoming politically astute and recognized the need to maximize their chances of their judicial success by demonstrating to the court that they were pursuing other routes to legality. MMA and MFOM quickly drafted a bill to present to the Joint Health Care Committee to define midwifery as separate from nursing and the practice of medicine. The first version of the bill attempted to establish a joint board of midwifery, including both nurse-midwives and lay midwives. Ironically, in this era, the major objection to the bill from the health care committee and many nurse-midwives was precisely the call for a joint board of midwifery. Seventeen years passed before a different social context emerged in which a joint board could be presented as a viable political strategy.

In 1984 the bill was redrafted to regulate lay midwives only, leaving nurse-midwifery regulations to the Nursing Board. However, the bill was not revised in time to be presented to the Joint Health Care Committee. This would have to wait until the following year. Subsequently, all attention turned to the impending Janet Leigh litigation. With a ruling in favor of the Nursing Board, especially with citation of *Commonwealth v. Porn*, lay midwifery could be interpreted as the practice of medicine. Such an action might nullify any legislative movement.

In June 1984, Leigh's lawyer presented her case to Massachusetts Supreme Court Justice Herbert P. Wilkins. In an innovative move, the lawyer used the current sociocultural context as grounds for negotiating and redefining the 1907 law in such a way that midwifery could be declared separate from the practice of medicine without overturning the law. He argued that the 1907 decision designating midwifery as the practice of medicine revolved around the use of obstetrical instruments by the midwife, and that this had no bearing on the present case. In addition, he emphasized that the court could make a legal distinction between lay midwifery and the practice of medicine. The 1907 decision could be interpreted as historically dated with little current relevance. For example, the court had used an outdated lexicon by referring to midwives as female obstetricians. This was bound to confuse issues in the present social and cultural terrain where standard terminology demarcates between midwifery and obstetrics. Consequently, current terminology makes it possible to separate midwifery from the practice of medicine while leaving *Commonwealth v. Porn* intact (Commonwealth of Massachusetts, Supreme Judicial Court of Suffolk county, Plaintiff's Memorandum in Support of Motion for Summary Judgment, June 1984). Regarding the Nursing Board's case that the midwife was practicing nurse-midwifery without a license, Janet's lawyer argued that lay midwifery must be seen as a profession in its own right separate from the practice of nursing; therefore, the board has no jurisdiction over nurses engaged in practices separate from nursing.

Judge Wilkins: Informal Judicial Support In September 1984, Wilkins announced a decision that was in keeping with the national milieu in which the courts were becoming reluctant to penalize alternative health-care providers. The official statement read as follows, "It is ORDERED and ADJUDGED, that the decision of the Board of Registration in Nursing is vacated and the case is remanded to that Board for further consideration" (Commonwealth of Massachusetts, Supreme Judicial Court of Suffolk County, *Janet Leigh v. Board of Registration in Nursing*, September, 1984, emphasis in original). In this action the judge avoided ruling on the distinction among medicine, nursing, and midwifery. Nevertheless, homebirth advocates considered his decision a major victory.

The midwifery community interpreted the ruling to mean that the sociocultural lexicon argument could be credibly used to reinterpret the 1907 law in their favor. In returning the case to the Nursing Board for further consideration, Judge Wilkins noted that the board's case was "cryptic" and offered insufficient explanation for disciplining the lay midwife. He made it clear that mere citation of the 1907 law did not make the Nursing Board's case evident. Further, the judge made several comments in support of the lay midwife in question by referring to the social situation in which the incident occurred. These comments illustrate how the nature of the case can have an enormous bearing on judicial attitude. His statements, while doing nothing to change the legal aspects of the case, succeeded in conferring informal judicial support and thereby enormous cultural legitimacy for lay midwifery and simultaneous chastisement for the BORN. He pointed out how the lay midwife had acted in an altruistic manner while the nursing board's actions appeared self-interested rather than health-oriented:

> If the matter were for me to decide on my own view of the record, I would conclude that the case had not been made by a preponderance of the evidence that the nurse misrepresented herself. . . . [In addition], the decision gives no consideration to the circumstances of that misrepresentation or whether it was the kind of 'deceit' that has ever been a ground of discipline of licensed professionals. . . . There was no personal gain intended to be derived from the misrepresentation. She was trying to help her patient who was being treated inappropriately by the paramedics. The procedures the nurse was recommending for the treatment of a prolapsed cord were correct. In such a situation, I would not have found fault if she had said she was head of the obstetrics department of every hospital in Boston or said

anything else that might have saved the unborn child's life. In its new decision the Board will have to explain why any discipline is warranted on the grounds of deceit. (Commonwealth of Massachusetts, Supreme Judicial Court of Suffolk County, *Janet Leigh v. Board of Registration in Nursing*, September 1984)

As for separating lay midwifery from the practice of medicine and nursing, Judge Wilkins suggested that this was an issue for the legislature. Here again, however, his statement was far from neutral and was sympathetic to the lay midwife while caustic toward the nursing board:

> The Board should explain its grounds of finding gross misconduct. What misconduct is inherent in failing to apply for authorization when the only authorization would have been as a nurse-midwife within medical facilities? The authorization would have done the nurse, engaged in home deliveries, absolutely no good. (Commonwealth of Massachusetts, Supreme Judicial Court of Suffolk Count, *Janet Leigh v. Board of Registration in Nursing*, September 1984)

Finally, when the judge alluded to the fact that distinguishing the practice of midwifery from the practice of medicine and nursing was a matter for the legislature and not the courts, he made reference to the recently revised midwifery bill, pending approval by the Joint Health Care Committee in its next hearing—the same bill redrafted by MMA and MFOM. This statement gave the judicial nod to the legislation.

The cultural and social capital that lay midwives obtained from the judicial ruling was considerable. Media coverage gave public credibility to lay midwifery. The most prominent local newspaper, the *Boston Globe*, ran a front-page article on the case entitled "Judge Reinstates License of Nurse Who Is Midwife" (September 11, 1984). The article included the judge's comment that he would not have found fault with her if she had claimed that she was the head of every obstetrics department in Boston. The impact of the court decision went beyond symbolic value when the midwives gained the allegiance of a powerful ally in the legislature. The chairman of the Joint Health Care Committee not only agreed to sponsor the lay midwifery bill, but also wrote a letter to the Nursing Board requesting that they defer any further action until the legislature had time to act.

Lay midwives and their supporters had won the first round in the battle to keep lay midwifery and homebirth a viable health-care option. Gaining legitimacy while retaining identity and autonomy appeared within reach, but in December 1984, the Nursing Board again suspended the lay midwife's nursing license, this time dropping the deceit charges but pursuing the gross misconduct charges. Undaunted, Leigh and her lawyer, encouraged by Judge Wilkins's ruling, began making plans to submit the case to Justice Wilkins once again; this time confident that they could prevail.

Midwifery Week in Massachusetts In the larger state context, the Nursing Board had lost so much credibility that this suspension appeared to have little impact on lay midwifery legitimacy. Lay midwifery was gaining momentum as a health-care option rather than losing it. In February, two bills pertaining to the status of lay midwifery came to the attention of the Joint Health Care Committee. One was the bill to set standards for and regulate lay midwifery; the other was a bill declaring lay midwifery illegal, imposing criminal penalties for this "illegal" practice. The health-care committee responded by giving a favorable report on the lay midwifery regulation bill and an unfavorable report on the bill outlawing lay midwifery. Shortly after these reports were made public, the administrative branch of government joined the judicial and legislative branches by adding even greater social legitimacy to both lay midwifery and nurse-midwifery when the governor declared Midwifery Week in Massachusetts.

In a relatively short period of time, the fate of lay midwifery in the state changed remarkably. The homebirth movement, relatively underground until it faced potential legal obliteration, had now gained recognition from all three branches of the government—judicial, legislative, and administrative. Despite the fact that midwifery had still not been separated from the practice of medicine or nursing, the social legitimacy that such recognition conferred on the movement made it unlikely that lay midwifery could be easily dispensed with in the future.

General encouragement of the lay midwifery option by political gatekeepers led to growing social legitimacy and organizational consolidation. Since its inception, the statewide midwifery consumer group (MFOM) had conceived of itself as a democratic organization with no official leadership. However, the viability of a leaderless organization became increasingly untenable as the membership proliferated (from sixty members in November 1983 to over 400 members by March 1985). The need for a more coordinated liaison with the legislature, media, and general public became paramount. Consequently, the group held a statewide meeting during which they elected officers for the purpose of facilitating internal and external communication. This consumer group focused on broadening its base of support by joining the Women's Statewide Legislative Network and intensifying fundraising, lobbying, and publicity campaigns.

Janet Leigh and the Massachusetts Supreme Court A setback came when Judge Wilkins passed Janet Leigh's appeal to regain her nursing license to the full bench of the Supreme Judicial Court, after determining that either side (i.e., the Nursing Board or Janet Leigh) would appeal his second ruling on the matter. This action had high stakes for all parties concerned. The court's decision would be final and binding. If the court ruled in Janet Leigh's favor, lay midwifery would be considered separate from nursing and medicine, thus legalizing lay midwifery. If the court ruled in favor of the Nursing Boards, lay midwifery would be considered the practice of nursing and/or the practice of medicine and thereby outlawed. In either case, the outcome would determine the long-term legal status of midwifery in Massachusetts.

In May 1985, Janet Leigh's case came before the full bench of the Supreme Judicial Court. Janet's lawyer invoked the same social and cultural argument he had successfully used earlier. He also stressed that the *Commonwealth v. Porn* decision was based on use of obstetrical instruments. In the current case before the court, the midwife did not use obstetrical instruments (*Janet Leigh v. Board of Registration in Nursing*, Hearing before Supreme Judicial Court for Suffolk County, Observation, May 8, 1985).

The assistant attorney general presented the case for the defendant (the Board of Registration in Nursing), arguing that the Nurse Practice Act authorizes only CNMs to engage in the practice of midwifery. She made the further point that the BORN has the jurisdiction to discipline a registered nurse for gross misconduct when the nurse engages in the unauthorized practice of lay midwifery. Again in the Nursing Board case, it was unclear whether the board included all midwifery under its jurisdiction or only nurses engaged in the practice of midwifery. When the Supreme Court justices asked the assistant attorney general to clarify the Nursing Board's interpretation of *Commonwealth v. Porn*, she replied that it would have a "chilling effect"[4] on all those practicing lay midwifery, regardless of whether they possessed a nursing license. However, she declined any further comment on the decision, leaving the Nursing Board interpretation of *Commonwealth v. Porn* undefined (*Janet Leigh v. Board of Registration in Nursing*, Hearing before Supreme Judicial Court for Suffolk County, Observation, May, 1985).

In August 1985 the court announced its decision. Making use of Leigh's lawyer's innovative reading of the law, the court refrained from overturning *Commonwealth v. Porn*, interpreting it in such a way that separated lay midwifery from the practice of medicine:

> There is no statutory prohibition against the practice of midwifery by lay persons. The Legislature has not regulated midwifery by persons other than nurses. Nor do we interpret our case law to prohibit the practice of midwifery as the unauthorized practice of medicine. In COMMONWEALTH VS PORN, this court upheld the conviction of a midwife for the unauthorized practice of medicine. However, the basis of her conviction was not her practice of midwifery per se but the fact that she used the 'usual obstetrical instruments'...Thus, 'ordinary assistance in the normal cases of childbirth' which we interpret to mean the practice of midwifery, would not be considered the practice of medicine. (*Janet Leigh v. Board of Registration in Nursing*, Supreme Judicial Court of Massachusetts, Decision, August 15, 1985)

Judicial Recognition for Lay Midwifery: Now What About Licensing?

In making this decision, the court judicially legalized lay midwifery and ended the long debate over whether the practice of lay midwifery is the practice of medicine in Massachusetts. This decision had the paradoxical effect of both legitimating lay midwifery and undermining this legitimacy at the same time. On the one hand, the court implicitly acknowledged lay midwifery definitions of reality by separating midwifery from the practice of medicine. This part of the decision was a major victory for lay midwifery legitimacy. On the other hand, the second part of the decision indirectly undermined this legitimacy by giving the Nursing Board the power to revoke the license of nurses engaged in lay midwifery on grounds of gross misconduct. This, in effect, meant that anyone *but* a nurse could legally practice lay midwifery. If anyone could now practice lay midwifery except a nurse, the legitimacy of lay midwifery was questionable: "it's absurd that your next-door neighbor and your hairdresser can practice midwifery legally, but a nurse can't" (*Boston Globe*, August 16, 1985).

Those in the homebirth movement received the decision with mixed reactions. The idea that lay midwifery would never be perceived as a legitimate profession without licensing divided the movement and brought to the forefront long-standing conflicts "smoldering beneath the surface" (homebirth consumer advocate, interview). Most midwives and consumers still favored licensing of lay midwives, but a significant minority of both believed that the recent "legalization" of lay midwifery made the need for licensing legislation less of a priority. Before the recent

Massachusetts Supreme Court decision, those who opposed licensing legislation campaigned and lobbied for it, despite their misgivings, because they believed that without it, lay midwifery could be outlawed at any time. Given the recent "legalization" of lay midwifery, opponents of licensing became more reluctant to support the licensing bill, arguing that licensing would make midwifery more akin to the medical model, as well as exclude many midwives unable to meet the stringent criteria. These are the same objections presently heard from the minority in Massachusetts who oppose the current licensing bill.

Discussions about the benefits and drawbacks of licensure focus on issues of legitimacy and co-option. Those who support licensing emphasize the marginal status of midwives when they practice without legislative jurisdiction. Those who oppose it stress the "high cost" of licensing—midwifery might become subsumed within the medical model and thereby lose integrity. For about five years after the Massachusetts Supreme Court decision, homebirth midwives and their supporters tried to pass legislation legalizing lay midwifery. Every session they reintroduced new legislation. The legislature responded by noting that passing a piece of legislation that pertained to so few people (the figure often quoted was about fifteen active primary midwives at any one time) was not a priority. What further dissuaded the legislative effort was the discovery by the midwives that they were now able to practice without harassment from the political-legal system. The dominant sentiment eventually became "why mess with a good thing?"

A UNIFIED MIDWIFERY MODEL[5]

In 1987, CNMs successfully achieved legislation that gave them formal legal rights to attend homebirths, but attending homebirths proved to be impossible in practice for CNMs. In the early 1990s, lay midwives came to prefer calling themselves direct-entry midwives in order to emphasize both their professional competence and their unique point of entry into midwifery. As mentioned above, the Massachusetts DEMs' legislative efforts became less and less of a priority until they were abandoned altogether in the early 1990s. A MFOM member who participated in the organization for almost seventeen years explained how the legislative effort faded out:

> Around 1990 the legislative focus shifted to emphasize the benefits of midwifery from a public health perspective. On the basis of midwives' demonstrated success in reducing infant mortality in high-risk populations, the legislation was rewritten to provide

reimbursement for midwives working with low-income women. Otherwise, its basic provisions remained the same. This initiative represented a great opportunity to support the work of urban midwives, but did not succeed in overcoming the inertia of state government. Legislative activity was discontinued in the early 1990s, and the independent practice of midwifery in Massachusetts is still unregulated.

Developing a Reputation for Direct-Entry Midwifery

As the years passed, Massachusetts DEMs continued to operate marginally but with a great deal of autonomy. Most midwives set their standards according to the Massachusetts Midwives Alliance (MMA) protocols. These midwives have been rigorous in supporting each other to adhere to these protocols rather than deviate too far from them and risk soiling the reputation of direct-entry midwifery. Their autonomy was augmented by increasing support from local hospitals when a homebirth required a transfer. In fact, for almost a decade, beginning in the 1990s, one nationally renowned hospital actively solicited homebirth clients who needed to be transferred. Over time the hospital staff came to respect the skill and competence of the direct-entry midwives. For example, a homebirth consumer recounts her experience when her baby was born with a terminal illness and they transported in to this hospital:

> My [direct-entry] midwife came in with us when my husband and I went meet with the neonatologist. My midwife addressed the neonatalogist and said, "'I need to ask you—is there anything that I or any of the other midwives did or did not do that has contributed to this baby's problems?" The neonatologist responded, "Absolutely not, this baby was in such great condition when it came in—we were expecting when we heard there was a homebirth transport that we were going to get a disaster. What this has done is really alter mine and my staff's view of what homebirth midwifery is and the level of care that is provided. We were incredibly impressed."

This was not an isolated incident. One of the busiest DEMs in Massachusetts commented on her unofficial yet close relationship with the chief of obstetrics and gynecology at this hospital:

> He heard from his staff and residents that they particularly liked how I practiced. So after hearing those reports several times and specifically after one birth where the resident and the staff were just raving . . . he said that his staff was willing to give me the

same privileges that outlying hospitals have. That is, if you were a doctor delivering at another hospital and you run into trouble that is bigger than your hospital can handle, you can call into this hospital and say, "I want to transfer my patient to you." Basically I was given the privileges to transfer my people as if I was a different hospital, so I got the beeper that these other hospitals have for transferring in their complicated cases.

Further, this midwife emphasized that this chief of obstetrics and gynecology maintained an open mind in his view of homebirth:

When I went to see him [the chief of obstetrics and gynecology] he said, "I don't know what is right. I know that one-half of everything that I believed to be right ten years ago in medicine I now know to be wrong. This means one-half of everything I hold now to be right I will probably find out to be wrong in the next ten years. I just don't know which one-half, and who knows, maybe everybody who possibly can, should be birthing at home. I don't know, so I am not about to go about telling people what they should be doing. What interests me is that whatever people are choosing, they can be as safe as possible. So, I want the people choosing homebirth to have the best possible help and backup when you come into the hospital—that is my interest."

My seventy in-depth interviews, conducted from 1999 to 2001 with midwives and women who had a homebirth in Massachusetts, indicate that such experiences were the rule rather than the exception. In other words, and generally, when homebirth mothers transported into Massachusetts hospitals in the 1990s and the early 2000s, they were either treated with support or with neutrality.[6] In marked contrast from transport situations in the 1980s, during which I often heard stories about hostile transports in which the mother was treated with open contempt and/or the midwife was verbally harassed, in the 1990s only in a few cases did the transporting situation turn openly hostile. Between 2002 and 2004, the transport situation became less open as some Massachusetts hospitals became more reluctant to accept homebirth transports. During this time a homebirth transport occurred in which, in the estimation of hospital personnel and many homebirth midwives themselves, the midwife waited too long before deciding to transport from home to hospital. As a result of this transport, a physician supportive of homebirth lost his hospital privileges and left the area. While the overall transport circumstances remain favorable, this event points to the vulnerability of midwifery in a state without legislative statutes.

Institutional support for homebirth transports will continue to fluctuate as long as direct-entry midwives lack positional authority. Without a legislative mandate, such midwives must base their authority on charisma. This type of power is personally based and inherently unstable as well as eminently mutable. The transition from personal to positional power via legal edict and the professionalizing project enables the "routinization of charisma" whereby administrative rules create stability and predictability based on institutional protocols (Hughes, Martin, and Sharrock 1995).

A New, Joint Legislative Effort

In the late 1990s, when support for the midwifery legislation was gaining momentum, the transport situation was more favorable and open than it had ever been in Massachusetts. In addition, two well-respected DEMs decided to become CNMs. This decision did not involve abandoning their commitment to homebirth and direct-entry midwifery. Both of these midwives continue to have great respect for DEMs and homebirth. They have served as a local bridge between Massachusetts DEMs and CNMs, consistently meeting with both groups and facilitating the ongoing dialogue between them.

Why then, under these favorable conditions for direct-entry midwifery in Massachusetts, did the DEMs spearhead a new legislative effort? The foremost reason they give is the shift in the larger social environment, which would eventually have negative ramifications for their practices. Their logic illustrates how the national political context can structure local policy.

The "shift in the larger social environment" to which Massachusetts DEMs were referring was the passage of the 1992 New York Midwifery Practice Act described in chapter 2. This law removed New York midwifery from the jurisdiction of nursing and placed it within the Department of Education under the Board of Regents, and resulted in a new direct-entry certification defined by the ACNM (American College of Nurse-midwives) as the Certified Midwife (CM). This midwifery designation makes it possible to become a midwife without becoming a nurse. In New York, CMs now exist alongside their CNM counterparts. The educational requirements for the CM closely mirror the qualifications necessary for becoming a CNM. To date, the New York Department of Education has refused to recognize the apprenticeship model as a legitimate pathway to midwifery. A direct result of this legislation was that around the country, homebirth midwives, including DEMs and CPMs, came to mistrust legislative cooperation with CNMs.

The Massachusetts DEMs at the forefront of the legislative drive for legalization and licensure have consistently stressed the need to take a proactive stand to avoid Massachusetts becoming "the next New York state." They point out that taking the legislative initiative gives them the advantage by making them the vanguards of action instead of trying to latch onto a legislative process that is not their own. Their strategy is similar to that of Janet Leigh's lawyer. Given a potentially hostile climate, he initiated the litigation instead of waiting to be caught in a defensive position. One of this core group of midwives discussed her motivations to start the legislative project. As she recounted the story in a stream-of-consciousness manner, she was jolted by the memory that a major impetus behind the legislation was the trepidation that Massachusetts had all the components for becoming "another New York":

> I was one of the first ones pushing for us getting into the legislation piece here. . . . I think we have to take the chance, I think we have to be proactive and on the offense instead of the defense. Because once you are on the defense you are just behind before you even start. Or no [she pauses and restarts her conversation], it is not that kind of defense. I became convinced that the nurse-midwives are going to get their certified midwives program here and they will kill us when they do. We will be dead by default. It was seeing that it happened in New York that really woke me up.
>
> The CNM who runs [a professional university-based] midwifery program—she is a dynamo. She is brilliant, powerful, energetic, as well as pro direct-entry midwives. She has always supported it and she is pro-alternative. However, at the same time she has also had a long-term goal of removing nurse-midwives from the control of the nursing board. She dislikes the nursing board jurisdiction over midwifery. And when I heard about New York removing midwives from under the umbrella of nursing, I thought, "This nurse-midwife will do it. Without question she will do it and she will try to protect us, she is nice and she is in favor of us but it if gets down to her program versus ours, guess who dies?"

The preceding quote shows the mutual admiration that is possible between the CNM and the DEM. While there are exceptions on both sides, I found this respect among Massachusetts midwives to be steadily growing. The DEMs who initiated the legislation wanted to increase the chances that both sets of midwives would not find themselves in structurally antagonistic positions and be forced to act against one another, and ultimately the Massachusetts CNMs have agreed.

Massachusetts midwives have gained considerable political savvy over the years and have recognized that an educational reorganization would have to be put in place before any legislative action could begin. In Massachusetts, where education is a critical element of state identity, many believe that no bill would pass without an accredited midwifery education program. Two changes were made in order to create a viable educational foundation for the planned legislative action. First, the MMA agreed to stop certifying its own midwives and asked them instead to apply for the CPM (the North American Registry of Midwives national credentialing process) so that the certification process would be based on nationally recognized standards. Second, the midwives transformed their informal education process into an organized two-part program. The first was a year-long program for aspiring midwives that would introduce the midwifery model of care, called Stepping Stones to Midwifery. The second was an accredited direct-entry school for committed students in New England that would meet the legislative criteria for education. After eighteen months of work, midwives were able to bring the MEAC-accredited Seattle Midwifery School distance-learning program to New England. Their Stepping Stones to Midwifery curriculum includes prerequisites and an accepted equivalent to the initial midwifery class at the Seattle Midwifery School. This two-part, three-year program encourages incipient midwives by aiding them to get an accredited education that will most likely be required by legislators (personal correspondence with B. J. Mackinnon, and Stepping Stones handout, 2004).

As the foundational education pieces were being put in place, a small group of individuals met to draft the midwifery licensing bill. This group included key direct-entry midwives from the MMA, including the two midwives who had recently become CNMs, and homebirth consumers, among whom was a dedicated lawyer whose daughter was born at home. From the onset, the bill was envisioned as pertaining to all nationally certified midwives—CNMs, CMs, and CPMs. The events in New York state motivated Massachusetts midwives to overcome professional rivalries in order to avoid becoming structurally opposed in future political activities. Seventeen years after the initial bill proposing a joint midwifery board, the time had finally come to propose establishing such a board. This newly formed alliance between the

CNMs and CPMs is the first of its kind in the country. (Although there are presently no CMs in Massachusetts, the potential for their existence in this state is included in the jointly proposed legislation.) As mentioned earlier, the original vision of both MMA and MFOM was to include all midwives. History has come full circle, and what was yesterday's impossibility is now today's (proposed) reality.

During these seventeen years, both CNMs and DEMs have been able to establish a solid foundation for their respective practices as well as a respect for each other's competence. Based on these years of experience, Massachusetts midwives have discerned both the advantages and disadvantages of their corresponding positions. Although occupying structurally distinct positions, each has experienced the negative consequences of physician dominance. Many in both camps believe that their most effective strategy for overcoming this dominance is by uniting their forces into one consolidated group of midwives. DEMs recognize that the New York State Midwifery Practice Act left them vulnerable. The lessons of their prior legislative attempt in Massachusetts were not lost on them: most acknowledged that they were too few in numbers to be able to pass a licensing bill on their own behalf. In order to be taken seriously they needed allies. Further, many Massachusetts DEMs have noted how remaining unlicensed, marginal practitioners keeps them out of the public domain and consequently, most women remain unaware of their existence. Further, the majority of DEMs find themselves working long hours with little financial reward. The jointly proposed bill would add social legitimacy to their practice by granting them licenses as well as positioning them favorably for insurance reimbursement.

Massachusetts CNMs have become frustrated with the tensions their structural position entails. These structural stresses and strains are largely due to problems inherent in the practice of nursing as it is presently organized (Clement 1998). CNMs are classified as advanced practice nurses. Despite an enabling statute that mandates collaborative relationships with physicians, the regulations that flow from older supervisory language are still in effect. In addition, CNMs' prescriptive authority requires physician supervision. In many cases midwifery and medical protocols diverge radically. Practicing midwifery under these conditions places considerable strain on the integrity and quality of the model. To practice the midwifery model of care, the midwife needs a collaborative rather than a supervisory relationship with the physician. The proposed legislation would rectify the structural constraints that have become an everyday reality for CNMs by removing them from the jurisdiction of nursing and the direct supervision of physicians.

Both groups of midwives agree that a central objective is independence. The jointly proposed board will recognize both the university and the apprenticeship models of midwifery. The DEMs want to make sure they keep as much of their current independence as possible in order to keep the integrity of the midwifery model intact. The CNMs want independence to gain full admitting privileges to hospitals. Currently, their dependent medical status prevents them from formally obtaining these privileges. While several nurse-midwives in the state have limited admitting privileges, under JCAHO (the Joint Commission on Accreditation of Healthcare Organizations), these midwives and hospitals could be formally cited for legal non-compliance. JCAHO regulations require that the admitting practitioner and the independent practitioner do not operate under direct supervision. Additionally, Massachusetts nurse-midwives are not always able to obtain independent provider numbers from insurance companies. When they do get a number as a result of consumer pressure, their reimbursement level is sometimes as low as sixty-five percent, far below physician compensation for the same activities.

Massachusetts CNMs have both philosophical and practical reasons for participating in a joint legislative effort with DEMs. These sentiments are expressed eloquently by one of my CNM interviewees:

> I think the certified nurse-midwives will benefit with being in collaboration with the direct-entry midwives. This collaboration will help nurse-midwives remember our roots. The CNMs will look at their own practices and be more careful about automatically turning toward medical interventions at birth. Most certified nurse-midwives have great respect for direct-entry midwives. We all wish we could practice with the same freedom. But currently there are no licenses, no standards, and no educational requirements for direct-entry midwives. This bill will be an assurance that everyone will be practicing within a certain standard of safety. This legislation will ensure that both direct-entry midwives and certified nurse-midwives will each be drawing more toward the middle. We can set a model for the nation. If we can do it in Massachusetts it can be done anywhere. (Certified Nurse-Midwife, interview)

To gain further understanding into why Massachusetts CNMs have become part of this legislative initiative, the national context must be referenced. The 1992 New York State Midwifery Practice Act has had reverberations far beyond Massachusetts. On a much larger scale, the national bodies that include both sets of midwives (ACNM and MANA) are actively working to create a liaison to promote midwifery unity in order to become a counterhegemonic force vis-à-vis the cultural, economic, political, and legal hegemony of professional physician organizations. Massachusetts CNMs have been quick to mention this united effort and the resulting spirit it has created, and many of them participate in the Bridge Club, a group of CNMs and CPMs dedicated to midwifery unity (described in chapter 1).

Further, it is impossible for Massachusetts CNMs to have a homebirth practice under the current state regulations. As noted earlier, homebirth practice for CNMs became legal in 1987, but that was a legal right in name only. A CPM who is also a CNM exemplifies the insurmountable obstacles involved in such an endeavor. With the exception of one other CNM who only briefly attended homebirths in Massachusetts, she has been the only CNM in the state to have a homebirth practice for an extended period of time. Other CNMs have watched and taken due note of her struggles. Here she recounts how incredulous she was when she encountered the difficulties in practically trying to exercise her legal right as a CNM to have a homebirth practice:

> As I was finishing up my CNM studies, I was aware that it would now be legally necessary for me to have a consulting relationship with the doctors in order to continue to practice. I believed that my best option was an obstetrician/gynecologist who had always been really good with homebirth over the years. The direct-entry midwives would send people to him and he would have them on his books if we had to transport and he was wonderful about it.
>
> He told me that now that I am a CNM and not a direct-entry midwife he can no longer be my unofficial consulting doctor. And I said, "I can't believe this." I was sure that he would say yes because all these years he had been [consulting with me as a direct-entry midwife]. Things changed radically when I became a CNM and he was advised not to put his name on a piece of paper that will make him vicariously liable. I was horrified because this is what I need in order to continue to do homebirth as a CNM. When he said "no," I said "I am sunk"—if I don't get him, what am I going to do? I had not taken my exam yet but it was coming up soon and after the exam I had to be legal.

This CNM highlights the lack of autonomy Masschusetts CNMs suffer in contrast to their DEM sisters. This midwife was now caught in an impossible position because once she passed her CNM exam and became licensed as a CNM, she would have to have a consulting physician oversee her practice in order to continue attending homebirths. In transitioning from a DEM/CPM to a CNM, she found that her freedom was severely curtailed. She gained legal legitimacy at the expense of independence. She had practiced as a well-respected direct-entry midwife in her local area for over twenty years, and in doing so had gained a solid reputation for her competence. Fortunately, her local reputation led to a surprising turn of events. She said:

> Most unexpectedly a group of local physicians said "Yes." I was shocked. Absolutely some of the reason they signed it is because I have a reputation and they know about me and they have known about me for twenty years and now I am a CNM. If I was a stranger to the community they would not have done it.

Unfortunately, she discovered that to have a truly autonomous homebirth practice was not possible without physician permission:

> I started jumping through hoops—I went straight to the Drug Enforcement Agency (DEA) and got the applications and called the insurance company and got the applications. The applications, both the DEA number and the insurance require the physician's number on them. I can't get a DEA number without the physician DEA number on my application. (That is the supervisory language of the current legislation.) And the insurance—I can't get insurance unless I have the physician's insurance number on my application, which makes them vicariously liable.
>
> Now with all my homebirth experience and as a CNM I can't have my own practice, but I can go out and do well-woman care because I can get my DEA number for the drugs that only cover well-woman care. I have to have doctor's signature for this. I happen to have a really good friendly physician who would do that for me. So I could do that part, but I can't do births. It is insanity. This is why I sit on the legislative committee.

By September 2004, this midwife had closed her homebirth practice, after almost two years of struggle, due to insurmountable obstacles under the current legislation. Her experiences highlight the frustration that Massachusetts CNMs experience in their current situation. That is, even though most are not trying to set up homebirth practices for obvious reasons, they have too often experienced the constriction of the midwifery model of care by the medical model. Most of them would like to know they could have an independent homebirth practice if they so chose. Their desire for independence has been a major force behind the nurse-midwifery interest in initiating new legislation.

The proposed Board of Midwifery will consist of equal numbers of CNMs/CMs and CPMs, in addition to one MD and consumers. The proposed legislation will require that every midwife be nationally certified according to ACC or NARM standards. The only exceptions will be those "grandmothered" in by the board for a specified time period or those who practice for religious reasons and do not accept pay. All other midwives will by law be illegally practicing midwifery. The punishment will be the same as that for a physician who practices medicine without a license—" a fine of not less than one hundred nor more than one thousand dollars, or imprisonment of not more than twelve months."

As time has passed, more of the minority of midwives on both sides who were originally opposed to the legislation have eventually come to believe that such a bill is in their best interest. Those midwives who still oppose the legislation point out that confining midwifery practice to licensed midwives will eliminate immigrant midwives and others who choose a less formal path. They believe that such a bill will unfairly exclude and narrow the range of practicing midwives. They couple this fear of "repeating New York" with the fear that apparently positive legislation may be sabotaged by the requirement of physician supervision, as it was in California, seeing this possibility as too much of a risk to take. They would rather leave things as they currently are.

The alliance in Massachusetts between DEMs and CNMs remains uneasy. In order to enable both groups of midwives to interact on an informal basis, MFOM organized various home parties where both groups could meet for dinner and conversation. The goal was to create a solid bond on a personal level and resolve differences in a private and informal setting. Many in the community believe that such interaction will make it harder for the midwives to sell each other out as the legislative effort gets more intense. In addition to these parties, MFOM has been involved in numerous public education events around the state. Most prominent among these activities have been showings of the film *Born in the USA*. These public premiers provide a unifying connection among midwives because both DEMs and CNMs join together as a panel following the film to answer audience questions. Further, a newly organized Massachusetts Coalition for Midwifery (MCM) was formed to promote midwifery consolidation. This group worked hard to support the legislation. This coalition integrated both sets of midwives and also included citizens. The makeup has been as follows: two CNMs, two DEMs, and two members of MFOM. For the first year, I served as one of the two MFOM representatives on the coalition.

Midwives, their consumers, and other supporters mounted an intense lobbying effort of the Health Care Committee to ensure that their bill would be solidly and prominently supported. The bill was introduced in December 2000 with a much larger number of supporters than expected; the chairman of the Health Care Committee sponsored the bill, which made its debut with forty-two sponsors. Following this, the midwifery legislation was heard before the Health Care Committee. Midwives and their consumers showed up in large numbers to demonstrate their support. In addition to attending the hearing, the midwifery supporters also lobbied their legislators to make their presence known.

As the midwifery legislation becomes increasingly visible, presenting a unified public midwifery presence becomes paramount. To achieve this end, both midwives and their supporters are reinterpreting and redefining their definitions of the situation. Rather than referring to DEMs or CNMs, the preferred term is simply *midwives*. When discussing the practice of midwifery, the new orientation emphasizes similarities rather than differences by referencing the midwifery model of care that all midwives share. Finally, rather than referring to homebirth, the preferred public terms are *out-of-hospital* and *in-hospital* births.

With a few exceptions, almost everyone agrees that a long and protracted struggle, measured in years, will be necessary to pass the jointly proposed midwifery legislation. Recent events have interacted to both promote and obstruct passage of the bill. On the one hand, medical dominance has been moderated as all health-care budgets have been moved into the Department of Public Health, including the Board of Registration in Medicine. The Board of Registration in Medicine fought hard to prevent being included in this health-care melting pot, but to no avail. On the other hand, a more formidable impediment to passage of the bill than medical opposition has now emerged. The Massachusetts legislature has become increasingly budget conscious, and is consequently loath to create an independent board of midwifery that will constitute an extra state expense. Consumer advocate mobilization will be necessary to mount a successful legislative bid. If past history is an indicator, there is every reason to believe that grassroots homebirth consumer support can be generated swiftly when the stakes are high relative to the fate of midwifery.

CREATING A WAY OUT OF NO WAY, AGAIN?

The historical efforts of Massachusetts midwives discussed at the beginning of this chapter illustrate the potential for creating new health-care spaces. Both DEMs and CNMs in Massachusetts have proven able to create a way out of no way in the past. It remains to be seen whether they can do it again, this time gaining their independence from medical jurisdiction. As was the case historically, the national sociocultural and political scene will have an important influence on the way events unfold in Massachusetts. Present events appear favorable for midwives. As the twenty-first century dawns, many large-scale institutions and traditions are being transformed at a core level. Nowhere is this truer than in American health care, where a market-driven system is replacing a physician-dominated system. Other recent structural changes, such as the increase in mind/body medicine, the emphasis on prevention, and the emergence of evidence-based medicine,[7] lend additional credibility to the midwifery model of care. To this end, the PEW Health Professions Commission and the University of California, San Francisco Center for the Health Professions published a joint report called "Charting a Course for the 21st Century: The Future of Midwifery." In this publication, the joint taskforce notes that it has "reviewed the available literature and analyzed recent market changes. It is the finding and vision of the taskforce that the *midwifery model of care is an essential element of comprehensive health care for women and their families that should be embraced by, and incorporated into, the health care system and made available to all women*" (1999: i, emphasis in original).

As the structural framework of health care is being reconstructed, midwives have slowly been increasing their presence in American maternity and women's health care. In Massachusetts the percentage of births attended by midwives is considerably higher than it is nationwide, with an overall rate of 13.2 percent (National Vital Statistics Reports 1999). At the very least, the Massachusetts midwives have a solid foundation from which to launch their joint legislative proposal.

TIMELINE OF MIDWIFERY HISTORY IN MASSACHUSETTS

1907 Massachusetts becomes the first state to declare midwifery the practice of medicine.
1973 Nurse-midwives initiate a bill to gain licensure.
1977 The legislature passes a midwifery licensing bill.
1977 The governor vetoes the midwifery licensing bill.

1977　The legislature overrides the governor's veto and Massachusetts becomes one of the last states to pass a bill legalizing CNMs. However, CNMs were legally prohibited from attending homebirths.

1982　A homebirth attended by a family practitioner/birth attendant team ends in a neonatal death.

1982　A homebirth attended by a direct-entry midwife who was also a nurse ends in a neonatal death.

1983　The Massachusetts Nursing Board brings a case against the direct-entry midwife revoking her nursing license and charging her with deceit, malpractice, and gross misconduct, and strongly implying that direct-entry midwifery is practicing medicine without a license.

1983　Massachusetts Friends of Midwives (MFOM) is created to support the direct-entry midwife and fight for the future of direct-entry midwifery in Massachusetts.

1984　In a strongly worded decision in favor of the direct-entry midwife, the judge reinstates the direct-entry midwife's nursing license.

1985　Midwifery is declared separate and distinct from the practice of medicine.

1987　CNMs win the right to attend homebirths.

2000　Massachusetts becomes the first state to submit and propose a bill with a joint board of midwifery including both direct-entry midwives and certified nurse-midwives.

2005　The joint midwifery bill continues to be resubmitted for legislative approval.

ACKNOWLEDGMENTS

My deep thanks to B. J. Mackinnon, Peggy Garland, and Robbie Davis-Floyd for their helpful comments on this chapter.

ENDNOTES

1. This portion of the paper is based on archival research and a four-year field investigation (1983 through 1987) completed by the author for her doctoral dissertation.

2. During the 1970s and early 1980s most midwives who attended births at home called themselves lay midwives. During the later 1980s and early 1990s they rejected this term with its pejorative implications in favor of the present term, direct-entry midwives.

3. MFOM formally supported both lay midwives and certified nurse-midwives, but the early group was largely a support group for lay midwives. The MMA also began by formally including both certified nurse-midwives and lay midwives, but their focus soon became oriented only toward lay midwives and has remained this way. During

this stage in Massachusetts history the interests of nurse-midwives and lay midwives did not coincide. Nurse-midwives aimed their efforts at establishing legitimacy within the medical arena. Supporting unlicensed marginal practitioners would compromise their hard-won professional status. Lay midwives were engaged in a pitched battle for survival that consumed all their efforts, and concerns about gaining professional status would have to come after their survival was assured.

4. This is a legal term meaning that a particular law has potentially dire, but as yet uninterrupted, consequences.

5. The research for this section is based on over seventy in-depth interviews (averaging five hours each) with midwives and their clients, physicians, health-care educators, lawyers, nurses, psychologists, and scientists. Further, over thirty additional informal interviews with the same population have supplemented the investigation.

6. This transport situation remains unofficial and as such it can change substantially at any time. For years, midwifery transports in Massachusetts had been gaining more and more hospital support. However, as I write this, the current transport context has begun to change. A couple of hospitals in the state have questioned recent transports by a midwife and as a result have become less receptive to future homebirth transports.

7. An international enterprise to systematically review the scientific evidence for current health-care practices.

REFERENCES

Annas, George. 1984. *A Practitioner's Guide to Birth Outside the Hospital*, 161–181. Rockville: Aspen Systems Corporation.

Board of Registration in Nursing. 1983. Adjudicatory Hearing in the Matter of Janet Leigh. *Board of Registration in Nursing.* May

Board of Registration in Nursing. 1983. Order to Show Just Cause. *Board of Registration in Nursing.* October.

Boston Globe. 1984. "Judge Reinstates License of Nurse Who Is Midwife." September 11.

Boston Globe. 1985. "SJC Approves Lay Midwifery." August 16.

Boston Magazine. 1982. "Midwife Crises." September.

Boston Sunday Globe. 1977. "Home Births." October 16.

Centers for Disease Control and Prevention. 1999. *Trends in the Attendant, Place, and Timing of Births and in the Use of Obstetric Interventions: United States, 1989–97.* Hyattsville, MD: National Center for Health Statistics, National Vital Statistics System. 47(27).

Clement, Grace. 1998. *Care, Autonomy, and Justice.* Boulder, CO: Westview Press.

Commonwealth v. Porn. 1907. Decision. Supreme Judicial Court of Massachusetts. October 15.

DeClerq, Eugene R. 1994. "The Trials of Hannah Porn: The Campaign to Abolish Midwifery in Massachusetts." *American Journal of Public Health* (84):1022–1028.

DeVries, Raymond G. 1985. *Regulating Birth: Midwives, Medicine, and the Law.* Philadelphia, PA: Temple University Press.

Edwards, Margot & Waldorf. 1984. *Reclaiming Birth.* New York: Crossing Press.

Hughes, John A., Martin, Peter J., and W. W. Sharrock. 1995. *Understanding Classical Sociology.* London: SAGE Publications.

Janet Leigh v. Board of Registration in Nursing. 1984. Decision. Division of Registration, Board of Nursing. January.

Janet Leigh v. Board of Registration in Nursing. 1984. Plaintiff's Memorandum in Support of Motion for Summary Judgment. Supreme Judicial Court of Massachusetts of Suffolk County. June.

Janet Leigh v. Board of Registration in Nursing. 1984. Judgment. Supreme Judicial Court of Massachusetts of Suffolk County. September 6.

Janet Leigh v. Board of Registration in Nursing. 1985. Decision. Supreme Judicial Court of Massachusetts of Suffolk County. August 15.

Midwife Advocate. 1987. Special issue, Vol. 3, No. 4, winter.

Pew Health Professions Commission and the University of California, San Francisco Center for the Health Professions (A joint report). 1999. *Charting a Course for the 21st Century: The Future of Midwifery.* San Francisco: University of California.

Sallomi, Pacia. 1982. "Midwifery and the Law." *Mothering,* summer 1982.

Sullivan, Deborah and Rose Weitz. 1988. *Labor Pains: Modern Midwives and Home Birth.* New Haven, CT: Yale University Press.

Thompson, Becky W. 1994. *A Hunger So Wide and So Deep.* Minneapolis: University of Minnesota Press.

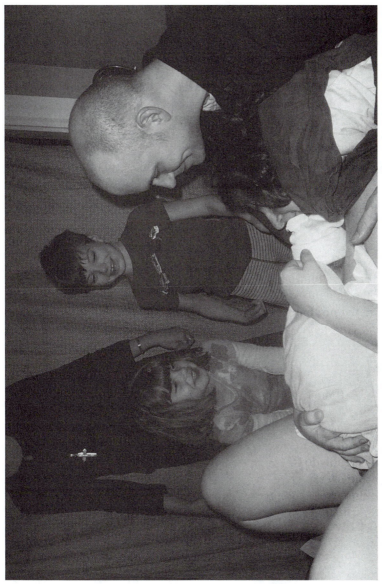

Fig. 9.1 Joyfully greeting the new arrival—a recent Massachusetts home birth. Photographer: Mikaela Walters.

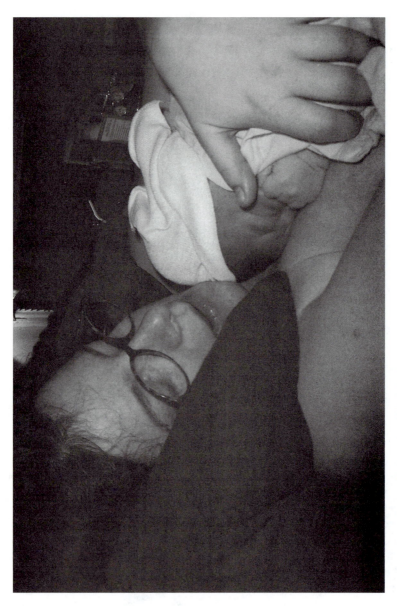

Fig. 9.2 Peacefully bonding in Boston. Photographer: Mikaela Walters.

Part III

Core Issues in Mainstreaming Midwives

These four chapters address core issues in mainstreaming midwives. Betty-Anne Daviss brings humor and wit to her sociological analysis of the tensions between the social change agendas of the midwifery and alternative birth movements, and midwifery's professionalization project. She describes standard professionalization theories (showing how midwives fit them and don't) and social movement theories, strongly suggesting that midwives' approach is most "nobly characteristic" of how social movements become institutionalized to create effective change.

Through poignant stories about "renegade" midwives and their clients, Robbie Davis-Floyd and Christine Barbara Johnson address the thorny issue of midwives who choose to violate professional protocols in favor of helping even high-risk women achieve their desires for natural births. The authors ask whether such midwives constitute assets or liabilities to midwifery, concluding that in a "can't live with 'em, can't live without 'em" paradox, renegade midwives, sometimes irresponsibly, do threaten the professionalization project while at the same time demanding, by example, careful consideration of the compromises that are made in the bid for social legitimacy. The authors note that whether at home or in the hospital, when faced with a dichotomy between what protocols dictate and what the mother wants, the midwife can call on her talent for "normalizing uniqueness"—taking information both from physical indicators and from deep intuition about what is right for this particular woman at this particular time. Trust in intuition can help midwives find the right balance between the needs of the woman and the needs of their profession—just beneath the surface of apparent conformity, to some extent every midwife is a renegade.

For midwifery to enter the mainstream, midwives attending homebirths must be able to transport to hospitals when necessary without encountering disrespectful treatment of the midwife or the mother from hospital staff—a core issue both for both homebirth midwives and medical practitioners, who must choose between stereotypical denigration and factual evaluation of the particular circumstances of the birth. The typical biomedical response to home-to-hospital transport is criticism of a "botched homebirth"—an attitude that disregards the responsibility and concern for safety homebirth midwives exhibit when they do transport. Johnson and Davis-Floyd address this core impediment to mainstreaming midwives through recounting transport stories during which mutual respect and accommodation came to characterize the homebirth/biomedical interface, a phenomenon the authors identify as a *magical transport mandorla*.

The final core issues addressed this section are *why midwives matter,* and if they matter so much, *what are the barriers to midwives becoming the primary care providers for the majority of American women?* Johnson and Davis-Floyd take on these issues, describing the essence of midwifery care, listing the primary barriers to its growth, and noting the multiple ways in which midwives and consumers are seeking to overcome these barriers.

10

FROM CALLING TO CAREER: KEEPING THE SOCIAL MOVEMENT IN THE PROFESSIONAL PROJECT

Betty-Anne Daviss

• **American Midwifery and Professionalization Theories** • **Jane and the Kids in Court: The Catch in a Capsule** • **The Four Theories of Social Movements: How Midwifery Fits** • **Conclusions**

An aspiring midwife of today, like her sisters of the Middle Ages, may enter childbirth circles through an enraptured "calling" to transform each mother and her own life during the sacred act of birth. Another may choose an infinitely more practical but no less rewarding path to ambitiously embark on a search for a professional career in midwifery, choose the "best midwifery school" and accreditation system, engage in medical research, and even dare envision a little brush with fame. In North America, the eager and willing coming from either point of entry stand to encounter major disappointment. The spiritual idealist commonly discovers that her chosen route of education or the mothers who "just want to have a baby" may not suitably measure up to the midwife's spiritual aspirations. The career builder will become disillusioned that in spite of scientific proof of the efficacy of midwifery care, even midwives graduating from prestigious schools have to defend their credibility, the right to insurance and hospital privileges, and indeed the right to practice.

In this chapter I challenge the dominant theories that suggest the dichotomy that midwifery is primarily either a calling or a profession—a common debate midwives have had for several decades. I contend that becoming a midwife is nothing short of a lifelong engagement in social activism. Whether you are promoting the call to spiritual enlightenment and saving womankind from counterfeit birth or trying to advance the midwifery profession in an increasingly technological landscape dominated by medicine, the essential career of the modern North American midwife is first and foremost that of social activist. She stands "with woman" to help empower her, in the context of her debilitating societal constraints, to do even more than she thought she was capable of doing.

In previous works I have pointed out that much social science literature about midwives has been devoted to their legislation and professionalization. Less analysis focuses on monitoring the social movement from which midwives gained their momentum because it is more difficult to gauge (Daviss 1999). I have demonstrated how the alternative birth movement (ABM) took its place among the social movements of our time—feminism, civil rights, the environmental and counterculture movements (Daviss 2001a:70–86). In the following pages, I will integrate social movement and professionalization theories to describe what midwives do. First, I will follow the trajectory of social science theories about how professions arise and maintain power, demonstrating where American midwives have converged on such a path and where they have not. As an example of midwives' social movement versus professionalization dilemmas, I will recount the story of a midwifery client who got herself into trouble—and out again—when she bumped up against the legal/mainstream world. Finally, I will demonstrate how the growth of the ABM fits each of the four theories of the development of social movements in order to suggest that the midwives' approach may be more nobly characteristic of how social movements become institutionalized than of how professions stake out their jurisdictions and create monopolies over a body of knowledge.

The experience of trying to maintain the ideals of the movement—heed one's calling and become a professional, often all at the same time—is taking midwives through a series of collision courses. Learning how to deal with these forces is an art form requiring understanding of infrastructures and processes much like the grammatical framework of a foreign language. This chapter intends to provide some frameworks with which to tackle this challenge, and thus I find it fitting to dedicate it to aspiring midwives. It is better, I contend, to take up the banner of enthusiasm riddled with reality than to be hit with the sudden surprises that can arise when midwifery myths confront sociocultural realities.

AMERICAN MIDWIFERY AND PROFESSIONALIZATION THEORIES

Does the development of American midwifery fit standard professionalization theory? The original *taxonomic* and *process* approaches to professionalization suggest that professions distinguish themselves from other occupations by core features or steps that they take: (1) becoming a full-time occupation; (2) establishing training programs, preferably at the university level; (3) developing a professional association; (4) attaining state licensure to protect their territory; and (5) establishing a formal code of ethics around community service (Barber 1963; Parsons 1954, 1967; Wilensky 1964). While the members of the American College of Nurse-Midwives (ACNM) have carefully taken steps to fulfill all of these requirements, the midwives in the Midwives Alliance of North America (MANA), who are trained in a variety of ways, have often intentionally deviated from such a course. Comparing these two major midwifery organizations in the United States can be deceptive or unfair because they have different functions. As MANA has seen opportunities to professionalize, it has generally deferred such tasks to other organizations such as the North American Registry of Midwives (NARM) and the National Association of Certified Professional Midwives (NACPM). The history behind this calculated strategy of avoiding professional encroachments on MANA's looser social movement style offers important perspectives on the trouble with professionalization.

First, many MANA members chose not to treat midwifery as a full-time job. They began midwifery after their own or a friend's homebirth, extended that opportunity to other mothers in their community, but coveted time at home with their own children. In the year 2000, even those MANA members credentialed through NARM as Certified Professional Midwives (CPMs) were doing on the average only eighteen births per year (Johnson and Daviss 2005a). While small, these numbers are significant: such midwives often provide more continuity of care because they are more available, take more time to debrief with each woman about her birth and the rest of her life, and are more prone to answer the "simple" questions that busy full-time midwives may find tiresome. Second, MANA members have continually questioned whether "higher education" necessarily creates better midwives than the apprenticeship approach (see chapter 1), especially given that a woman ambitiously distracted by a university career path may lack the patience or aptitude to provide the kind of grunt work required to get a woman through her labor. Third, midwives in MANA have heavily debated for two decades about how or whether to form a professional association (one that requires national certification for membership), not wanting to exclude from their organization consumers, doulas, students, and those midwives not interested in becoming evaluated or registered under accredited schools or evaluation systems such as the ACNM Certification Council (ACC) or NARM. Fourth, legislative rulings have also been challenged more by MANA than ACNM members (see part II and chapter 11 of this book) because interventive procedures espoused by the legal medical monopoly turn up in statutes to "protect the public," but become unethically imposed on women whether they want them or not (e.g., cesareans required for all breech deliveries). And fifth, the two common professional characteristics deemed critical by both MANA and ACNM have been the creation of core competencies and a code of ethics. Providing informed choice for women has become a major component of those ethics for all midwifery organizations.

A second professional theory, the neo-Weberian approach, departs from the simplistic theory that professional qualification is merely stipulated by certain traits or processes. Neo-Weberian theorists study how professions create and maintain power structures, arguing that a profession generates *collective pretensions*, monopoly over a body of knowledge, and exclusionary closure over the right to practice in a jurisdiction by the creation of self-government and legal sanctions (Hughes 1971; Parkin 1979; Saks 1983). The ultimate stage of social closure in establishing a profession is control over other professions, such as medicine over midwifery (Freidson 1970a,b).

The third theory, the *neo-Marxist* approach, notes that the neo-Weberian approach attributed the power of professionals to knowledge but ignored the social conditions that make some kinds of knowledge more powerful than others. Neo-Marxist theorists suggest that the capitalist system provides a context in which certain divisions of labor become more important economically. For example, physicians acquired and maintained authority by establishing themselves in those privileged positions and becoming incorporated into the upper classes (Johnson 1977:93–110; Boreham 1983:693–718). Then acting for the dominant class, physicians could obscure or exclude social causes of illness, mask the economic patterns of activity that damage health, and prescribe antidotes to the problem that can be accessed only through the medical profession.

A fourth theory integrates the neo-Marxist approach with the neo-Weberian one, suggesting that an occupation seeking professionalization must develop exclusive control and standardization over the tasks it designates as important through professional licensing, certification, and monopoly over the market. Since the invention of forceps and their lure for mothers to get the job done faster through somebody else's power, midwives' efforts to maintain a monopoly in the market of childbirth have been usurped. One of midwives' best negotiating tools for self-preservation during the nineteenth century was the indignity of having a medical man at the birth. Today, midwives' strength usually lies in their ability to facilitate the process of pregnancy and birth with as little intervention as possible. But this is a hard sell in a society increasingly obsessed with the modus operandi that important tasks require technology. Establishing a midwifery monopoly on birth would require an overhaul of the American value system.

The fifth approach to professionalization theory incorporates gender (Grandjean and Bernal 1979; Hearn 1982). Anne Witz integrates the Marxist, Weberian, and gender approaches, noting that "men engaged in occupational professionalism will have access to the resources of class as well as gender privilege" (1992:37). She illustrates the gendered occupational imperialism that results when a male-dominated profession "encircles" and "subordinates" women "within a related but distinct sphere of competence" (47). This encirclement and subordination occurred in the United States between 1908 and 1918 (Donegan 1978; Witz 1992) when the obstetric nurse began to become the norm instead of the midwife. As in Britain during the nineteenth century, however, midwifery survived in the United States in part because physicians were not interested in doing births for the poorer classes—a task continued by the "black granny midwives" of the South and nurse-midwives in both inner cities and rural settings. Nevertheless, the medical profession was careful to demarcate specific duties for the nurse-midwife, and to attempt to *de-skill* her by guarding anything considered "abnormal" as the exclusive prerogative of the physician.

Witz's prescription for midwives to negotiate their way out of a subordinate role to physicians would be to take what she calls a "revolutionary" rather than an accommodating stand—to *re-skill* themselves in instrumentation, intervention, and the use of medicine. The ACNM followed this path, negotiating nurse-midwives' way into hospitals and even, in 1973 and 1976, making a statement against homebirth (rescinded in 1981) (Rooks 1997:66). Taking an entirely different approach, MANA midwives chose not to demarcate themselves from their consumers. Rather than re-skill the midwife with instrumentation, they decided to ignore the patriarchal monopolistic tendencies of the professions and to re-skill the client in learning how to control her own birth. While the CNMs were making important inroads into helping women gain access to midwifery care in hospitals, the supreme act of the revolution was to take birth out of the domain of the professionals altogether and return it to the home. Challenging the hospital professionals' monopoly over birth was strategic for the movement.

Some theorists suggest that the dominance of medicine among health-care professionals—chiropractors, midwives, nurses, psychologists, naturopaths, and so forth—is period-based and that the reemergence of modern allied health professions has been a regeneration of nineteenth-century health-care pluralism (Cant and Sharma 1999). I would contend that while there has been some reaction to medical attempts at monopoly over the last forty years, the threat to medical licensing laws is not as widespread as it was in the 1840s, when the Jacksonian democratic era allowed widespread distrust of elite monopoly privilege (Starr 1982). Particularly with respect to childbirth, the relative monopoly physicians have today is relentless. It is still clear that it will take a huge societal shift outside of professional spheres to make the changes necessary to bring a sense of normalcy back to birth.

The "collective pretentions" that have been amassed by professions in order to create and maintain jurisdictions (Hughes 1971:338–347), and certain ideologies that may not reflect reality but are nevertheless successful (Rushing 1993:46–47), are used by professional groups to project an image that will win them status. Hughes and Rushing agree that a substantial amount of delusion—some deliberate, some circumstantial—is required to attain the professional goal. In sum, since the early taxonomic theorists, all of the analytical approaches to professionalization (neo-Weberian, neo-Marxist, and gendered) have questioned how admirable and ethical the motivations of professional projects actually are. By the time Witz wrote in 1992, the prevailing paradigm in professionalization theory was that professions develop an elitist and self-serving approach to win status over other professions. Meanwhile, the typical defensive norm among professions has been to cling to illusory, historic adages like "Do no harm."

Midwives in the 1970s and 1980s recognized the importance of acknowledging the strategies of delusion and denial used by professions to stake out and retain jurisdictions (Hughes 1971; Rushing 1993). Nevertheless, as they re-create midwifery in the United States, midwives are often beguiled by the structures that give them the credibility they deserve, yet adorn them with the patriarchal persona they so disdain. Because their struggle resonates with the struggles of many idealists in other social movements, I offer the case of Jane, a midwifery client, as an appropriate segue to understanding the legacy midwives inherit as they develop their social movement. Jane's experiences of betrayal and reemergence when she bumped up against the system typify the plight of the idealist/social activist.

JANE AND THE KIDS IN COURT: THE CATCH IN A CAPSULE

I'll provide some fictitious names to protect identities, but this is a true story (with a little added color) about a midwife client's interaction with the mainstream world. Jane and Malcolm threw out their TV, moved to the country, and ate a lot of peaches. Particularly under Malcolm's spirit of brazen independence, they took up composting, grew as much as they could on their own, heated with solar energy, had their kids at home with a neighbor who had apprentice-trained and attended 135 births, and tried to raise children in an antiracist environment. They stayed away from a diet of anything white—white bread, white pasta, white sugar, white eggs—and avoided anything plastic except Frisbees. While looking up at the stars during her menstrual cycle, I'm sure Jane squatted over moss. But somewhere along the way, Malcolm got tired of the fieldwork, met a city-wiser maiden, and left the woman with whom he had frolicked in the fields. When he decided to sue for custody of the kids, his story was that she was "weird" and shouldn't really take care of the kids because she ran around with them in the nude in the woods and "must be a witch or something." Suddenly and conveniently he was concerned about convention. But he didn't know the power of his supposedly gullible ex, whom he underestimated in her ability to handle other social contracts.

Supported by her midwife, who went to court with her, Jane got on the stand in a red suit and pearls. When the man in a black suit and tie asked Jane about witchcraft, she produced a brochure that demonstrated that, yes, she had been asked to create a dance for a gathering of women. Was this what Malcolm was trying to say was witchcraft? Even the judge and the other suits realized the young man was twisting the story for his own purposes, and let *her* have custody of the kids. His strategy backfired on him. This wasn't Salem, and it was 1992—not 1692. Jane had new rules—not necessarily ones she thought judicious, but she learned quickly how to play the game under a different paradigm and a new box of behavior codes. She kept the kids in the country and kept up her lifestyle, but she also made sure that the kids learned about the city and its enticements, and about parents whose value systems change as they grow up. Jane's out-of-the-system bubble had to expand to encompass that other reality called society and social norms, with its changing rewards and ethics.

Many midwives of the 1970s and early 1980s, enjoying the counter-culture and influence of their own clients, worked their way into their own small circle of creative norms. Reviewing theories about how social movements arise is one of the best ways to explore the reality these midwives have created as they have wandered in and out of the mainstream. While many CNMs were part of this process, the history of the major experiments of the social movement among midwives is best illustrated not through the ACNM, but through organizations like MANA, Midwifery Today, and Birthing the Future, which epitomize the effort to debunk any sniff of the patriarchy, embrace every possible birth modality, and consider every tangential diversity of thought. However, the recent firings in large numbers of CNMs in Austin, San Antonio, New York, Cleveland, and many other cities around the United States have sparked CNMs as well to seriously consider the question: Where have all the flowers and placards gone? What was started in the 1970s may just have been cut short by the mass practical strategy of legislation. Let us revisit why we started our social movement in the first place, through the analytical lens of social movement theory.

THE FOUR THEORIES OF SOCIAL MOVEMENTS: HOW MIDWIFERY FITS

The four theories of social movements are infinitely instructional with respect to the dilemmas of the alternative birth movement.

Classical or Strain Model Theory: From the 1960s to the Present in the United States ABM

Classical *strain theory* holds that social movements arise in response to some breakdown in society (Lang 1961; Smelser 1962). The breakdown studied by *collective behavior* theorists had its roots in the post-World War II world of the 1950s. As the American administration increasingly engaged in imperialism around the world—getting rid of Arbenz in Guatemala in 1954, dividing Korea (1950 to 1953), backing a military coup in the Dominican Republic (1965), and tracking down and assassinating Che in Bolivia (1967)—people at home were building inspiration from the civil rights, women's liberation, and anti-Vietnam-war movements. Women were experiencing the imperialism of the medical profession over their health care, especially in childbirth.

The "breakdown" they sensed was a disconnection from their own bodies and their ability to perform a normal bodily function. Prevailing obstetric techniques seemed to be the cause of the alienation. During the 1970s, a growing discontent with the medical profession paralleled the counterculture spirit and sparked the natural healing movement, which thrived not only on bee pollen and granola, but also on its key ingredients: self-help, self-discovery, and self-transformation. The 8,000 ways to self-actualize in America created an uninhibited group of women who took things into their own hands. The optimism was high and dictatorial: make love not war, focus on female support for life instead of avoidance of death, and have your baby in your own bed, not on someone else's turf. As with Jane's neighbor midwife, the essential reason why many midwives in North America in the 1970s began their work was merely as an extension of other things they were doing with their lives. They incorporated assisting at other women's births as part of a code of behavior through which they connected and promoted their lifestyle. Should one among them feel "called" to attend births, the others supported her. They used feminist language: "the personal is political."

A characteristic stressed by classical strain social movement theory is that participants must go through a conversionlike experience. Social movements mobilize consumers in a transformative fashion. True to this genre, mothers and fathers busy with newborns create space for hours of volunteer work, and natural birth practitioners spend passionate and inordinate hours at meetings, all "for the cause." Job satisfaction among midwives becomes a moot point when the stakes and rewards are far beyond any "job." Jane and her midwife were part of this movement.

The Resource Mobilization Model or Theory (RMT): The Early 1980s to the Present in the United States ABM

In well-articulated, at times fierce opposition to classical strain theory, *resource mobilization* theorists argue that breakdowns happen on a pretty regular basis now in modern society and are often unaccompanied by any social movement. There must be some other critical factor that facilitates a social movement to emerge (Olson 1965; McCarthy and Zald 1973). I find the various slants available for explaining this theory best encapsulated in three interpretations:

Social movements succeed when beliefs are transformed into concrete action (Diani 1992:4). ABM members share the common goal of "changing childbirth by minimizing medical intervention and maximizing women's choice," heralding birth as a normal physiologic event and women's role in their own decision making as paramount (Daviss 2001:74–75). The concrete results produced in the 1970s and 1980s by ABM members included: near-universal access to childbirth education; the presence of partners and family during labor and birth; alternative birth centers in hospitals; increased rates of breastfeeding and VBACs; and making it possible for laboring women to be "awake and aware," to drink and eat lightly, to stay in the same room for labor, delivery, and recovery, and to keep the baby in their room after birth. ABM members also provided the options of homebirth, birth in freestanding birth centers, and water birth.

Social movements respond to conditions that facilitate the constitution of their organizations as well as the dynamics of cooperation/competition among them (Diani 1992:4). The ABM shone in its ability to rally all those who believed in the importance of keeping birth normal and reclaiming it from the clutches of medical men and technology. Various joint consumer/midwifery groups arose in the 1970s, such as the National Association of Parents and Professionals for Safe Alternatives in Childbirth (NAPSAC), which joined professionals and parents together in the common cause. Unlike the nursing, medical, and nurse-midwifery professions, the ABM was consumer-based and consumer-driven. MANA was created in 1982 to unify all midwives, but MANA did not connect as well as its members had hoped with the ACNM, which had pulled away in the 1970s and 1980s from any connection with what many nurse-midwives perceived as those rabble-rousing, anti-establishment, irreverent midwives of questionable integrity and training.

In the 1980s, the countercultural and New Age midwives who felt at home in MANA found common ground with indigenous and ethnic groups, religious groups, and feminists. Yet in spite of the fact that the counterculture midwives were attracted to serving aboriginal, African-American, and Hispanic groups, the ABM has not reached these groups on a wide scale. It is hard to motivate women still striving to have rights to health care to reclaim the natural childbirths they were forced to have because they were denied full access to hospitals and their technologies. Shortly after the Alabama state health department took away the license of a black granny midwife, I asked her whether or not her daughter would want to become a midwife. "Oh no," she said. "She wants to get an education."

It has been the sad irony of the ABM that some African-American women assume that "midwifery" and "education" are somehow oxymorons. At an affirmative action meeting in the 1980s at MANA,

African-American midwives called attention to the fact that they weren't interested in wearing the secondhand clothes adorning the white hippie middle-class midwives in the room. They said they wanted "to look nice" and avoid the social stigma of appearing unable to afford new clothes. Concomitantly, it is entirely understandable that African-American women might equate "granny midwifery" and homebirth with low social status.

As the homebirth movement of the 1970s was beginning, some religious groups, such as the Amish and the Mennonites, had already intentionally divorced themselves from mainstream medicine and were using their own midwives. These groups began to make use of midwives outside their religious circles as they became available. Mennonite and Amish women still account for an astounding 33.5 percent of all CNM-attended homebirths and for 12.3 percent of CPM-attended home-births (Murphy and Fullerton 1998; Johnson and Daviss 2005a). Other fundamentalist Christian groups like Seventh Day Adventists, Mormons, and Christian Scientists also believe in the importance of keeping birth as natural as God intended. Most ABM members who do not identify with organized religion do identify with a sense of the sacredness of birth and the value of a spiritual kind of midwifery (Gaskin 1975, Arms 1975). As various social movement theorists have shown, this kind of shared belief can create a group consciousness so strong that it overcomes competing differences of class, religion, and age (Lawn-Day 1994).

The ABM has not yet overcome the factors of race and ethnicity: ninety percent to ninety-five percent of women having homebirths attended by CNMs and CPMs in America are white Caucasians (Murphy and Fullerton 1998; Johnson and Daviss 2005a). The many women in religious groups who birth at home rarely attend the sociopolitical conferences organized by groups like MANA and Midwifery Today. In contrast, while few native and African-American women birth at home African-American and native midwives, often sponsored by these organizations, both attend and speak at their conferences. Some African-American midwives have felt that their white sisters hang out with them because they are "exotic," but don't really understand their unique dilemmas. Their initiation of their own midwives' association has been a liberating move; in Portland in October 2004, they were in the fitting position of inviting MANA members to *their* meeting, the third annual Black Midwives and Healers Conference, a herstoric one for the midwifery sisterhood. In inner-city hospitals, many dedicated CNMs/CMs serve minority women. In 1985, MANA created the Sage-Femme award for "Grand Midwives," who have worked for many years for their community; women in minority groups are usually honored with this award. Such ongoing exchanges with minority groups through birth attendance and conference participation continue to inspire and ground the members of the ABM in an important history and shared social cause.

When the counterculture midwives first joined with the feminists, they were strange bedsisters. An early feminist stand embodied in such works as *The Dialectic of Sex* (Firestone 1970) argued that bearing children is the root of women's oppression by men, class, and race, and that the solution freeing women from this biology is the use of technology, which eliminates biological reproduction. Feminists have long struggled with concepts of birth, mothering, and work in the home. In 1977, Adrienne Rich's *Of Woman Born* distinguished between two meanings of motherhood—one superimposed on the other: The *potential relationship* of any woman to her powers of reproduction and to children; and the *institution* of motherhood, which aims to ensure that the potential (and all women) remain under male control (xv). During the 1970s and 1980s, *Mothering Magazine* became popular among women searching for a way to deal with a new age in mothering, new reproductive technologies, and a career, with solutions like house husbands. While engaging in these discussions, midwives and midwifery consumers often espoused home schooling along with homebirth, creating a tension between feminist philosophy and midwifery. As the first midwife ever asked to speak at the National Women's Studies Conference (Chicago, July 1987), I was told quite directly that this organization's lack of interest in midwives was a result of midwives' leanings toward "enslaving women to the home setting" and promoting the traditional role of the wife and values of motherhood in the biological reductionism of bearing children.

There was another, perhaps more subtle difference in the way the counterculture and New Age ABM members functioned compared to the feminists. They were more pacifistic. Spiritual idealists often dislike the concept of "tainting true midwifery" with too much organizational or political talk, even too much analytical academic work. For many years, even the notion of charging for services was considered outside the realm of "real midwifery." When researchers proposed the notion of amassing statistics on birth outcomes by having homebirth midwives fill out data forms, there were those midwives who said, "Birth is magical. Why adulterate it with statistical analysis?" Such midwives have often been considered by feminists to be "stuck," while their counterparts move on.

The issues that eventually galvanized the counterculture midwives *and* the feminists were the imperatives of reproductive rights and informed choice for women. During the MANA convention of 1984 in Toronto, Canada, Michele Landsberg, a well-known Canadian journalist, appealed to a large audience to get rid of the "many petty divisions amongst women, especially in the area of motherhood vs. feminism" because "both the feminist and midwifery movements are about freedom of choice for women" (Worts 1985). Consensus was the modus operandi for MANA, an ambitious undertaking when the counterculture/ethnic/religious/feminist groups were all so individualistic.

Midwifery attracted several other groups that had difficulties in the early days in associating with each other. Caucuses developed and met at each MANA conference—Christian midwives, lesbians, Wiccans. (Some Christians left MANA in 1987 when Starhawk was a featured speaker; others stayed to make sure such things didn't happen again, squelching a move to present Ina May Gaskin with a broomstick or a big black cauldron, choosing instead an electric skillet.) There were frequent discussions about whether having all these caucuses wasn't disruptive, polarizing, and a distraction from the issues rather than the desired expression of diversity. At one point Maggie Bennett, legal dwarf and revered California midwife, stood up and asked, "Shouldn't there be a caucus for short people?" Nevertheless, such caucuses have enabled midwives to articulate their identities with likeminded sisters, and have constituted an acknowledgment that midwifery is tied to culture.

The dynamics between MANA and ACNM are much discussed in other chapters in this volume. Suffice it to say that MANA midwives alienated ACNM members not only because MANA midwives refused to embrace university education, but also because they did not create an image deemed professional enough—they engaged in too many "wild" behaviors at their conferences and in public presentation, and they based a large amount of their practice on feeling and intuition, which could be easily interpreted as conjecture. Equally discouraging, because ACNM members created the statement against homebirth in 1973, internationally spoke out against lay homebirth midwives at the International Confederation of Midwives (ICM) conference in The Hague (1987), excluded them from the New York 1992 legislation, tried twice to discredit the right of MANA to be a member of the International Confederation of Midwives, and denigrated the validity of the CPM credential for years after its creation, they in turn alienated many members of MANA. Such difficulties between ACNM and MANA caused two groups that could have been working together for many years for the same cause to instead waste precious time on turf wars. As Davis-Floyd describes in chapter 1 of this volume, the tensions and alienations between these two American groups prompted Canadian nurse- and lay midwives to unite to avoid similar problems in Canada.

Social movements succeed when there is economic growth and prosperity (Marx and McAdam 1994). The period between the 1960s and 1990s was generally a prosperous time in the United States, with an increasing emergence of alternative therapies (Cato Institute 1995). During Clinton's term there was genuine hope, with the White House Commission on Complementary and Alternative Medicine Policy (White House 2002), that there would be increased access to these alternative therapies with third-party billing, but it did not produce the hoped-for major changes. With the Bush administration's focus on war rather than health care at home, there have been fewer resources to divert to social movements.

ACNM has been relatively successful at accessing resources because its members are often on the faculty at nursing or nurse-midwifery schools affiliated with universities, or in established positions with hospitals. In contrast, MANA midwives have spent many of their waking hours trying to help women escape institutions and what they perceive as the disempowering belief and categorical contradiction that laboring women require ivory and glass towers to be helped to perform a natural bodily function. At the MANA conference in Lake Tahoe in 1999, a group of MANA members metaphorically enacted this belief in a performance of "The Wizard of Os" (*os* is the medical term for cervix.) In this skit, Dorothy wanders down the yellow brick road looking for some way to help women understand that "there is no place like home to open your os." The Scarecrow (a midwife who was told by the obstetricians that she didn't have a brain because she didn't know how to manage birth), the Tinman (an obstetrician whose medical school forgot to give him a heart), and the Lion (an obstetrician too cowardly to back up homebirth midwives), reach their goal—the Wizard's domain—only to find that he lives in a make-believe Ivory/Emerald Tower of little use, and that Dorothy and her troupe had "the power" within themselves all along.

The metaphor is apt and well articulates the common concerns of MANA members, but it doesn't propose solutions about how to institutionalize midwives' idealism. Homebirth midwives in the United States have often lacked confidence that their own belief system could change the character of national institutions, and have worried that exposure to such domains will irreversibly change their ideals. Such concerns have compromised both their willingness and their ability to access the financial, academic, and political institutions that provide bureaucratic power. In order for the ABM to flourish, certain criteria must be met: access to education for both midwives and the public so that alternative types of care can be procured; recognition of midwifery as a credible profession and social closure on its acceptability; research into the reasonableness of consumer demands and the efficacy of midwifery care; and positive media coverage of women's choices in childbirth, including midwifery care. All of these would benefit from financial backing.

In each state and nationally, once midwives have been able to override their own inertia at *wanting* to access funding mechanisms connected with large institutions, other problems emerge. Accessing funding for research into therapies that use *less* technology proves difficult in a health-care system in which increasing technology use represents financial gain for the big business of birth. Thus, when research demonstrates that minimizing technology in birth improves outcomes, such advice is rarely heeded because the system does not stand to benefit from a decrease in health care costs. CEOs, hospitals, and physicians *do not* make money from natural childbirth. They *do* make money from using interventions like oxytocin to speed labor, which besides its pharmaceutical costs, increases the predictability of labor and the more efficient use of staff and space. The increased complications that result from the overuse of technology in birth are also financially lucrative for the system because more use is made of the laboratory, the ultrasound unit, the neonatal intensive care unit, and the long hospital stay (Perkins 2004). In the economic context of the resource mobilization theory, as long as the American people continue to support corporate America in considering health care to be a business run for profit rather than a citizen's right, the ABM will remain marginalized.

Political Process Theory and the ABM
from the 1980s to the Present

Political process theory suggests that social movements develop in response to an increase in political opportunities in a changing political system (McAdam 1982; Tilly 1978, 1984). In this conception, social movements are made up of groups performing organized political activity that lack the necessary leverage to pursue their goals through "proper political channels." Society is seen as a system of power relations that grants some groups routine access to power while denying it to others (Marx and McAdam 1994). This theory takes the resource mobilization theory one step further because it suggests that in a democracy, money certainly talks, but political clout institutionalizes your ideas.

Canadian feminists Vickers, Rankin, and Appelle (1993:45–46) point out that whereas English Canadian feminists in the 1970s and 1980s tended to be pro-state and politically proactive, American feminists of the same time period tended to reject the ordinary political process and replace politics with individual consciousness-raising. In other words, American feminism has had more of a focus on the individual transformation typified in the classical strain theory of social movements, while Canadian feminism has focused more on mobilizing resources and political structures. In parallel form, American homebirth midwives have tended more often to embrace the kind of spiritual focus described in Ina May Gaskin's *Spiritual Midwifery* and Elizabeth Davis's *Heart and Hands* than Canadian midwives (Daviss 1999, 2001a).

There is another, broader reality that has played out here. As Scott points out (1990), social movements, in contrast to interest groups, deal with previously unmobilized populations and have more ability for mass mobilization than do political parties and pressure groups. American midwives were tired of patriarchal politics and saw feminism as fundamental both to their philosophy and the very infrastructure with which they set up their organizations. They replaced the usual patriarchal structures with their own. Much attention has been devoted, especially at MANA, to consensus and process, inclusion rather than exclusion, and unity in diversity.

However, as with Jane, reality struck when American midwives observed how their legal system and mass media handle inquests and court cases over homebirth deaths. They watched in horror the creation of the nefarious illusion that homebirth deaths result from not being in the hospital. They watched the baby deaths from intended homebirths (one to three in 1,000) spread across the newspapers while the same ratio for in-hospital births went unreported by the mass media. They also watched how the successful ABM reforms of the 1970s and 1980s were accompanied by dramatic rises in electronic fetal monitoring, cesarean section, and the use of pain-relieving drugs, especially the epidural. With this realization, the preservation of independent midwifery and out-of-hospital birth became even more important to the members of the ABM, many of whom felt that their efforts to transform hospital birth had been co-opted by the dominant system (Rothman 1981). These concerns provoked DEMs to look more seriously at developing evaluation systems to prove the value of the kind of midwifery that would give women choice, gain more mainstream support politically, and make midwives "legal." Some midwifery organizations, like Midwifery Today, continue to provide cultural and educational focus on experimenting and converting people's minds through colorful conferences. For state midwife associations and MANA, however, it began to be clearer in the 1980s that feminist slogans like the "personal is political" did not go far enough. Better strategies were needed in order to access structures that would change government policies. Politics is about creating the proper image, especially one that will fit with the mainstream. This has been difficult for a group whose historical business is to question mainstream integrity and values. It is obvious where Jane and her midwife fit in Table 10.1.

CNMs have been able to access legislation more easily. This is partly historic, partly because they have carefully cultivated a highly professional image so that they are not as associated with the radical social movement elements in the left column of table 10.1. In a similar way, Canadian homebirth midwives were already trying to change their image, pursuing legislation in the early 1980s and gaining ground in part because their legislators have tended to be more open to the feminist rights and responsibilities approach (Daviss 1999). To further their legislative efforts, American DEMs found it necessary to develop a national certification—the CPM—that would create an accessible evaluation system and a professional image without compromising their commitment to apprenticeship and their holistic approach (see chapters 1 and 3).

NARM offers a competency-based certification process credentialing primarily direct-entry midwives who do homebirths. While NARM intentionally avoided attaching itself to already established universities and colleges, the Canadians did precisely the opposite. With the exception of Manitoba, which chose to use NARM's certification system, Canadian midwives deemed their clientele to be from a population that wanted university graduates. No Canadian provinces, however, chose nurse-midwifery. At about the same time, in the early 1990s, ACNM also changed its former requirement of nursing training and opened itself up to university-educated direct-entry midwives with the creation of the new CM credential. But the categorical dismissal of apprentice-trained midwives persists among some CNMs, as evidenced by the debate described in chapter 1.

According to vital statistics reports (Martin, Hamilton, Sutton, Ventura, Menacker, and Munson 2003) only 1.1 percent of the births that CNMs attend take place at home. However, CNMs have always been far ahead of direct-entry midwives in publishing in academic journals, and had already published two homebirth studies (Murphy and Fullerton 1998; Anderson and Murphy 1995) demonstrating their successful outcomes before the DEMs began their first major homebirth study.

Table 10.1 Stylistic Comparison of Social Activists and Health Professionals

	Alternative Counterculture and New Age Birth Activists	Health Professionals
1. Characteristics of gatherings.	Rallies, marches, demonstrations, goddess gatherings, mothers' activist groups with kids.	Professional association meetings, conferences on clinical research and liability concerns, in-service workshops, rounds, no kids allowed (except nursing infants).
2. What is recorded.	Dedication to recording history of human rights violations, spiritual revelations and incidents that bear meaning to humankind. Newsletters include poetry.	Strict adherence to charting and documentation of clinical interaction with patient/client. Professional journals that are peer reviewed, and association newsletters.
3. Diet regimen.	Vegetarian or at least the option thereof at potluck lunches. Tofu, raw veggies, and herb tea. Attempts to recycle at all gatherings.	Coffee and muffins. Recycling if the hotel has the interest.
4. Dress.	Dress in anything colorful, ethnic preferred. Birkenstocks, thongs, no shaving allowed. Carry knapsacks. Tams (beatniks), floppy and broad-brimmed hats (hippies), little hats (punk rockers). Long hair or no hair. Earrings that dangle.	Suits or surgical greens. High heels, hard shoes, no toes showing. Shave any body part or hide it. Carry briefcases. Starched hats (nurses, although no longer in the United States). Styled hair. Small earrings that attract no attention.
5. Seating arrangements.	Often sit on the floor, but preferably on the grass. Like seating arrangements in circles and hug trees.	The longer the table, the better, especially if there is someone who can sit at the head of it. In offices, chairs that roll. At larger meetings, like microphones and speakers in a line facing an audience on a lower level.

(Continued)

Table 10.1 Stylistic Comparison of Social Activists and Health Professionals (*Continued*)

	Alternative Counterculture and New Age Birth Activists	Health Professionals
6. Lighting and props.	Candles or soft ambient lighting, drumming, real flowers, bumper stickers (e.g., "meconium happens"). Hate anything plastic except frisbees.	Fluorescent lights, machines that go beep, fake flowers, insignia and diplomas wherever possible. Artificial accoutrements are used to keep up the image.
7. Language.	Singing, chanting, praying, political slogans. Sensational and catchy if possible.	Medical language, the more daunting the better. The more reserved and unimaginative the better.

Between 1994 and 2000, more than 500 midwives from across the United States and Canada earned NARM certification as CPMs. A large cohort of midwives defined by a common certification process was precisely what was needed in order to create a homebirth study on a defined group over a defined time period. Epidemiologist Ken Johnson and I persuaded the NARM Board that such a scientific study would be prudent to demonstrate the worth of NARM's certification. CPMs must be recertified every three years. The NARM Board agreed to make participation in the study that Ken and I proposed a requirement for recertification, so that all CPMs would participate. The stakes were high. Would a group of individuals concerned about the impingement of bureaucratic structures cooperate with such a study? How would the funding be obtained? And what of the ultimate concern—what if the statistics were bad? With our hearts in our hands and our computers buzzing, we undertook a large, prospective study of all births attended by CPMs in the United States and Canada in the year 2000. As coauthor of this study (Johnson and Daviss 2005a), I was both pleased and saddened to find out that it is the largest prospective homebirth study ever conducted anywhere.

The purpose of the CPM2000 study was to provide reliable, detailed, systematic information on the clients, care, and outcomes of planned homebirths with CPMs; to provide feedback to consumers, the CPMs themselves, and their education accreditation organization; and to inform health professionals, policymakers, and the general public. Its size created the stable perinatal figures that other smaller studies had been unable to provide, and its results provided the necessary validation of the safety of homebirth. Because the perinatal mortality rate for CPM-attended planned homebirths was similar to that of both low-risk hospital birth and CNM-attended homebirths, the CPM2000 study also demonstrated something that was not its expressed purpose: apprentice-trained midwives who complete this certification process recognize when to transfer, what their limitations are, and have good outcomes. (The study's results [Johnson and Daviss 2005a] are provided in chapter 3 of this volume and can also be found at www.bmj.com, volume 330, issue 7505.)

The outcomes of the CPM2000 study suggest that arguments about university training creating better midwives—if defined as better perinatal outcomes—may be off base. MANA and ACNM will probably continue to argue about the advantages of university training (supposedly more technical and research-based) versus apprenticeship (supposedly more woman-centered). But political process theory suggests that the argument promoting university education is focused on the wrong issue. It's not about creating better midwives—it's about accessing resources and credibility. Jane had figured that out when she put on her red suit and pearls. The question remains, does university education necessarily mean that the ideals of the movement will be obliterated by a monster bureaucracy that has no idea what birth is really about?

Benoit, Wrede, and Maclean-Alley (1997) noted that practitioners' abilities to balance life-world and scientific ways of knowing can be impeded or enhanced by the type of training they receive, as well as by the general organization of the health-care system in which they practice. The ideologies of both the ABM and the early feminist movement tended to develop outside both of those spheres—outside the programs where health care practitioners are trained and outside the health-care system in which they work—just as other social movements have usually developed outside of established institutions. It behooves the aspiring North American midwife to understand this *outsideness* of her history and its grassroots connection to the inside realities of women's lives, because this history has entailed the effort to move this out-of-system consciousness into the system without losing that sense of connection.

It was an important part of the political process to have the methodology of the CPM2000 study scrutinized by the epidemiology division of the American Public Health Association (APHA) before it was carried out. When the preliminary results emerged, the association's epidemiologists, privy to the quality of the data, were supportive of a joint statement, wisely proposed by both the ACNM and MANA, to increase access to out-of-hospital birth attended by direct-entry midwives (American Public Health Association 2002:453–455).

This was a major victory, not only for homebirth, but also for the unification of midwives from a variety of backgrounds across the United States. MANA and ACNM had taken an important step forward, together.

The politics of professionalization are not always so rewarding. In 2004 the senators of South Dakota requested evidence that CPM certification would produce good outcomes, but when they discovered that such data actually existed, they ignored it and blocked the proposed legislation anyway. (Some similar unfortunate politics of individual state legislative processes are recounted in various chapters of this anthology.) The new rewards some DEMs have achieved in the legal and political arenas, like those Jane achieved in court, have been put under strain when the local legislature is heavily lobbied by physicians or by CNMs trying to prevent direct-entry homebirth midwives from achieving licensure or moving into positions of power. As well, the *Journal of the American Medical Association* (*JAMA*) rejected the CPM2000 study when we sought publication there, stating that "it would not be of interest" to their readers (physicians). This statement highlighted the sad truth: the important socioeconomic solutions, reduction of interventions without compromising outcomes, and empowerment to women that homebirth provides (see chapter 13) are undervalued by the American medical profession, which often chooses to perpetuate its own ignorance. Fortunately for midwifery, the *British Medical Journal* (*BMJ*) did not share *JAMA*'s view, and after rigorous review, all the *BMJ* editors who reviewed the article accepted it unanimously for publication (Johnson and Daviss 2005a).

In Canada, midwifery legislation pushed physicians' organizations to come around on the homebirth issue and create statements acknowledging the rights of women to make choices for midwifery and homebirth (Society of Obstetricians and Gynecologists of Canada 2003; College of Physicians and Surgeons of Ontario 2001). In contrast, the American College of Obstetricians and Gynecologists (ACOG) has not been as responsible in dealing with the evidence. ACOG has emphasized instead a single and highly misleading homebirth study conducted in 2002 (Pang et al. 2002). This study was based on vital statistics forms, did not include the planned place of birth, was highly publicized even before it was published, and generated multiple responses pointing out obvious problems (see for example Johnson and Daviss 2003). ACOG placed the questionable results on its website, and they remain there to this day. With its present attitude, ACOG is not expected to acknowledge what the rest of the world is increasingly realizing: being anti-homebirth is *so* last century!

ACNM is years ahead of MANA in research matters, attempting to prudently apply research to changes in practice, erring on the side of safety in their concern for the woman and her baby. MANA members have been less likely to produce research or accept any research validating increased intervention without assuming foul play. While as a researcher this latter attitude could make me nervous, I have found myself, on three occasions in the last four years, publishing letters in medical journals protesting research on homebirth or VBAC that has led to unjustifiable conclusions (Daviss 2001b; Johnson and Daviss 2003; Johnson and Daviss 2005b). On all three occasions, CNMs seemed more accepting of this flawed research than MANA members. I would submit that somewhere between reactionary suspicion and uncritical acceptance would be a happy middle ground for the advancement of the ABM.

In spite of the fact that there are now in the United States over 1,000 CPMs practicing in almost all states, and MANA members in all states, the national rate of homebirths has remained relatively stable since 1989, at around 0.6 percent (Martin et al. 2003). Politics and economics have served to get midwives legislated, as seen in many chapters in this text, but they do not appear to be working to support the ABM with respect to homebirth choices.

The New Social Movement Theories (Hopefully, the Mainstay of the United States ABM of the Future)

The New Social Movement theories attributed originally to Touraine (1978, 1981, 1995) and Melucci (1985) have tackled the larger contextual understanding of how social movements have become vehicles of transition to a new, more egalitarian postindustrial society. They distinguish between labor movements concerned with issues of economic distribution and political power, and *new social movements* (NSMs) that arise out of large-scale structural and cultural changes. NSMs are organized around new identities and new communities, and are concerned with replacing old jaded views with more ethical ones. They include the civil rights and feminist movements, the antinuclear and ecological movements, the animal rights and gay rights campaigns, Native American movements, and others.

Touraine said that inherent in these NSMs is a mandate to understand and save the historicity of human function and interaction. He thus offers some explanation for the ABM's attraction to understanding the cultural norms of the indigenous peoples of North America, and why many midwives have embraced an unabashed connection with the history of witchcraft. Connecting the medical establishment with the Inquisition does not produce positive local public opinion or win favor in legislatures, but this type of historic connection galvanizes the spirit of the ABM. Even some Christian midwives acknowledge the burning of the witches during the Inquisition and in Salem as a take-over of evil forces, recognizing with candor their connection with the healing women of the Middle Ages. In the "Wizard of Os" skit mentioned above, the Good Witch asks midwife Dorothy whether she is a good witch or a bad witch. Dorothy's response is a politically correct denial that midwives have any connection with witchcraft at all. The Good Witch overrides Dorothy's apparent ignorance by stating:

> I'm an anthropologist and I know a postmodern witch when I see one! You fit because you don't like the hospital. And you don't like sending in your statistics but you know you should. And you have the audacity to think every woman should be allowed to do what she wants in labor!

I suggest that it is within NSM theory that the alternative birth movement resides best. While NSM theorists understand that the microelements of the organizational, financial, and political processes are important, they focus on the larger ethical issues, the importance of looking at the big picture, and the possibilities of all of the social movements working together to make large-scale cultural changes. NSM theorists give a certain dignity to the classical strain theories, making them appear less haphazard. Thus, Jane's adoption of the clothes and behavior necessary to convince the judge of her social fitness becomes a noble strategy connected with her comprehensive ethics. She plays the game in order to prevent her kids from having to move to the city away from their mother and the family's original ideals.

While resource mobilization and political process theories may support the importance of making midwives legal and connecting with prevailing hierarchies, classical strain and NSM theories focus on the possibilities of more fundamental changes resulting from the cultural struggle, including actual changes in the way institutions function. Like apologies made by various national governments to some indigenous groups for their mistreatment, John Paul II's apology in 2000 for the sins of Roman Catholic abuses during the Inquisition could only be considered a victory for NSM aspirations—a sign of hope that institutions are beginning to understand human rights.

Because NSM theories tackle the importance of interconnectedness, they may present some answers to why consumer movements have been so essential to midwives. Social movements are by definition inclusive, increased "citizen surges" being a means of measuring success (Lofland and Johnson 1991:1–29). They want to expand through an ethic of consciousness-raising, relegating "being exclusive" to a trait equated with snobbery and with disrespect for diversity. Midwives recognize that they are only a small part of a much grander project. Professions, on the other hand, form exclusive clubs with strict criteria for entry and heavy discipline if a member does not live up to standards. Professions tend to set up structures and use established colleges and institutions. Social activists tend to be iconoclastic and break down established institutions. In a changing system with changing rules, like the one in which Jane found herself, differing ideologies among midwives become more salient. Antagonisms build up between those who work for legislation and those who don't. The voices of the pacifists and anarchists clash with the voices of those wanting more political strategizing and structure. Looking at the larger historic context, as NSM theorists do, can give midwives the stimulus to recognize the relevance of their actions, and to incorporate both the visionaries and the left-brained organizational types. While organization is always necessary in a social movement, bureaucracies can easily subsume the original vision and commitment needed to remain effective.

As it takes gall to stand up and be counted, I suggest we borrow a term from Kodak and menopause and become conscious and proactive each time we have the opportunity for a "social activist moment." This would be the moment we see a physician about to perform an unnecessary episiotomy, the moment we are told a midwife has been unfairly treated by her regulatory body, the moment a media commentator twists something to make a good story at the expense of homebirth, the moment an obstetric organization misrepresents a study to suit its own purposes, and the moment professionalizing tendencies within midwifery run the risk of subsuming the social movement spirit. Seizing these moments usually requires personal risk to the midwife's professional reputation, but a connection with the universal code of social movement ethics can give her the stimulus and the courage to wrench the situation around. Like the motto of Physicians for Social Responsibility, the motto of the ABM should be "Never whisper in the presence of wrong."

The changing questions of the NSM theorists, as time has marched on, parallel the changing vision and stresses of the ABM. By 1992, Touraine was asking, "Can the 'new' social movements in fact play the role assigned to them and change the entire society?"

CONCLUSIONS

I began with an interest in helping the aspiring midwife avoid the temptation of putting all her potential eggs into either a spiritual or professional basket. The tour of professionalization theories I have presented in this chapter is useful both for understanding prescribed routes to professionalization and for clarifying how midwives have not precisely followed these routes and have rejected the impulse to engage in developing the "collective pretensions" of professionals. While midwives have realized the importance of attending births safely and developing an ethical code of behavior, their understanding of ethics varies somewhat from the average health professional. Many midwives and their clients continually find fundamental problems in the professional tendency to respond more to bureaucratic and legal concerns than to concerns about the patient/client herself. The DEM's relationship with expectant mothers has also been traditionally different from other health professionals because of her interest in re-skilling her client rather than in super-skilling herself. The midwife who is interested in using her everyday work activity as a means of living out her ideology is probably better able to survive the intense conflicts she faces on a daily basis.

Midwives truly trying to reform their society are frustrated by patriarchal political models, now promoted as much as ever in spite of (and often fully supported by) medical school student populations that are approximately fifty percent female. The midwives' problem with becoming regulated stems from a distrust of the corrupt professionalization system of medical maternity care providers, built on creating the illusion that pregnancy is like a malignant tumor requiring high-tech extraction. Midwives can best reconcile becoming professionals if they can find a way to take the "lies" out of "professiona-lise," and institutionalize such concepts as informed choice. Like Jane and other idealists and social activists, midwives have had to learn the tools of the legal/mainstream world without allowing it to change their vision.

The passion of Jane and her midwife, along with many others, is to be involved in an amorphous movement to establish better values than those evidenced through the prevailing professional tendency to be exclusive and hierarchical. Opening up the classification of the midwife as a social activist allows for the use of academic literature that can broaden such a role rather than limit it to the pursuit of the professional engaged in an exclusionary project. Midwifery organizations like ACNM, NARM, the Midwifery Education Accreditation Council (MEAC, which accredits direct-entry midwifery schools), and the NACPM have emerged as the groups designated to take care of the professional project, exemplifying RMT and political process theories. MANA, Midwifery Today, and Birthing the Future form harbinger groups watching out for the social movement, exemplifying classical strain and new social movement theories. Put another way, while there are individuals in both types of organizations who think similarly and do not necessarily fit in the box of their respective groups, organizations like MANA seem to attract more midwives drawn to midwifery through a spiritual kind of calling, whereas groups like ACNM attract midwives more interested in professional development. It has become increasingly clear to those of us working between these organizations that their meeting point has been the work that members of both types of organizations are doing as social activists. We see that homebirth midwives and their clients are prioritizing *how to get the values of their social movement institutionalized* more than how the midwifery profession can stake out a jurisdiction and create a monopoly over a body of knowledge. In an ideal world, one can do both.

Highlights of some of the principles that have been discussed in this chapter are found in table 10.2.

From the 1970s to the year 2000, we midwives felt that we were changing the world because our own little world, like Jane's, was in fact changing—but so was that of the wider society. Here, in conclusion, I will name only six of the most recent and most disturbing change vectors.

1. Disturbing trends in obstetric research have adulterated the spirit of the Cochrane Collaboration, which since 1989, has benefited the ABM via scientific identification of the problems with technological birth through systematic epidemiologic reviews. American obstetric societies have answered the call for evidence-based practice by selectively isolating and utilizing individual studies of questionable merit, especially when these studies support increased instead of decreased intervention: cesareans for breeches (Hannah 2000), decreased choice in VBAC (Lydon-Rochelle et al. 2001), elimination of the birth center option for VBACs (Lieberman et. al 2004), and discrediting of homebirth (Pang et al. 2002).

2. It is the sad truth that in the United States, homebirth has not proportionately increased for thirty years, in spite of the fact that the ABM has been going strong since the 1970s and there are homebirth practitioners in virtually every state. Women's choices continue to mirror the values and beliefs of the wider technocratic society (Davis-Floyd 2004).

Table 10.2 Comparing Social Movement Principles to Health Professional Principles

Social Movement Principles	Health Profession Principles
1. **Goal: To create change** (Brandwein 1985). Usually a save-the-planet orientation (peace, environment, equality), returning to "normal"—the way it was before the destruction wrought by economics and bad politics.	1. **Goal: To provide good service, usually defined by the profession.** To create and maintain their profession. Ultimately to achieve professional dominance (Freidson 1970a and 1970b; Larkin 1983; Abbott 1988).
2. **Development of historicity** that embraces concepts perceivable as negative, such as witchcraft and "spiritual" midwifery.	2. **Selective historicity** based on what image one wants to develop for the profession, and therefore what history one wants to remember.
3. **Exploring full potential,** concern about public image, but dedication and integrity of the cause held to be the ultimate driving force. Love to use the mass media. In fact, thrive on it.	3. **Exploring potential with qualifiers** on what kind of potential: dedicated to upholding proper comportment and image, as well as legal status of the profession. Going to the media is generally considered unprofessional, but is done selectively.
4. **The ethic of inclusion.** By definition, want to include as many members as possible, and success based on how large a citizen surge will rally to support the movement (Lofland and Johnson 1991). Social movements actually cultivate inclusiveness (Scott 1990). Exclude by default those not willing to take a stand for the principles of the particular movement (e.g., peace, composting, homebirth). However, do not require a high degree of ideological agreement or agreement on ultimate ends (Scott 1990).	4. **The ethic of exclusion.** In order to fulfill the goal of creating and maintaining a profession, and the ultimate goal of acquiring professional dominance over other professions, a profession must create a monopoly over a certain body of knowledge and maximize rewards and privileges by limiting access to them (Weber 1978; Witz 1992). One has to compete to get into the university program of a profession, and work to live up to established protocols and guidelines to guard one's status.
5. **Emphasis on good process**, especially in the feminist movement (Carr 2003).	5. **Emphasis on "the end justifies the means"** to promote the profession.
6. **Solidarity based on common ethical alignment,** interest in support, and the common cause. Fear and concern about repercussions less cultivated. A belief cultivated in the ability of truth and justice to prevail.	6. **Solidarity should be based on service to the clients/patients,** according to ethical codes. Often, much of the solidarity and unity is based on fear from the threat of liability (Perkins 2004).

3. The commodification of birth as a service to be sold to the highest bidder, and the closing of small hospitals and subsequent centralization of birth in larger institutions, are both patterns contrary to the kind of birth the ABM has sought to foster.
4. While ACNM is making great strides internationally, MANA lacks the same amount of funding or womanpower to carry out international projects. Neither MANA nor ACNM are taking action with respect to larger political strategies like GATS (General Agreement on Trades and Services), which can affect midwives around the globe—a move that their country's administration promotes.
5. CNMs have been experiencing increased hostility and territorial encroachment from physicians resulting in the firing of many nurse-midwives or the loss of their hospital privileges; as a result, CNMs are demonstrating more fiercely than perhaps they ever have before. At the time of this writing (February 2005), they have not yet claimed their social activist moment to fight the injudicious exclusion of VBAC from birth centers, but they are beginning to see the ironic power CPMs have won in some states: brand new legislation in Virginia, for example, gives CPMs the ability to practice without the physician supervision under which the CNMs still suffer (see chapter 7).
6. Elective cesarean section has been ethically accepted by ACOG, and more women are choosing this option for birth. Executive director of ACNM Deanne Williams and past president Mary Ann Shah have cowritten letters to the *New York Times, Boston Globe, Los Angeles Times, and Washington Post* debunking the notion that elective primary cesarean is associated with perineal integrity. Unfortunately, their letters remain unpublished beyond midwifery publications. The feminist rhetoric of choice appears to be an adulterated way for women to bypass their biological privilege of giving birth naturally. The obstetrical borrowing of *informed choice* may force the ABM to move beyond working to give women whatever they want and return to a more fundamental issue: creating a major drive to raise consciousness. Perhaps the most important social activist moments of this century will be the moments in which we have the boldness to suggest to women planning hospital births that they have homebirths, and to provide women planning medically unnecessary cesareans with lists of risks regarding their choice. We ourselves have generally been afraid to do so because of liability, but the data is in: for low-risk women, the chance of having a successful unmedicated, low-intervention birth with an excellent outcome is far greater if

they choose homebirth with a CPM or CNM. CPMs' homebirth cesarean rate is 3.7 percent, CNMs' 2.3 percent; their perinatal outcomes are similar to those of low-risk hospital birth (Johnson and Daviss 2005a; Murphy and Fullerton 1998).

With current acute needs inherent in all of these changes, the need for midwives to do strategic planning has increased. Midwives are moving from fighting for individual women's rights to taking on the responsibilities of saving women's reproductive historicity and accepting nothing short of changing the world. Accessing the political power of official recognition and licensure is one thing; it is quite another to mobilize women not already outside of the mainstream to see the need for midwifery services.

The new midwives coming into practice are Jane's and her midwife's kids, having learned from their weird parents that living on the idealistic margin is not all it is cracked up to be, but neither is the mainstream world. Once an aspiring midwife swims on the other side of the ocean as a social activist, it is pretty hard to return to a hospital job unless change is part of the institutional vocabulary. While many midwives have tired of the politics, are burned out from doing too many births in too little time, or feel burned in the courts like their ancestors at the stake, fortunately, various midwifery groups are moving on to new initiatives with renewed vigor.

The "calling" of the midwife has taken on new dimensions beyond preserving birth's sacredness. It is now a call to prepare women to walk through the health system labyrinth with their integrity and faith in themselves unscathed. The credibility of the "professional" part of each midwife hovers in her abilities, through research and clinical skills, to delicately portray for a woman how she can use less technology while the rest of the health-care establishment is telling her she needs more. Since the dawn of our legislative efforts, we have been politically correct as midwives to suggest that our role is *complementary* to other health professionals. At this stage of my career, I dare to state that this tricky role as social activists in professional clothing entails an ethic superior to that of the self-serving health professions—one that the medical establishment would do well to adopt.

Consensus decision making, refusal to censor diversity of thought or values—midwives have experimented with it all. Concern with licensure and regulation for "the public good" suggest that the goal of mainstreaming midwives should be to fit them into the medical system where they will buckle under new practice protocols and manage technocratic births. But I suggest a much higher goal for the mainstreaming of American midwives: to continue to work to change the system even as they work to fit into it—a critical challenge to their vital responsibility as social activists. Through politics, preservation of their ideals, savvy utilization of resources, judicious research and use of scientific evidence, efforts to create a major cultural shift through consumer and legislator education, and the individual seizing of social activist moments, midwives and all members of the alternative birth movement should continue to undo an image of being on the fringe when they are really the frontier.

ACKNOWLEDGMENTS

I appreciate the editorial support and constructive suggestions provided by Robbie Davis-Floyd, Mary Ann Shah, Ken Johnson, and Diane Holzer.

REFERENCES

Abbott, Andrew. 1988. *The System of Professions: An Essay on the Division of Expert Labor.* Chicago: Chicago University Press.

American Public Health Association. 2002. Increasing access to out-of-hospital maternity care services through state-regulated and nationally certified direct-entry midwives 2001–2003. *American Journal of Public Health* 92(3):453–455.

Anderson, Rondi., and Patricia Murphy. 1995. Outcomes of 11,788 planned homebirths attended by certified nurse-midwives. A retrospective descriptive study. *Journal of Nurse Midwifery* 40(6):483–492.

Arms, Suzanne. 1975. *Immaculate Deception.* Boston, MA: Houghton-Mifflin.

Barber, B. 1963. Some Problems in the Sociology of the Professions. *Daedalus* 92(4):669–688.

Benoit, Cecilia, Sirpe Wrede, and Beverly Maclean-Alley. 1997. The midwifery knowledge debate in three countries: Life-world versus scientific ways of knowing. A paper prepared for SFAA/SMA Joint Meetings, Seattle, Washington.

Boreham, P. 1983. Indetermination: Professional knowledge, organizational control. *Sociological Review* 31 693–718.

Brandwein, R. A. 1985. Feminist thought-structure: An alternative paradigm of social change for social justice. In *A Conference in Search of Strategies for Social Change: March 23–25, 1984,* ed. D. Gil and E. A. Gil. Cambridge, MA: Scheakman Publishing.

Cant, S., and U. Sharma. 1999. *A New Medical Pluralism, Alternative Medicine Doctors, Patients and the State.* New York: Garland Publishing.

Carr, E. Summerson. 2003. Rethinking empowerment theory using a feminist lens: The importance of process. *Affilia* 18 (1):8–20.

The Cato Institute. 1995. Cato Policy Analysis, 246.

College of Physicians and Surgeons of Ontario. 2001. Reports from Council. Home Birth Policy Rescinded.

Davis, Elizabeth. 2004 (5th edition, orig. pub. 1987). *Heart and Hands: A Midwife's Guide to Pregnancy and Birth.* Berkeley: Celestial Arts.

Davis-Floyd, Robbi. 2004. *Birth as an American Rite of Passage,* 2nd edition. Berkley: University of California Press.

Daviss, Betty-Anne. 1999. From social movement to professional midwifery project: Are we throwing out the baby with the bath water? M.A. Canadian Studies diss., Carleton University, Ottawa, Canada.

Daviss, Betty-Anne. 2001a. Reforming birth and (re)making midwifery in North America. In *Birth by Design: Pregnancy, Maternity Care, and Midwifery in North America and*

Europe, ed. Raymond Devries, Cecilia Benoit, Edwin Teijingen, and Sirpa Wrede, 70–86. New York and London: Routledge.

Daviss Betty-Anne. 2001b. Study's focus on induction vs. spontaneous labour neglects spontaneous delivery, Letter to the editor re Vaginal delivery after caesarean section. *British Medical Journal* (323):1307.

Diani, M. 1992. The concept of social movement. *Sociological Review* 40(1).

Donegan, J. 1978. *Women and Men Midwives: Medicine, Morality and Misogyny in Early America*. Connecticut and London: Greenwood Press.

Firestone, S. 1970. *The Dialectic of Sex*. New York: Morrow.

Freidson, E. 1970a. *Profession of Medicine: A Study of the Sociology of Applied Knowledge*, 2nd ed. Chicago, IL: University of Chicago Press.

Freidson, E. 1970b. *Professional Dominance. The Social Structure of Medical Care*. New York: Atherton.

Gaskin, Ina May. 1975. *Spiritual Midwifery*. Summertown, TN: The Book Publishing Co.

Grandjean, Burke and Helen Bernal. 1979. Sex and centralization in a semi-profession. *Sociology of Work and Occupation* 6:84–102.

Hannah, Mary, Walter J. Hannah, Sheila A. Hewson, Ellen D. Hodnett, Saroj Saigal, Andrew R. Willan, for the Term Breech Trial Collaborative Group. 2000. Planned caesarean section versus planned vaginal birth for breech presentation at term: a randomised multicentre trial. *Lancet*. 356:1375–83.

Hearn, J. 1982. Notes on patriarchy, professionalization and the semi-professions. *Sociology* 16(2):184–202.

Hughes, Everett. 1971. The sociological eye: Selected papers on work, self, and the study of society. Chicago: Aldine Atherton.

Johnson, Kenneth C., and Betty-Anne Daviss. 2003. Outcomes of planned homebirths in Washington State: 1989–1996. *Obstetrics and Gynecology* 101(1):98–200.

———2005a. Letter to the Editor concerning Results of the National Study of Vaginal Birth after Cesarean in Birth Centers. *Obstetrics and Gynecology* 105(4): 897–898.

———2005b. "Outcomes of Planned Home Births with Certified Professional Midwives: Large Prospective Study in North America.." *British Medical Journal* 330(7505): 1416, June. www.bmj.com.

Johnson, T. J. 1977. The professions in the class structure. In *Industrial Society, Class, Cleavage and Control*, 93–110. London: George Allen and Unwin.

Lang, K., and G. Lang. 1961. *Collective Dynamics*. New York: Thomas Crowell.

Larkin, G. 1983. *Occupational Monopoly and Modern Medicine*. London: Tavistock.

Lawn-Day, G. 1994. Using institutionalized social movements to explain policy implementation failure: The case of midwifery. Ph.D. dissertation, University of Oklahoma.

Lieberman, E. Kitty Ernst, Judith Rooks, Susan Stapleton, B. Flamm. 2004. Results of the National Study of Vaginal Birth After Cesarean in Birth Centers. *Obstetrics & Gynecology* 104(5):933–942.

Lofland, J., and V. Johnson. 1991. Citizen surges: A domain in movement studies and the perspective on peace activism in the 1980's. In *Research In Social Movements, Conflicts and Change*. 13:1–29.

Lydon-Rochelle M., V. L. Holts., T. R. Easterling, D. P. Martin. 2001. Risk of uterine rupture during labor among women with a prior cesarean delivery. *N Engl J Med*. 345 (1): 54–5.

Martin, Joyce, Brady Hamilton, Paul Sutton, Stephanie Ventura, Fay Menacker, Martha Munson. 2003. *Births: Final Data for 2002*. Hyattsville, MD: National Center for Health Statistics, National Vital Statistics Reports 52(10).

Marx, G., and D. McAdam. 1994. Collective behaviours and social movements. In *Process and Structure*. Upper Saddle River, NJ: Prentice Hall.

McAdam, D. 1982. *Political Process and the Development of Black Insurgency 1930–1970*. Chicago and London: University of Chicago Press.

McCarthy, J., and M. Zald. 1973. *The Trend of Social Movements in America: Professionalization and Resource Mobilization*. Morristown, N.J.: General Learning Press.

Melucci, Alberto. 1985. The symbolic challenge of contemporary movements. *Social Research* 52(4):789–816.

Murphy, Patricia, and Judith Fullerton. 1998. Outcomes of intended homebirths in nurse-midwifery practice: A prospective descriptive study. *Obstetrics and Gynecology* 92(3):461–470.

National Institutes of Health. 2002. White House commission on complementary and alternative medicine policy. NIH Publication 03-5411. 2002.

Olson, M. 1965. *The Logic of Collective Action: Public Goods and the Theory of Groups.* Cambridge, MA: Harvard University Press.

Pang, Jenny, James Heffelfinger, Greg Huang, Thomas Benedetti, and Noel Weiss. 2002. Outcomes of planned homebirths in Washington State: 1989–1996. *Obstetrics and Gynecology* 100(2):253–259.

Parkin, F. 1979. *Marxism and Class Theory: A Bourgeois Critique.* London: Tavistock.

Parsons, T. 1954. The professions and social structure. In *Essays in Sociological Theory,* ed T. Parsons, 34–49. Glencoe, IL: The Free Press.

Parsons, T. 1967. *Sociological Theory and Modern Society.* New York: Free Press.

Perkins, Barbara. 2004. *The Medical Delivery Business.* New Jersey: Rutgers University Press.

Rich, Adrienne. 1977. *Of Woman Born: Motherhood as Experience and Institution.* New York: Bantam Books.

Rooks, Judith. 1997. *Midwifery and Childbirth in America.* Philadelphia: Temple University Press.

Rothman, Barbara K. 1981. Awake and Aware, or False Consciousness? The Co-option of Childbirth reform in America. In *Childbirth: Alternatives to Medical Control,* ed. S. Romalis 150–180. Austin: University of Texas Press.

Rushing, Beth. 1993. Ideology in the re-emergence of North American midwifery. *Work and Occupations* 20(1):46–47.

Saks, M. 1983. Removing the blinkers? A Critique of recent contributions to the sociology of professions. *Sociology Review* 31(1):1–21.

Scott, A. 1990. *Ideology and the New Social Movements.* Controversies in Sociology series. London: Unwin Hyman.

Smelser, N. J. 1962. *Theory of Collective Behavior.* New York: The Free Press.

Society of Obstetricians and Gynecologists of Canada. 2003. Policy Statement No. 126. Midwifery. Journal of Obstetrics and Gynecology of Canada 25(3):5.

Starr, Paul. 1982. *The Social Transformation of American Medicine.* New York: Basic Books Inc.

Tilly, Charles. 1978. *From Mobilization to Revolution.* Reading, MA: Addison-Wesley.

———. 1984. Social movements and national politics. In *Statemaking and Social Movements,* ed. C. Bright and S. Harding, 297–317. Ann Arbor: University of Michigan Press.

Touraine, Alain. 1978. *The Production of Society.* Chicago, IL: University of Chicago Press.

———. 1981. *The Voice and the Eye: An Analysis of Social Movements.* New York: Cambridge University Press.

———. 1992. Beyond social movements? *Theory, Culture and Society* 9(1):125–145.

———. 1995. *The Critique of Modernity.* Oxford: Blackwell.

Vickers Jill, Pauline Rankin, and Christine Appelle. 1993. *Politics as If Woman Mattered.* Toronto, Ontario: University of Toronto Press.

Weber, Max. 1978/1922. *Economy and Society: An Outline of Interpretive Sociology.* Berkeley: University of California.

Weimer, Jon. 1999. Breastfeeding: Health and Economic Issues. *Food Review* 22(2):31–35.

Wilensky, Harold. 1964. The professionalization of everyone? *American Journal of Sociology* 70:137–158.

Witz, Anne. 1992. *Professions and Patriarchy.* London: Routledge.

Worts, D. 1985. Report on 1984 MANA Convention. ISSUE Newsletter of the Midwifery Task Force in Ontario 6(9).

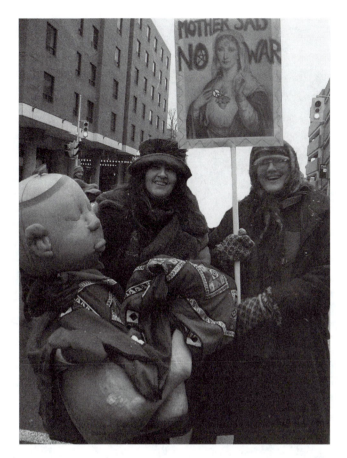

Fig. 10.1 Placard carrying midwives participating in an anti-war demonstration. Photographer: Kenneth C. Johnson.

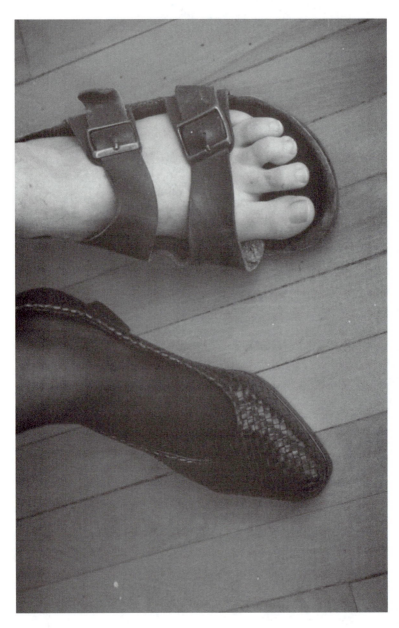

Fig. 10.2 A midwife wearing two hats on one head, as demonstrated by her feet! Photographer: Kenneth C. Johnson.

11

RENEGADE MIDWIVES: ASSETS OR LIABILITIES?

Robbie Davis-Floyd and Christine Barbara Johnson

- **Renegade Midwives' Stories** • **Stories from Women Choosing to Give Birth with Renegade Midwives** • **Normalizing Uniqueness: How Far Should It Go?** • **The Role of the Stranger** • **Living into the Answers**

Scratch any midwife, and you'll find a renegade.

—**Richard Jennings, CNM**

RENEGADE MIDWIVES' STORIES

A homebirth midwife in Massachusetts receives a knock on the door in the middle of the afternoon. She opens it to find a woman she has never met before in early labor and in tears. She had planned to give birth in a birth center run by nurse-midwives, but was refused at the last minute because she was two days past the forty-two-week deadline the nurse-midwives by state regulation were obliged to comply with. They had officially transferred her to the hospital, but instead she drove to the home of this particular midwife because she was known as a *renegade* who would sometimes ignore protocols in the interests of serving

447

the woman. The homebirth midwife conducted an exam, concluded that the baby and mother were fine, and proceeded to assist the mother to give birth in the midwife's home, with an excellent outcome.

A nurse-midwife in California attended homebirths in her community for many years; in so doing, she was practicing outside the protocols of nurse-midwifery in the state because she had no physician backup. She was honored and revered by the women she served, and by many California midwives who saw her as a courageous, skilled, and compassionate midwifery pioneer. One day she had a mother with an obstetric emergency and transported her to the hospital appropriately. Both mother and baby were fine, and the birth turned out well. But the hospital and the state prosecuted the nurse-midwife for illegally attending births at home; she was not supported by the local or national nurse-midwifery associations, some of whose members had long considered her a renegade. She was forced to stop practicing. A few years later she died both of cancer and of grief. Her name was June Whitson.

A young nurse-midwife in Washington state opened a highly successful homebirth practice. One day she made an appropriate transport for an emergency; the baby died in the hospital. She experienced immediate ostracism from the hospital-based nurse-midwives, but was supported during the trial by the homebirth midwives. Her license was revoked; nevertheless, she continues to practice.

A highly experienced direct-entry midwife in southern California, who had been in practice for twenty years and had trained many of the younger homebirth midwives in her community, was attending over ten homebirths a month, a huge stress factor in itself. When the births happened back to back, she was going without sleep for days at a time, and she was taking on cases that even the midwives she had trained as apprentices felt were "way too far out of protocol." (At the time, all of the DEMs in California were illegal, but they had formed a state association and created their own set of protocols and their own peer-review process.) Several peer reviews of this particular midwife's practice resulted in censure, but she paid no heed. Then she was approached by a woman with two previous cesareans who asked her to attend a VBAC at home. The midwife went to the library and did some research, and warned the couple that there was approximately a three percent risk that the woman's uterus would rupture. The couple declared their willingness to accept this risk. In early labor the woman's uterus did rupture. The midwife transported her immediately, but the baby died. On this and several other counts, the midwife was prosecuted by the state. None of the midwives in her community would testify on her behalf. Even though they loved her and many of them had been trained by her, they were angry that she had not heeded their warnings, which they had repeated over four or more years. She was convicted and spent four years in prison. The letters she sent from prison to her supporters and friends were published in newsletters and widely distributed. They revealed her enormous courage, strength of will, compassion for other prisoners, and her openness to learning and growing as much as she could from the often devastating things she experienced during her imprisonment (from extreme verbal abuse to leg chains). Finally she was released, returned home to her family and friends, and as far as we know has not gone back to attending births.

A couple in one state, deeply committed to homebirth, received their prenatal care from a direct-entry midwife. Toward the end of the pregnancy, she diagnosed the position of the baby as footling breech. This condition is perceived as dangerous, but breeches often change their status from footling to complete to frank at the end, as well as during, the delivery. The client insisted that she did not want a cesarean and did not want to go to the hospital. A straightforward breech (bottom first) only occurs in about three percent of all births, and is medically considered a risk condition. In states where they are licensed and regulated, homebirth midwives are usually prohibited from attending any kind of breech birth. In this particular state, homebirth direct-entry midwives are illegal anyway, and so their practice is entirely unregulated and autonomous. This midwife felt that she had the skills to handle a breech birth, so she agreed to go ahead and attend the birth at home. She successfully delivered the baby's feet, but there was a significant delay between the emergence of the feet and the emergence of the baby's head. The baby did not breathe upon birth. The midwife attempted resuscitation, which failed. The baby died. The couple remained supportive of the midwife, but she was put on trial by the state.

At the time she attended this birth, she was already on probation because the state had discovered that she was attending home-births illegally. Her attendance at this birth constituted a tremendous risk for her, for the parents, for the baby, and for the efforts of the direct-entry midwives toward legalization. The birth was videotaped, and the tape was widely circulated to midwives for legal purposes.

Some months later, Robbie attended a meeting of highly experienced midwives involved in the national midwifery movement. This case came up for discussion. Some of these midwives had seen the videotape and had concluded that the midwife was guilty of irresponsible practice: (1) she should not have taken on the birth in the first place, given the risks of footling breech and her own already probationary status; (2) she waited too long between the delivery of the feet and the head, when she could and should have intervened to make the birth happen faster; (3) they believed her neonatal resuscitation skills were not up to par, as her efforts as recorded on the videotape seemed to them to be inadequate and inappropriate. There was general agreement at the meeting that her care had been substandard, and that she had not only been responsible for the baby's death, but also had enormously impeded the legalization efforts of the midwives in her state. But the discussion did not focus on the issue of footling breech in itself.

So, ever the anthropologist, Robbie asked these experienced midwives how many of them had attended footling breech births at home. About half of the hands in the room went up. Then she asked, "Have any of you experienced a bad outcome as a result?" No one had. Her next question was, "How many of you would do it again?" and the same midwives who had raised their hands in the first place did so again. For them, the issue was not attendance at a footling breech per se, but the *particular instances of this particular birth*: a challenging delivery position, known about in advance, and attended anyway by a midwife already on probation in a state currently in the midst of legislative procedures involving midwifery in general. ("Too many tensions and risks all in one basket," one midwife noted.)

A bit shocked that footling breech, considered an immediate indicator for a cesarean in the hospital, was not per se the issue for this group of experienced midwives, Robbie was forced once again to realize how much these midwives' philosophy, practice, and experience differed from American norms, how deeply reliant and confident they were in their hands-on skills, and how willing some of them were to take what any obstetrician, most nurse-midwives, and about half of all homebirth midwives, would consider a totally unacceptable risk. Further questioning revealed that the midwives who had raised their hands both times had attended, over twenty or thirty years of practice, dozens and sometimes over 100 breech births, footling and otherwise, and considered themselves the preservers and guardians of this skill, which they pointed out, the vast majority of American obstetricians do not have because they are taught simply to do a cesarean for any type of breech.

STORIES FROM WOMEN CHOOSING TO GIVE BIRTH WITH RENEGADE MIDWIVES

Mary's first birth by cesarean section had taken place years before, but she still lived with the deep psychological scarring that she sustained as a result of this experience. In fact, for close to a year after the birth she was deeply depressed and unable to function, a recluse in her house. Before this birth she had been vibrant, active, and professionally and personally successful. Eventually, she began to sense that she had mostly put this tough birth experience behind her, and was feeling more and more like her old self. Then Mary discovered that she was pregnant again. She did not feel ready to handle a hospital birth, as she was still in the final stages of completing her recovery from the first one. A number of midwives she approached declined to attend her, due to her VBAC status. Finally, she located a renegade midwife in her state who agreed to attend her. This homebirth was deeply healing and nurturing for her; afterward she felt that all the scars from the first birth had healed. She emerged from this second birth with an enthusiasm and strength that she "had never experienced before."

Celene was pregnant and planning to give birth at home when she and her midwife determined that she was carrying twins, which made her ineligible for a homebirth because her midwife was unwilling to jeopardize her professional standing in the community by risking a bad outcome in what most would consider a risky birth. Celene was beside herself; she was terrified of hospitals and believed that if she were to be forced into this option she would have a very difficult birth and an even more difficult time recovering. She called midwife after midwife, but they all said the same thing: "It's not worth the risk."

Celene was desperate to find someone who would attend her at home; finally, some midwives referred her to a midwife willing to fly in to attend her. Ultimately, two midwives came. The birth of the first twin went smoothly, but the second one was stuck and the midwives urged hospital transport. They transported, with one midwife from the team remaining behind and another accompanying Celene to the hospital to ensure that she was supported. The second baby was delivered by cesarean section and emerged healthy and well. The hospital staff was aghast and gave Celene many severe looks and lectures, but Celene herself was ecstatic that she was able to labor and have the first baby at home. She was sorry about the hospital birth, but was grateful that she had her midwife there to support her through it. She feels very empowered and is most grateful that this alternative was available to her, certain that had she been forced to start out in the hospital she would have been discounted and disempowered in ways that would have been difficult to recover from, and would have adversely affected her parenting.

A woman whose first homebirth ended in cesarean section was so emotionally traumatized by this birth that no midwife in her state would agree to attend her second birth at home. The mother was a highly respected professional with a demanding career, a commitment to social activism, and an enthusiastic attitude for life, but the scars from her first birth ran deep. This emotional baggage, coupled with a VBAC at home, seemed just too risky for the midwives in her state. Some were willing to assist at the birth, but refused to be the primary midwife in charge. Rather than leave the woman stranded, these midwives suggested a midwife from out of state who would fly in and attend her at home. The woman elected this option and the result was a healthy baby born at home. This birth was deeply healing, and in the aftermath she noted that her parenting improved immensely as well as her overall emotional well-being. She stresses that if she had been forced to enter the hospital, she is not sure what shape she would be in today.

A mother in Connecticut was diagnosed with severe schizophrenia and depression. She believed that part of the cause lay in the highly medicalized hospital birth she had endured a few years earlier. She was pregnant again and desired a homebirth, not only for the experience but also because she believed it would help her to heal. No homebirth midwife in her state would take her on because they all considered her "crazy" and therefore high risk. Finally she found a doula in another state who was willing to fly to her city to assist her, and the doula found a midwife who was also willing to fly in from another state. She successfully gave birth at home to twins, and her psychological health improved enormously. She became a birth activist, organizing various conferences and meetings in her community, and advocating for midwives to expand their definitions of *normal*.

After Robbie completed a talk on humanistic childbirth at a university in Michigan, she was approached by a student/mother with tears her eyes, who spoke of the trauma of the cesarean birth of her first baby. Pregnant with her second child, this woman deeply desired a homebirth, but had been told that no homebirth midwife in Michigan would attend a VBAC at home. Certain this was not the case, Robbie made a few calls to various homebirth midwives, and was assured that some of them would attend home VBACs. She gave their phone numbers to the mother, who went away radiant with the hope that her dreams of an empowering birth might yet be achieved. Robbie was close to tears herself: her certainty had been reaffirmed that these professional Michigan midwives, although prohibited by protocols to attend VBACs at home, would not deny the option to this mother who so deeply desired it and had nowhere else to turn.

NORMALIZING UNIQUENESS: HOW FAR SHOULD IT GO?

Licensure is not something that should be forced on recalcitrant midwives by a paternalistic government. It is something that should be created by midwives; it is the next step in self-actualization.

—**Ida Darragh, North American Registry of Midwives Newsletter, 2004**

All midwives can be considered renegades to some extent. Just to be a midwife, any kind of midwife in the United States, is to constitute a radical critique of the dominant obstetrical system in which physicians attend ninety percent of all births. But there is a special category of *renegade midwives*, illustrated in the preceding stories, which we wish to specifically address in this chapter because they are very important to American midwifery in both positive and negative ways.

The term *renegade midwife* is used by midwives themselves. Sometimes they use it pejoratively, as a criticism of the midwife who practices, in the majority peer opinion, too far outside the protocols of her peer group or state regulations. Some midwives apply the term to themselves, using it to acknowledge the fact that they often practice outside of protocols, and to emphasize that their doing so constitutes a very conscious critique of those protocols.

The midwife who calls herself a renegade believes that other midwives adhere too strictly to protocols and standards of care and do not go far enough to serve the birthing woman. She believes that a woman's desire to give birth naturally, even in conditions that others would regard as adverse to homebirth, should be primary and that the midwife should serve the client and not the regulatory system. Thus, renegades are often highly skilled and experienced midwives who feel confident in their abilities to handle such conditions as VBACs, breeches, and sometimes even twins at home. Unless there are signs of fetal distress or insufficient amniotic fluid, they are often willing to let a woman go two or three weeks past her due date and still attend her at home (most protocols state that women should be induced after forty-two weeks). They will take on women whom other midwives might screen out because of gestational diabetes (which many midwives think is a medical myth), or, as the preceding stories illustrate, because of odd psychological characteristics or even complications as extreme as footling breech. These midwives believe they are placing the desires of the client first, and that doing so is appropriate. When there is a condition that they truly believe they cannot handle, even renegade midwives refer the woman to a physician in advance or transport her if the condition develops during labor. What makes them "renegades" is usually not ignorance, arrogance, or lack of training, but rather the fact that they will take on women whom most other midwives would reject. Thus they constitute both a liability to other midwives, and an asset.

The asset has to do with the services renegade midwives provide. Licensed professional midwives who are not renegade, who do practice within agreed-upon peer protocols or within established state regulations, often feel conflicted when confronted with a woman who deeply desires an out-of-hospital birth but should, according to protocols, be screened out in advance or transported if certain conditions develop during labor. As we have seen in earlier chapters, homebirth midwifery itself began as a renegade social movement in which midwives and mothers together agreed to flout obstetrical norms and to jointly take responsibility for conducting births in radically alternative ways. Many homebirth midwives are still loyal to the flavor and force of this movement, and feel a strong pull to place the interests of the client first, as "lay" midwives (in the beginning) tended almost always to do. But those were the days (the early 1970s) when lay midwives had little experience with birth complications and risk management. Because homebirths attended by midwives turn out fine for the vast majority of the women who plan them, it took years for some of the early homebirth midwifery pioneers to encounter enough complications and dangers to begin to take more seriously their responsibility to acknowledge and deal with risk. When they did begin to get together to discuss and establish protocols, it was usually in individual regions or states where they were illegal anyway, so any protocols they set were ones they themselves agreed on. Herein lies the liability: in spite of the fact that babies die in the hospital too, because homebirth is so culturally marginal, all it takes is one death at home that would most likely have been prevented in the hospital, or one "botched transport," to undo years of goodwill.

As the battle for legality and licensure in various states got underway, the homebirth midwifery movement in some states became deeply divided over the issue of the renegade midwife. On one side were the professionalizing midwives who were willing to accept regulations (such as prohibition from attending VBACs, breeches, and twins) in return for legality and the benefits of not having to live in terror of arrest or prosecution and of opportunities to serve many more women. On the other side were midwives who refused to accept any restrictions on their practice and preferred to remain illegal or alegal, completely outside the system, because as long as they were not regulated they were fully autonomous and able to practice in any way they pleased. In Pennsylvania and a few other states, such midwives refer to themselves as "plain midwives." This rhetoric constitutes a deep critique of labels such as "direct-entry midwife" or "nurse-midwife," which these plain midwives perceive as restrictive. For the sake of clarity, in this chapter we will use the term *plain midwife* to refer to midwives who reject legalization, licensure, and the usually resultant restrictions on practice.

In *The Rhetoric of Midwifery: Gender, Knowledge, and Power* (2000), Mary Lay thoroughly described this divide as it occurred in Minnesota, where the professionalizing midwives developed a rhetorical strategy that stressed accountability, protocols, and regulation, and the plain midwives stuck to their insistence on keeping the woman central and not being restricted in any way. This rhetorical strategy on the part of the professionalizing midwives impressed state legislators; at the same time, it clarified and magnified the gap between the professionals and the "plains."

Some plain midwives are so because of religious reasons. There are hundreds of Christian midwives practicing in various states completely outside the law and the health-care system; their belief system revolves around the concept that "God is the real midwife," that God's will should and will prevail, and that any complications that develop during birth can be resolved through prayer and openness to the Holy Spirit. Christine has interviewed a number of these midwives who are deeply committed and can recount story after story about the practical results of relying on divine intervention at birth. One recounted her own birth story—she had an unassisted birth with her husband because she could not find anyone willing to attend her. This was in the 1970s when the homebirth movement was in its nascent stages. During her ninth month she sensed that something "felt funny," but she did not know what it was and this filled her with fear. At this time she was not yet a full-fledged midwife. She stayed in prayer almost constantly for three days. During labor, she could feel that "something was in the way"; again she was not sure what it was and she continued her prayer vigil. (See Klassen 2001 for a cogent analysis of the various types of spirituality that influence the choices of homebirthers and the midwives who serve them.)

Eventually a healthy baby girl emerged. The mother's subsequent midwifery experience showed her that what she experienced was placenta previa. Many professionalizing midwives do believe in God and do pray during birth, but tend to take the more pragmatic approach that "God helps those who help themselves." Thus they transport to the hospital when they believe they do not possess the necessary knowledge and skills to handle complications at home. Such professionalizing homebirth midwives are the ones who have worked hard to create CPM certification and to lobby for legalization and licensure of the CPM (achieving it in twenty-one states to date; see chapter 1). Their nurse-midwifery counterparts worked hard in earlier decades to achieve the same thing for the CNM.

It would be easy to say that the plain midwives are the renegades while the professionally oriented midwives, most of whom are CNMs or LMs or CPMs, are not, but reality is not that simple. As we noted previously, renegade midwives are often highly skilled and experienced. Many of them practice outside of protocols because they believe that they can handle the complications the protocols would instruct them to avoid. They observe that such protocols are often set by regulatory boards or state legislators who understand little about the knowledge base of homebirth midwives. And they know from statistics and from long experience that their services are the only means by which women with complications defined obstetrically as "high risk" can avoid a cesarean. (Most obstetricians will automatically do a cesarean for breeches or twins, and often for VBACs; many younger OBs have no experience with vaginal delivery in such situations.) Many such midwives achieve CNM or CPM certification and state licensure. In the process, they fight for regulations that will allow them the broadest possible scope of practice. But if they lose the regulatory battle and are forced to accept narrow protocols, they deal with this failure by occasionally flouting the state regulations they resisted in the first place. In this way, they distinguish themselves from midwives who stick carefully to such regulations. Such midwives place a higher priority on protecting the profession of midwifery in their state than on putting the desires of the client first. They believe that protecting midwifery is essential to maintaining out-of-hospital birth as an option, at least for women who do meet protocols, and that endangering it by taking obvious risks is irresponsible. They are often angry and resentful of renegade midwives who threaten the status of professional homebirth midwifery. But these same professionally oriented midwives are often grateful for the existence of the renegades (who are often also licensed or certified), because when a professionally oriented midwife is confronted with a potential client whom she has to screen out, she does not have to let the woman down utterly by telling her that her only option is the hospital birth she dreads. Instead, she can refer the mother to the renegade midwife who lives down the road or perhaps many miles away, who is more likely to go out on a limb to honor the mother's wishes.

At the 2001 MANA conference in Albuquerque, New Mexico, Robbie was asked to moderate a panel entitled "When Clients' Wishes Conflict with Midwifery Protocols." The room was packed—obviously this was an issue of great import to MANA members because, as we mentioned above, it places the social movement of midwifery in direct conflict with the professionalization process (see chapter 10), leaving many midwives in a quandary that they are often unable to philosophically resolve. If they refuse care in high-risk cases, they are letting the woman down. If they grant care, they are endangering the profession they have worked so hard to build. Quite a dilemma!

On the panel was a mother who had two previous cesareans and wanted a home VBAC, her husband (who had fully supported her choices), the midwife she had originally approached but who had refused to take her case because it was out of protocol, and an obstetrician who is very supportive of homebirth. The woman described how devastated she was when the professional midwife refused to take her on for a homebirth, and how relieved she was when that same midwife provided her with the option of going to an illegal, unlicensed (and therefore unregulated) midwife who lived over 100 miles away in an adjacent state. The woman and her husband went to talk with that renegade midwife, who agreed to take them on. The result was a "fantastic" birth experience for the couple, who had such faith in their choice that they gave birth in a remote desert location.

The professional midwife who had originally refused homebirth care keenly felt her responsibility to her profession, and did not regret making this her priority. At the same time, she was thrilled that the renegade midwife had been able to provide the birth experience the woman had so deeply desired. (The alternative would have been giving birth completely unassisted. Some women do choose this option [Moran 1981; Shanley 1994], but because this book is focused on midwives, we do not fully address such choices here.) Again paradoxically, the gratitude of the professional midwife to the renegade midwife was accompanied by the fear that the renegade would eventually have bad outcomes that would then endanger the status of midwives everywhere.

The obstetrician on the panel at first spoke about the importance of risk management and of appropriate referral. She noted with regret that this would mean that women like the mother on the panel might not be able to have the birth experience they longed for, but felt that this was the price that had to be paid for assuring safety in birth. She was challenged by several homebirth midwives in the audience, and toward the end of the discussion did a complete about-face. In essence, she acknowledged her fears, noted that they were inappropriate and that they reflected her socialization as an obstetrician, and apologized to all the midwives present for forgetting that "trusting birth and a woman's ability to give birth is the most important ingredient in a successful birth outcome."

Near the end of the scheduled time for this session, Robbie noticed that the audience was about to be left with an irreconcilable conceptual split between sticking to protocols for the sake of the profession, and flouting them for the sake of the woman. Seeking to provide the midwives on the panel and in the audience with another way of thinking about this opposition, Robbie attempted to provide a deeper, less oppositional approach. She reminded the audience of her study of midwives' use of intuition during prenatal care and birth (Davis-Floyd and Davis 1997), noting that midwives themselves had told her that one of their greatest skills is listening to the inner voice that can inform them which woman is truly at risk and which woman can actually achieve the homebirth she wants. She spoke of the importance of individualization, as opposed to standardization, of care, reminding them that whereas obstetricians are taught to standardize (Davis-Floyd 1987, 2004; Davis-Floyd and St. John 1998), midwives ideally are taught to individualize—to "normalize uniqueness" (Davis-Floyd and Davis 1997).

As an anthropologist who had studied midwives for over a decade, Robbie was able to speak a truth that every midwife in the audience recognized. Almost all homebirth midwives, and many nurse-midwives, will respond to the individual beliefs, desires, and circumstances of an individual woman in individual ways. The standards and protocols of midwifery care and of evidence-based medicine are there in front of them. But for midwives, standards are only "standard" (in other words, representative and expressive of the hegemonic obstetrical system), and research that compares two groups within a hospital can be irrelevant and often actually misleading and detrimental to homebirth practice.

For example, the famous *Friedman's curve*, which has for many years set the standard for how long women should be allowed to labor, was based not on normal, natural childbirths but on women drugged on scopolamine and whose labors were often augmented with pitocin. In spite of this extreme deficiency, obstetricians still utilize Freidman's curve to justify radical interventions to speed up labor (from pitocin to episiotomy to forceps to cesarean section). Midwives' experiences of homebirths teach them that Friedman's curve is not a reliable standard but rather a detriment to successful homebirth outcomes, because labors with no medical intervention can vary in time from a few hours to a few days without danger to mother or baby. Thus every midwife who practices outside the hospital has good reasons to ignore, even to scorn, obstetrical standards that many midwives who practice in the hospital are obliged to heed. In some cases, their scorn results from the inadequacy or misuse of medical "evidence." In other cases, such as VBACs, breeches, and twins, homebirth midwives acknowledge that the evidence does indicate increased risk, but they also note that the risks are small, and that hospital birth entails its own set of risks, which include unnecessary cesareans and iatrogenic damage to mother and/or child.

Thus, homebirth midwives who look carefully at the data come to understand that negative outcomes can occur as much or more from inappropriate obstetrical interventions as from deficiencies of nature.

Thus when confronted with specific women with specific complications, their only viable option becomes individualization of care. Sometimes a homebirth midwife's intuition tells her that *in this particular case, this particular woman* needs, and can achieve, natural birth even if her condition does not meet protocols, and consequently the midwife will accept the risk of attending the woman at home. Conversely, when everything seems normal and totally within protocol, that same homebirth midwife may transport simply because she intuits that something is wrong (for potent examples see Roncalli 1997). In other words, midwifery care tends to be individualized, not standardized, and some of that individualization comes from the deep reliance many midwives come to develop on their inner knowing and that of their clients.

As Robbie spoke, every midwife in the audience nodded her head; some were sobbing. What we noted at the beginning of this chapter was displayed in that moment—the spirit of the renegade lives in every midwife, whether she acts on it or not. And in fact, every midwife either of us has ever interviewed (over 400 practicing midwives of all types) admits or is overtly proud of the fact that she will sometimes practice out of protocols in any setting in order to protect a woman from unnecessary intervention.

It is important to note that hospital midwives too have a whole myriad of strategies for subverting the system: they fudge charts to keep the laboring woman off of Friedman's curve and thus give her more time, let her family members slip in food and drink although the hospital prohibits it, avoid the monitor when they can, break amniotic sacs covertly (and/or stretch the cervix) with their fingers to speed labor when the threat of pitocin looms, and sometimes even lock the door to the labor room to give the couple the privacy they need to make love and thus strengthen labor through nipple and clitoral stimulation (which naturally increases oxytocin levels) instead of through a pitocin drip. As the quote from Richard Jennings (director of the Bellevue Birthing Center and the midwifery practice in Bellevue Hospital, New York City) with which we began this chapter was intended to express, many hospital-based midwives are closet renegades; they just do subtly what homebirth midwives do much more overtly.

The great myth about themselves that nurse-midwives have created is that they only attend low-risk, normal births—an area in which they are the experts. In truth, from the beginning of their entry into hospitals in the mid-1950s, nurse-midwives have been attending the births of poor, inner-city, malnourished, and therefore high-risk women—and they have been doing an excellent job, as all their studies show (see

Rooks 1997 for summaries). But their attendance of these high-risk women is in contrast to the public image of themselves they have sought to create, an image they hope makes them appear to be less of a threat to physicians and safe practitioners for normal women. Their frequent attendance of poor, relatively high-risk women, in tandem with the many subversive strategies they develop in the hospital, reinforces our point that CNMs are often closet renegades, flouting the system while appearing to comply with it, and expanding the choices for their clients while appearing to normatively conform to medical protocols and state regulations.

We acknowledge that Robbie's take on homebirth renegade midwives is necessarily influenced by her 1984 experience of a home VBAC at forty-three weeks with a three-day labor and a ten-pound baby. This birth would not have been allowed to take place naturally in any hospital in the United States. In her written birth stories (Davis-Floyd, n.d.), Robbie notes that the pain was stunning but the accomplishment was far more so. Her deep intuition that her choice was right and that the baby was safe all the way through seemed to Robbie and to her midwives to be far more meaningful than "risk factors." Robbie's experience of pushing through the pain to give birth with her own psychological strength and physical power was utterly life transforming. Had she not been able to find two renegade midwives in Austin, Texas, in 1984, who were willing to attend her VBAC at home even though their state regulations made that illegal, she could not have experienced the empowerment of that birth, but would have had to relive the devastating disempowerment of her previous cesarean.

Is the price of the risk worth the value of the reward? Robbie is, in effect, in the same dilemma as the midwives she studies. She supports and has actively aided the professionalization of lay midwifery and the development and implementation of national certification for direct-entry midwives and national recognition for direct-entry schools, which perforce has entailed some degree of standardization of skills and care. At the same time, she is also keenly aware (through her own experience and her interviews with over 100 women about their birth experiences) of the importance of normalizing uniqueness though with individualized, intuitive care—the kind of care that in some cases can only fully be offered by those midwives who proudly claim the term "renegade."

Renegade midwives acknowledge that their existence and praxis threaten the tenuous toehold in the technocracy that their professional compatriots, and often they themselves, are working so hard to establish. They are also aware that their existence and praxis help to keep the spirit of the homebirth midwifery movement alive and the full range of options open to American women. Here again the differences between plain and professional midwives come into play. Plain midwives have made it clear that they prefer to practice completely outside the law; they desire neither national certification nor state licensure. Thus plain midwives who are renegades can at least be rhetorically excluded (Lay 2000) by the professionally oriented CNMs, CPMs, and LMs, who have both worked for the creation of, and have themselves obtained, national certification and/or state licensure. But when one of these professional midwives practices as a renegade, she cannot be rhetorically excluded or differentiated from licensed or certified midwives who do (usually) stick to protocols (or at least try to appear to) in the interests of protecting their profession. Thus the overtly renegade professional midwife constitutes the greater liability. And yet the fact that she has achieved licensure or certification as a CNM, CPM, LM, or CM at least demonstrates that she has obtained the requisite knowledge, skills, and experience to practice safely and presumably to trust her own judgment, and thus is perhaps more qualified to be a renegade than the plain midwife who has not been formally tested.

Many midwives have noted that "the CPMs remind the CNMs about the dangers of overmedicalizing, and renegades remind both groups of the same danger." One very experienced CPM reaffirmed this perception: "I'm glad there are people out there pushing the envelope—if they didn't, people like us would be on the edge. I don't want to put mothers and babies in danger to be on the edge." Another longtime midwife who had been somewhat of a renegade in her early years, responded, "I don't want to go out on a limb anymore. My heart can only handle so much stress. You end up on the edge often enough without knowingly, premeditatedly going there."

Our awareness of the existence of various renegade CPMs in the United States is the reason why we waited with baited breath for the outcomes of the CPM2000 statistical study. When the data finally did become available, our fears were allayed. To recap from chapter 3, eighty-eight out of every 100 women who planned a homebirth with a CPM did give birth at home successfully and safely. CPMs transported twelve out of every 100 women to the hospital during labor, and only 3.6 percent of the time was it considered urgent. The cesarean rate for CPM clients was 3.7 percent, and the perinatal mortality rate was two in 1,000 (1.7 in 1,000 if breeches are not included)—equivalent to what it is for CNMs attending out-of-hospital births and for physicians attending low-risk women in hospitals (in other words, exactly what it should be given optimal care) (Johnson and Daviss 2005).

We are certain that the data submitted by 350 CPMs for this study included data from a number of known "renegades." And we are grateful that their willingness to practice outside of regulations and protocols does not statistically generate negative data, but rather reinforces the point that CPMs attending homebirths have outcomes as good as, and often better than, other kinds of birth practitioners. But the results of this study are not yet widely known; thus *one* bad outcome from a CPM-attended birth still has the detrimental effect of reinforcing cultural stereotypes and making midwives of all types appear incompetent to the general public. Such stereotypes constitute part of the reason why these midwives, after decades of practice, still attend less than one percent of American births. Combating such stereotypes through an emphasis on professionalization and professionalism has been a dominant ethos of nurse-midwifery from its inception; such an emphasis only became important to the former lay midwives in the 1990s. Now they too wish to change the cultural image of midwifery, but at what price? This is a question many nurse-midwives also pose to themselves.

And so we repeat at the end of this section the thought with which we began this chapter: all midwives are, to some extent, renegades. Yet there is a *spectrum of renegadeness,* and those at the further end of it threaten the cultural acceptance of professional midwifery. Every midwife must decide for herself to what extent and under what circumstances she will adhere to regulations and protocols, and to what extent and under which circumstances she will flout those protocols in what she believes are the best interests not of her profession, but of her individual client. And every midwife must also keep in mind that protecting the profession is also ultimately in the best interests of mothers and babies, because it is the existence of midwifery that keeps the options of safe, non-interventive, and nurturant birth open to all who choose midwifery care.

THE ROLE OF THE STRANGER

The stranger does not share the local assumption and so becomes essentially the one who has to place in question nearly everything that seems to be unquestionable to members of the approached group.

—Zymunt Baumann

Renegade midwives are to professional midwives what midwifery is to biomedicine—a challenger to everything that appears evident and beyond question. This is the role the "stranger" has played from time immemorial. Without exception, all societies produce strangers, and most subgroups in society produce their own unique set of strangers. Knowledge systems are self-evident as long as no one from a contesting ideology is around to ask questions "about their grounds and reasons, point out the discrepancies, lay bare their arbitrariness. This is why the arrival of the stranger has the impact of an earthquake. The stranger shatters the rock on which the security of daily life rests" (Baumann 1997:9). Such outsiders make life uncomfortable. Encounters with the stranger stir things up and produce uncertainty, anxiety, and questions about boundaries. One of the most exasperating things about this state of affairs is the difficulty in creating definitive guidelines for action when "the stranger exhales uncertainty where certainty and clarity should have ruled" (Bauman 1997:18). The stranger impedes the professionalization effort at every turn by stimulating this uncertainty. In so doing the very ground of professionalization—building methodical and secure knowledge systems—is undercut.

In confrontations with the stranger, one of two options is usually chosen: assimilation or banishment. In the case of the renegade, no matter how many are assimilated, there will always be more who refuse and resist this assimilation. Is banishment a viable alternative? With banishment the lines of communication are broken and there is precious little chance to develop shared meanings leading to constructive dialogue and transformation (as we point out in chapter 12, on home-to-hospital transport).

There is a third alternative—a middle way between these two extremes that involves recognizing the key point that "social actors can and do play a crucial role in creating new combinations of compliance and commitment, power and autonomy, control and trust" (Reed 2001:13). This third and most radical alternative is remaining in dialogue and keeping the channels of communication open. Nothing meaningful can be accomplished if trust is not established. Midwives have the opportunity to chart new territory in today's world, not only with respect to their systems of knowledge, but also with respect to innovating new typologies for collegial conduct. They have the chance to pioneer groundbreaking forms for staying in discourse despite ferocious disagreements with one another. This effort will take a tremendous commitment of time and energy, but what is the alternative? Keeping these lines of communication open can only add to the rich heritage and contemporary viability of midwifery.

Judith Rooks (1998) discusses three possible models for future relationships between nurse-midwives and direct-entry midwives. We can extend her analysis to include the relations between protocol-oriented and renegade midwives. The first path involves co-option, which is akin to assimilation; the second path is remaining isolated from one another with minimal contact—a path where hostility and competition prevail. The third alternative calls for a convergence of views in which the best of both are combined into a unified whole. While renegade midwives and protocol-oriented midwives will continue to reside in separate domains, a great deal more convergence between the two models can be accomplished. This convergence can only add to the vitality of the midwifery knowledge system.

The renegade's very existence can contribute to clarifying the boundaries and parameters of the midwifery knowledge system. As mentioned earlier, homebirth midwifery itself arose as a renegade movement that captured society's attention with regard to the need for reforms in biomedical birth practices. At her best, the renegade can serve as check and balance that professional homebirth midwives do not stray too far from the heart of their commitment to women.

During one of Christine's conversations with a CNM, the nurse-midwife explained that she remained in continuous contact with a renegade midwife to keep her from straying too far from her midwifery origins. Plain and renegade midwives can sharpen the edges of midwifery social change by imploring careful consideration of the compromises that are made in the bid for social legitimacy. In addition, renegade midwives serve as keepers of alternative knowledge, which thereby remains available to both protocol-oriented midwives and their clients to provide alternatives that formal regulations deem unacceptable. Given enough evidence over time, VBAC, breech, and twin births may become acknowledged as variants of "normal," and thereby become viable candidates for both homebirth and vaginal births in the hospital.

The potential for radical change in institutional views about midwifery with respect to issues such as breech birth became evident in a California court case in which a renegade licensed midwife was sued by the medical board for vaginally delivering a breech birth at home. The court brief noted that "the medical 'standard of care' for breech birth is to do a cesarean section in most cases," however, the court also emphasized that "the medical model's applicability to midwifery is inappropriate and summarily dismissed" (Department of Consumer Affairs, State of California 1999:3,11). The tribunal hearing the case allotted the midwifery model the same level of authority as the medical model:

> Midwives employ a midwifery model of practice distinct from the medical model of practice. . . . Unlike physicians, physician's

assistants, physician assistant midwives, registered nurses, or certified nurse-midwives who practice within the context of a medical model, licensed midwives practice within the context of a midwifery model. Complainant contends that the medical model should function to define the scope of a midwife's practice. This issue arises because the ACT provides that a licensed midwife is authorized by his or her license, "under the supervision of a licensed physician and surgeon to attend cases of normal childbirth.... "Normal" within the context of the medical model specifically excludes, inter alia, breech presentation because of the risk for complications. *Within the context of the midwifery model, breech presentation is merely a variant of normal childbirth.* (Department of Consumer Affairs, State of California 1999:11,14)

This case is noteworthy and instructive in that it dramatically illustrates how important renegade midwifery can be for mainstreaming midwifery practices often sacrificed in the name of state sanction.

At her worst, the renegade midwife can go too far with resultant bad outcomes either at home or in a hospital transport. These incidents do considerable damage by spoiling the reputation of midwifery and requiring years to reestablish the legitimacy of midwifery in a given community. In a tit-for-tat way, protocol-oriented midwives can provide a check and balance for renegade midwives by reminding them of the larger context in which they practice. Much as the renegade would prefer the luxury of only considering the needs of the individual woman she is attending, the renegade acts in a larger context and is responsible for this whether or not she chooses to acknowledge it. Ongoing dialogue with professionally oriented midwifery groups will give the renegade midwife a stronger sense of orientation.

Battles between professionally oriented and renegade midwives over the proper domain of midwifery invoke larger philosophical issues of choice and responsibility. "The acceptance of responsibility does not come easy—not just because it ushers in the torments of choice (which always entails forfeiting something as well as gaining something else), but also because it heralds the perpetual anxiety of being—who knows?—in the wrong. . . . The snag is, though, that foolproof recipes are to freedom, to responsibility, and to responsible freedom what water is to fire" (Bauman 1997:202–203). Creativity comes through the courage to engage the tension of opposites until a new synthesis can be fashioned.

LIVING INTO THE ANSWERS

Trust is not something out there but rather a social process that is constructed for and by people and a matter of the choices and actions of individuated subjects.

—**Christine Garsten (2001)**

In ending this chapter we propose that each midwife ask of herself the following question: What is my responsibility to the "other" midwife? What is the best way to address this issue from a position of higher consciousness rather than a position of lower consciousness? The answers to these questions cannot be intellectually crafted or analytically developed, but rather must be lived into. How each midwife decides to answer these questions involves nothing less than the quality and integrity of the legacy contemporary midwives bequeath to the future.

ACKNOWLEDGMENTS

Our thanks to Betty Anne Daviss for her careful reading of, and corrections to, this chapter, and to Barbara Katz Rothman and Raymond DeVries for their helpful comments.

REFERENCES

Baumann, Zymunt. 1997. *Postmodernity and Its Discontents.* New York: New York University Press.

Boston University Corporate Education Center. 2003. *Management Development Programs.* Boston, MA: Trustees of Boston University.

Davis-Floyd, Robbie. Nd. "Knowing: A Story of Two Births." Unpublished manuscript.

———. 1987. "Obstetric Training as a Rite of Passage." *Medical Anthropology Quarterly* 1(3):288-318.

———. 2004. *Birth as an American Rite of Passage,* 2nd edition. Berkeley: University of California Press.

Davis-Floyd, Robbie and Elizabeth Davis. 1997. "Intuition as Authoritative Knowledge in Midwifery and Home Birth." In *Childbirth and Authoritative Knowledge: Cross-Cultural Perspectives,* pp. 315-349. Berkeley: University of California Press.

Davis-Floyd, Robbie and Gloria St. John. 1998. *From Doctor to Healer: The Transformative Journey.* New Brunswick, NJ: Rutgers University Press.

Department of Consumer Affairs, State of California. August 16–20, 1999. *In the Matter of the Accusation Against Alison Osborn, Case No. 1M-98-83794.*

Durkheim Emile. 1933, *The Division of Labor in Society.* New York: The Free Press.

Garston, Christine. 2001. "Trust, Control and Post-bureaucracy." *Organizational Studies.* March.

Johnson, Kenneth C. and Betty Anne Daviss. 2005. "Outcomes of Planned Home Births with Certified Professional Midwives: Large Prospective Study in North America." *British Medical Journal* 330(7505): 1416, June. www.bmj.com.

Klassen, Pamela. 2001. *Blessed Events: Religion and Home Birth in America.* Princeton: Princeton University Press.

Lay, Mary M. 2000. *The Rhetoric of Midwifery: Gender, Knowledge, and Power.* New Brunswick, NJ: Rutgers University Press.

Moran, Marilyn A. 1981. *Birth and the Dialogue of Love.* Leawood, KS: New Nativity Press.

Reed Michael I. 2001. "Organization, Trust and Control: A Realist Analysis." *Organizational Studies.* March.

Roncalli, Lucia. 1997. "Standing by Process: A Midwife's Notes on Storytelling, Passage, and Intuition." In *Intuition: The Inside Story,* eds Robbie Davis-Floyd and P. Sven Arvidson, pp. 177–200. New York: Routledge.

Rooks, Judith. 1997. *Midwifery and Childbirth in America.* Philadelphia: Temple University Press.

Rooks, Judith. 1998. "Unity in Midwifery?: Realities and Alternatives." *Journal of Nurse-Midwifery* 43 (5): 315–319.

Shanley, Laura Kaplan. 1994. *Unassisted Childbirth.* Westport, CT: Bergin and Garvey.

12

HOME TO HOSPITAL TRANSPORT: FRACTURED ARTICULATIONS OR MAGICAL MANDORLAS?[1]

Christine Barbara Johnson and Robbie Davis-Floyd

- **Disparate Knowledge Systems and Magical Mandorlas** • **The Nature of a Crisis** • **Mandorla Transport Stories** • **Contextualizing the Mandorla Transport** • **Articulating Transport Mandorlas**

The Mandorla signifies the place . . . where miracles arise. It is beyond our ordinary way of seeing . . . where two irreconcilable opposites are over-lapped into a sublime whole.

—**Robert A. Johnson,** *Owning Your Own Shadow*

DISPARATE KNOWLEDGE SYSTEMS AND MAGICAL MADORLAS

Ideologies and institutions are not smoothly functioning monoliths. Rather, they form amalgams of internally contested and inconsistent ideas. In complex societies, for each cultural ideology, parallel knowledge systems exist. Throughout history a selected few gain cultural ascendancy while numerous others are marginalized and disappear or survive on the cultural fringe. The cultural ascendancy of a particular knowledge system must not be mistaken for truth, but rather seen as an outcrop of social power. As Bauman (1997:13) notes:

> The dispute about the veracity or falsity of certain beliefs is always simultaneously the contest about the right of some to speak with authority which some others should obey [and] about the establishment or reassertion of the relations of superiority and inferiority, of domination and submission, between holders of beliefs.

The biomedical model and the midwifery model characterize two parallel, often conflicting, and sometimes overlapping knowledge systems (Giddens 1991; Jordan 1993). The biomedical model is culturally ascendant while the midwifery model is culturally marginalized and devalued. Both systems of knowledge encapsulate vital truths about birth, which all too often remain fragmented from one another, especially in states where midwifery is illegal or unlicensed.

In this chapter we explore what happens when the ascendant knowledge system (biomedicine) and the devalued one (midwifery) are forced to confront one another on today's postmodern terrain. The postmodern technocracy offers an unprecedented opportunity for deconstructing and reconstructing knowledge systems. Postmodernism dismantles and disembeds traditional institutions by popularizing the principles of relativity and radical doubt. In this venue, "all knowledge takes the form of hypotheses: claims which may very well be true, but which are in principle always open to revision and may have at some point to be abandoned" (Giddens 1991:4). These postmodern developments have particular importance for the health-care arena. Alternative health-care models that directly challenge the biomedical model have gained widespread public support. This public acceptance, coupled with the modern emphasis on consumer needs, puts enormous pressure on the biomedical environment to innovate new health-care systems that combine standard and alternative care (Best and Kellner 1997). In the United States, midwifery transport to the hospital exemplifies a place where conflicting ideologies, hegemonic and alternative, are forced to encounter one another during a crisis to resolve a problem. These compulsory interactions have the potential to heal the split or further solidify the division.

In "Home Birth Emergencies in the US and Mexico: The Trouble with Transport," Robbie Davis-Floyd (2003) presented and compared transport stories told by American homebirth midwives and Mexican traditional midwives. She noted that:

> biomedicine and home-birth midwifery exist in separate cultural domains and are based on distinctively different knowledge systems.

> When a midwife transports a client to the hospital, she brings specific prior knowledge that can be vital to the mother's successful treatment by the hospital system. But the culture of biomedicine in general tends not to understand or recognize as valid the knowledge of midwifery. The tensions and dysfunctions that often result are displayed in midwives' transport stories, which I identify as a narrative genre and analyze to show how reproduction can go unnecessarily awry when domains of knowledge conflict and existing power structures ensure that only one kind of knowledge counts. (Davis-Floyd 2003:1912)

Robbie's article analyzes "*dis-articulations* that occur when there is no correspondence of information or action between the midwife and the hospital staff," and "*fractured articulations* of biomedical and midwifery knowledge systems that result from partial and incomplete correspondences," contrasting these two kinds of disjuncture with the "*smooth articulation* of systems that results when mutual accommodation characterizes the interactions between midwife and medical personnel" (Davis-Floyd 2003:1912). Her focus in that article was primarily on the fractures in care that result when the midwife's knowledge and recommendations are discounted in the hospital. Such fractured articulations between the medical and midwifery systems can and do result in the unnecessary death of mother or child. Robbie's article recounts numerous examples of such fractures, in which the midwife's knowledge about the mother's history, prior labor status, and present needs is ignored by medical staff, and the midwife, in spite of giving good care and transporting appropriately, may be threatened with a lawsuit for a "botched" homebirth—certainly a detriment to her willingness to transport in the future and a cementing of further alienation between the medical and midwifery worlds.[2]

In this chapter, we will extend Robbie's work through a primarily positive focus on what Robbie termed "smooth articulations" between the medical and homebirth midwifery systems. From the outset of the medical-midwifery encounter, the power differential becomes evident as the midwife is usually forced to cross the threshold into the biomedical world and act within its institutional and ideological parameters. Despite this power divide, genuine reconciliation between these separate worlds and their reconstruction into a unified whole does occur on many occasions, which we seek to exemplify here in the interests of presenting a more positive set of possibilities for mother, child, midwife, and hospital staff, and a further pathway to the mainstreaming of midwifery care.

We will use the mandorla as a conceptual ideal type to investigate the nuances of these more positive transport sagas. The *mandorla* is an ancient symbol for the place where opposites can meet and honor one another, and in this reconciliation forge a new reality that is greater than the sum of its parts. "A mandorla is the almond-shaped segment that is made when two circles partly overlap" (Johnson 1991:98). Inside the overlap, separate domains are united and merged into innovative structures, within which effective solutions can emerge. This perspective can offer us a conceptual prototype for transcending the bounds of ordinary consciousness by overlapping opposites and integrating them into a transcendent whole in which everyone's interests and concerns are appropriately addressed. This chapter takes an in-depth look at what conditions facilitate a transport mandorla in states where midwifery is either illegal or allowed to exist, but remains unsanctioned by a legislative mandate. In these cases, the individual actors must transcend the limits of their knowledge systems without benefit of structural guidelines. Studying such smooth articulations between systems provides an opportunity to view how, when, and under what circumstances mutual accommodation by opposing parties become the predominant theme. These mandorla encounters embody what Grossberg (1992:57) calls the recasting of separate spheres into "active structures . . . that cut across domains and planes."

THE NATURE OF A CRISIS

Dialogues among homebirth midwives and physicians are uncommon, especially in states where homebirth midwives remain unlicensed. Most often, these practitioners inhabit separate worlds that only intersect when a homebirth goes awry and a transport is the necessary

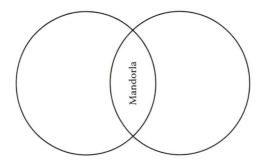

Fig. 12.1 The Mandorla.

result. Most home-to-hospital transports are preventive, but some take place during genuine crises. Such crises can create important opportunities. The Chinese depict a crisis as an "opportunity riding on dangerous wings." (The Chinese pictograph for *crisis* incorporates both the character for *danger* and the character for *opportunity*.) A homebirth transport is a threshold moment in which the seeds for the new are present but not yet manifest. ·Vulnerability and its potential for lowering of defenses can make crises a fertile ground for creating new ways of understanding and forging innovative structures. In meeting the "other" during such intense and vulnerable encounters, alliances that might never otherwise be made can be forged. The inertia that typically supports alienation from one another can be transformed into creative amalgamation.

Analyzing the crisis scenario has another advantage. Institutional behavior constantly reaffirms itself through regularized patterns, rituals, and routines that take on the appearance of being "evident." These regularized encounters promote a trust founded on predictability. The predictable nature of the environment masks the dynamic and active process of maintaining trust. A crisis breaks the routine and exposes the often forgotten fragility of social processes, and in so doing allows the unmasking of the social processes that undergird daily reality and the degrees of freedom that exist for reconfiguration. "In circumstances of uncertainty and multiple choice, the notions of trust and risk have particular application" (Giddens 1991:4). By exploring the interplay of risk and trust, constellations that promote social integration or disintegration can be clarified.

Hospital transports capture the interactive and dynamic processes through which meaning structures are generated and regenerated by the actors themselves. By analyzing these events, we can observe how the meaning of a particular transport situation is actively constructed—created and recreated through shared interaction, whether or not the actors are conscious of this process. While it is true that institutions generate unspoken rules that tend to regularize encounters between biomedical and "outside" practitioners, their interaction during a crisis can nevertheless generate a sense of freedom from these rules in the interests of serving the mother and child. What emerges from the mandorla transport narratives presented in this chapter are the ways in which everyday life interactions carry within them not only the possibility of conformity to stereotypes, but also the possibility of transformation of those stereotypes into systems of mutual understanding and trust. These narratives reveal the potential for *flow*, in which involved individuals participate through acting, reflecting, adjusting their opinions to input from others, and negotiating in order to achieve a shared meaning of the situation (Wallace and Wolf 1995).

All midwives who practice out of the hospital must occasionally transport. In the United States, homebirth midwives have a transport rate of twelve percent (Johnson and Daviss 2005). In other words, eighty-eight percent of their clients give birth safely at home, while twelve percent are transported to the hospital during or after labor for various reasons (see chapter 3). In only 3.6 percent of intended homebirths does the midwife consider the transfer urgent. The transport stories we have culled from our interview data and selected to recount cluster inside that three to twelve percent. We ask our readers to keep in mind that the circumstances they recount are rare and not representative of the vast majority of births. These experiences are often encoded in narrative because they are so unusual, and because of their heavy emotional charge. Stories give meaning and coherence to experience. Midwives who transport under frightening circumstances often need to find that coherence and to evaluate through narrative, with the benefit of hindsight, their own actions and those of the mother and the biomedical personnel.

As we describe in the Introduction to this volume, both of us have conducted extensive interviews with midwives and their clients. During the course of this research, which involved hours of formal interviewing and even more hours of "hanging out" with midwives and mothers, we both heard many transport stories. Over time, these transport stories began to emerge for both of us as a narrative genre that richly encapsulates the continuum of possibilities that result when a subaltern system encounters a dominant system.

We chose the particular stories we present here primarily because they represent and typify the integrated mandorla type of transport we seek to highlight in this chapter, illuminating the ground upon which opposite systems find their reconciliation. The stories thus embody both the collision of worlds and the merging of worlds, portraying integrated mandorla transports as positive models of smooth articulation between the medical and midwifery knowledge systems. (All names used here are pseudonyms.)

MANDORLA TRANSPORT STORIES

The stories Robbie presented in her article on transport were all told by midwives. Here we present primarily stories told by mothers who elected to give birth at home with a midwife, so that we can see how an integrated mandorla transport looks and feels from the birthing woman's point of view. We also include one midwife's story because we want to highlight the significance of the mandorla transport for the midwife and her relationships with the technomedical system. Because we have no way of ascertaining the truth or untruth of these stories, for the purposes of this chapter we take them at face value and unpack them for what they reveal about midwives' and women's perceptions of, and meanings they attribute to, events as they unfold. We seek to elucidate the social processes through which adherents of a dominant knowledge system sometimes dismiss what adherents of a marginalized system have to say, and other times honor and include them.

Mothers' Stories

> Gradually, the two disparate circles begin to overlap and the mandorla grows.

—**Robert A. Johnson,** *Owning Your Own Shadow* (1991:106)

The following stories illustrate the wide variety of transport problems that can culminate in a creative amalgamation of the biomedical and midwifery models. These narratives unmask the process through which boundary renegotiation occurs. The first story shows how even a neo-natal death can provide fertile ground for forging connections. The next account is from a woman interviewed both before and after her first birth, and demonstrates how a transport ending in a cesarean can strengthen the connection between opposites. The final story in this section is also from a woman who was interviewed both before and after her second birth. This woman became the first in her family to give birth without a cesarean. Were it not for the emerging respect and appreciation of the "other" that took place in the hospital after transport, this woman would have been the next in a long line to give birth by cesarean. This particular story is illustrative of how a transport that begins with strained communication can end with a mutual respect that enlarges the worldview of all those involved.

Kate's Story: The Long Journey   Kate Sims, a white female in her early forties who straddles the fence between lower-middle and middle-class, has a BA in social science and owns her own small business. She has been married for over ten years and has given birth three times. Her first child was born in a hospital by cesarean in 1991. Her second child was born at home in 1995, was transported to the hospital in critical condition, and died shortly after the transport. Her third baby was born at home in 1996, healthy and well, without hospital involvement of any kind.

Kate's first birth, which took place in a large teaching hospital, left her devastated. At the time she was unaware of the difference between the midwifery and the biomedical model of birth. Against her better judgment, Kate agreed to have her labor induced. As her contractions became increasingly intense, she was left alone for most of her labor. Even when she felt that the biomedical suggestions she received were in error, Kate had no point of reference from which to evaluate them. Lacking access to alternative information, Kate felt that the least risky option was to capitulate, but she left this birth experience convinced that a trusted support person would have transformed its nature and that the outcome would have been radically different. We recount the following narrative of her first birth to demonstrate the extent of her aversion to the hospital at the time of her second birth transport, and to show that despite Kate's negative predisposition and the critical nature of her second birth, the subsequent transport encounter paved the way for new understandings and an embracing of the cultural other.

As Kate's labor intensified, the force of the pitocin-induced contraction "frightened me and no one reassured me that I was okay. And that would have made a huge difference to me." Eventually, Kate asked for an epidural, and soon after:

I was numb from my breasts to my toes. . . . And I remember my blood pressure dropping right after I got the epidural—it was eighty over something. I felt woozy, breathless, and I was passing in and out of consciousness. It was very clear that the hospital staff was worried and someone came in and gave me an injection to stimulate things. I began to stabilize and they turned out the light. I remember waking up after about an hour and looking around and feeling that "this is no way to have a baby. Now I can't even tell that I am in labor. This is the most momentous day of my life and I am not even able to participate in the experience. I have all these machines that are keeping an eye on me so no personal contact is necessary." I just remember feeling so disappointed and so let down. After a while they started to prep for a cesarean section and it hit me that I was about to have major abdominal surgery. The only surgery I had ever had in my life was a tonsillectomy when I was a child. I was just beside myself and I totally forgot I was having a baby and I started shaking. They put an oxygen mask on me and I just remember being so claustrophobic and terrified. Eventually I noticed the physician standing there holding a baby and I thought, "Why is he telling me to look?" I was so disoriented. This birth was an awful experience and not something I would wish on anyone.

After this devastating experience, Kate launched an extensive investigation into her birthing options. Eventually she decided to give birth at home with a direct-entry midwife. Three years later she became pregnant. During this pregnancy Kate immersed herself in building solid and trusting relationships with her caregivers. In addition to her one-hour prenatal care visits, she elected to take an independent childbirth course with another direct-entry midwife she met during her research endeavors. This childbirth class was instrumental in leading Kate through the tragedy of her second birth:

> In one of our childbirth classes, we explored our worst-case scenario. During this class, my husband and I felt that we really needed to become settled in taking responsibility for a home-birth even with the possibility of a poor outcome. Not that we were being cavalier about our baby's health. We had already completed a copious amount of research and became convinced that homebirth was a safe option. So in this childbirth class my husband and I wrote out our worst nightmare to bring it down to size and make it manageable. Both my husband and I had a very similar worst case: the baby might be severely compromised and wind up on a lot of machines with a medical limbo status with always more that could be medically done with unknown consequences. This process was very powerful for us. It had a huge impact on how we addressed all our fears about a worst-case scenario birth outcome. So when it actually happened I was never afraid. I was frustrated, angry, excited, elated, joyful, and sad, but I was never afraid.

This narrative makes it clear that Kate now felt empowered to trust herself and the midwifery model of care with respect to what kinds of risks were acceptable to her and what kinds were untenable.

Kate was well prepared for her second birth by the time she went into labor. She had a complete trust in the midwifery model of birth and was ready to fully embrace any risks involved. On the other hand, she distrusted the biomedical approach to birth and perceived it to be fraught with a greater set of risks. This unwavering faith in the midwifery model helped to promote an integrated transport.

As her labor began, Kate felt a multitude of emotions: happy, excited, comfortable, and relaxed, knowing she was well prepared and attended to by midwives she trusted. These feelings were augmented by the awareness that she didn't have to go anywhere because she would give birth in her own haven—her home. She called a few family members and friends to join her as her labor began. As the contractions became more intense, the midwives arrived. Kate commented:

> I got what I asked for. I was not detached from my experience—I was very present and connected. The result was a real family experience with a couple of friends there as well. This time I had all the support that was lacking in the first birth. I got into this labor rhythm and I remember feeling very connected in particular with my friend. It was so important to me just to know that she was there. Suddenly I let out a roar and felt this uncontrollable urge to push. My baby came out really fast, she just pushed out and I only had a tiny little tear because the midwives did perineal support, massage, and stretching.

Kate's second birth unfolded exactly as she had dreamed it would. The birth began and ended at home with the support of family, friends, and supportive and competent caregivers she trusted completely. As a result of this birth, Kate gained a new appreciation of her own strength. Her extensive research had been well worth it, culminating in a joyful, empowering birth experience. But Kate had little time to assimilate and savor this moment.

> After about ten minutes we noticed that his ribs were starting to retract. At this point I began thinking, "This is starting to look like the worst-case scenario." The midwives called the hospital and they told us to bring the baby in. We had been in the hospital for a while when finally the neonatologist came out to meet with us. The neonatologist and all the staff were very gracious and included my midwife in all the professional conversations.

Here we see that the inclusion of the midwife in the lines of communication laid the foundation for the reconciliation of opposites.

> As we all met (my husband, myself, our midwife and the neonatologist), our midwife Maria [said to the neonatologist] "I need to ask you, is there anything that I or any of the other midwives did or did not do that contributed to this baby's problems?" I must say that is the greatest act of personal courage I have ever witnessed in my life. The doctor responded immediately, saying

"Absolutely not. This baby was in such great condition when it came in! We were expecting to get a disaster when we heard that it was a homebirth transport. Instead, this baby was in terrific condition given what is wrong." After an initial exam the doctor noted that our baby had severe lung and heart problems, and she suspected a fatal genetic disorder and that there wasn't anything that could really be done. The neonatologist talked about how strong he looked and what a great job we had done with the prenatal health and that most babies with this condition don't grow to be this big and strong. The temp was normal, the baby was pink—"This baby is doing really, really well."

As illustrated in Kate's words, in the mandorla transport, two opposites meet, and in the encounter see for the first time who the "other" really is, devoid of stereotypes. In the process, these opposites renegotiate the boundaries of their own worldviews. The meaning of homebirth was profoundly redefined by the biomedical team as the physician herself openly acknowledged the validity of homebirth midwifery care. At the same time, Kate and her midwife changed their definition of the hospital as hostile territory as it became increasingly obvious that they were being met with honor and respect. Kate's narrative documents how the trust between the biomedical team and the midwifery team was a cumulative process with each interaction building and reconstructing the nature of trust between these separate cultural spheres. From the onset, both the midwife and the neonatologist were able to accommodate one another and thereby establish a mutually beneficial line of communication. Each communication solidified and built upon the previous communication, as if each side were feeling the other out and only too happy to respond in kind when met with respect. The hospital team initiated the contact in a respectful and honoring manner. The midwife in turn responded by exposing herself to a potentially scathing critique from the biomedical system. The neonatologist followed this response by emphasizing the high quality of midwifery care that she observed, while stressing that her own evaluation of midwifery was being reconstructed to accommodate this new evidence. If one or both parties had insisted on devaluing the proverbial "other," this transport could easily have resulted in a further entrenchment of the alienation each had previously felt. Instead, through this transport such a strong connection was made that homebirth transports by this midwife became welcomed at this hospital, and the midwife became more willing to transport earlier in the labor rather than later because of this receptive environment.

The nature of the infant's condition was a major contributing factor promoting the trust and the reverence that each party exhibited toward the other. The baby was genetically fatally ill and there was nothing anyone could do medically to alter this fact. Rather than blaming the midwife and the couple, the neonatologist kept her mind open to recognizing the midwife's quality of care. And the midwives kept their minds open to learning from the neonatologist. This psychological openness on the part of both parties is essential to the emergence of a mandorla transport: we have both recorded stories of similar genetic problems becoming evident at homebirths, yet in these other stories when the midwife transported, she was not received with openness but with blame. Kate said:

> The neonatologist told us that "this transport has really altered mine and my staff's view of what homebirth midwifery is and the level of care that is provided. We were all incredibly impressed." Since then our midwife Maria has had to transport several times and has brought them to this doctor because this team developed a respect for homebirth midwifery as a result of this transport. The result has been a friendly transport environment.
>
> After the geneticists looked at him they were very sure that he had a genetic disorder that was fatal 100 percent of the time. We said, "Okay, now it is time to take out the tubes so we can be with our baby without all the tubes and wires." We were in the neonatal care unit at that point, but once we made the decision to unhook everything, they moved us to what they call a family room so we could have privacy. Our midwife stayed with us the whole time. The hospital staff was very supportive and they brought in a camera and took numerous photographs. Thank God! I would not have thought of doing that and I am so grateful to have them. The whole experience was really peaceful and powerful and the nurses came in very quietly and one kneeled down next to me and just put her hand on the baby's foot. They were so caring and supportive.

At this point in the encounter Kate and her midwife have actively reconstructed their concepts about hospital care to incorporate the idea of the hospital as an environment where their needs could be met in a supportive and respectful manner. As trust and respect became the framework for the communication between parties, each side became increasingly accommodating to the other. Each side engaged in countless versions of "perhaps this, perhaps that, maybe it follows that, I wonder if . . ."(Johnson 1991:106), which broke the bounds of ordinary consciousness to heal the split and recombine biomedicine and midwifery into parts of an innovatively emerging whole.

> I remember the neonatologist saying to us after this experience how moved the hospital staff was by the way we had just embraced the baby's passing and how we were able to be with her through everything. The neonate told us that this outcome is not something people want to think about so they are usually just totally unprepared to deal with it. She went on to say, "The fact that the two of you could just look at each other and know that you needed to take the tubes out and just be with your baby is so powerful." My husband and I had already come face to face with this worst-case scenario in our childbirth class and knew that we wanted the human connection and did not want to use the technology to avoid it.

Here we see the growing respect by the hospital staff for Kate's choices. Kate is not blaming medicine for the death of her baby, but rather understanding the limits of medical technology and welcoming the emotional support. Recognition of the limits of medical technology, and the accepting presence by both the biomedical team and the midwifery team at an impending death, created an opportunity for communicating through shared symbols that allowed an overlap in worlds. There were no angry accusations on either side, and each party was stretched to new depths by this encounter with the other.

Kate, her family, the midwife, and the nursing staff attended the baby until she died in Kate's arms. She was more grateful than ever that she had so diligently prepared for this birth, including facing her worst-case scenario much prior to it actually happening. After the baby's death, Kate and her family had an added burden that most bereaved parents do not face: the need to assure her community that the baby's death had nothing to do with being born at home. Consequently, they held a neighborhood memorial service for their infant about one week after the birth/death. The midwife, her apprentices, and a few of the hospital staff attended, including the neonatologist, who spoke about how unusually healthy the baby was given the genetic condition, and how there was nothing anyone could have done, emphasizing that the death was "definitely not the result of a homebirth." Her words turned this newly created transcendent whole (integrating biomedicine and homebirth midwifery) into a public announcement. Kate's transport is an extraordinary example of how stereotypes can be demolished and a new integration of formerly conflicting ideologies can then become possible. The "other" is embraced as companion. One year later Kate gave birth again at home with the same midwifery prenatal care team. This birth was ideal from start to finish, and on this occasion Kate "felt like the sun came out again and a cycle had been completed."

This transport story illustrates how even a fatal outcome, if evaluated objectively by the dominant knowledge system and met openly by the midwifery model, can lead to expanding the boundaries of both the dominant and the alternative ideological systems.

Rose's Story: The Best-Laid Plans We recount the following birth story for two major reasons: (1) to include both a before and after birth sequence to avoid using only retrospective accounts of situations; and (2) to illustrate the wide-ranging effects that accumulate over time when opposites are united into a transcendent whole. Christine interviewed Rose both before and after her first birth.

Rose was a white, upper-middle-class woman in her late thirties and pregnant for the first time. While she never felt an intense biological drive to give birth, she decided to get pregnant because she sensed that her opportunity to have a family would soon disappear if she did not act. At the time of her birth, she had been married for almost a decade and felt very securely grounded both economically and emotionally. Her husband had a successful business as a consultant and she was the president of a thriving corporation. Rose was a participant in an eight-week childbirth course that Christine attended as a research participant observer. Consequently, Christine was able to witness Rose's struggle to define the set of risks she was willing to accept and the concomitant levels of trust she accorded to the biomedical and midwifery models of birth. Rose initially planned to give birth in the hospital, but eventually opted for a homebirth in 2000.

Prior to her pregnancy, Rose was familiar with homebirth and midwifery. While she was attracted to the idea of homebirth, she was initially not ready to make that choice because she perceived it as too risky. On the other hand, she also knew that hospital birth entails another set of risks. Unable to fully trust either model, Rose decided to straddle the fence between models in order to reduce her set of risks. She engaged the services of both an obstetrician and a direct-entry midwife for prenatal care. Her initial plan was to use the midwife as labor support in the hospital, but also to provide for the possibility that if she changed her mind, she would have already established a relationship with a midwife. This arrangement had the additional advantage of enabling Rose to evaluate closely the level of trust she was willing to invest in each caregiver and a more extensive knowledge about the risks endemic to each situation. Rose's story exemplifies the advantages of holding the tension between opposites until a greater and more unified reality can be formed.

As her pregnancy progressed, Rose became increasingly knowledgeable about the many aspects of pregnancy and birth. About eight weeks before Rose was due to give birth, she was able to choose where her allegiance would lie. She discovered that having her questions answered in a way that suited her needs was an essential ingredient for trust building and risk reduction. Rose experienced the obstetrician as increasingly defensive and began to wonder just what kind of a birth she would have with this woman when communication was already so strained. The obstetrician exhibited minimal willingness to incorporate midwifery tools and techniques that Rose desired. If the obstetrician had been more flexible, Rose would have felt secure in the boundary-spanning behavior she was attempting to generate between the biomedical and midwifery worlds, and probably would have opted for a hospital birth. Simultaneously, Rose was feeling more and more comfortable with the care and expertise of the midwife, who was not only willing to answer her questions, but also embraced the value of the biomedical model. Rose opted for the model that was more inclusive rather than less, as this choice reduced her efforts to stretch between worlds. In addition, Rose and her husband had been doing a lot of research into the safety of hospital and homebirth and had come to the conclusion that homebirth was a well-considered and safe alternative. Before the birth, Rose said:

> We started out with an obstetrician because we were not sure that homebirth was for us. At the same time, we had been seeing [this midwife who was to be our labor support] from the beginning and really got to know her and developed a lot of trust and confidence in her. She had already done over 800 homebirths. And we feel that she has a really great approach to transport; if there is an issue she has no problem bringing us into the hospital and that is what we need in a midwife. I also know that I want to be fully present for my birth. My choice of homebirth is interesting because several years ago a few of my family members had homebirths and I thought they were crazy. I thought, "They are really taking a risk." I had no facts on which I based this judgment. And now based on our own very thorough research it really is clear that the decision to give birth at home is a safe one. This has been a major concern of mine all along.

At this point, after checking all the options and exhaustively doing all the research, we can't imagine not being at home.

So Rose decided to stay home to have her baby—a decision made with relative ease given that she already had developed a strong and trusting relationship with the midwife. If Rose had not chosen the unique path of utilizing the services of both models from the outset, she would have had a more difficult time exiting the hospital structure because she would not have fully understood the alternatives. Building trust takes time, and the eighth month of pregnancy is a difficult time to begin a new relationship with prenatal care provider. As Rose recounts below, an unexpected hospital visit during her pregnancy became a primary factor nudging Rose toward a homebirth:

I had tightness in my leg and I went to the hospital to check if it was a blood clot. I was anxious the moment I walked in the door. The whole culture was awful and I knew that I did not want to give birth in a culture like this. But I also want to make it clear that I am not at all anti-mainstream medicine. There are places for it and there are places not to use it and birth is one place not to use it if it is a healthy normal pregnancy. We want a safe, easy, and relaxing birth. We would also like a spiritual experience and this was the final piece that convinced us to do a homebirth.

Two months after her homebirth ended in a hospital transport and a cesarean section, Christine again spoke with Rose:

As labor began we had all these candles in my bedroom and the lights were down. It was great. My husband was with me as well as another midwife. When the midwives said "it is time to push," I said "I don't feel like I have to"—I had no urge to push. I pushed for four hours but nothing was really happening. At this point we decided to transport for failure to progress. I was then at the hospital for another four hours without any real progress before we decided to go forward with the surgery.

During this time the midwives were welcomed as an integral part of Rose's caregiving team. This relationship between the hospital staff and the midwife had been built over varied and numerous previous transports by this midwife during which each side had gained an increasing respect for the other.

This background was one of the major factors contributing to Rose's midwife's willingness to transport earlier rather than later. While the presenting situation is substantially different from Kate's birth, the perceived level of risk is similar, in that through mutual agreement, the risk was judged to be minimal. Kate's healthy home-birth of a genetically unviable baby forged an opening between worlds. In contrast, Rose's trail toward an overlap in worlds had already been blazed by the time of she gave birth. Rose's midwife reported that her initial rapport with this hospital had been established previously, when she brought in a high-risk mother and the exemplary nature of her midwifery care was so obvious that the biomedical team substantially reconstructed their concepts of homebirth. The postmodern influence (see Introduction) in promoting this reconstruction became salient when someone from the hospital requested a meeting with this midwife shortly after the birth. In this meeting the hospital representative elucidated the postmodern theme of relativity by noting that expert knowledge is continually changing and that in today's world it is entirely possible that medical definitions of the situation can be supplanted by midwifery definitions. This openness to the smooth articulation of knowledge systems could only take place in a post-modern setting, where all knowledge is potentially open to question and continual revision.

Rose had an epidural and pitocin but still no progress was evident. After four hours in the hospital, it became obvious that that baby was stuck in a position that made delivery very difficult.

> At this point I just made a decision to have cesarean section. The midwife came into the surgery with the hospital staff. It was a really hard time for me. My husband and I were crying before the section because it was so disappointing. We had worked so hard and had really been committed to the homebirth.

Because the relationship had already been solidified, the hospital staff did not judge Rose for choosing to initially give birth at home. In fact they did just the opposite—they openly embraced her decision and supported her, even as she elected for the cesarean section. This care changed Rose's view of birth in the hospital. In this example, it is possible to see how trust continued to build and deepen on both sides over time:

> In the hospital we were just so surrounded by love—that is the best way for me to describe it. I felt so connected to the nursing

staff, especially the one who came in and kissed me on the check and held my hand. We received so much support because people knew how disappointed we were not to have had a homebirth. Everyone knew that we started off with a homebirth and so there was just this outpouring for us. The head of obstetrics and gynecology came down to see me for a couple of days in a row. He was wonderful and he asked me why I chose a homebirth. He wanted to know. As for my decision to have a homebirth, I definitely feel that I got more of a spiritual intensity by starting out at home—there is no way I could have had that at the hospital. I have to say though that I was absolutely treated very well in the hospital.

While Rose's story does not have the drama of Kate's, her narrative depicts how attitudes can continue to be profoundly and subtly changed in the direction of increased wholeness and seamlessness over time. The transport provided an opportunity for Rose to see another, more compassionate side of hospital culture, and a chance for the chief of obstetrics to interact with a couple who chose homebirth and in the process soften stereotypes on both sides.

Jane's Story: Against All Odds   The following integrated mandorla transport story was recounted by Jane, an upper-middle-class Hispanic female in her early thirties who had been married for four years at the time of the first interview. Both Jane and her husband have advanced degrees. Jane's first child was a planned hospital birth in 1997, and her second a planned homebirth in 1999. Christine interviewed Jane both before and after her second birth. Jane was so traumatized by her first hospital birth that she was certain she could not withstand another hospital encounter during labor. Nevertheless, her second birth required hospitalization. Jane's narrative unpacks the process through which a transport that begins as fractured can morph into integration. Jane's before-birth interview was inundated with references to her first birth to illustrate exactly what she hoped to avoid with the second birth, which began at home:

I had a bad experience with my first birth—I didn't have an empowering idea about birth. I had a vision of what I wanted from my birth but no one around me was mirroring that vision back to me. I went to the doctor I chose because it was easy to get to him and close to my house. I didn't like the doctor but I thought, "He is competent—it doesn't really matter if I like him or not." The doctor told me, "People make such a big deal out of the birth—it is the baby that matters." I got the impression . . . that it was almost as if my contribution to the birth did not matter. In my family all the women had had cesarean sections. I wanted to be the first one in my family not to have a section. A lot of people around me, including my family, gave me a sense that this attitude was ridiculous. They told me that the baby is all that really matters, not the birthing experience itself.

Lines of shared communication between Jane and her physician were nonexistent, but because Jane was unaware of any other options, she felt constrained to operate within the bounds of the biomedical encounter. This lack of trust made it impossible for Jane adequately to assess her birthing risks and discern those she was willing to accept and those she was unwilling to engage. Without any symbols of shared meaning, Jane entered the hospital for her first birth feeling isolated and alone.

My first experience in the hospital—I was always trying to protect myself emotionally while trying to relax and have my baby. My water broke and nothing happened for about twelve hours. The doctor came in and said, "We can put you on pitocin." I told him, "No, I want to wait and give it more time." I waited about a half-hour and then I started to cry. I told the doctor that I was scared. He promptly replied, "I know what your problem is—you need to let go of control." The nurse said, "Honey, you gave up control when you got pregnant." I felt so unsupported and unheard at that point that I just withdrew into myself.

In an ironic twist, Jane came to believe that the only way she could have any power at all in the hospital was to demand what she did not want, a cesarean section, before she was informed that she had to have one.

Twelve hours later they started the pitocin and they told me that I had to be continually monitored. They put me on the non-portable fetal monitor because the portable one was broken. What this meant is that I only had a three-by-three area that I could walk in because I had to be plugged into the electronic fetal monitor. And it was awful—the little room to move about and I kept hearing the noise of the monitor. Finally I asked for an epidural. After I got the epidural the doctor said that he was going to take a nap. At that point I said "No, don't take a nap, I want a c-section." Asking for a c-section was my way of taking control of the situation and getting some of my power back. They had told me before that I was a on a timetable and the baby had to be out within twenty-four hours. All I was thinking about was the clock and they had told me about the twenty-four-hour time limit because of the risk of infection after the water had broken. But I had no fever and no indication of a problem.

Jane had no reference point to dispute the necessity of a cesarean after a prescribed time period. Although Jane did not trust her caregivers, under the circumstances she felt forced to comply with the hospital definition of risk.

This whole terrible birth changed my life in a wonderful way. I was just not informed the first time I gave birth. The second time I got pregnant, I eventually found a direct-entry midwife. When I spoke with her on the phone for the first time I really liked the connection. As I learned more I thought, "I want a homebirth." I was so happy with my direct-entry midwife, I thought, "she is emotionally connected with me. . . . At this point in my life I cannot imagine giving birth with a stranger."

For my birth this time I have bought bouquets of flowers in every room and I am making soup that I love. I can smell it when people are on my side. I dislike the nursing mentality more and more. Everything is about shutting you down and managing you.

This time I am totally prepared. I have chosen a homebirth because I don't want to go back into the hospital . . . because I don't want to be physically guarded while I am trying to let go while giving birth. I am hoping to be really present and that my midwives will help me be present and I want it to be a life-changing spiritual event. I don't want it to be just something I have to get through.

Jane and Christine spoke again a few months after her second birth and subsequent hospital transport. As will be seen in her postbirth narrative, through an extended hospital transport stay Jane modified her view and eventually came to trust the biomedical team and develop a shared language and dialogue about the nature of risk.

This time [second birth] my water broke early in the morning and by the afternoon I was feeling surges. And all the next day the same thing again—every hour I would have a few contractions and that would be it. My water had been broken for twenty-four hours. In addition to my direct-entry midwife, I also had asked another labor support person who knew about relaxation therapy to come. She just was really good at helping me focus and would say things like, "Let your birthing body take over." She put her hand on my belly and told me to breathe into her hand and breathe up the surge and then she would breathe with me and it was about taking really slow deep, deep breaths and slowly letting them out. I would let my birth team know a contraction was coming—"It is intense, help!" You can see it in the video when my direct-entry midwife kneels down and helps me and talks me through it and I really felt I needed connection during surges. That whole period from about 5 to 10 centimeters was so hard. I had been doing this for two days and I felt it was never was going to end.

This scene is radically different from the one described in her first birth. In this second birth, the trust and connection with her caregivers are solid.

Eventually the midwives said, "We think the baby is turned the wrong way and we are going to try and turn her and it will hurt," and I said, "Whatever you have to do." They couldn't turn her and so they said, "Sorry honey, you are going to have to go to the hospital." I just started crying and wailing—I was so upset and I did not want to go to the hospital and I had no backup plan. Then I said, "Okay it is over—I give up." I was now sure that I would have a cesarean section.

At this stage, Jane perceived going into the hospital as entering enemy territory where all hope of connection and getting her needs met would be lost.

The transport began with strained relationships between the hospital staff and the midwifery team. When the hospital insisted on separating Jane from her trusted support team, Jane's fear escalated because she had no basis for trusting the care she would receive.

We went to the hospital and I wanted my support team to be with me and with the initial evaluation they made me wait alone. For me the mind–body connection was so clear, but the relaxation exercises went out the window because I stopped being attentive to relaxing. I was just so tense and focused on all my fearful and scary thoughts and this cut off all the blood supply to my uterus and everything tensed up and I was a wreck. It was not so excruciating physically in the car, now that I think of it, it was more the emotional piece that was excruciating.

This particular hospital had been the recipient of many prior home-birth transports, in which lines of communication and nexuses for smooth articulation had been established. In fact, in response to the challenging economic climate, this hospital actively solicited home-birth transports. The reasons why the initial contact between the mid-wife and the hospital team was strained are unclear. Eventually, however, the midwife was allowed to share her information with the attending physician and the hospital staff. As a result of previous expo-sure to the midwifery model, the hospital staff exhibited a willingness to work more within the parameters of the midwifery model than the biomedical one by allowing Jane to continue her labor, despite the fact that she was considerably over the twenty-four-hour limit that the hospital allows for broken waters.

And then the doctor came in and said, "We realize that you don't want to be here and we are going try and work with you, but let's be very clear. Your water has been broken for three days—this is a very serious situation and we are going to monitor you very closely and as long as there are not signs of infection we are going to work with you. But if we say that we have to prep for a cesarean section, we expect your cooper-ation."

This accommodation on the part of the hospital staff was tainted by the subsequent devaluing and discounting of the midwife's account of Jane's labor progress. The transfer of knowledge from midwife to hospital staff was partial and disjointed, with distrust mounting on both sides. Nevertheless, due to the prior positive experiences with other homebirth midwives at this hospital, the entire midwifery team was allowed to remain with Jane in her room.

The willingness of both teams to remain in contact and dialogue, disjointed though it had been, proved to be key in eventually paving the way for a smooth and mutually transforming mandorla transport.

As my midwife relayed her information to this physician, she also told him that I had been to ten centimeters twice. [In the midwifery model, it is accepted knowledge that a cervix can dilate and then retract, usually as a result of emotional tension. The biomedical model does not recognize this possibility.] At this point he rolled his eyes to one of the other women there like my midwife was crazy. And I thought, "I am supposed to relax and trust this doctor when he doesn't believe my midwife," and that was hard. They gave me an epidural and pitocin.

Despite the rift in communication on both sides, there was enough rapport for Jane to make requests and have them heard and acted upon.

I made them turn off the monitor because I did not want to hear it and they could have turned it off last time but I didn't know that. The doctor told me, "we are not going to check you a lot because of the risk of infection" and when he checked me I was at six centimeters and he looked at me and said, "You are at six," and he said it in such a way that was like, "Don't delude yourself—ten centimeters!" I didn't like him at the beginning but it got better later.

The biomedical expertise of the anesthesiologist and his eventual willingness to open the lines of communication began to alleviate Jane's fear and distrust of the hospital. Trust was established as the dialogue ensued:

When the anesthesiologist came in we were talking about the possibility of a cesarean section. I told the anesthesiologist that I had to have a general before because there was a window in my back and I was terrified of it. He explained to me that, "There are many things we can do short of a general." He kept trying to brush me off and move on and I told him, "I need to know so I can move on." Finally he got engaged in the conversation and he explained to me what other things could be done to numb you short of a general. Then I started to feel a little better being here at this hospital—"At least these people know what they are doing, at least they have modern technology here." I was pissed—why didn't my other doctors know this?

After spending all day in the hospital, my contractions were not getting closer together. They said, "You will have to think of what you want to do—we can keep upping the pitocin but there is a limit to how far we can go and at that point we will need something else"—obviously the something else was a c-section.

On the basis of prior experience with other homebirth clients who had transported into this hospital, the staff, wherever possible, was willing to honor the decision-making power of the woman who was giving birth. Almost all women electing to give birth at home become very knowledgeable about the process of birth and risks and benefits of each intervention. Hospital exposure to these homebirth clients created options for Jane that would not have been possible without this accumulated experience.

The attending physician had given Jane and her midwifery team time to confer with one another.

> After they left I said to my team, "Huddle up, huddle up," and they surrounded the bed—and said, "What are we going to do?" It was a major group decision for me—I needed to hear what they thought. My direct-entry midwife said, "Let's keep trying with the pitocin and see what happens." Her assistant said, "Well I am looking at this and thinking the baby is doing great and your uterus is tired and not performing the way it should, why wait until the baby is not doing great, now would be the time to stop and have a c-section—you are tired." And to me her assistant made more sense than pushing the limit. I was so focused but tired and I thought, "I don't want to wait until code red." And I said, "Okay, let's do it" [the c-section] and I started to cry again and I said to my midwifery team, "Help me have peace about this."

At this point, with everyone in agreement, Jane would have received a cesarean section if not for an emergency situation that occupied her obstetrician for a time.

> We called the doctor in and he said, "I hear you want a c-section but I can't do it right now. Why don't we just keep the pitocin going and we will see what happens. I have an emergency down the hall I have attend to now." I fell asleep at this point for the first time.

When the attending physician returned about one and one-half hours later and found Jane ready to give birth, he was happy to support her in a vaginal birth. At this point he took the lead from Jane and honored her wishes without insisting that he direct the show.

> I slept until midnight when he came in and checked me. I was totally dilated and his face was just totally shocked, happy shocked, and he said, "Well you are ten and you can push now," and the whole room lit up. Suddenly everyone got up and got ready and got me positioned. My midwife said, "You can turn off the epidural if you want to, it might make you feel more and make your pushes more efficient." I agreed. Before doing this the physician asked, "Are you sure? A lot of women have a hard time when doing this." I said yes.

As the midwifery team and the hospital team interacted during the intimacy of the moment, they become more integrated. The physician facilitated their integration by making himself vulnerable and becoming interested in the outcome. He personalized his care, saying that he would treat Jane as his sister and give her the best care he could. In time, the midwives and Jane came to trust him to such an extent that they saw him as part of the birthing team. This created a space for Jane to respond in kind and share an intimate detail about birth:

> I told the physician that I wanted my husband and myself to be the first ones to touch the baby. He replied, "Okay, but that might be kind of hard for me—I get really excited when the baby comes out." At that point we all actually liked this doctor. He had made himself very human and he had been so patient.

It later became clear that the doctor's prior exposure to the midwifery model had been a major factor in his willingness to accommodate Jane's wishes and to do all he could to facilitate her vaginal birth.

After several hours of pushing with a great deal of unified support from her midwifery team and the physician, her baby was born vaginally. By this time the biomedical team and the midwifery team had bonded to the point of becoming a united, close-knit team with everyone enjoying the miracle of the moment.

> I told [here she calls her physician by his first name] I wanted the baby put on me immediately with the cord cut when the baby is on me. I don't want my baby taken away and I don't want her to be given a bath. I want her just to be with me and I asked him to do whatever he had to do to make this happen.

> He said "Okay." There she was and she was born and she was on my chest and we were all around her. Then [again she calls the physician by his first name] came in and said, "It has been five minutes, we have to cut the cord." I will never forget it—I just wanted to say no and then I said, "Fine." They cut the cord and kept her with me for a while and then they took her away.

The doctor was able to convey the effect that this birth had on him and some of the transformation he had undergone as a result.

> He came in the next day and he was really beaming and he said, "Wow, that was a really great experience. It was really good for me." I didn't quite know what he was referring to then, so I went back to see him a couple of weeks after the birth and talked to him about it. He said that it was really nice the way we cut the cord and that we waited a little bit. He had to really push it to do that because the hospital demands that it be done right away and that he was glad we waited. And he really liked that we cut the cord on top of me. Hospital protocol is to hold the baby down and cut it below the mother's body, which he said he thought was ridiculous and that he thought it should be done just the way it was done. The way we did it—he thought that that is the way birthing should happen. It felt really good.

Jane's story illustrates how individuals who inhabit separate conceptual worlds, when forced into an encounter, often begin the initial communication reluctantly and with resistance—with uneasy toleration rather than acceptance. But a generous amount of time spent together in a potentially critical situation can allow the possibility for establishing the rapport essential to a mutually satisfying and transforming, and eventually smooth, articulation of psyches and knowledge systems. Jane came away with a respect for biomedicine and trust in the care provided by the physician. The physician, in turn, allowed himself to be positively influenced by midwifery ideologies of birth, and initiated a reconstruction of his former concepts. Each made allowances to accommodate and adjust to the "other" along the way. In this case, extensive prior rapport with other homebirth midwives was the backdrop that facilitated the mandorla. Jane's transport illustrates how institutional protocols can be significantly and continually altered in individual situations as cultural opposites sustain continued contact with each other over time. We will return to the power of this theme in the conclusion of this chapter.

"A Home Birth in the Hospital" We close this section of midwifery homebirth client stories by briefly describing a transport that occurred a few months ago and was recounted to Christine. Both the midwife and the woman who gave birth shared their narratives. Christine conducted before and after birth interviews with the mother.

Prior to her birth, the one thing the woman most wanted was to stay at home. However, she was eventually transported for failure to progress. Upon arrival at the hospital, the midwife and laboring couple were greeted respectfully and warmly. The midwife showed the staff the woman's chart and answered any questions asked. The mother stated that she wanted an epidural, as she had been laboring throughout the night and was ready for some relief. She was given the epidural and pitocin. During her hospital stay, the mother noted that for the most part, they were treated respectfully and midwifery knowledge was honored to such an extent that when the time came for her to push, the doctor invited the midwife to massage the mother's perineum with oil. As she massaged, the midwife remarked to the parents that this was "a homebirth in the hospital." She said, "There we were, I was attending the birth, her husband was holding one leg and the nurse the other, as peaceful as can be, just as we had planned, only in a different location. We were grateful for the epidural and pitocin— it facilitated the success of this birth."

At the point of crowning, the hospital staff gathered around. The midwife recounted how she kept waiting for the doctor to say, "Okay, you can move aside now," but that didn't happen. Much to the contrary, as the baby was arriving, the attending chief resident stood back and asked the midwife if she needed anything else. The midwife asked for gauze and promptly a table with the necessary obstetrical equipment was brought over to her. The staff watched as the midwife received the baby and put him on his mother's chest. Soon after this, the hospital staff left to give the midwife, parents, and the baby time alone.

Both the mother and midwife enthusiastically expressed how positive this experience was for them. The mother emphasized that while she was previously very anti-transport, she has now changed her mind and realized that sometimes it is necessary. In retrospect she noted that the epidural and pitocin were welcome aides. In this transport we can witness the profound and extensive mandorla transformations that can occur from the bottom up to reconstruct the meaning of birth from both the biomedical and the midwifery perspectives.

A Midwife's Stories: Bridging Worlds

The following story comes from Carrie, a certified professional midwife (CPM) who has practiced in Georgia for almost twenty years, attending during that time over 850 births. Her practice is "unlawful" (meaning that it is punishable in the misdemeanor category in her state). Most of the homebirths she attends are for white middle-class couples. She does prenatal care out of her own home in an Atlanta suburb. She began her birth career in the late 1960s working as a volunteer in labor and delivery, and then took training as a biomedical assistant, working in labor and delivery and for a pediatrician for several years. Starting in 1977 she began attending the homebirths of friends; in the early 1980s she undertook an apprenticeship (1.5 years) with another homebirth midwife who later became her partner.

A mother pregnant with her second child, whose first birth had been very fast, started bleeding during mild early labor with contractions six to eight minutes apart. Carrie had sent her for an ultrasound at thirty-four weeks, which had been normal, so she knew she was not dealing with a placenta previa (the placenta does not move after thirty-four weeks). Carrie noted that "If the mother had not had the ultrasound, there is no way I could have checked her with that much bleeding at home." (In a case of true placenta previa, doing a cervical check can cause harm.) Carrie checked the baby's heart tones, which sounded good. Carrie was concerned by the dark red color of the blood, which indicated that it was not from a superficial cause. She called the hospital and talked to the nurse-midwife who works for Carrie's backup doctor, telling her it looked like some kind of placental abruption might be occurring. They drove the mother to the hospital, where the nurse welcomed them into the labor and delivery unit and put the mother on an electronic fetal monitor, hooked up an IV, and drew blood to type and screen in case she had to have a cesarean. The baby's heart tones remained steady and strong. The doctor came in about ten minutes after they arrived and said to Carrie and the nurse, "It looks like you have everything under control." Carrie expressed her concern about the color of the blood, but the doctor was not worried. He stayed for only about five minutes. After he left, the mother labored for another three hours. She spent time in the Jacuzzi, sat on the toilet, and then on the birth ball for a while; eventually she got in bed to try to rest. Carrie and the nurse-midwife turned all the lights off in the room. When pushing contractions kicked in, the mother pushed for about ten minutes, as Carrie recalls, and delivered on her hands and knees while the nurse-midwife caught the baby. The baby stayed with the mother. The placenta came fairly quickly after the birth; when Carrie and the CNM examined it, they could see a five centimeter clot on it—an indication that the placenta had partially detached in that area and had been bleeding from that place for a while. (If a placenta detaches uniformly after the birth, there will not be many clots on it unless it has been sitting in the uterus for quite a while, but if there is a partial separation, there will be clotting or additional clotting at the site of the partial separation.) The mother and baby went home the next morning. After the birth, the doctor told Carrie that she probably could have stayed at home for this one. And Carrie told him, "You have to realize that it's important for me to transport sooner rather than later when I have the option." And he said "You are right—I don't always see it from your side."

In the hospital, a partial placental separation is not cause for major alarm because facilities for a cesarean are there at hand. But homebirth midwives like Carrie prefer to err on the side of caution—if you see too much bleeding to feel okay about it, you transport. A primary ingredient in Carrie's willingness to transport early rather than late was the trust she had established over time with this doctor and this particular hospital. This trust has evolved into a smooth articulation of knowledge systems in which risk assessments can be mutually understood. She said:

> Since the early years of my practice, over time we have built up a lot of really good rapport, so that we have a lot of unofficial backup [it can't be official as Carrie's practice is not legal or licensed in Georgia]. We now have a doctor who is providing backup for us in that during the pregnancy he will see the mothers if we need him to—if we need an ultrasound he'll do one in the office. He says he doesn't like homebirth, but also he doesn't like the fact that many doctors are refusing to see homebirth mothers. He says everybody deserves good medical care when necessary. And if something comes up in labor, we can call the nurse-midwives who are always in-house. They listen to what we have to say on the phone and have everything set up when we arrive—the operating room ready, the doctor already in-house. So it is a really good situation—there are no animosities or repercussions or "attitudes" toward homebirth mothers. The doctors aren't exactly thrilled—they have said to the CNMs, "I wish you'd quit being so nice to these midwives so they'll quit bringing women in." And the CNMs have answered, "Would you rather leave them at home?" And the hospital is wonderful! It has no newborn nursery—I would consider them mother-baby friendly.

> The babies are never taken away from the moms unless they are really in trouble and need to be in the NICU.

Carrie's experiences point out that different kinds of articulations can happen in the same location as the actors come to know and develop trust in each other over time.

In 1978 with the publication of *Birth in Four Cultures*, Brigitte Jordan issued a call for the replacement of top-down, culturally inappropriate obstetrical systems with models of mutual accommodation between biomedical and indigenous systems—a plea that is equally significant for all homebirth midwifery systems. The stories recounted above illustrate the positive results of this sort of mutual accommodation. These mandorla transports can reconstruct institutional knowledge and protocols from the bottom up. Nurse-midwives are especially well placed to achieve such relationships, as they inherently straddle and bridge (and occasionally fall into the fissures between) biomedicine and homebirth midwifery. Establishing close relationships with homebirth midwives who are not legal is simultaneously a transgressive and a boundary-spanning act.[3] The prior communication between Carrie, the nurse-midwives, and the supportive physician certainly facilitated the smooth articulation of systems illustrated in these stories. Carrie feels that the key to this sort of smooth articulation is mutual respect and a cooperative attitude on the part of all concerned. Carrie's long and safe practice in her community has earned her this kind of respect from the hospital practitioners who know her best. She notes that it can take years to build this kind of relationship, especially with physicians who start out mistrusting midwives. Once established, though, such relationships tend to last. Many homebirth midwives do presently enjoy mutually accommodating relationships with one or two supportive physicians, which they have worked hard to build over the years. But they note that such smooth articulations are jeopardized when the supportive physician moves away or retires and is replaced by a younger doctor "with an attitude," as Carrie puts it, and then the midwife has to start all over again on the process of building trust. Midwives cannot always count on the availability of the physicians who support them, and even those who have spent years building good reputations and good relations with certain physicians sometimes still have to deal with fractured articulations during transport.

But in Carrie's case, because of her long-term relationship with the nurse-midwives in her local hospital, the articulation between her knowledge system and that of the hospital and its practitioners is so smooth that she is more than willing to transport even for situations that have nothing to do with risk, but rather with the mother's comfort alone, as the following short story shows:

A primapara (mother giving birth for the first time) had pulled a muscle in her back at the end of her pregnancy and was in a lot of pain as a result; she called Carrie to her home in the middle of the night. Carrie arrived to find the mother was in very early labor, at two centimeters dilation, but with close to unbearable pain from the back spasms. Carrie spent hours trying to relieve the pain in her back with showers and warm compresses and massage. She said:

> After a while we were running into brick walls as far as pain relief for the spasms, so we decided to go into the hospital where they have Jacuzzis in the labor rooms. By the time we got there, she was six centimeters. The nurse-midwives who received us told her she was doing great. The jets did good counterpressure on the back pain. They never started an IV and she had no pain medication. The baby's heart tones always sounded great. I was able to catch the baby as "the grandmother" on the chart—the nurse working with us had had her babies at home, and the nurse-midwife was very supportive and felt this mom really deserved the continuity. The baby was fine and the family went home twelve hours after the birth.

As these two stories illustrate, smooth articulation between knowledge systems proceeds through points of overlap, transition, and communication, which facilitate the seamless flow of information and linked, imbricated decision making in which the actions taken by one person or group build on the information supplied by another. The relationships between Carrie and the hospital-based CNMs encompass such points. This kind of bottom-up decision making within the top–down biomedical system requires a rejection of its tendency to discount or dismiss as irrelevant other ways of knowing. Such rejections can and do take place at the level of the individual even when the system as a whole remains dismissive. The process of forging connections between practices and effects across the midwifery/biomedical divide can produce not only safer transfers but also a merging of the best of midwifery and the best of biomedicine.

CONTEXTUALIZING THE MANDORLA TRANSPORT

What motivates or inspires a physician to reject the top–down system and give credence to homebirth midwifery knowledge? In our experience, the ingredients key to an individual's rejection of biomedical hegemony in favor of mutual accommodation include: (1) exposure to midwifery care, (2) exposure to midwives, and (3) attention to the scientific evidence. We will briefly deal with each of these in turn.

Exposure to midwifery care. Some doctors train in hospitals where nurse-midwives practice and thus are able to observe first-hand the benefits of midwifery care. Physicians we have interviewed are often awed by the midwife-attended births they witness, which are often visually and aurally nothing like the births they have seen. Women attended by midwives in hospitals are more likely than women attended by physicians to give birth in upright positions, with lots of vocalization, without an episiotomy, and with a great deal of hands-on support. Nurturance and consideration tend to characterize the midwife's approach to the mother; shared decision making takes place in a context of mutual respect. Physicians who do not ordinarily witness this kind of birth can find the experience transformative, can become imbued with a desire to incorporate this kind of respectful, humanistic approach into their own practices, and will be more likely to work with nurse-midwives in the future from a partnership, rather than a hierarchical, perspective. Occasionally a brave physician will venture outside hospital bounds and observe a midwife-attended homebirth—an experience that tends to be emotionally evocative and ideologically transformative (see for example Wagner 1997).

More profoundly, it is important to note that clinicians judge other clinicians as individuals, not just as members of a class or category; individual judgments can overcome prejudices based on subcultural differences. Does a practitioner give good care, make good decisions, and communicate accurately? Individual practitioners make decisions on the basis of experience. All clinical practitioners constantly gather experience and information, and react differently to a comment, order, or action from someone they trust as opposed to someone whose judgment has been faulty in the past or whom they do not know. Midwives work best with the doctors they have come to trust as a result of experience, and vice versa. But most doctors have little or no experience working with homebirth midwives; the experience they do have may be skewed if it comes only during emergency transports. Lack of experience with working together creates problems that exacerbate and perpetuate lack of experience with working together (Judith Rooks, personal communication, 2002).

Exposure to midwives. We can say without overstatement that American homebirth midwives tend to have huge hearts, impressive personalities, a strong sense of commitment and dedication to serving women, a secure sense of their own self- and professional worth, and a large fund of knowledge about parturition that seamlessly permeates their conversation. Simply spending time with them can turn a hospital practitioner from an opponent to a supporter. In U.S. communities where smooth articulation characterizes transport, home and hospital midwives, and sometimes physicians, occasionally participate in periodic potluck dinners where models of mutual accommodation begin to emerge over casseroles and drinks. Hospital midwives who develop respect for, and good relationships with, homebirth midwives often transmit this trust to the physicians with whom they work in a kind of spillover effect that paves the way for future smooth articulations during transport.

Attention to the scientific evidence. There is increasing emphasis these days on "evidence-based medicine" (Rooks 1999). As we have seen, midwifery tends to be more evidence based than obstetrics because midwives are generally less interventive than physicians (Frye 1995; Davis 1997; Gaskin 1990; Rooks 1997) and the scientific evidence (Rooks 1997:345–384; MacDorman and Singh 1998; Goer 1999; Enkin et al. 2000) shows that many common interventions do more damage than good. Any doctor who actually looks at the evidence, instead of relying solely on what he is taught by biomedical tradition, will take note of the benefits of midwifery care, will thus be less likely to assume a blanket superiority for obstetrics, and will be more open to learning in the moment, "going with the flow."

ARTICULATING TRANSPORT MANDORLAS

> Articulation is the production of identity on top of difference, of unities out of fragments, of structures across practices. Articulation links this practice to that effect, this text to that meaning, this meaning to that reality, this experience to those politics. . . . And these links are themselves articulated into larger structures.
>
> —**Lawrence Grossberg,** *We Gotta Get out of This Place: Popular Construction and Postmodern Culture*

While trust is only possible when individuals continually form and reform institutional structures, it is equally true that it is difficult to keep trust sustainable among individuals without the contextual coordination enabled by social organizations. Action and structure are inextricably interlinked into different aspects of the same whole and cannot be disconnected from one another. The best guarantees of mandorla transports are legislative statutes that institute and clarify the rules and resources available to midwives, and in so doing greatly reduce uncertainty and stabilize transport encounters.

Today in most developed countries, the homebirth rate hovers around one percent. That homebirth might be more widely chosen in the developed world if it were more readily available is indicated by the Netherlands experience, where the homebirth rate has never dropped below thirty percent (DeVries 2004); and by New Zealand and the Canadian province of Ontario, where in recent years it has risen significantly as the result of acknowledgement of the scientific evidence supporting homebirth and a strong alliance between midwives and consumers, which has generated active government support. These three regions stand as models of what Davis-Floyd calls *seamless articulation*—their midwives practice, and their health-care systems fully support, birth in all settings, creating ease of choice and continuity of care across what in most other countries can only be seen as the home/hospital divide (DeVries, van Teijlingen, Wrede, and Benoit 2001). In the United States, we find few examples of institutionalized seamlessness, but as we have shown in this chapter, *smooth articulation* that leads to an integrated individual birth experience can be manifested in the mandorla transport. The more such transports occur, the thicker will be the webs of articulation mandorla transports build between individuals across biomedical and midwifery knowledge systems and worlds. Until and unless institutional systems of seamless articulation can be created, the further mainstreaming of American midwives will depend on the continued weaving of these fragile, easily ruptured, but always reweavable webs.

ENDNOTES

1. Portions of this chapter are adapted from Davis-Floyd 2003.
2. Medical practitioners who only see problematic homebirths that are transported to the hospital tend to think that all homebirths are "botched." The rate of problems derives as a function of a numerator (number of cases with problems) and a denominator (total number of cases—the majority—that have good outcomes). If one only sees the numerator, it is impossible to realize that the rate of transports is actually very low compared to the number of successful homebirths (Johnson and Daviss 2005).
3. About 200 nurse-midwives attend homebirths in the United States. Ideally, their transport experiences should be smooth but often are not. While there is excellent data on the statistical *outcomes* of nurse-midwife-attended births in the U.S., including home to hospital transports (MacDorman and Singh 1998), we know of no research on American nurse-midwives' transport *experiences*. Further research should also include thorough quantitative and qualitative studies of the treatment of transported women and the specific outcomes.

REFERENCES

Baumann, Zymunt. 1997. *Postmodernity and Its Discontents.* New York: New York University Press.

Best, Steven, and Douglas Kellner. 1991. *Postmodern Theory: Critical Interrogations.* New York: The Guilford Press.

Davis, E. 1997/1983. *Heart and Hands: A Midwife's Guide to Pregnancy and Birth,* 3rd ed. Berkeley, CA: Celestial Arts.

Davis-Floyd, R. 1998a. "From Technobirth to Cyborg Babies: Reflections on the Emergent Discourse of a Holistic Anthropologist." In *Cyborg Babies: From Techno-Sex to Techno-Tots,* ed. R. Davis-Floyd and J. Dumit, 255–283. New York: Routledge.

———. 1998b. "The Ups, Downs, and Interlinkages of Nurse- and Direct-Entry Midwifery: Status, Practice, and Education." In *Getting an Education: Paths to Becoming a Midwife,* ed. J. Tritten J. and J. Southern, 4th ed., 67–118. Eugene, OR: Midwifery Today. Also available at http://www.midwiferytoday.com.

———. 2000. "Global Issues in Midwifery: Mutual Accommodation or Biomedical Hegemony?" *Midwifery Today,* March, 12–17, 68–69.

———. 2003. "Home Birth Emergencies in the US and Mexico: The Trouble with Transport." In "Reproduction Gone Awry," ed. Gwynne Jenkins and Marcis Inhorn. Special issue of *Social Science and Medicine.* 56(9): 1913-1931.

———. 2003. "Qualified Commodification: Consuming Midwifery Care." In *Consuming Motherhood,* ed. J. Taylor, D. Wozniack, and L. Layne.

DeVries, Raymond. 2004. *A Pleasing Birth: Midwives and Maternity Care in the Netherlands.* Philadelphia: Temple University Press.

DeVries, R., E. van Teijlingen, S. Wrede, and C. Benoit, eds. 2001. *Birth by Design: Pregnancy, Maternity Care and Midwifery in North America and Europe.* New York: Routledge.

Enkin, M., M. J. Kierse, J. Neilson, C. Crowther, L. Duley, E. Hodnett, and J. Hofmeyr. 2000. *A Guide to Effective Care in Pregnancy and Childbirth,* 3rd ed. New York: Oxford University Press.

Frye, A. 1995. *Holistic Midwifery: A Comprehensive Textbook for Midwives in Homebirth Practice, Volume I, Care During Pregnancy.* Portland, OR: Labrys Press.

Garston, Christine. 2001. "Trust, Control and Post-bureaucracy." *Organizational Studies.* March.

Gaskin, Ina May. 1990. *Spiritual Midwifery, 3rd ed.* Summertown, TN: The Book Publishing Company.

Giddens, Anthony. 1991. *Modernity and Self-Identity.* Stanford, CA: Stanford University Press.

Goer, Henci. 1999. *The Thinking Woman's Guide to a Better Birth.* New York: Penguin Putnam/Perigree.

Grossberg, Lawrence. 1992. *We Gotta Get Outta This Place: Popular Conservatism and Postmodern Culture.* New York: Routledge.

Johnson, Christine Barbara. 1987. Normalizing Birth. PhD diss., Boston University.

———. 2000. "The Public Face of Midwifery in Massachusetts." Paper presented at the May American Anthropological Association, San Francisco, CA.

———. 2001. The Ethic of Care and the Ethic of Autonomy. Paper presented at the May Pacific Sociological Association, San Francisco, CA.

Johnson, Christine Barbara, and Priscilla Galvin. 2001. *Transforming the Health Care System with On-Line Technology.* United States National Library of Medicine Information Infrastructure Program, Contract N01-LM-6-3539.

Johnson, Kenneth C. and Betty Anne Daviss. 2005. "Outcomes of Planned Home Births with Certified Professional Midwives: Large Prospective Study in North America." *British Medical Journal* 330(7505): 1416, June. www.bmj.com.

Johnson, Robert A. 1991. *Owning Your Own Shadow.* San Francisco: HarperSanFrancisco.

Jordan, Brigitte. 1993. [originally published in 1978] *Birth in Four Cultures*, revised and updated by Robbie Davis-Floyd. Prospect Heights, IL: Waveland Press.

MacDorman, M., and G. Singh. 1998. "Midwifery Care, Social and Biomedical Risk Factors, and Birth Outcomes in the USA." *Journal of Epidemiology and Community Health* 52:310–317.

Rooks, Judith P. 1997. *Midwifery and Childbirth in America.* Philadelphia, PA: Temple University Press.

———. 1999. "Evidence-Based Practice and Its Applications to Childbirth Care for Low-Risk Women." *Journal of Nurse- Midwifery* 44(4):355–369.

Ventura S. J., J. A. Martin, S. C. Curtin, R. Menacker, and B. E. Hamilton. 2001. Births: Final Data for 1999. *National Vital Statistics Reports* 49(1). Hyattsville, MD: National Center for Health Statistics.

Wagner, Marsden. 1997. "Confessions of a Dissident." In *Childbirth and Authoritative Knowledge: Cross-cultural Perspectives,* ed. R. Davis-Floyd and C. Sargent, 366–396. Berkeley, CA: University of California Press.

Wallace, R., and A. Wolf. 1995. *Contemporary Sociological Theory: Continuing the Classical Tradition,* 4th ed. Upper Saddle River, NJ: Prentice Hall.

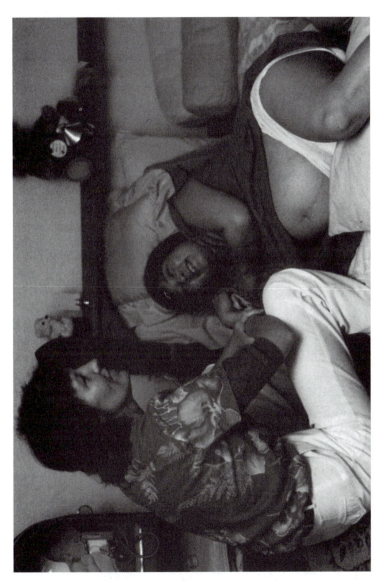

Fig. 12.1 A birth that began at home in California with midwife Faith Gibson in attendance. Photographer: Jennifer Gates.

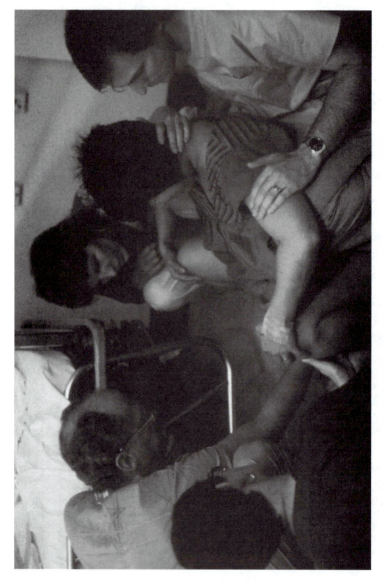

Fig. 12.2 A magical transport mandorla in which the homebirth midwife remains in supportive attendance and full cooperation with the hospital team. Photographer: Jennifer Gates.

13

WHY MIDWIVES MATTER: OVERCOMING BARRIERS TO CARETAKE THE POWER OF BIRTH

Christine Barbara Johnson and Robbie Davis-Floyd

• **Fostering Autonomy through an Ethic of Caring** • **Barriers to Midwifery Care and Efforts to Overcome Them** • **Conclusion: Integrating Care and Autonomy**

The art and science of midwifery are characterized by these hallmarks:

1. Recognition of pregnancy, birth, and menopause as normal physiologic and developmental processes
2. Advocacy of non-intervention in the absence of complications
3. Incorporation of scientific evidence into clinical practice
4. Promotion of family-centered care
5. Empowerment of women as partners in health care
6. Facilitation of healthy family and interpersonal relationships
7. Promotion of continuity of care
8. Health promotion, disease prevention, and health education
9. Promotion of a public health care perspective
10. Care to vulnerable populations
11. Advocacy for informed choice, shared decision making, and the right to self-determination
12. Cultural competence
13. Familiarity with common complementary and alternative therapies
14. Skillful communication, guidance, and counseling

15. Therapeutic value of human presence
16. Collaboration with other members of the health-care team

Excerpted from the ACNM Core Competencies for Basic Midwifery Practice

The midwife provides care according to the following principles:

Midwives work as autonomous practitioners, collaborating with other health and social service providers when necessary.

Midwives understand that physical, emotional, psycho-social and spiritual factors synergistically comprise the health of individuals and affect the child-bearing process.

Midwives recognize that a woman is the only direct care provider for herself and her unborn baby; thus the most important determinant of a healthy pregnancy is the mother herself.

Midwives synthesize clinical observations, theoretical knowledge, intuitive assessment, and spiritual awareness as components of a competent decision-making process.

Excerpted from the MANA Core Competencies for Midwifery Practice

This book has focused on the historical relationships between nurse- and direct-entry midwives, on the creation of two new direct-entry midwifery certifications during the 1990s—the CM and the CPM, on the political struggles of direct-entry midwives for legalization and licensure, and on the fractures and fissions within American midwifery that have complicated those struggles, most especially the ideological differences among midwives over appropriate types of education and practice. We hope that our analyses of these divisions will lead to a deeper understanding of the real and reasonable motivations for the actions of various individuals and groups of midwives as they have struggled to mainstream their marginalized profession. In this concluding chapter, we wish to clearly identify the reasons why, no matter what their struggles, we believe that *midwives should become the primary caregivers for most American women throughout pregnancy and birth.* We base this statement on both qualitative and quantitative data. In *Midwifery and Childbirth in America* (1997: Chapter 10), midwife and epidemiologist Judith Rooks thoroughly documents the many quantitative studies demonstrating the excellence of nurse-midwifery care, as did, among others, a comprehensive study published in 1998 by MacDorman and Singh and a smaller study (Davidson 2002) on the outcomes of high-risk women cared for by CNMs. Generally speaking, these studies show that CNMs both in and out of hospital achieve outcomes equal to or better than those of physicians attending low-risk births. The only thorough and methodologically sound study conducted to date of the outcomes of CPM-attended births is the CPM 2000 study, conducted by Canadian epidemiologists Kenneth C. Johnson and Betty Anne Davis (2005). Its results definitively show the good outcomes achieved by CPMs and are presented in chapter 3. In this chapter, we will take the excellent quantitative outcomes of midwifery care as a given, and will make our argument through an ethnographic analysis of the common and unifying qualitative elements that make midwifery care so precious and meaningful to the women who receive it (see also Kennedy 1995, 2000, 2004).

Much has been written about the theory and ideology of the midwifery model (see chapter 3 for a discussion of the difference between "midwives" and the "midwifery model of care"), but often this work focuses on comparing the midwifery model with the medical model, and thus cannot give full attention to the unique merits of the midwifery model. In this chapter, we examine the midwifery model per se by focusing on the elements of care common to almost all midwives in the United States, making clear *why midwives matter*, and describing the unique characteristics of their invaluable contributions to the care of mothers and babies. Purposefully, we make as few distinctions as possible between home- and hospital-based midwives; they are all *midwives*, and the elements we identify below are common and crucial to the care midwives in general seek to provide.

This chapter is based primarily on the seventy interviews that Christine conducted with midwifery clients from 1999 through 2003, and more peripherally on the many interviews Robbie has conducted with birthing women and midwives as described in the Introduction. In the first section of the chapter, we describe how the midwifery model creates an ideological and practical space within which what Grace Clement (1998) terms an "ethic of care" and an "ethic of autonomy" can emerge as interdependent elements of health-care interaction. Christine has adapted these concepts to elucidate their interdependence and how they form essential elements of the midwifery model of interaction between the midwife and the woman she is serving (Johnson 2001). Her adaptation of these concepts forms a unique analytical contribution to explaining the benefits of midwifery care. We give special attention to how pregnancy and birth are actively constructed on an ongoing basis as normal life events in which the midwife cares the pregnant woman into a sense of autonomy, which culminates in an embodied sense of power following the act of birth.

FOSTERING AUTONOMY THROUGH
AN ETHIC OF CARING

Christine has identified seven major elements of what she terms "the ethic of midwifery caring" that foster a strong sense of autonomy in women; this is initially established during prenatal care visits (Johnson 2001). The *ethic of midwifery caring*, as Christine defines it, acknowledges that midwives:

1. realize that context is not neutral but rather sets the stage for connection or disconnection;
2. build a personal dimension into the professional relationship;
3. recognize that emotional well-being is as important as physical well-being;
4. offer concrete, particular information as an essential criterion for creating a shared knowledge base;
5. encourage critical thinking in their clients;
6. promote the woman's belief in body efficacy and body integrity through conversation;
7. value and respect the woman's desires and definitions of the situation, and honor her intuition and their own as important adjuncts to rational knowledge.

During labor and birth, midwives add three further dimensions to this ethic of caring. They:

1. hold a conceptual space within which the woman can give birth according to her desires and needs;
2. keep the woman center stage as the main actor, supporting her in remaining there even when she doubts her ability to continue;
3. *normalize uniqueness* (Davis-Floyd and Davis 1997)—that is, within the parameters of safety, midwives affirm that what is happening in the labor in question is normal for that particular woman in that place at that time in her life, thereby helping the woman to avoid perceiving individual peculiarities of her birthing process as pathological and thus maintaining her sense of ability and self-confidence.

Christine's in-depth interviews revealed that midwives' application of this ethic usually "cared women into autonomy" by generating in them a sense of *embodied power*, which has four major components:

1. The mother's body image, if previously negative, shifts toward a more positive view and an enhanced sense of intrinsic self-worth.

2. If the mother chooses to labor without pain relief, even for only part of the labor, she is facilitated by the midwife to understand pain in many dimensions of life as potentially transformational—as not necessarily to be avoided but rather to be used as a guide to obtaining a level of consciousness and power she had not previously realized.
3. The mother develops a strong sense of confidence in her mothering skills.
4. The mother learns to take more responsibility for her own health-care choices and for those of her family.

Of course, the midwifery model of care as practiced by individual midwives does not always fulfill these potentials. A woman may not be cared into autonomy with a resulting sense of power for various reasons. The emotional bond between the pregnant and/or birthing woman and the midwife may be insufficiently developed (e.g., within a hospital, the woman might have been arbitrarily assigned to midwifery care and thus may come to the care experience with expectations that do not include this kind of relationship; within home care, the mother might have come to the midwife late in the pregnancy); a home to hospital transfer (or a transfer of care within the hospital) may result in the midwife being discounted or discredited; the midwife or midwives with whom the mother has a strong relationship may not be available to attend her labor and birth; or there may be a disconnect between the mother's desires and the midwife's responses to them. Like other professionals, midwives can have their off days; act in a petty, self-serving, self-centered manner; or simply be exhausted and stressed out during any given client encounter. Midwives are not perfect, but their standards of care and aspirations for relationship-centered caring are very high. In our many interviews with mothers, we have found that while a few of them were disappointed by or angry with their midwives, the vast majority did feel cared into autonomy and embodied power by the midwives who attended them. In the following section, we describe their experiences of this process.

Fostering Autonomy through the Ethic of Caring during Prenatal Visits

The following sections describe the multiple ways in which midwives foster autonomy in their clients through their ethic of caring and the ways in which they implement that ethic.

Context is not neutral but rather sets the stage for connection or disconnection. Most midwives attempt to arrange the prenatal examination room to meet the woman's needs as well as the needs of the institution, if any. In the following quote, a blind woman describes how the environment felt to her and how it helped her feel cared for and increased her sense of safety.

> My midwife . . . has a day bed and she gives you these pillowcases and sheets and there are designs that you pick. Each time you visit her you use your own personal pillow and sheet. And I can't even see these things and [my husband] describes them to me—she tries to make it so comfortable and a loving experience. She tells me, "I really want you to look forward to coming here."

A personal dimension is interwoven into the professional relationship. Prenatal visits with midwives almost always involve more than the clinical details of the pregnancy. The nature of the interaction offers a personal dimension in which mutual disclosure can take place. When asked what one word they would use to describe their relationship with their midwife, the overwhelming majority of woman use the word *friend*. Often the visits are family affairs with the spouse and/or children present. Many women note that they feel a loss when they do not go to prenatal visits anymore. They miss the relationship they have built with the midwife over the past nine months. The following quote demonstrates not only how personal and intimate the relationships can become, but also how the interaction contains mutually revealing elements. This personal relationship establishes the trust that will be necessary during the birth, when the woman needs to rely on the midwife's assessment of the birth process:

> Sometimes we would be talking in prenatal visits about something that had nothing to do with childbirth. We would be talking about some other medical issue or some other social event that was mentioned in the paper that day. You get to know each other as people. This is important because then when you are in the middle of labor this person is standing by your bed—you believe what they tell you because you know them. I knew her children's names, I knew her experience and how she had come to where she was practicing, I knew her as a person.

Often the relationship gets established with other family members who have participated in the prenatal visits. In many cases even the husbands note that they will miss their visits with the midwife. For example, "When I went in for my checkup, my husband took the morning off from work to go with me. He said, 'I am going to miss the midwife. What are we going to do when we don't go visit her anymore?'" In many cases, this meaningful relationship can remain over a lifetime, as the woman can continue to visit the midwife for further pregnancies or for the well-woman gynecological care that many midwives provide.

The woman's emotional and physical well-being are equally promoted through her encounters with the midwife. During prenatal care visits, many things are talked about and the woman's overall well-being is considered an important part of having a healthy pregnancy. For this reason the midwife administers emotional as well as physical care:

> It is a wonderful feeling to walk into the prenatals and have them say, "Hello, how are you feeling?" and not just how am I doing physically but how am I doing emotionally—"How is your other child adjusting, how are your days going, how are things with your husband?"

The following quote illustrates how far this emotional care can extend:

> I felt very comfortable with my midwife. I told her we were going to a funeral and I was feeling emotional— my pregnancy brought waves of emotionalism. I was nervous going to a funeral and I was afraid it would harm me in some way, but my husband really needed me there. And I told [our midwife] this. I cannot believe the difference she made for me in this instance. She said, "You know that one way I look at it is that a birth is very similar to a funeral—you have a lot of people around and you are celebrating that person's life in a sense and there is a lot of commonality." That perspective really helped me and I told her later, "You helped me go there and have it be okay."

Concrete, particular information is an essential criterion for creating a shared knowledge base. The midwife makes a decision based on particularized knowledge of each woman rather than making decisions based on statistical normality alone. The following account demonstrates how the midwife uses this knowledge to interpret the definition of risk in a way that the mother can understand and work with to help her combat the fear of childbirth that is pervasive in this culture.

In prenatal visits, I told my midwife how scared I was that something would go wrong during the birth and that I wouldn't have
enough information to know what to do—that the hospital
would just start doing stuff to me as they had done before. Then
during labor, when I started feeling the urge to push, a lot of
meconium started coming out and my husband got worried that
this was a sign of a serious problem, so I started to get scared as
well, and I just kind of shut down and the urge to push went
away. I did not understand what was happening or what it
meant—I just felt this overwhelming terror. The midwife
explained to me that the meconium was thin, watery, that the
baby's heart tones were good and strong, and that there was
time for me to go ahead and give birth if I would just go for it.
She was so clear and straightforward that my fear just vanished
and I pushed with my whole will and within minutes the baby
came out. There was thin meconium everywhere, and the midwife continued to explain that she was aspirating the baby and
that she would not cut the cord until she was sure the baby's
lungs were clear so that the baby would get plenty of oxygen
until he was ready to breathe. And sure enough, he breathed and
cried a little, and my feeling of confidence returned and I just
held him and talked to him and then I realized that I knew he
was fine, he was *fine*. And then I realized, I did it! I was scared,
but I did it, I gave birth to a healthy baby on my own. No one
took my power away like the time before. It was the clear information the midwife gave me that got me through my fear.

Critical thinking by the client is encouraged. Ensuring that women
and their families understand the details of the situation is key, and
often this takes a lot of critical thinking. As illustrated in the previous
quotation, rather than try to brush over difficult issues, midwives tend
to openly address them on both rational and emotional levels until the
matter is resolved. Most of their clients highly value the midwife's
veracity as a part of the trust-building process. In the following
exchange, the woman's husband is with her as they put some tough
questions to the midwife regarding a document the mother needed to
sign, which clearly stated that in some situations a planned homebirth
might have a better outcome in the hospital, while in others a planned
hospital birth might have a better outcome at home:

We read through the legal document she asked us to sign.
Unfortunately my midwife had to deal with my [being] upset

about this and I am glad that this was told to me because this is the truth. We are still discussing this—it was brought up last time and we just started discussing it. What I am learning is that there is a balance about when to use medical technology and when to not use it. We felt very satisfied with our midwife's competence and signed the document. I actually found it very truthful. I felt that my midwife's honesty about the letter put more trust in her rather than less.

Through conversation, the woman's belief in body efficacy and body integrity is established and reestablished. The following quote illustrates how interaction with the midwife transformed this woman's body image. Note how she stresses that her encounters with the midwife changed her self-talk and hence her own subjective meaning of giving birth:

> My main midwife, instead of saying, "This could go wrong or that could go wrong," she was saying, "The likelihood is that everything is going to go well. The high percentage is that everything is going to be fine"—nobody had been saying that. She did a physical exam and said, "How beautiful you look!" and all these positive things about my body. For somebody who had always felt that their body was inferior and didn't do things right, this was very empowering. And I started thinking, "Maybe my body is going to really work, maybe I can really do this." So there was that real paradigm shift and the focus was not on the process of birth as a physiological mechanical event, the focus was on me, on me giving birth. It wasn't that the midwives were saying, "We have to work hard to get you prepared," it was that they provided an atmosphere and a supportive place where I could grow into being ready to give birth and I could ask them questions.

This woman illustrates how midwives put themselves in the supporting role, give the woman the starring role, and in so doing, encourage the woman to take responsibility for herself. The following encounter communicated to the client that she had authority over her own body:

> Just the level of respect of having you put your clothes back on [right after the exam] like a human being so there was not this authority person—that just made such a difference to me—and it was very clear that she was saying, "I am not in charge here. This is *your* body, I am here to support *you*."

The woman's subsequent experience is indicative of how the process of prenatal care is as important as the content. She specifically comments on the midwifery technique of respectfully asking permission rather than giving orders:

> My midwife asked permission to do things—"May we?" instead of just telling me to stick my arm out. And it is things that you don't realize that you have a choice about in a conventional practice because they just say you are expected to submit to these things. They were very careful to say, "This is why I'd like to do this but if you really don't want to there are other options. Asking your permission before they touch your body—it just made me glow almost—"May I take your blood pressure now?" "I am going to touch your belly, is that okay—may I start now?" I thought, "Wow, my body is my own body, they are letting *me* decide."

The midwife values and respects the woman's desires and definition of the situation, and honors the woman's intuition as an important adjunct to rational knowledge. We previously gave an example of how the concrete information a midwife provides can change a woman's perception of danger, giving her the courage to go forward. Here we call attention to the ways in which midwives can use the woman's own definition of the situation and her intuitions about her condition to facilitate her birth process. This midwifery approach includes acknowledging intuition as an important adjunct to rational knowledge. Some women are accustomed to validating their feelings and intuition as important aspects of their everyday lives. Others, like the woman quoted below, take longer to define feelings and intuition as legitimate complements to rational knowledge. Her case is instructive for two reasons. First, her account illustrates the general manner in which the midwife can validate a woman's knowledge. Second, her experience gives insight into how the midwife, in this case also a neighbor, can help the woman make the paradigm shift from the medical-rational model to trusting her own definition of the situation:

> My neighbor, who later turned out to be my midwife, supported me in my intuition—she gave me faith in myself, she trusted me, she validated my voice, my internal voice that was emerging as a woman in this pregnancy. When they told me at my HMO where I was doing my prenatals that I had to take a genetic screening test, I thought, "I am just beginning to establish trust

in my body that I am normal. What will taking this test do to disrupt this trust?" [My midwife encouraged me to research the pros and cons of the test, and based on this research I decided not to have the test because it has a high rate of false positives, which can lead to further testing or to a decision to abort a baby that is perfectly healthy. I was at very low risk of having this condition and my intuition was strong that my baby was fine]. This was a very important step for me and as the pregnancy progressed, I continued with that assertive self. I started reading books and I started learning about birth and I started discovering what it was that I wanted for birth experience and my neighbor midwife was right there with me all the way. I found my voice and found myself. I saw a new side of me. My neighbor midwife—she was right there for me the entire time.

As many social scientists have shown (see for example Browner and Press 1995, 1997), the mere existence of genetic screening tests generates a cultural expectation that women should have such tests in order to give their babies "the best care." Yet as this woman's words acknowledge, such tests can undermine a woman's confidence in the integrity of her pregnancy and her baby, and the test results can be misleading. Her midwife's encouragement to do the research and make the decision for herself empowered her to think critically and at the same time to factor her intuition into the final decision.

Fostering Autonomy through the Ethic of Caring during Birth
Midwives hold a conceptual space within which the woman can give birth according to her individual desires and needs. By *conceptual space* we mean an ideology of flexibility that allows the woman room for variation in her movements, the progress of her labor, and her desires. Many women doubt their ability to give birth, yet find that ability enhanced when external cues convey that birth is not a medical condition but rather a normal life event. Some examples of this are when women are able to walk about, labor in the hot tub, and respond to their body messages:

I remember laboring in the hot tub. My husband was in the tub with me. I felt like my birth was being sanctified in a natural environment where other people care. Candles and music were present. . . . Then I started waking up every couple of minutes because I was having contractions every couple of minutes.

> Finally, I got up and started walking around. This gave me a needed sense of freedom.

Midwives themselves often experience a steep learning curve with respect to their ability to hold this conceptual space for normal birth. One of the student midwives Robbie interviewed described being sent in to attend the hospital birth of a woman she had not previously met. She said,

> By the time I got to this woman, her labor was kind of stalled and she was just wild, writhing around, pulling out her IV. I didn't know what to do with her, I simply didn't know what to do. So I called in the OB, who pitted her and got her contractions stabilized, got her under control and her labor back on track. Once she was back on track and pushing, I felt like I could handle the birth.

The student went on to say that if she had felt more confidence, she would have "held the woman, soothed her, gotten her up, given her something to drink, helped her take a shower or walk around." But, she continued, "The circumstances didn't allow it—there was no space for me to connect with her at that level." In contrast, another midwifery student in a similar situation did do all of the above because her preceptor encouraged her to follow the midwifery model and to have confidence in what we would call its ethic of caring. She said, "My preceptor backed me up—she held a space for me as a student within which I could trust myself, my intuition, and the woman's ability to give birth when she felt safe and supported. And it was a beautiful birth, and it taught me, when I was on my own, how to hold that space myself, that precious space in which the woman can do what she needs to because she has the support she needs." In our terms, the preceptor fostered a sense of autonomy in the student so that the student could foster that same sense in the mother.

Midwives keep the woman center stage as the main actor, supporting her to remain there even when she doubts her ability to continue. Midwives make a very clear point: The woman is the one giving birth. Although they are often tempted to talk about the babies they "delivered," when they really think about it, they change that language into "catching the baby" or "assisting" or "attending" the birth—their way of acknowledging that the mother is the one who does the hard work of labor and delivers the baby to the world. One woman was filling out a form after the birth with a space that required her to fill in who delivered the baby. She thought, "Well, that would be me," and she put her name on the dotted line. The woman is center stage and the midwives are there to support her and provide guidance or care as needed. One of the forms this takes is remaining in tune with the birthing woman and being conscious of her needs at all times. The following quote shows how all interactions are centered on the needs of the birthing woman rather than those of her caregivers.

> And one of the things that I really distinctly remember was the two midwives would be talking about things. Then, when I was having a contraction, everybody could tell and the talking stopped and nobody moved and that was so important to me because anything was really distracting to me. But because they did that, I was really able to stay with my contractions. And they were very intense and it was like a volcanic energy—those contractions were such that I just had to go with them, I couldn't resist them, if I resisted them it was terrible.

Most birthing women can manage the contractions if they can get into and sustain a rhythm. Such a rhythm can be easily disturbed and is contingent on the birthing woman's needs remaining paramount:

> I could almost see the contractions like waves. I saw myself body surfing over them. I remember at the peak it was so intense I just kept thinking, "This is almost more than I can stand, but this means that it is almost over." And I just got into this rhythm. I didn't want anybody to talk with me. I didn't want anybody to touch me or touch the bed or move anything. I wanted nobody to move around in the room. I wanted no stimulation whatsoever and my friend was really great, she was really protective, if the midwives came in she would say in a whisper, "She doesn't want anybody to talk to her."

The following midwife explains the importance of artfully navigating the boundary between care and autonomy to achieve a woman-empowering outcome when the birthing woman loses faith in her ability to accomplish the birth. In this case, rather than take it as an indication of failure, her birth team cares her into remaining autonomous and reminding her that she has everything she needs to complete the process. Her personal care is intimate—even when she is falling down, she has a group of people who care enough about her to help her come back up again and get through it. The mother and midwife we quote, speaking jointly, use a sports metaphor to help them express how the homebirth team loves the woman into fully manifesting her power:

> If you want to be an Olympic skier, or if you want to be on the basketball team in high school, you get this drive to do it and you wind up with a support system. When you fall down and you miss a basket or you blow it on the ski slope, your support team rallies around you and gets you together and gets you back out there to do what you need to do to be at your best. When you miss a basket, your support team would never think of saying, "You are really losing it, here let me get a ladder to help you make the basket." Rather, your support team rallies around you. Homebirth is that way.

This woman eloquently describes how she was supported both physically and emotionally during the birth:

> When the contractions got really intense I [wondered if I could really do it]. At these times I was sitting on the side of the bed and the apprentice midwife was sitting behind me so her back was up against mine and supporting my back. My husband would be sitting in front of me holding my hands or holding my head and the apprentice midwife had her back right up against me so I didn't fall backwards—I didn't have to use any of my muscles to hold myself up—I was literally being held up by everyone around me instead of trying to hold myself up and get through a contraction. I could completely relax and let my body go limp and everybody else made sure that I was supported—not just emotionally supported but they physically supported me through all of this. This was demanding on all of them—they were up all night long.

This woman discusses how she was having trouble dealing with the pain—it felt overwhelming to her, and her midwives' response altered her internal experience of the pain in such a way that it became manageable:

> The contractions got really intense. At that point, the midwives were gathered around us singing songs to encourage me. It was music. This helped me to see that the pain was not just pain—it

was a special kind of happening. It was something very unusual and very sacred.

This woman's experience of midwifery care illustrates how midwives negotiate the boundary between care and autonomy by providing full-on, attentive care without taking autonomy away from the mother. Rather, their care enhances her ability to remain autonomous.

Midwives normalize uniqueness. Within the parameters of safety, midwives affirm that what is happening in the labor at hand is normal for that particular woman in that place at that time in her life, thereby keeping the woman from identifying individual peculiarities of her birthing process as pathological (if they are not), and thus maintaining her sense of ability and self-confidence:

> I experienced tremendous pressure during my homebirth to "do it right" because I felt a responsibility to midwives and the entire birth activist community to prove that they were right. I wanted to be the exemplar of everything that they were saying and that I also believed in. I think that's why I needed to have such a long labor—three days! At any point after the first twenty-four hours the midwives could have said, "That's it, it's been too long, you are way out of protocol, you've been at four centimeters forever and we need to transport you. But they didn't. Instead, they asked me, "What do you think is going on?" And I said, "I think I just need time—this birth is making me process my previous cesarean, and I'm trying so hard to prove something, and I think I just need time to get beyond all that and just get into this labor and birth on its own terms. I want to do this, I believe that I can do this—I just need time." They were monitoring the baby's heart tones, and he was fine the whole time. And so they said, "Then that's normal for you, that's what you need to do, and we are here for you—take the time you need." And their trust and support were fundamental—once I knew in my bones that they weren't going to take this birth away from me the way the doctor had before, I relaxed, forgot about the pressure, got into the experience, and ended up doing it all on my own, the way that I had hoped, dreamed, prepared, and planned that I would. I knew that a three-day labor with a VBAC was way out of protocol for them, but they understood that it was normal and right and necessary for *me*. And it worked, and I gave birth, and their faith in the abnormal as normal and right for me at that time in my life was right on!

Embodied Power

Midwife-attended women develop or reaffirm a positive body image.
A very common experience for women who receive midwifery care during birth is the development (or reaffirmation) of a positive body image—one not based on cultural ideals but on the personal power they experience from discovering that their bodies are capable of such feats:

> I had not felt that great about my body before that—it was not the conventionally attractive body. And through this experience I fell in love with my body! Bearing children has changed my whole feeling about getting older—having babies is a huge and important experience that I wouldn't trade for anything. And my body shows I did this and my body can do this, and the more I do things like this the more wise I get and the more powerful I get and the more competent I get. And every wrinkle and gray hair and everything else I get says, "I am becoming wiser and stronger."

"If I gave birth I can do anything": Midwife-attended women learn to experience pain as transformational. This woman's experience is illustrative of the majority of women in Christine's sample who gained a great deal of personal empowerment from giving birth. For her, the empowering value of the experience has not diminished but has grown stronger over time:

> When the baby came out of me, I thought, "I can do anything!! I did this, my body worked, my body is wonderful and I am strong and I can do *anything*—that incredible sense of empowerment of almost being bigger than life. And since that time I still get energy from remembering that experience. My birth experience has built on itself. That kind of intense purpose and conviction and that kind of inner power—that comes from giving birth. That feeling that nothing is going to stop me is from giving birth and it carries over into my work life. I am accomplishing things in my work life that I would never have attempted prior to birth.

Most women say they have gained an enormous sense of personal power from the knowledge that they gave birth themselves rather than having someone else do it for them. As a result of this experience, they have a new way of being in the world—knowing they possess the power to accomplish difficult tasks. This woman sums up the general feeling:

You come out in a different place after birth. It felt like a major life change was occurring and I was being present for it. *I* was going through it. I was walking that path and I hadn't been carried. I *walked*—I hadn't been drugged or I hadn't been cut open. I walked that path and came out the other end conscious and fully present. And that felt good. It wasn't like waking up on the other end wondering how I got there, and I knew very well how I had gotten there. And there was a lot of support to get there—it wasn't a one-woman show.

Many women consciously invoke the birth to talk themselves into knowing that they can accomplish other difficult tasks. For example,

A couple of weeks ago I was jogging. I hadn't jogged for ten years and I was starting up again. I found myself thinking, "I don't know if I can do this." Then I thought, "Wait a minute—I went through that long birth. My body did this incredible thing. I can do this! I can do any physical thing that I put my mind to."

Another woman said,

About a year after giving birth to my daughter in hospital with a midwife, with no drugs and no episiotomy and twenty hours of labor, I went skiing again. And when I got off the lift, I took a wrong turn and ended up on a really difficult slope full of moguls. At first I freaked out, and thought about retracing my steps. And then I thought, "Hey, I gave birth even in the face of pain and fear—this is nothing compared to that." So I tackled those moguls, and I'm sure it wasn't the most graceful of descents, but I found myself surrendering to the realities of the mountain the way I surrendered to the realities of labor—I kind of just flowed with those moguls, down and around, down and around, my knees swallowing their eddies, my body leaning into the strength of the mountain while swaying with its flows and depths. I discovered that I could trust the mountain to be there the way I had ended up trusting that the pain of labor would be there as long as I needed it. I had never been an athlete, and every muscle in my body was aching and I almost cried from the pain, but somehow that mountain and I became one, just exactly the way the equally reliable pain of labor and I became one. And I made it to the bottom and had lots of thrills doing what would have absolutely terrified me and taken me down before I gave birth.

Midwife-attended women tend to develop confidence in their competence as mothers. Many of the women Christine interviewed noted that they often found that their response to a crying baby evoked the birth experience. To the extent that they experienced themselves as competent and powerful, they had immediate access to this feeling as a foundation for exploring how to care for their child. To the extent that they felt frustrated and disempowered, these feelings translated into uncertainty and frustration in dealing with their child. In these cases they had to work hard to overcome the negative birth experience. Usually, a positive birth experience was sufficient to reinterpret the first birth and heal a parenting style with the first child that had become troublesome. This woman discusses how her second birth, which was midwife attended, allowed her to redefine and reinterpret the meaning of the first birth:

> This homebirth was my way out of that first birth, and I did it beautifully and I know that I have a fabulous relationship with my new baby. This birth changed my relationship with my oldest son. It sounds weird to say but I forgave him for his birth. I feel closer to my oldest son after this birth, and I also feel like I can handle it. He would throw these temper tantrums before and I would just get so frustrated and now it is like, "I can do this." My first baby came into the world with my sense of frustration attached—my anger, my frustration, my feeling of being out of control. From the time he was a newborn and started crying—the first place I went was, "I am frustrated, I am angry, I can't handle this"—this is absolutely how I felt at the birth. . . . From the moment this second baby was born the tape in my head says, "This is fabulous, this is beautiful, I can do anything. I can handle anything. I am strong enough and I have the tools and if I don't have the tools I know who to call." My work colleagues, my friends, and husband tell me that I am different after the birth—that I am not the same person that I was before the birth. They say that there is something calmer, gentler, more laid back. The consensus is that I have turned a corner somewhere—I have passed a milestone, on a spiritual level.

Midwife-attended women learn to take responsibility for their own health-care choices and for those of their families. In the technocracy (Davis-Floyd 2004), people in general, and women in particular, are socialized to depend on physicians for health care. Physicians in general are trained in a technocratic model of health care that stresses aggressive intervention and reliance on drugs and technologies that often cause more harm than good. Moving away from this dependence requires that women develop the sense of embodied power we address here as an outgrowth of midwifery care. While technocratically oriented physicians tend to be comfortable with their authoritative role, holistic physicians, who make a paradigm shift toward seeing themselves as supporters and facilitators of individual choice and responsibility, often express a sense of frustration that their clients come to them for a quick fix that requires no responsibility or informed choice on the part of the consumer (Davis-Floyd and St. John 1998). Like holistic physicians, midwives work hard to foster in their clients that sense of autonomy and individual responsibility that can lead them to making informed decisions on their own. As this woman describes, midwife-assisted births can be transformative in this regard:

> My first birth—an unnecessary cesarean in the hospital—left me feeling disempowered and helpless. I realized this most fully when my baby girl's eye outlets did not open properly and so her eyes would get filled up with gunk. I took her to a pediatrician and I let him strap her down in a Velcro body bag and kick me out of the room while he pierced her outlets and she screamed the whole time. If I had insisted, he would have let me be there with her to comfort her during the procedure. My sense of powerlessness and victimization increased. By the time I was pregnant with my second child, I was determined to have a homebirth as a way of learning the meaning of autonomy. When I pushed out my ten-pound son, I realized that I could in fact do anything—I did not need to kowtow to authorities for my children's care. From then on, every health-care decision I made for myself and my family was well considered, well researched, and was my own. I realized my own responsibility in allowing that first cesarean—I just let it happen—and that I didn't need to just succumb anymore. So I read everything I could about self-help in health care, and from that time on, I made the right decisions about how to heal every time anyone in my family was sick. Giving birth on my own changed my life, and I know that it happened because of me, but also because my midwives held the space in which I could learn and grow into taking responsibility.

In homes or hospitals, urban cities or rural communities, culturally comfortable or disjunctive situations, rich environments or poor, midwives work hard to hold this kind of space for women and to deliver them into their own power and autonomy as they give birth. All of the political, ideological, and personal conflicts that midwives face pale in comparison to what they give to the women they attend.

BARRIERS TO MIDWIFERY CARE AND EFFORTS TO OVERCOME THEM

> More and more the wisdom of midwifery is confirmed by epidemiology, and more important, social and historical research is providing new understandings of the forces that prevent the wisdom of midwifery from being realized. The re-establishment of independent midwifery in the United Kingdom and Canada and the use of nurse-midwives by managed care organizations in the United States are preparing the cultural soil needed to sustain a new obstetric system, a system that is characterized by love and justice, a system that makes prudent use of our resources, a system that supports women, babies, and families.
>
> **—Raymond Devries, Making Midwives Legal: Childbirth, Medicine, and the Law**

The above reasons why midwives matter would indicate that instead of 40,000 obstetricians attending ninety-one percent of American births and around 8000 midwives attending nine percent, there should be 40,000 midwives attending at least eighty-five percent of American births (this figure is based on the WHO [World Health Organization] estimate that even in high-risk tertiary care hospitals, the cesarean rate should not be more than fifteen percent) with around 5,000 obstetricians giving care to high-risk women and attending birth emergencies, as is the comparative situation in most European countries. So why is this not the case in the United States? In the introduction and part I, we discussed some of the historical factors that led to midwives' near-elimination in the United States during the first half of the twentieth century, and the enormous efforts midwives have made to achieve their American renaissance through the growth of nurse- and direct-entry midwifery and the development of two new national direct-entry certifications, the CM and the CPM. The chapters in part II illustrate the struggles of direct-entry midwives to achieve legalization and licensure in various states. And the chapters in part III illuminated some of the complexities midwives encounter in their attempts to practice autonomously and holistically in a technocratic society, and to balance the competing demands of their social movement and professionalization projects. Here, in summary, we provide a list of the barriers that continue to prevent American midwives from realizing their full potential, along with descriptions of efforts to overcome these barriers.

The first and most salient barrier to women's widespread utilization of midwives is *the general public assumption that obstetricians are the best attendants for pregnancy and birth*, and the concomitant lack of awareness of midwives' knowledge, skills, and competence. Certainly there has been some progress here. When Christine and Robbie first began to study midwifery around sixteen years ago, hardly anyone we spoke to in public arenas even knew that midwives still existed in the United States. Today that situation has dramatically changed—almost everyone we speak to out there in the world at least knows that midwives exist. Some people understand the difference between hospital and home-based midwives, yet many only know about one kind or the other and have little understanding of what midwives have to offer. To address this barrier, both ACNM and MANA, as well as many midwifery state organizations and dedicated consumer groups, have written books and articles; printed and distributed thousands of brochures; given public talks in all kinds of places, including classrooms; held rallies; given interviews to the press; and hired marketing firms and lobbyists—all to increase public awareness of midwives and what they do. (Certainly, national advertising campaigns on television would help, but midwifery budgets do not extend to such endeavors.)

In some places these efforts have begun to pay off, as evidenced by increased utilization of midwives. The percentage of births attended by midwives has increased every year since the National Center for Health Statistics began to gather and keep track of that information from birth certificates, and presently stands at around nine percent. CNMs attend approximately eight percent of all births nationwide, and ten percent of vaginal births. Many practicing CNMs have solid jobs with good salaries, and many DEMs, who attend around one percent of American births, have well-established home or birth center practices (see Davis-Floyd 1998 for a more detailed discussion of the nuances of midwifery economics). But even when midwives are able to find jobs or establish relatively successful independent practices with sufficient client loads to make a living, they are confronted with the other major barriers our technocratic and legalistic society imposes.

One of the most significant and challenging of these barriers is *hospital and physician resistance to midwives*, which is sometimes purely economically motivated, and sometimes motivated by an erroneous belief that midwives are not really competent professionals—at least not as competent as the doctors themselves. CNMs experience physician or hospital administrator resistance when they are overscrutinized (usually when someone is looking for a reason to get rid of them) or fired outright in large numbers, or when physicians refuse to provide backup for their birth center, homebirth practices, and even hospital practices, and/or harass the few physicians that do. Two recent books—*Critical Condition: How Health Care in America Became Big Business* (Barlett and Steele 2004) and *The Medical Delivery Business: Health Reform, Childbirth, and the Economic Order* (Perkins 2004) thoroughly document the distorted economic priorities of our current health-care system, which fails to support midwives and natural childbirth because the low intervention approach to birth brings no economic benefit to hospitals or doctors. Susan Hodges (personal communication 2005) offers an enlightening metaphor to explain why:

> Midwifery care, with its individualized patience and respect for each unique woman and her birth process, is like the work of an artist—painstaking, patient, unique. Hospital birth is more like a factory, with economic analyses etc. to ensure operating as efficiently as possible to make money. How many factories mass-producing some product for money would consider changing to artisans creating the objects by hand? When we want to have midwives providing midwifery care with the qualities you list above, we are essentially expecting the efficient, mass-producing hospital factory/institution to make space for hand-crafted, one-of-a-kind births that don't get done on a schedule and are not efficient at all from the hospital's point of view. So, besides all the philosophical, power, etc. issues between MDs and midwives, there is also a misfit between hospital culture and value systems and *any* other way of "managing" labor and delivery.

DEMs experience physician resistance in the form of the same refusal of backup care, insulting treatment in the hospital when they transport a patient, investigation of their practices by physicians determined to shut them down in what midwives all over the country refer to as "the witch hunt," and heavy lobbying by professional medical organizations against legislation to legalize and regulate DEMs in various states. In chapter 10, we described three ways in which formerly antagonistic physicians may become midwife supporters; to recap, these are (1) exposure to midwifery care; (2) exposure to midwives; (3) attention to the scientific evidence.

While most CNMs do have liability insurance and insurance reimbursement for their services, those who practice out of hospital, like DEMs, may not be able to obtain them in many states. *Lack of insurance reimbursement and malpractice coverage* often limits midwives' abilities to grow their out-of-hospital practices, as does the *high cost of insurance* when it can be obtained. Like many obstetricians, some midwives are leaving their practices because of liability concerns and an inability to pay increases in insurance premiums (Fennell 2003). Insurance companies may fail to see the overall savings from less interventive midwifery care, focusing only on the fact that if a midwife consults with an obstetrician or a planned midwife-attended birth ends up with a cesarean, the insurance company may be charged for the services of both the obstetrician and the midwife. And CNMs are often not reimbursed for their services at the same rates as physicians. (For example, Medicare reimburses CNMs at only sixty-five percent of the Medicare physician fee schedule, while nurse-practitioners and PAs are reimbursed at eighty-five percent.) The ACNM has been actively promoting national legislation that would redress that situation, and actively seeking to educate insurance companies about the value of midwifery care. DEMs have been able to obtain insurance coverage in several states, and are working hard to do so in others. Yet like many alternative health-care practitioners, many DEMs are able to succeed financially because their (mostly middle-class) clients are willing to pay out-of-pocket for their services.

Lack of educational programs is an enormous obstacle in particular for the new Certified Midwife. While there are forty programs for students who want to become CNMs, twenty or so private vocational schools for DEMs that can help them achieve CPM certification (half of which are accredited by MEAC), and hundreds of midwives who precept apprentices who can then go on to become CPMs, there are only two programs in the country for training the CM (see chapter 1). This situation is unfortunate because one of the goals of the New York nurse-midwives who worked to create the CM was to increase access to midwifery education by eliminating the nursing requirement. Around the country there are probably hundreds or thousands of women who would become CMs if there were laws in their states legitimizing the CM and educational programs to meet the demand. But passing such laws requires money, effort, and time, as demonstrated by the ten-year process the New York CNMs went through to pass their legislation legitimizing the CM (see chapter 2), and by the chapters in part II of this book, which show how hard and how long DEMs have had to work to achieve their own laws, with variable success. With so many other problems to deal with, CNMs in most states don't give high priority to legalizing CMs, given the expense and effort required to create new statutes and new educational programs for them. Judith Rooks (personal communication 2004) notes that:

> Many CNMs would like to get out from under nursing, but some think nursing is just fine and few have the time and energy, consensus and leadership, to prioritize this issue in any state. States are also likely to resist the CM, as her legal existence would require the development of a separate midwifery board, and most states adamantly refuse any new professional boards because they are expensive. Most states require the members of the regulated profession to pay for the costs of regulation through their licensing fees, which can be exorbitant.

Thus we cannot expect any kind of rapid growth in the number of CMs in the near future, in spite of the fact that the CM represents an important opportunity for the future of American midwifery, and that she is an ACNM (ACC)-certified midwife qualified to provide both maternity services and primary health care who does not have to spend the years (and the psychological toll) it takes to become a nurse first. From any educational route that entails a baccalaureate degree, she can go on to become a midwife qualified to practice in hospitals, where the vast majority of American women chose to go for birth. Her services are needed across the nation, and we fervently hope that someday the vision of the nurse-midwives of New York, who created the CM, will be realized with her legalization and licensure in every state, and with the concomitant creation of educational programs that will be needed to accommodate the many women who would choose to become CMs if that option were available in their states.

Of course, *lack of legalization and licensure in many states also creates a huge barrier for non-CM direct-entry midwives.* Although homebirth direct-entry midwives do practice in all of the states in which they are not legal, their growth in numbers in unlicensed states is often inhibited by fear of persecution and arrest, and their legislative attempts may be limited for the same reasons. (This situation varies by state; for example, in Michigan and Maine, unlicensed DEMs are able to practice rather openly because they are not hunted by state agencies, while in Ohio they are aggressively pursued.) In addition, the lack of visibility resulting from the underground nature of their practice can make them hard to find and thus limit their accessibility. DEMs, aided by consumer groups and others, are addressing this barrier through legislative efforts in almost every state in which they are not yet legal and licensed, some of which we have documented in part II of this book. They have been greatly aided in this endeavor by NARM's creation of the CPM credential in 1994, NARM's subsequent membership in the National Organization for Competency Assurance (NOCA) and certification by the National Commission for Certifying Agencies (NCCA), and by MEAC's official recognition as an accrediting body for direct-entry midwifery schools by the U.S. Department of Education in 2000 (reaffirmed in 2003). Such national recognition for these direct-entry certification and accreditation processes impresses legislators. Yet MEAC's government recognition brought with it what many DEMs perceive as the danger that some states may accept CPMs only if they graduate from MEAC-accredited programs (as is currently the case in several states), thus threatening the ongoing viability of the apprenticeship learning that the CPM certification was, in part, designed to protect.

Further protection for the CPM credential, with all the educational routes it supports, now exists through national standards for CPMs created and adopted in 2004 by the National Association of Certified Professional Midwives (NACPM) (see chapter 1). Until now, CPMs have lacked clear national practice standards. (MANA has had such standards since the mid-1980s, but not all CPMs belong to MANA, and not all MANA members are CPMs.) The codification of such standards constitutes another step forward in the CPMs' professionalization project; the mere fact that these standards were under development has already helped midwives' legislative efforts in the states of Utah and Wisconsin, and has been of immediate benefit in Massachusetts as well, where legislators made it clear to the CPMs that their law stood no chance of passage without such standards. Indeed, it was in response to the situation in Massachusetts that the NACPM was created, so that CPMs could have a national standard-setting organization more structurally similar to the ACNM than MANA. (To recap from chapter 1, MANA is inclusive, requiring only the statement that one is a midwife, any type of midwife, for voting membership; in contrast, the NACPM requires the CPM for membership, just as members of the ACNM must become either CNMs or CMs.) If all or most CPMs eventually come to join the NACPM (the professional organization) and leave MANA (the social movement organization), the NACPM may eventually come to threaten MANA. At present, such an occurrence appears unlikely (see chapter 1). NACPM incorporates its meetings into MANA's annual conferences and urges its members to join MANA as well. For the foreseeable future, it appears that MANA, to which hundreds of DEMs hold a twenty-year allegiance, will continue to serve as the umbrella organization and the ideological anchor for NARM, MEAC, and the new NACPM.

Ironically, as we showed in chapter 11 on renegade midwives, the very legalization midwives seek in order to avoid legal harassment and increase their public visibility and accessibility, and which NARM, MEAC, the NACPM, and many DEM state organizations and consumers are working so hard to provide, can create barriers to homebirth midwifery care once state laws are passed. *Licensure and regulation can compromise midwives' autonomy* by, for example, prohibiting their attendance at VBACs and breech births, which some very experienced homebirth midwives feel more qualified to attend than obstetricians who nowadays tend to deal with such births by performing a cesarean. In addition, licensure and regulation can result in a requirement that midwives obtain malpractice insurance—another complication, as we have seen. Most of the midwives we interviewed prefer licensure to illegality; they deal with the possible restrictions that can result by doing their best to write their own state regulations (not possible in some states, where regulations for midwives are written by others). Once those regulations are in place, most DEMs who achieve licensure are careful to abide by them, checking themselves and each other through ongoing peer review processes in their states. But as we saw in chapter 11, when confronted with certain situations, midwives must make difficult individual choices about abiding by or choosing to lay aside those regulations to serve a particular mother.

A further barrier to midwifery care has to do with *the negative publicity that occurs almost every time there is a bad outcome at a homebirth.* Deaths in the hospital of baby or mother are rarely publicized because the hospital constitutes the cultural standard for safety, and physicians tend to protect their own from public view. Thus a death at home rings loud cultural alarm bells, sounding the culturally ingrained message that homebirth is an irresponsible choice for mothers, and that homebirth midwives must be far less competent that hospital-based practitioners. The case presentations in our chapter on home to hospital transport, and in the Massachusetts chapter on the harassment that a midwife (who in fact delivered exemplary care) received during transport, highlight this fact. This barrier can only be overcome by increased public education, which as we mentioned above, is an ongoing effort on the part of midwives and consumers.

In some of the states that do offer licensure for direct-entry midwives, where the situation can appear rosy, there is often *insufficient financial support for state midwifery boards.* Most state governments want such boards to be supported financially by the fees the midwives themselves are required to pay, but realize that there are not enough midwives to sustain the board by paying reasonable fees, and that if the fees are too high, they will put midwives out of business. Thus, some state midwifery boards run deficits that have to be paid from the state's budget—a precarious situation.

This is not a problem in New York, where around 1,000 CNMs and around fifty CMs provide enough income at reasonable fees to sustain the board, but it is a serious problem in other states whose midwifery boards regulate only direct-entry midwives relatively few in number, especially when the board faces complaints or other legal actions for which it must pay, as has happened in Oregon and Washington. A potential solution to this problem is presented by the Massachusetts midwives, who seek to create a midwifery board that would regulate CNMs, CMs, and CPMs; collectively, their numbers should be high enough to sustain the board they want the state to create. Because many CNMs around the United States would like to "get out from under the thumb of nursing," and many CPMs seeking independent licensing boards need greater numbers to sustain their boards, we can hope that future collaborations between such groups in various states might lead to a transcendence of this barrier. If CPMs continue to grow in number and establish successful practices, they might alone become more able to sustain the fees necessary to sustain the boards that regulate them. This, of course, would require more women to choose homebirth—again, the midwives hope, a question of public education.

A barrier particular to the growth of organized midwifery, which midwives can easily eliminate, is the fact that *many midwives do not choose to belong to their national organizations.* Seventy-five percent of CNMs are members of ACNM (some are retired and others don't feel that ACNM supports their individual needs and concerns). About one-third of CPMs belong to MANA (the NACPM is too new for specific numbers to be available); the other two-thirds, who do not, tend to feel that their state organizations do more for them than MANA. ACNM, MANA, and the NACPM are dependent on membership numbers, dues, and active participation for their annual budgets and the projects they aim to achieve. Each national organization is actively campaigning for increased membership, and *we personally urge every midwife to join at least one of them.* As the midwives of Europe discovered some time ago, there is power in numbers and national organizations that cannot be achieved to the same extent at a local level.

A barrier to the ability of CPMs to serve more women is their inability (with a handful of exceptions) to obtain hospital privileges. On this note, let us return for a moment to the Ontario midwives discussed in chapter 1 of this book, who created ways to evaluate the competence of their direct-entry midwives along with the means to empower those same midwives (who had previously never practiced inside a hospital) to maintain their competence inside the hospital system. American CPMs, who are as knowledgeable about normal birth as CNMs and CMs, could be equally empowered to attend hospital births if medical systems would choose to allow it. Clients choosing CPMs could then also have the choice of a CPM-attended hospital birth. We can find no valid scientific, educational, or ideological reason why such options should not be created in our homeland. The current for-profit, specialized, and bureaucratic structure of health care remains the problem (Barlett and Steele 2004, Perkins 2004).

The following barrier will be controversial among midwives, but the need for its transcendence is made obvious by the *splitting of midwifery care* generated by the fact that most CPMs can only practice outside the hospital and most CNMs and CMs can only practice inside of hospitals. Thus, as we discussed in chapter 1, to choose a particular kind of midwife is also to choose a particular place of birth. In the interests of eventually healing this divide (as the midwives of Ontario were able to do), we suggest that having three national organizations instead of one (or two) entails a splitting of energy and resources, and generates conflicts of interest in which midwives sometimes work against each other. At the very least, it might eventually behoove MANA and the NACPM to merge (if their members can ever agree that the CPM should be a requirement for membership). At the very most, we envision a time in which ACNM, MANA, and the NACPM might, in the social movement sense, unite behind the midwifery model of care to promote all nationally certified midwives. The longer these organizations remain separate in their concerns, the more vital energy may be drained away from the real source of the conflict: the hegemonic obstetrical system. A united American midwifery movement might well gain enough momentum and power to pose formidable obstacles to medical definitions of birth, and to vastly increase birth options available to women.

Midwifery consumer Susan Hodges, president of Citizens for Midwifery, adds the following suggestion:

> My own thought, as an alternative, would be for MANA, NACPM and ACNM to acknowledge the contributions of each to the survival of midwifery—because of the ACNM, at least in part, most people have heard of the word *midwife*, while the DEMs, whose laws for the most part do not require any agreement from any

doctor in order to practice, have demonstrated that midwives can practice safely and effectively without "permission" or oversight from doctors. DEMs benefit from the generally excellent reputation of CNMs, but CNMs can benefit from the independence of DEMs to make their own case for autonomy. I would think this coming together could happen to everyone's benefits without even entertaining the idea of merging and losing one or more of these organizations, certainly for a long time to come. (Personal communication 2005)

New potential barriers for CNMs come from nursing. There are a number of specialties in advanced practice nursing, and each of these requires program accreditation. The deans of nursing of various schools, impatient with the bureaucracy of these accreditation processes, are considering eliminating them in favor of the same process for advanced practice nurses of all types. CNMs perceive this potential action as a core-level threat to their identities as midwives, as it might take away ACNM/DOA's power to accredit programs, which lies at the heart of nurse-midwifery's identity, in part because the DOA has to date been able to require that nurse-midwives be taught by nurse-midwives. Another potential threat from nursing lies in a decision made by the American Association of Colleges of Nursing (a national alliance of nursing organizations) to require a Doctorate in Nursing Practice (DNP) for all advanced practice nurses by 2015. This would be a clinical degree distinct from, but equivalent in prestige to, the academic Ph.D. (One argument used in favor of this move is that the number of hours earned to get a master's in many advanced practice nursing programs, including nurse-midwifery programs, is not far short of what is required for a Ph.D.) While ACNM as yet has no official position on this issue, many CNM leaders have expressed feelings ranging from "concern" to "dismay" (Deanne Williams, personal communication, 2005), as they are very aware that advanced degrees do not equate to better practitioners (see chapter 1). One ACNM leader proposes a preemptive strike: she suggests that ACNM create a Doctor of Midwifery (a clinical degree like a Doctor of Medicine or a Doctor of Chiropractic that focuses on clinical practice more than academic research) to enable CNMs and CMs to maintain their identity as midwives. These two nursing initiatives are too new for us to be able to evaluate their eventual impact; all we can do here is point to them as potential problems for nurse-midwives that indicate even more sharply some of the reasons why many midwives wish to "get out from under the thumb" of nursing.

To summarize, the barriers to midwives becoming the primary attendants at birth in the United States include:

1. the general public assumption that obstetricians are the best attendants for pregnancy and birth, and the concomitant lack of awareness of midwives' knowledge, skills, and competence;
2. physicians' resistance to the competition midwives present, in combination with the economic structure of U.S. health care, which makes natural childbirth and midwifery care money losers for hospitals and OBs;
3. lack of sufficient insurance reimbursement and malpractice coverage;
4. lack of educational programs and legalization for CMs in forty-eight states;
5. lack of legalization and licensure for DEMs in twenty-nine states;
6. the restrictions on autonomous midwifery practice that can result from legalization and licensure when midwives do not have enough authority to write their own regulations;
7. the negative publicity that occurs almost every time there is a bad outcome at a homebirth, while negative hospital outcomes are often hidden from public view;
8. insufficient financial support for some state midwifery boards;
9. the fact that many midwives do not choose to belong to their national organizations;
10. the inability of CPMs to attend births inside of hospitals and the inability of most CNMs and CMs to attend births outside of hospitals (because of lack of physician backup and insurance restrictions);
11. three national midwifery organizations that do not present a united front to the public in favor of the midwifery model of care, due to their internal differences;
12. recent nursing initiatives to eliminate specific program accreditation and to require a Ph.D. for all advanced practice nurses by 2015.

For every barrier we presented above except the last one, which is too new to fully evaluate, we also presented possible routes for overcoming these barriers that midwives and their consumer and legislative supporters are trying, or might try in the future, to create. Their struggle is ongoing and deserves the support of every American citizen and resident who cares about better birth for mothers and babies.

CONCLUSION: INTEGRATING CARE AND AUTONOMY

As we have seen in this chapter, the midwifery model provides both an ideology and a method through which care and autonomy can become integrated. Without the ethic of care, the client may have a difficult time remaining or becoming autonomous. Without a sense of autonomy, the client has little chance of developing an embodied sense of power through the birth process. Our analysis of these interrelationships, which we offer as an important subject for further research, suggests that care and autonomy should not be conceptualized as competitors but rather as inseparable allies for building new professional models that are equally conducive to excellent outcomes *and* to human well-being. Midwives matter because they are specialists in the conscious development of these interrelationships between care and autonomy, paving the way toward the kind of integral health care that must come to characterize and facilitate the human future.

ACKNOWLEDGMENTS

We wish to thank Judith Rooks, Ida Darragh, Susan Hodges, Katherine Camacho Carr, and Deanne Williams for their extremely helpful editorial contributions to this chapter.

REFERENCES

Barlett, Donald L., and James B. Steele. 2004. *Critical Condition: How Health Care in America Became Big Business—and Bad Medicine.* New York: Doubleday.

Browner, Carole, and Nancy Press. 1995. "The Normalization of Prenatal Diagnostic Testing." In *Conceiving the New World Order: The Global Politics of Reproduction,* ed. Faye Ginsburg and Rayna Rapp, 307–322. Berkeley and London: University of California Press.

Browner, Carole, and Nancy Press. 1997. "The Production of Authoritative Knowledge in American Prenatal Care." In *Childbirth and Authoritative Knowledge: Cross-Cultural Perspectives,* eds. Robbie Davis-Floyd and Carolyn Sargent. Berkeley: University of California Press.

Clement, Grace. 1998. *Care, Autonomy, and Justice.* Boulder, CO: Westview Press.

Davidson, Michele R. 2002. "Outcomes of High-Risk Women Cared for by Certified Nurse-Midwives." *Journal of Midwifery and Women's Health* 47(1):46–49.

Davis-Floyd, Robbie. 1998. "The Ups, Downs, and Interlinkages of Nurse- and Direct-Entry Midwifery." In *Getting an Education: Paths to Becoming a Midwife,* ed., Jan Tritten and Joel Southern. Eugene, OR: Midwifery Today.

Davis-Floyd, Robbie. 2004, 2nd edition. *Birth as an American Rite of Passage.* Berkeley: University of California Press.

Davis-Floyd, Robbie, and Elizabeth Davis. 1997. "Intuition as Authoritative Knowledge in Midwifery and Home Birth." In *Childbirth and Authoritative Knowledge: Cross-Cultural Perspectives,* ed. Robbie Davis-Floyd and Carolyn Sargent. Berkeley: University of California Press.

Davis-Floyd, Robbie, and Gloria St. John. 1998. *From Doctor to Healer: The Transformative Journey.* New Brunswick, NJ: Rutgers University Press.

DeVries, Raymond G. 1996. *Making Midwives Legal: Childbirth, Medicine, and the Law.* 2nd ed. Columbus: Ohio State University Press.

Fennell, Karen S. 2003. "The Professional Liability Crisis: Access to Obstetrical Care at Risk." *Quickening* 34(6):8.

Johnson, Christine Barbara. (2001). "The Ethic of Care and the Ethic of Autonomy." Paper presented at the May Pacific Sociological Association, San Francisco, CA.

Kennedy, Holly Powell. 1995. "The Essence of Nurse-Midwifery Care: The Woman's Story." *Journal of Nurse-Midwifery* 1995(40):401–407.

Kennedy, Holly Powell. 2000. "A Model of Exemplary Midwifery Practice: Results of a Delphi Study." *Journal of Midwifery and Women's Health* 45(1):4–19.

Kennedy, Holly Powell. 2004. "The Landscape of Caring for Women: A Narrative Study of Midwifery Practice." *Journal of Midwifery and Women's Health* 49(1):14–23.

MacDorman, M., and G. Singh. 1998. "Midwifery Care, Social and Biomedical Risk Factors, and Birth Outcomes in the U.S.A." *Journal of Epidemiology and Community Health* 52:310–317.

Perkins, Barbara Bridgman. 2004. *The Medical Delivery Business: Health Reform, Childbirth and the Economic Order.* New Brunswick, NJ: Rutgers University Press.

Rooks, Judith. 1997. *Midwifery and Childbirth in America.* Philadephia: Temple University Press.

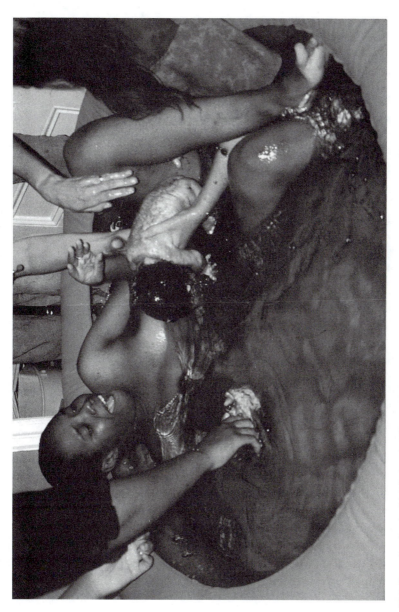

Fig. 13.1 Midwife-assisted water birth in hospital. Photographer: Kenneth C. Johnson.

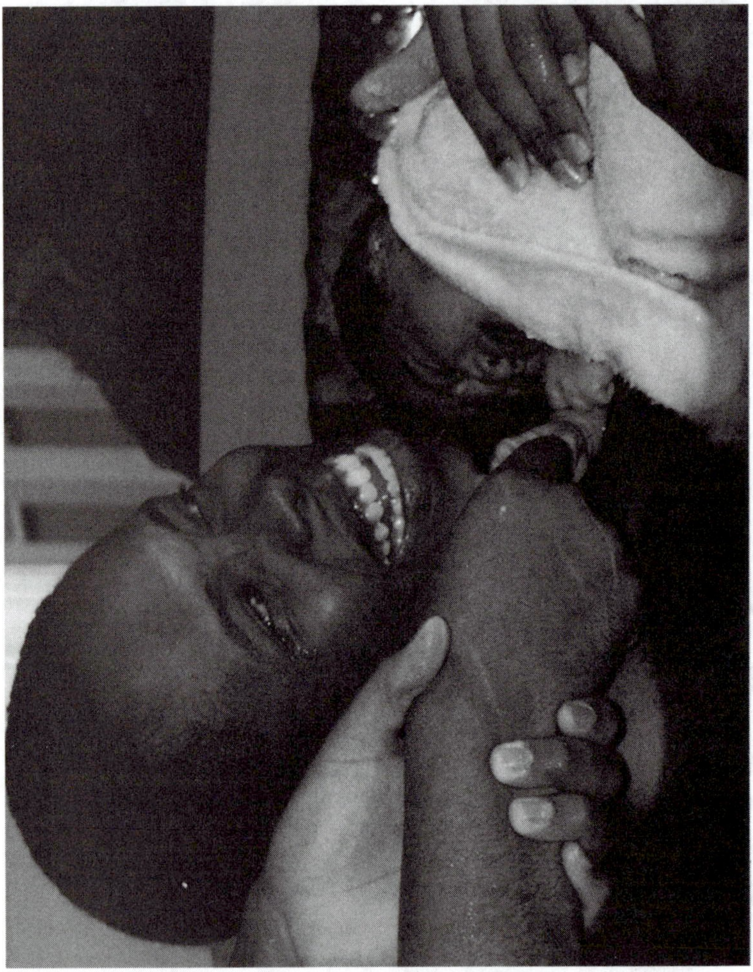

Fig. 13.2 Midwife-assisted water birth in hospital. Photographer: Kenneth C. Johnson.

CONTRIBUTORS

Amy Colo, RM, has been attending homebirths in Colorado since 1989, practicing as a registered midwife for eight years. She has a BA in Comparative Religious Studies from Amherst College. Her training in midwifery was accomplished solely through apprenticeship in Colorado as she raised her two children. She was active in the legalization of midwifery in the state, and served on the board of the Colorado Midwives Association for five years during the transition. Though her "wouldn't it be nice" list for the future includes midwifery as the standard of care in the United States, and a pervasive acceptance of homebirth and direct-entry midwives, she struggles with what she believes would be the cost of going public in this way. Stubborn and independent, she is happy to hold the light of the normal, natural, and sacred in birth for the twenty or so families she serves each year.

Christa Craven, Ph.D., teaches cultural and medical anthropology at the University of Mary Washington in Fredericksburg, Virginia. Her research focuses on the politics of holistic health care in the United States, including work with massage therapists, acupuncturists, chiropractors, herbalists, and midwives. Her doctoral dissertation focused on the shifting meanings associated with motherhood, political action, and citizenship among midwifery advocates struggling for access to homebirth practitioners in Virginia. A strong proponent of activist anthropology, she remains active in efforts to promote midwifery care. She has served on the Executive Board of Virginia Friends of Midwives and as a Legislative Advisor to the Commonwealth Midwives Alliance.

Robbie Davis-Floyd, Ph.D., is Senior Research Fellow in the Department of Anthropology at University of Texas Austin. She is a medical anthropologist specializing in the anthropology of reproduction and alternative health care, and a longtime childbirth activist. An international speaker, she is the author of over eighty articles and of *Birth as an American Rite of Passage* (1992, 2004); coauthor of *From Doctor to Healer: The Transformative Journey* (1998); and coeditor of eight collections, including *Childbirth and Authoritative Knowledge: Cross-Cultural Perspectives* (1997), *Cyborg Babies: From Techno-Sex to Techno-Tots* (1998), *Reconceiving Midwifery* (2004), and *Birth Models That Work* (forthcoming). Her research on global trends and transformations in health care, childbirth, obstetrics, and midwifery is ongoing. Her website is www.davis-floyd.com; many of her articles are available there.

Betty-Anne Daviss, RM, MA, is an apprentice-trained midwife who has worked on five continents in thirty years. As adjunct professor at the Pauline Jewett Institute of Women's Studies, Carleton University in Ottawa, Canada, she teaches social movement theory and midwifery history. She was involved with midwifery legislation in Canada, particularly in Quebec and Ontario, after her work as a midwife in the United States for three years in Alabama, giving her a unique Canadian and American perspective. Her ethnographic work has documented the traditions of Inuit childbirth in northern Canada, but she is just as happy out of academia, exchanging and strategizing with the traditional midwives in Guatemala, Afghanistan, and among Eastern European midwives, particularly in Hungary. Among her epidemiologic investigations, she considers the largest prospective homebirth study yet to be published (*British Medical Journal* 2005) one of her proudest achievements. The first midwife to be hired by the International Federation of Gynecology and Obstetrics (FIGO), she is presently acting as Project Manager for their Safe Motherhood and Newborn Health Initiative.

Melissa Denmark, CPM, MA, received her BS in biology and a minor in chemistry from the University of North Carolina in Chapel Hill in 1993. Using her molecular biology background, she moved to Seattle where she worked at the University of Washington doing research and clinical work on herpes viruses. Feeling isolated from patients in the lab setting and desiring to travel, in 1995 and 1996 she participated in a study-abroad program with the University of Minnesota, which took her to Kenya to live with a Maasai family and learn about their beadwork and herbal medicine. In 1998 she began graduate school in anthropology at the University of Florida and focused her attention on female reproductive health, birth, and midwifery. She conducted her master's research on the history of direct-entry midwifery in Florida, and subsequently desired to become a midwife herself. With her thesis not yet written, in 2000 she moved back to Washington and started the Seattle Midwifery School (SMS). While in midwifery school she had a beautiful homebirth, completed her master's in anthropology, and spent six weeks attending births in Vanuatu in the South Pacific. In 2004 she graduated from SMS and became a licensed midwife in Washington state, and gave birth to her second child at home. Currently she is busy with motherhood and eagerly anticipates practicing midwifery again.

Kerry Dixon, CPM, LM (retired), RN, is currently a student at the Frontier School of Midwifery and Family Nursing in the Community-based Nurse-midwifery Educational Program (CNEP). She is a former President of the Minnesota Midwives Guild (MMG) and of the Minnesota Council of Certified Professional Midwives (MCCPM), having spent many years working to help bring about the legal recognition of midwives in Minnesota. She is a member of both MANA and ACNM and will continue to work passionately to bridge the ends of the midwife rainbow. She is the mother of six children, four of whom were born into the hands of midwives and two blessings who were born in China. She is pursuing graduate studies to work internationally in an underserved area on behalf of mothers and children.

Susan L. Erikson, Ph.D., is a medical anthropologist interested in globalization and health. Her own birthing philosophies were formatively shaped while working as a Peace Corps volunteer with Mende people in Sierra Leone, where pregnancy, childbirth, and infant care were normative everyday events. Anomalous among her peers for having had one homebirth and one car birth, she remains unfailingly curious about the ways in which laws and policies shape women's notions of "normal" birth. In addition to working in prenatal care clinics in Sierra Leone, she conducted comparative research on prenatal diagnostic technology use in former East and West Germany. Susan is currently director of Global Health Affairs at the Graduate School of International Studies at the University of Denver.

Carolyn A. Hough, MPH, is completing her Ph.D. in anthropology at the University of Iowa, where she also recently completed a master's in Public Health. She carried out her doctoral fieldwork in Gambia, West Africa and is writing her dissertation on the role of *kanyaleng kafos* (organizations of women united by problems with infertility and/or child mortality) in contemporary Gambian social and political life, as well as in development and public health strategies. Her ongoing research interests include women's reproductive health, local/community-level involvement in international health initiatives, and immigrant and refugee health.

Christine Barbara Johnson, Ph.D., is a sociologist, an advocate of midwifery for over twenty years, and a national speaker who has presented numerous papers on normalizing birth. Christine has been an adjunct professor at Boston University and Boston College teaching medical sociology, and a research consultant on a National Library of Medicine study that included a key component on midwives. She sat on the board of directors of Massachusetts Friends of Midwives for many years, and has been an active participant on many committees supporting the midwifery model of care. Presently, Christine offers change management and conflict resolution seminars as well as executive and leadership coaching. She has recently been selected for inclusion in the 2005 *Who's Who in Executives and Professionals* .

Mary M. Lay, Ph.D., is a Professor in the Department of Rhetoric, a Faculty Fellow in the Law School, and a former Director of the Center for Advanced Feminist Studies at the University of Minnesota. She has been studying direct-entry midwifery in Minnesota since 1991, and is author of *The Rhetoric of Midwifery: Gender, Knowledge, and Power* (Rutgers University Press, 2000); "Midwifery on Trial: Balancing Privacy Rights and Health Concerns after *Roe v. Wade*," *Quarterly Journal of Speech* 89 (February 2003): 60-77; and "The Rhetoric of Midwifery: Conflicts and Conversations in the Minnesota Home Birth Community in the 1990s," with Billie Wahlstrom and Carol Brown, *Quarterly Journal of Speech* 82 (November 1996): 383-401. She has written an educational case study for decision making on the Minnesota direct-entry midwives, located at http://www.hhh.umn.edu/centers/wpp/midwifery_homebirth.htm. Professor Lay also volunteers for WATCH, a court-monitoring and research organization that follows cases of family and sexual violence and provides feedback to the justice system. In collaboration with WATCH, she is now studying how judges weigh victim impact statements in determining sentences in domestic violence cases.

Maureen May, CNM, WHNP, MSN, is a Ph.D. candidate at Syracuse University with an academic emphasis on childbirth, midwifery, organizational culture, social change, and ethnographic research. Having practiced in a variety of clinical settings as a women's health nurse practitioner (MSN, University of Rochester) and a certified nurse-midwife (Certificate of Midwifery, Frontier School CNEP), homebirth is now her clinical focus. She is also at work establishing a public policy nonprofit—The Childbirth Reform Project. Maureen's professional career began with an associate degree of nursing from a community college. "I entered nursing like so many women—for work. Spending my early adult life trying to change the world, I found myself with a baby and the need for a marketable skill. But it was through nursing that I found my life's calling, midwifery." Maureen lives in Tempe, Arizona, with her husband of twenty-seven years, Kurt Krumperman. They have one child, William (Bill) Sampson Krumperman.

INDEX

A

Abeler, Jim, 276
Abu-Lughod, Lila, 353
Adorno, T., 170
Advocates for Choices in Childbirth, 119
Alternative birth movement (ABM), 414–427
American Association of Colleges of nursing, 535
American Association of Nurse-Midwives (AANM), and frontier nurse-midwives, 36
American College of Midwifery (formerly American College of Nurse-Midwives), 59, 250
American College of Nurse-Midwivery (ACNM), 2
  accreditation process, 37–38, 49, 54, 437
  Certification Council (ACC), 28, 416
  conferences, national and regional, 2
    formality of, 50–51
  credentials for certified midwife (CM), 5, 56, 59, 415
  direct-entry midwives, educational proposal for CM, 134–136
  Division of Accreditation (DOA), 58
    definition of core competences, 38
    guidelines, 6
  Doctorate in Nursing Practice (DNP), 535
  educational training and standards, 41, 55–56
    conflicts with MANA on, 425
  embrace of distance learning programs, 50
  inclusion of gynecological practice, 51
  initial goals, 36–37
  and International Confederation of Midwives, 44
  Journal of Midwifery and Women's Health, 59–60
  and MANA, current efforts to create liaison, 401
    dynamics of, 8
    and irreconcilable differences with, 64–66
  membership growth, 182, 255
  membership limitations, 44
  nurse-midwives, 292
  representation of certified nurse-midwives (CNM), 5
  response to New York state licensure of CNM, 134
  revised criteria, 50
  timeline of events, 66–69
  training, affiliation with universities, 6
  trend toward professionalism, 51
American College of Obstetricians and Gynecologists (ACOG), 433, 440
  and elective cesarean section, 440–441
American Nurses Association (ANA), 36
American Public Health Association, 66, 181, 432–433
Appelle, Christine, 428
Arms, Suzanne, 67, 214
Association for the Promotion and Standardization of Midwifery, 91
Association of Women's Health, Obstetrical, and Neonatal Nurses (AWHONN), 2
Austin Area Birthing Center, 188

N